Contemporary Cardiology

Series Editor
Peter P. Toth, Ciccarone Ctr Prevent. Cardio. Disease
Johns Hopkins University, Sterling, IL, USA

For more than a decade, cardiologists have relied on the Contemporary Cardiology series to provide them with forefront medical references on all aspects of cardiology. Each title is carefully crafted by world-renown cardiologists who comprehensively cover the most important topics in this rapidly advancing field. With more than 75 titles in print covering everything from diabetes and cardiovascular disease to the management of acute coronary syndromes, the Contemporary Cardiology series has become the leading reference source for the practice of cardiac care.

George S. Abela • Stefan Mark Nidorf

Editors

Cholesterol Crystals in Atherosclerosis and Other Related Diseases

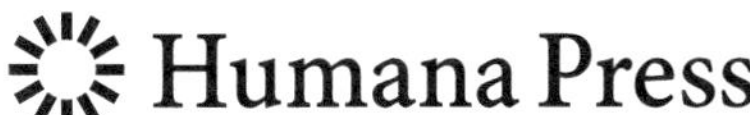 Humana Press

Editors
George S. Abela ⓘ
Department of Medicine
Division of Cardiovascular Medicine
Michigan State University
East Lansing, MI, USA

Stefan Mark Nidorf
The Heart and Vascular Research Institute
Sir Charles Gairdner Hospital
Perth, WA, Australia

ISSN 2196-8969   ISSN 2196-8977   (electronic)
Contemporary Cardiology
ISBN 978-3-031-41194-6   ISBN 978-3-031-41192-2   (eBook)
https://doi.org/10.1007/978-3-031-41192-2

This Humana imprint is published by the registered company Springer Nature Switzerland AG
The registered company address is: Gewerbestrasse 11, 6330 Cham, Switzerland

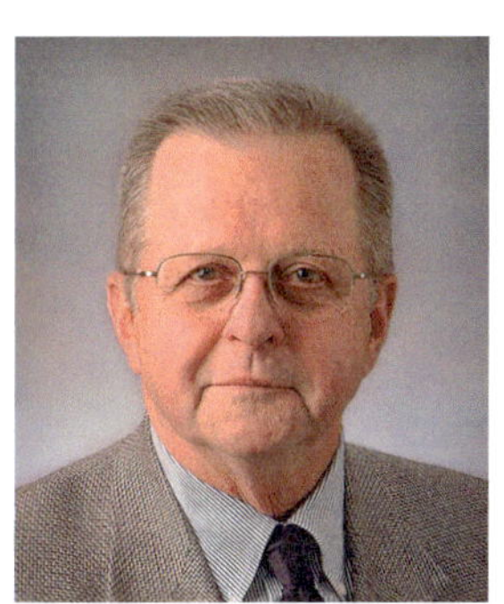

This book is dedicated to the memory of C. Richard Conti, MD, a great mentor and friend who paved the way for others to succeed and was always receptive to new ideas. He was the first to recognize the value of the cholesterol crystal concept and work.

"If I have seen further it is by standing on the shoulder of giants."

– Sir Isaac Newton

Preface

The purpose of this book is to shed light on of *the role of cholesterol crystals (CCs) in atherosclerosis and other medical conditions* by providing insight into how microscopic and macroscopic crystals can induce injury that is critical in the development and progression of several common diseases.

Although it is hard to conceive that micron-sized structures can lead to direct and potentially catastrophic injury, it is helpful to reflect that when wheat seeds stored below deck in closed compartments are inadvertently dampened, they can expand and rupture the hull of solid steel ships leading to their rapid demise.[1] Similarly, when a bottle of water is inadvertently forgotten in the freezer, the water that is converted to ice crystals will shatter the glass (Fig. 1). We have started with these dramatic examples of various capacity because they highlight how in the same way the dynamic process of CC formation, growth, and aggregation in cells and tissues especially in tight spaces can cause consequential microscopic and macroscopic injury wherever free cholesterol accumulates in the body. These fundamental physical principles are essential to understanding the process of plaque rupture.

Cholesterol crystals have been detected by pathologists using standard histologic techniques for over 100 years. In fact, what pathologists actually saw were not true crystals, but imprints of empty spaces (clefts) that formed where the crystals were deposited in vivo, and then etched away ex vivo by lipid-dissolving agents used to process tissues for histology. Most histologists and pathologists were aware that this phenomenon was caused by ethanol that they used as a dehydrating agent during tissue preparation to ensure the tissues would become sufficiently stiffened to be trimmed by a microtome, mounted on a slide, stained, and then examined by light microscopy. To our knowledge no one ever ventured to change this method of tissue processing to determine how CCs formed or behaved in vivo, because the long-standing dogma was that CCs and clefts were mere artifacts of tissue preparation.

---

[1] https://www.atlasobscura.com/articles/the-ship-wrecked-by-wheat-forgotten-on-the-california-shores.

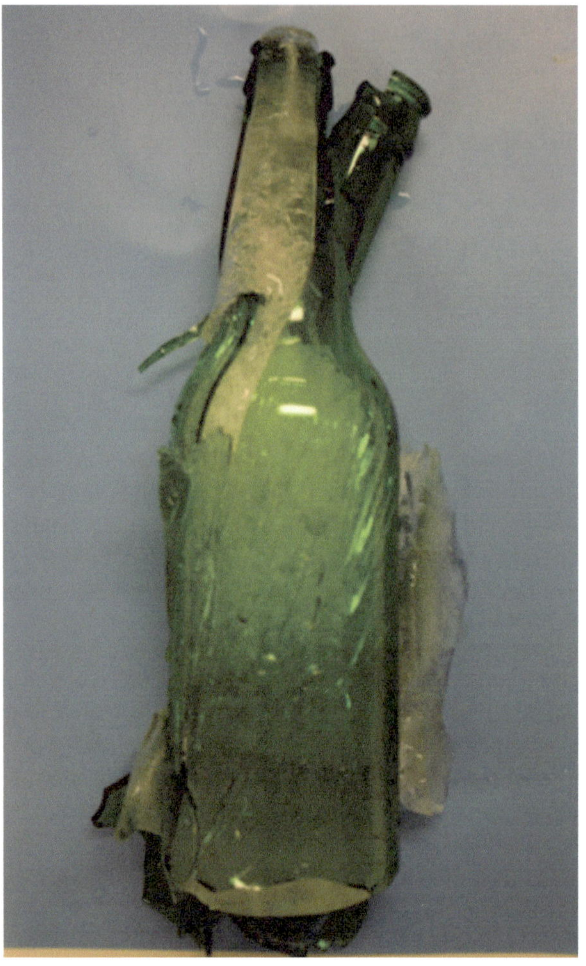

Two subsequent advances changed that dogma. First, the advent of scanning electron microscopy and confocal fluorescence microscopy made it possible to perform imaging without using ethanol, which allowed CCs to be directly imaged for the first time. Second, studies examining how CCs form and grow under different physiochemical conditions led to the clear understanding that as cholesterol transforms from a liquid to a solid it expands just as water expands when it crystallizes into ice.

Thus, it was reasoned that as liquid and semi-liquid cholesterol within the confined space of a lipid-rich atherosclerotic plaque transforms into CCs, they would expand the core and stretch its cap causing it to thin and become vulnerable to direct puncture and rupture or erosion that in turn would lead to athero-thrombosis. Moreover, CC embolization can lead to further tissue injury by microvascular occlusion or spasm with distal ischemic injury. Furthermore, it was subsequently proven that when CCs are "spilled" into the atherosclerotic bed in the plaque they can trigger acute and chronic inflammatory injury that promotes plaque growth and instability. *This dynamic view of CCs led to the proposition that when they form and aggregate in atheroma, CCs act to drive the atherosclerotic process.*

Interestingly, it now understood that there are similarities between atherosclerosis and other crystal-induced diseases such as gout, and that just as CCs induce vascular injury, they may play a similar role in other conditions ranging from cancer, diabetic retinopathy, degenerative valve disease, infective endocarditis, and even preeclampsia.

With the support of many of our colleagues who have also examined the role of CCs and other crystalloids in a range of diseases, the idea to write a book based upon our collective insights has finally been crystallized in this edition, which is divided into several parts.

Part I provides an overview of how the role of CCs was discovered and introduces the central CC paradigm. Part II describes how CCs can be imaged in vitro and Part III describes how they can be imaged in vivo. Part IV summarizes how cholesterol is trafficked in the circulation and arterial wall, and how CCs form in the vascular endothelium. Part V examines how CC-induced trauma leads to myocardial infarction, CC embolism, and sclerosis of heart valves. Part VI covers various aspects of CC-induced inflammation. Part VII highlights the potential role of CCs and other crystalloids in several diseases, touching on the common features of gout and atherosclerosis, vascular calcification, diabetic retinopathy, diseases of the central nervous system, cancer, infection, and preeclampsia. Finally, Part VIII describes how it may be possible to reduce the consequences of CC-induced injury by either inhibiting their formation, dissolve them, or dampening various aspects of crystal-induced inflammation.

In closing, we would like to thank our colleagues who have worked to advance this field of research and contribute to this edition. We trust it will serve as a reference for both clinicians and basic scientists to help guide their understanding of the role of crystals in a range of diseases including cardiovascular disease, cancer, gout, infection, diabetic retinopathy, and possibly other diseases yet to be formally investigated where free cholesterol accumulates, and CCs may form.

East Lansing, MI, USA   George S. Abela
Perth, WA, Australia   Stefan Mark Nidorf

Acknowledgments

The editors would like to acknowledge and thank Careen Loos, graphic artist, for much of the artwork, Elizabeth "Beth" Moore, academic assistant, for the help in securing permissions for using many images and Zain ul Abideen for technical support.

Recognition is due to Mary Dekker Nettleman, MD, former Chairperson of the Department of Medicine, the College of Human Medicine at Michigan State University, E. W. Sparrow Hospital, Lansing, Michigan, and the National Institutes of Health, Bethesda, Maryland, who supported this pioneering work.

Contents

Part I
Overview

Atherosclerosis as a Crystalloid Disease: The Discovery of the Role of Cholesterol Crystals in the Formation and Rupture of Atherosclerotic Plaques

Stefan Mark Nidorf, George S. Abela, and James E. Muller

1 Historical Views of the Mechanism of Plaque Rupture

The earliest recognition of atherothrombosis as the cause of myocardial infarction dates back to 1912 when Herrick found a thrombus in the coronary artery at autopsy of a man who had died suddenly following the onset of acute chest pain [1]. Herrick proffered that the thrombus he observed in the coronary artery was the cause of the man's death, however, as thrombi were not commonly found in coronary arteries during routine autopsy most of his peers disagreed, believing the thrombus had likely developed post-mortem [2]. Thus, for most of the last century pathologists continued to hold the view that myocardial infarction was caused by coronary artery spasm or hemorrhage into a plaque due to "spontaneous" rupture of the vasa vasorum rather than atherothrombosis [3, 4].

In 1963, Paris Constantinides, a pathologist in Vancouver Canada, demonstrated fissures (plaque ruptures) at the site of coronary artery thrombosis in patients dying from myocardial infarction [5]. Subsequently Michael Davis at St. George's Hospital in London, United Kingdom, demonstrated that plaque ruptures typically occurred at the edge of the fibrous cap [6, 7]. Notably, these and other investigators

S. M. Nidorf (✉)
Heart and Cardiovascular Institute, Perkins Research Institue, Perth, WA, Australia
e-mail: smnidorf@gmail.com

G. S. Abela
Department of Medicine, Division of Cardiovascular Medicine, Michigan State University, East Lansing, MI, USA
e-mail: abela@msu.edu

J. E. Muller
Division of Cardiovascular Medicine, Department of Medicine, College of Medicine, Harvard Medical School, Boston, MA, USA

G. S. Abela, S. M. Nidorf (eds.), *Cholesterol Crystals in Atherosclerosis and Other Related Diseases*, Contemporary Cardiology,
https://doi.org/10.1007/978-3-031-41192-2_1

3

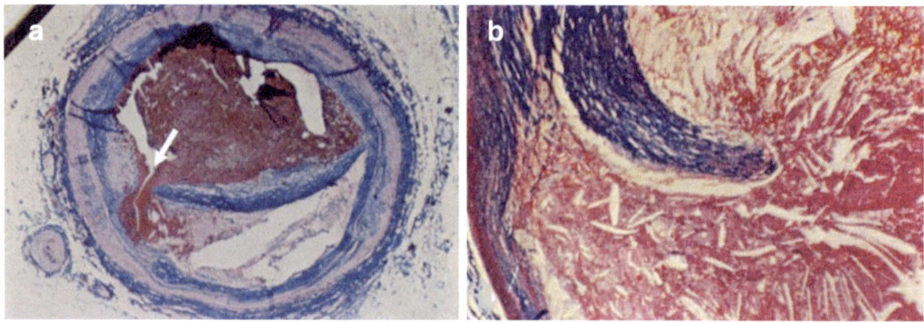

Fig. 1 Preliminary description of plaque rupture. (**a**) Occlusive thrombus over a crack (arrow) at the left margin of an atheroma at the junction of the atheroma capsule with the original coronary wall. Some bleeding has occurred through the fissure into the left part of the atheroma. Mallory stain. (**b**) Thrombus over a wide gap in the capsule of an atheroma. Thrombus has developed over the exposed gruel. Mallory stain. (Reproduced with permission [5])

frequently observed large quantities of cholesterol crystals (CCs) extruding from ruptured plaques but made little or no reference to them as they were thought to be inert incidental post-mortem artefacts [8, 9] (Fig. 1).

It was not until 1980 when DeWood et al. in Seattle, Washington, USA, performed coronary angiography within hours after the onset of myocardial infarction and confirmed that in most instances thrombotic occlusion of the infarct related artery was common at bypass surgery [10] that research turned in earnest towards understanding the causes of plaque rupture that led to atherothrombosis.

In 1989, it was hypothesized that the early morning surge in blood pressure associated with the circadian rhythm might increase shear stress on the arterial wall sufficient to trigger plaque rupture [11]. However, subsequent studies using finite element analysis methods at Massachusetts Institute of Technology revealed that it would require blood pressures well beyond those attainable in humans to rupture plaque [12].

In 1990, James Muller, a Nobel Prize Laureate at Harvard Medical School, put together a team of experts in cardio-atherosclerotic disease to form the Institute for Prevention of Cardiovascular Disease. This group, which included Geoffrey Toffler, Richard Nesto, Victor Gurewich and George Abela, introduced the lexicon of the "Vulnerable Plaque" to define plaques most prone to rupture [13]. Based on expert consensus at that time, it was accepted that the plaques most likely to rupture were those with a lipid-rich core, a thin fibrous cap, evidence of inflammatory cells with lymphocytes and macrophages surrounding their edge and decreased smooth muscle cell content that typically occurred in association with expansive remodeling of the artery [14]. However, while these characteristics appeared to define plaques most at risk of rupture, they did not explain how and why rupture actually occurred.

In 1993, the search for the cause of plaque rupture shifted the focus back to the role of vascular inflammation when Peter Libby and Zorina Galis at Harvard

Medical School, Boston, Massachusetts, proposed that the release of metalloproteinases and other lytic enzymes from macrophages in vulnerable plaques were responsible for plaque rupture [15]. This was based on the earlier work of Henney et al. that demonstrated localization of stromelysin gene expression using in situ hybridization in plaques that could cause plaque remodeling [16].

However, while there was broad agreement that inflammation played a central role in atherosclerosis and that it could contribute to plaque rupture, the *primary* trigger for vascular inflammation remained elusive. Furthermore, it was evident that inflammation could not explain why in some instances the fibrous cap of a ruptured plaque appeared as if it had been *primarily* torn and fibrous cap edges tethered as by a sudden traumatic event [17, 18].

2 Seeing Cholesterol Crystals in Atherosclerosis in a New Light

In 1995 George Abela's team moved from Harvard to Michigan State University where they re-instituted the modified atherosclerotic rabbit model developed by Paris Constatinides to explore the cause of plaque rupture and atherothrombosis. The model used a cholesterol rich diet to enhance the development of atheroma and utilized histamine to induce coronary vasospasm and Russell's viper venom as a prothrombotic agent to promote atherothrombosis [19].

While working with this model it became evident that the rabbits developed corneal opacities similar to arcus senilis in patients with hypercholesterolemia, and that CCs formed within the corneal deposits [20, 21] (Fig. 2). More importantly they also observed CCs perforating the internal elastic laminae of arteries associated with atherothrombosis at the sites of rupture of lipid-rich atherosclerotic plaques (Figs. 3 and 4) [22]. This was a unique observation, and while discussing how CCs might puncture the plaque surface with Kusai Aziz, his cardiology fellow at the time, Abela posed a simple question *"Does cholesterol expand as it transitions from a liquid to a solid state in the same way as water expands as it transitions into solid ice?"*

Abela and his team subsequently confirmed that cholesterol does indeed expand as it evolves into its solid crystalline form. This was demonstrated in bench studies in which CCs were formed by melting synthetic cholesterol powder and allowing it to cool to room temperature (Fig. 5) [23]. With this in vitro model, it was possible to observe and measure volume expansion during cholesterol crystallization in a test tube, and by placing a thin rabbit pericardial membrane over the mouth of the tube it was also possible to demonstrate the ability of growing CCs to perforate this fibrous tissue.

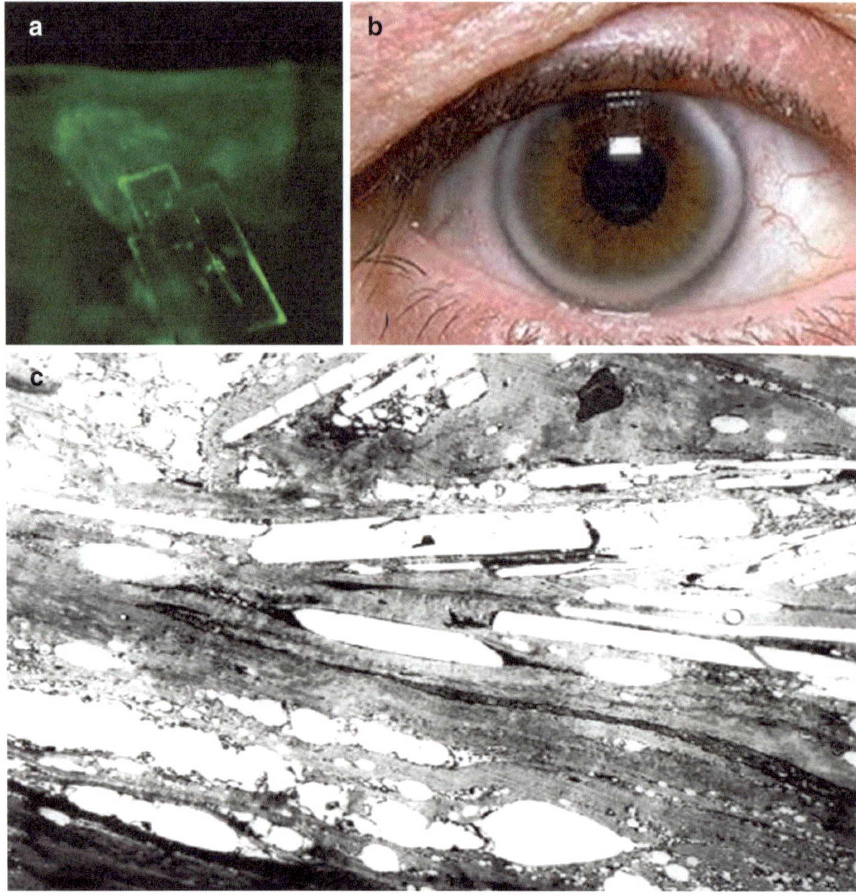

Fig. 2 Cholesterol crystal deposits in the rabbit and human corneas. (a) By confocal microscopy, atherosclerotic rabbit cornea with crystal cluster, (b) typical human arcus senilis, (c) crystals in human cornea. (Reproduced with permission [21])

Abela and his team subsequently used this model to evaluate the ability of various pharmaceutical agents including statins, aspirin, and colchicine to impair the process of cholesterol crystallization [24, 25], (Chapter Agents that Affect Cholesterol Crystallization and Modify the Risk of Crystal Induced Traumatic and Inflammatory Injury).

In addition, Abela used another bench approach, dissolving cholesterol powder in corn oil, placing the mixture in tubes in a water bath at 37 °C and then allowing the crystals to form over 24–48 h, [26, 27] to evaluate various physical and environmental factors that can affect crystal formation including; cholesterol concentration, temperature, and the degree of hydration of the cholesterol molecule, as hydrated cholesterol is most abundant in atherosclerotic plaques [28].

Perhaps one of the Abela's lab most important innovations, however, was the discovery that it was only possible to visualize CCs in these experiments by

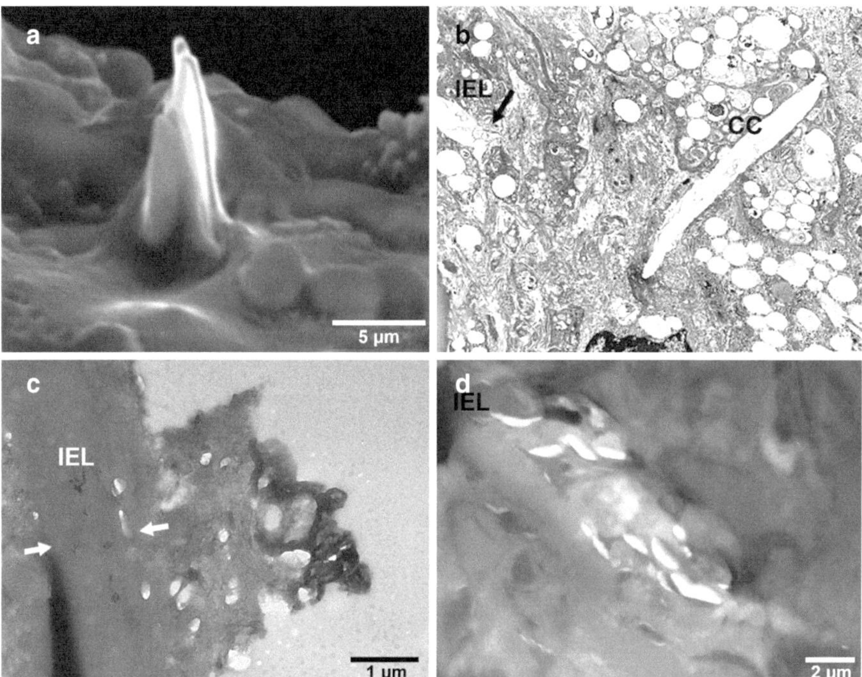

Fig. 3 Cholesterol crystals protruding from intima and internal elastic lamina. (**a**) Scanning electron micrograph with crystal perforating the intimal surface in coronary artery of patient who died with acute myocardial infarction. (**b**) Transmission electron micrograph of crystal crossing the internal elastic lamina (IEL) in atherosclerotic rabbit model (black arrow). (**c, d**) Crystals infiltrating the IEL lamina (white arrows). (Reproduced with permission [17, 22, 33])

avoiding the use of ethanol when processing tissue (Chapter Fig 5. The Innovation in Tissue Preparation and Imaging Revolutionized the Understanding of the Role of Cholesterol Crystals in Atherosclerosis) (Fig. 5) [17, 24, 29]. This insight was gained after it was noted during the in vitro experiments, crystals perforating the membranes which were clearly visible by the naked eye *before* tissue preparation *were no longer evident after using ethanol during tissue preparation* for scanning electron microscopy. Realizing that ethanol had dissolved the CCs, they avoided using it during tissue processing in subsequent in vitro and ex vitro studies of the coronary arteries of patients who had died following acute myocardial infarction [17]. In each scenario avoiding ethanol during tissue preparation made it possible to clearly see CCs perforating pericardial tissue and the fibrous cap of ruptured plaques. Importantly, these later features were not present in patients with advanced coronary disease who died from other causes (Chapter "Role of CCs and Their Lipoprotein Precursors in NLRP3 and IL-1β Activation"). *Thus, for the first time these studies confirmed that CCs were not inert or incidental post-mortem artefacts, but rather were capable of causing traumatic plaque injury and rupture independent of inflammation.*

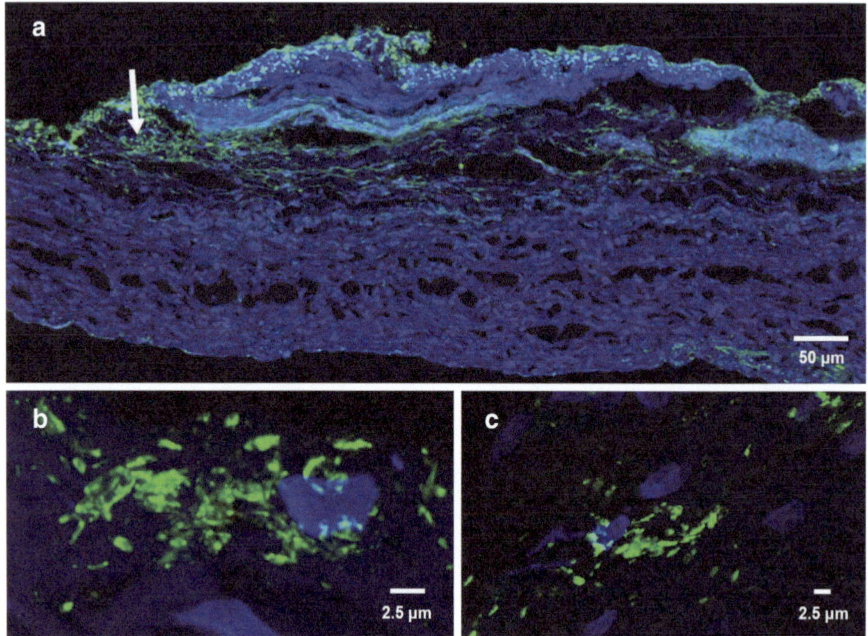

Fig. 4 Cholesterol crystals stained with Bodipy. (**a**) Fluorescence microscopy of atherosclerotic rabbit aorta with crystals present in the plaque and the elastic tissue (arrow). (**b, c**) High magnification of cholesterol crystal clusters from different sites. (Courtesy of GS Abela)

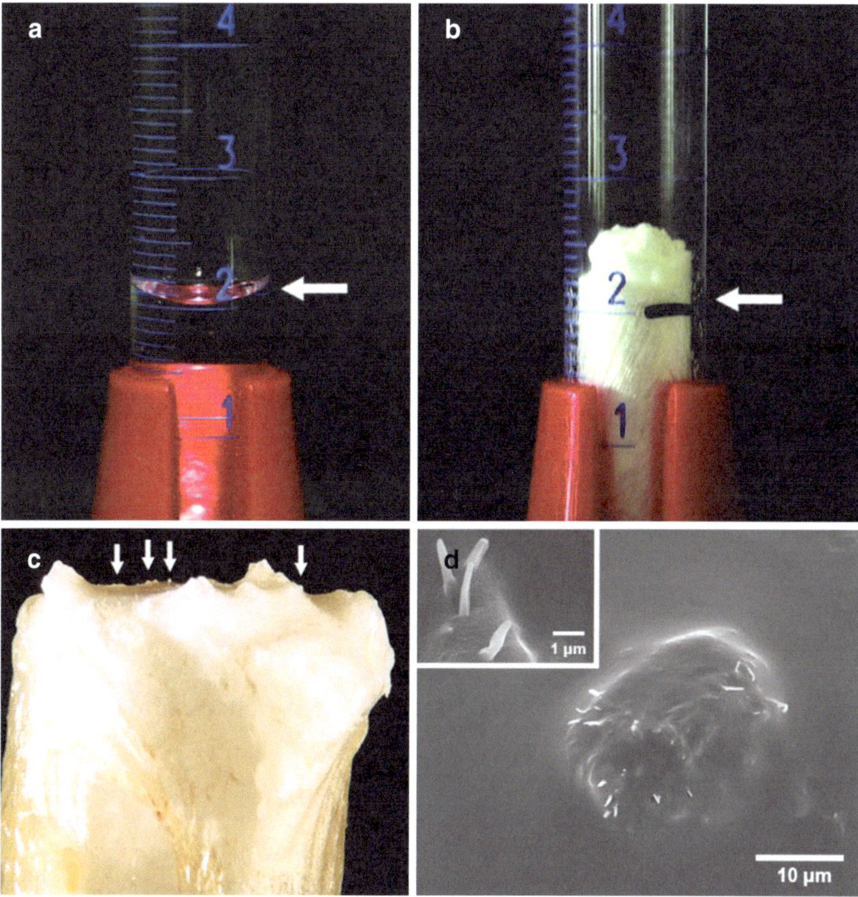

Fig. 5 Volume expansion of cholesterol with crystallization. (**a**)Test tube with melted cholesterol powder before and (**b**) after crystallization demonstrating an increase in volume above the meniscus level (arrows). (**c**) Test tube with pericardial membrane covering the mouth of the test tube and visible crystals perforating the membrane surface (arrows). (**d**) Scanning electron micrograph demonstrating peroration of membrane covering the test tube following crystallization. The sharp tips of cholesterol crystals are seen cutting through and disrupting the membrane. (Reproduced with permission [23, 38])

3 First Insights in the Pro-Inflammatory Potential of Cholesterol Crystals

In 2006 at the SCANNING conference in Washington DC, Abela presented his team's work related to the potential of CCs to cause of plaque rupture [30]. During the presentation he suggested that CCs might be the primary trigger for inflammation in atherosclerotic plaque by inciting the same inflammatory pathways as uric acid crystals in acute and chronic gout. By chance, Eicke Latz, an immunologist from Bonn, Germany, picked up on these comments and suggested that they explore this possibility in more detail as it was known that uric acid crystals could activate the NLRP3 inflammasome [31]. As a result, Abela sent Latz CCs to work with and in 2010, in collaboration with Eric Latz, Peter Düewell, and others they reported that CCs did indeed activate NLRP3 resulting in the production and release of IL-1β [32].

In 2014 Abela went on to demonstrate the development of CCs within atherosclerotic plaque in vivo using an atherosclerotic rabbit model [33]. These studies confirmed that CCs develop and aggregate within atherosclerotic plaque in association with macrophage infiltration, systemic markers of inflammation including C-reactive protein and an elevation in metalloproteinases (Chapter "Role of CCs and Their Lipoprotein Precursors in NLRP3 and IL-1β Activation").

Collectively, these new insights; that CCs can form within atherosclerotic plaque in-vivo *and that they may cause direct injury and incite inflammation, were profound. For the first time since Virchow opined about atherosclerosis, they provided an elegant paradigm that explained how cholesterol within atheroma could trigger inflammation and cause acute plaque rupture that were the hallmarks of the disease.*

4   Cholesterol Crystals May Contribute to Diseases Other Than Atherosclerosis

Abela's work has also provided new insights into how CCs released into the circulation following spontaneous and iatrogenic plaque rupture can cause distal tissue injury due to ischemia (induced by vasospasm and occlusion of the distal microvasculature) and local inflammation (Fig. 6) [34–37].

In addition, he and others have found CCs to be present and may play a role in a wide variety of diseases including *Bacterial infections*; with evidence that *Staphylococcus aureus* and *Pseudomonas aeruginosa* may selectively attach to and degrade CCs (Chapter "The Interaction Between Infection, Crystals and Cardiovascular Disease"), *Valvular heart disease*; with evidence that CC may perforate the intimal surface of sclerotic valves (Chapter "The Role of Cholesterol Crystals in the Development and Progression of Degenerative Valve Disease"), *Diabetic retinopathy*; with evidence that CCs appear in the retinal pigment epithelium, photoreceptors and within the neural retina (Chapter "Cholesterol Crysals in Cancer and Atherosclerosis"), *Solid cancers*; with evidence that CCs are present in a variety of solid cancers (Chapter "Cholesterol in the Central Nervous System in Health and Disease"), and in *Brain injury*, with evidence that CCs are found in the brains of patients with Alzheimer's disease (Chapter "Cholesterol in the Central Nervous System in Health and Disease").

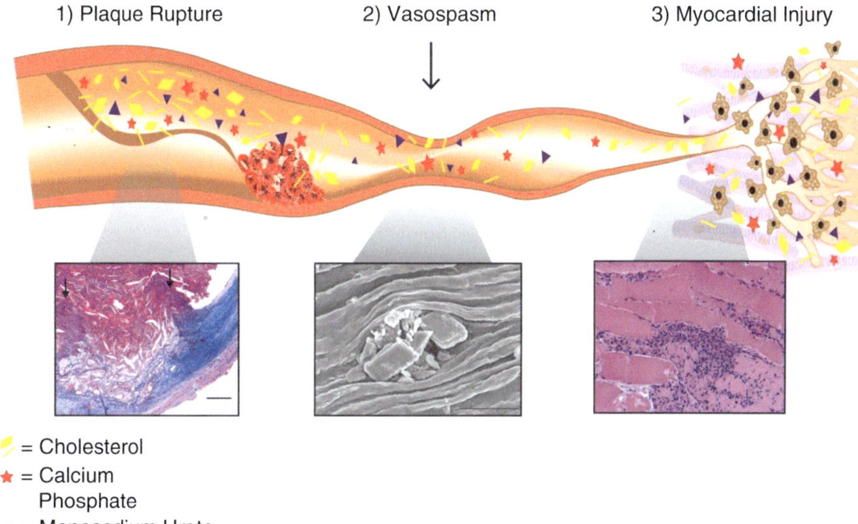

Fig. 6 Schematic of multiple steps of crystal related arterial injury. (*1*) Plaque rupture with tethered edges of torn fibrous cap; (*2*) Released CCs traveling downstream disrupt endothelium and trigger vasospasm; (*3*) CCs lodged in muscle induce inflammatory injury. (bar = 200 μm light micrograph; bar = 50 μm scanning electron micrograph). *CCs* cholesterol crystals. (Modified with permission [37])

5 A New Paradigm for the Treatment of Atherosclerosis

Appreciation of how CCs form (Chapter "Atherosclerotic Plaque Morphology and the Conundrum of the Vulnerable Plaque") trigger vascular trauma and incite inflammation provides a useful paradigm for the development of therapies for atherosclerosis. Specifically, it provides insight how the disease may be slowed by *reducing the propensity for CCs formation;* by reducing serum cholesterol and thus reducing cholesterol accumulation within vascular macrophages, or promoting its cellular efflux, *by dissolving CCs*, and by *reducing inflammatory injury* by inhibiting specific interleukins or "cellular players" incited by crystals (Chapter "Agents that Affect Cholesterol Crystallization and Modify the Risk of Crystal Induced Truamatic and Inflammatory Injury"). A small group of Dr. Abela's lab team present in 2009 (Fig. 7).

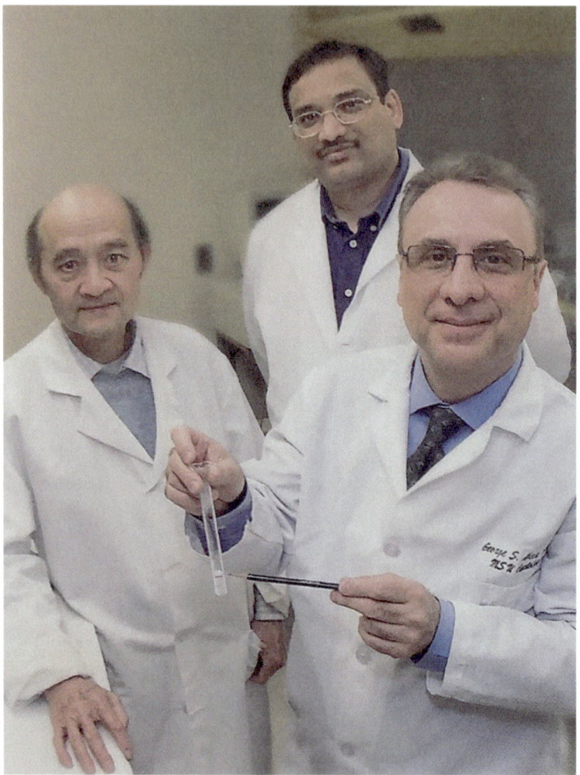

Fig. 7 Abela laboratory team at Michigan State University in 2009. (left) Ruiping Huang, Phd, (middle) Umesh Tamhane, MD and (right) George Abela, MD, MSc, pointing to expanded cholesterol in test tube

6 Summary

In the last few decades, the search for the cause of plaque rupture has led to the development of an elegant thesis that *the transition of cholesterol into its crystalline form is central to the development of atherosclerosis and plaque rupture.*

The purpose of this book is to delve deeper into how these insights were gained due to innovations in tissue preparation and imaging; to explain the process of cholesterol crystallization; to highlight how CCs ability to cause plaque trauma and incite inflammatory injury may contribute to a range diseases; and to demonstrate how "seeing atherosclerosis through a crystal lens" provides a paradigm that should help direct the development of treatments for one of the most common afflictions of humankind.

References

1. Herrick JB. Clinical features of sudden obstruction of the coronary arteries. JAMA. 1912;59:2015–20.
2. Roberts WC, Buja LM. The frequency and significance of coronary arterial thrombi and other observations in fatal acute myocardial infarction: a study of 107 necropsy patients. Am J Med. 1972;52:425–43.
3. Maseri A, Chierchia S. Coronary artery spasm: demonstration, definition, diagnosis, and consequences. Prog Cardiovasc Dis. 1982;25:169–92.
4. Barger AC, Beeuwkes R 3rd, Lainey LL, Silverman KJ. Hypothesis: vasa vasorum and neovascularization of human coronary arteries. A possible role in the pathophysiology of atherosclerosis. N Engl J Med. 1984;310:175–7.
5. Constantinides P. Plaque fissures in human coronary thrombosis. J Atheroscler Res. 1996;6:1–17.
6. Davies MJ, Thomas AC. Plaque fissuring: the cause of acute myocardial infarction causing sudden ischaemic death, and crescendo angina. Br Heart J. 1985;53:363–73.
7. Davies MJ. The pathophysiology of acute coronary syndromes. Heart. 2000;83:361–6.
8. Small DM. George Lyman Duff memorial lecture. Progression and regression of atherosclerotic lesions. Insights from lipid physical biochemistry. Arterioscler Thromb Vasc Biol. 1988;8:103–29.
9. Virmani R, Kolodgie FD, Burke AP, Farb A, Schwartz SM. Lessons from sudden coronary death: a comprehensive morphological classification scheme for atherosclerotic lesions. Arterioscler Thromb Vasc Biol. 2000;20:1262–75.
10. DeWood MA, Spores J, Notske R, Mouser LT, Burroughs R, Golden MS, Lang HT. Prevalence of total coronary occlusion during the early hours of transmural myocardial infarction. N Engl J Med. 1980;303:897–902. https://doi.org/10.1056/NEJM198010163031601.
11. Muller JE, Tofler GH, Stone PH. Circadian variation and triggers of onset of acute cardiovascular disease. Circulation. 1989;79:733–43.
12. Loree HM, Kamm RD, Stringfellow RG, Lee RT. Effects of fibrous cap thickness on peak circumferential stress in model atherosclerotic vessels. Circ Res. 1992;71:850–8.
13. Muller JE, Abela GS, Nesto RW, Tofler GH. Triggers, acute risk factors and vulnerable plaques: the lexicon of a new frontier. J Am Coll Cardiol. 1994;23:809–13. https://doi.org/10.1016/0735-1097(94)90772-2.
14. Schaar JA, Muller JE, Falk E, et al. Terminology for high-risk and vulnerable coronary artery plaques. Eur Heart J. 2004;25:1077–82.
15. Galis ZS, Sukhova GK, Lark MW, Libby P. Increased expression of matrix metalloproteinases and matrix degrading activity in vulnerable regions of human atherosclerotic plaques. J Clin Invest. 1994;94:2494–503.
16. Henney AM, Wakeley PR, Davies MJ, Foster K, Hembry R, Murphy G, Humphries S. Localization of stromelysin gene expression in atherosclerotic plaques by in situ hybridization. Proc Natl Acad Sci U S A. 1991;88:8154–8.
17. Abela GS, Aziz K, Vedre A, Pathak DR, Talbott JD, DeJong J. Effect of cholesterol crystals on plaques and intima in arteries of patients with acute coronary and cerebrovascular syndromes. Am J Cardiol. 2009;103:959–68.
18. Frink RJ. Parallel cholesterol crystals: a sign of impending plaque rupture? J Invasive Cardiol. 2010;22(9):406–11.
19. Abela GS, Picon PD, Friedl SE, Gebara OC, Federman M, Tofler GH, Muller JE. Triggering of plaque disruption and arterial thrombosis in an atherosclerotic rabbit model. Circulation. 1995;91:776–84.

20. Walton KW, Dunkerley DJ. Studies on the pathogenesis of corneal arcus formation II. Immunofluorescent studies on lipid deposition in the eye of the lipid-fed rabbit. J Pathol. 1974;114:217–29. https://doi.org/10.1002/path.1711140406.

21. Klintworth GK. Corneal dystrophies. Orphanet J Rare Dis. 2009;4:7. https://doi.org/10.1186/1750-1172-4-7.

22. Ma H, Aziz KS, Huang R, Abela G. Arterial wall cholesterol content is a predictor of the development and severity of arterial thrombosis. J Thromb Thrombolysis. 2006;22:5–11.

23. Abela GS, Aziz K. Cholesterol crystals rupture biological membranes and human plaques during acute cardiovascular events—a novel insight into plaque rupture by scanning electron microscopy. Scanning. 2006;28:1–10.

24. Abela GS, Vedre A, Janoudi A, Huang R, Durga S, Tamhane U. Effect of statins on cholesterol crystallization and atherosclerotic plaque stabilization. Am J Cardiol. 2011;107:1710–7.

25. Fry L, Lee A, Khan S, Aziz K, Vedre A, Abela GS. Effect of aspirin on cholesterol crystallization: a potential mechanism for plaque stabilization. Am Heart J Plus. 2022;13:100083. https://doi.org/10.1016/j.ahjo.2021.100083.

26. Vedre A, Pathak DR, Crimp M, Lum C, Koochesfahani M, Abela GS. Physical factors that trigger cholesterol crystallization leading to plaque rupture. Atherosclerosis. 2009;203:89–96.

27. Jandacek RJ, Webb MR, Mattson FH. Effect of an aqueous phase on the solubility of cholesterol in an oil phase. J Lipid Res. 1977;18:203–10.

28. Lundber B. Chemical composition and physical state of lipid deposits in atherosclerosis. Atherosclerosis. 1985;56:93–110.

29. Nasiri M, Janoudi A, Vanderberg AFM, Flegler C, Flegler S, Abela GS. Role of cholesterol crystals in atherosclerosis is unmasked by altering tissue preparation methods. Microsc Res Tech. 2015;78:969–74.

30. Abela GS, Aziz K. Plaques are ruptured by cholesterol crystals during myocardial infarction. Scanning. 2006;28:59.

31. Martinon F, Pe'trilli V, Mayor A, Tardivel A, Tschopp J. Gout-associated uric acid crystals activate the NALP3 inflammasome. Nature. 2006;440:237–41.

32. Düewell P, Kono H, Rayner KJ, Sirois CM, Vladimer G, Bauernfeind F, Abela GS, Franchi L, Nunez G, Schnurr M, Espevik T, Lien G, Fitzgerald KA, Rock KL, Moore KJ, Wright SD, Hornung V, Latz E. NLRP3 inflammasomes are required for atherogenesis and activated by cholesterol crystals. Nature. 2010;464:1357–61.

33. Patel R, Janoudi A, Vedre A, Aziz K, Tamhane U, Rubinstein J, Abela O, Berger K, Abela GS. Plaque rupture and thrombosis are reduced by lowering cholesterol levels and crystallization with ezetimibe and is correlated with flurodeoxyglucose positron emission tomography. Arterioscler Thromb Vasc Biol. 2011;31:2007–14.

34. Pervaiz MH, Durga S, Janoudi A, Berger K, Abela GS. PET/CT detection of muscle inflammation related to cholesterol crystal emboli without arterial obstruction. J Nucl Cardiol. 2018;25:433–40.

35. Ghanem F, Vodnala D, Kalavakunta JK, Durga S, Thormeier N, Subramaniyam P, Abela S, Abela GS. Cholesterol crystal embolization following plaque rupture: a systemic disease with unusual features. J Biomed Res. 2017;31:82–94.

36. Gadeela N, Rubinstein J, Tamhane U, Huang R, Pathak DR, Hosein H-A, Rich M, Dhar G, Abela GS. The impact of circulating cholesterol crystals on vasomotor function: implications for no-reflow phenomenon. J Am Coll Cardiol Intv. 2011;4:521–9.

37. Nidorf SM, Fiolet A, Abela GS. Viewing atherosclerosis through a crystal lens: how the evolving structure of cholesterol crystals in atherosclerotic plaque alters its stability. J Clin Lipidol. 2020;14:619–30. https://doi.org/10.1016/j.jacl.2020.07.003.

38. Abela GS. Cholesterol crystals piercing the arterial plaque and intima triggers local and systemic inflammation. J Clin Lipidol. 2010;4:156–64.

The Cholesterol Crystal Paradigm: Overview of How Cholesterol Crystals Evolve and Induce Traumatic and Inflammatory Vascular Injury

Stefan Mark Nidorf and George S. Abela

1 Introduction

Cholesterol crystals (CCs) are ubiquitous in the human body. They are found in atheromatous plaques, the lens, in fluid filled cavities including synovial sacs and the pleural cavity, pericardium, and on body surfaces including the skin, periodontal tissue, and in the biliary and urinary tract [1–10]. Their presence speaks to either disordered production, uptake, handling, or clearance of free cholesterol that is unable to be solubilized by binding to phospholipids. While their mere presence may not be a harbinger of imminent danger, their propensity to form indicates the potential of ongoing crystal induced injury that is dependent on where they form, the rate at which they grow, their size, and their ability to aggregate.

It has long been understood that atherosclerosis is a disease in which there is an ongoing attempt to sequester cholesterol as it unrelentingly transits from the intra-cellular compartment in foam cells into the extra-cellular environment of the arterial wall. In recent times evidence has accrued to indicate that as this process occurs free cholesterol accumulates within endothelium, macrophages, and the plaque core and forms into crystals that initiate and drive the atherosclerotic process by virtue of the trauma they cause and the inflammatory processes they incite [11–13] (Fig. 1).

The purpose of this chapter is to provide a brief overview of the "cholesterol crystal paradigm" as a prelude to subsequent chapters that explain in more detail

S. M. Nidorf
The Heart and Vascular Research Institute, Sir Charles Gairdner Hospital, Perth, WA, Australia
e-mail: smnidorf@gmail.com

G. S. Abela (✉)
Department of Medicine, Michigan State University, East Lansing, MI, USA
e-mail: abela@msu.edu

© The Author(s), under exclusive license to Springer Nature Switzerland AG 2023
G. S. Abela, S. M. Nidorf (eds.), *Cholesterol Crystals in Atherosclerosis and Other Related Diseases*, Contemporary Cardiology,
https://doi.org/10.1007/978-3-031-41192-2_2

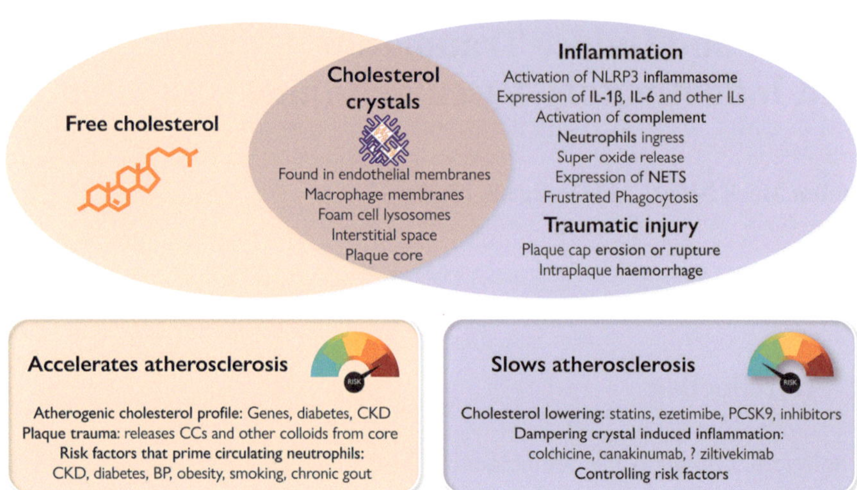

Fig. 1 The "crystal cholesterol paradigm" explains how and why cholesterol crystals that form in the vascular bed are the nexus between cholesterol deposition and atherosclerosis. As free cholesterol accumulates within endothelium, macrophages, and the plaque core and forms into crystals they initiate and drive the disease by virtue of the trauma they cause and the inflammatory processes they incite. Factors that modify the accumulation of cholesterol in the plaque and the inflammatory response to cholesterol crystals can modify the natural history of the disease. (Reproduced with permission [44])

how the lifelong accumulation of cholesterol and formation of CCs causes traumatic and inflammatory injury that leads to atherosclerosis and potentially plays a role in the range of other diseases as well.

2 Formation of Cholesterol Crystals

No matter where they form, the process of CC formation is dependent on the presence of sufficient free cholesterol mono-hydrate molecules and is sensitive to several factors in their local environment including the size of the free cholesterol pool, the amount of phospholipid, the extent of hydration of cholesterol, the presence of excess calcium, regional pH, and ambient temperature. In some environments such as bile, the rate of nucleation of cholesterol can be slowed by various glycoproteins [14–16].

As free cholesterol molecules dissociate from lipoproteins and phospholipid structures in situ they begin to spontaneously associate under favorable circumstances to form flexible meta-stable structures [17]. Initially the meta-stable CC takes the form of elongated string like filaments, and as the process continues the

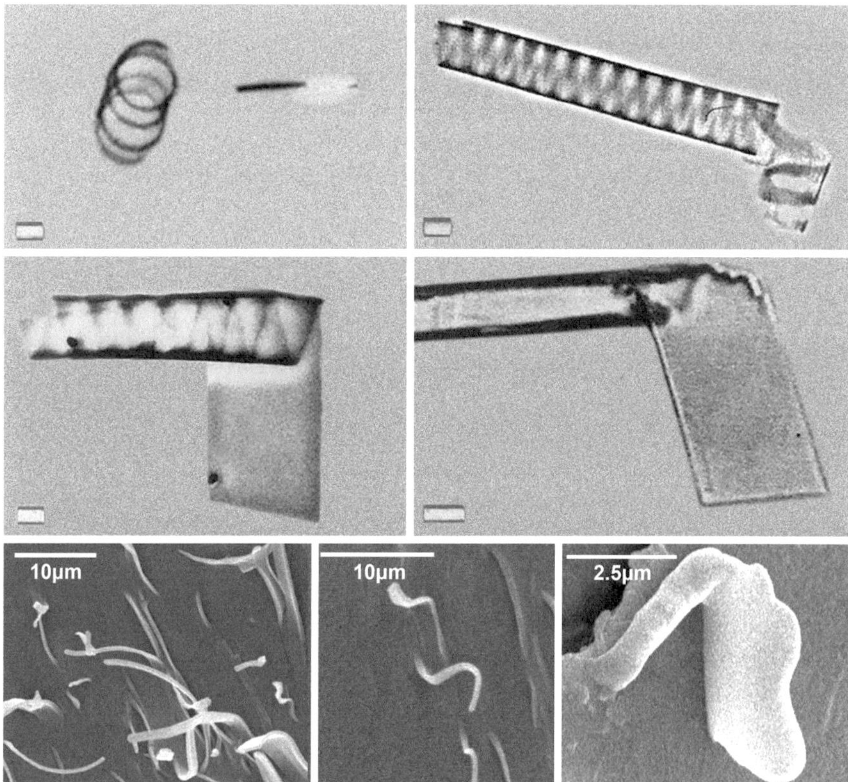

Fig. 2 Transitional phases of meta-stable to stable CCs. (upper panel) in vitro phases of crystal formation are seen to form over weeks (bars = 10 µm). (lower panel) In an in vivo atherosclerotic rabbit model, ribbons of cholesterol crystals appear transiently to be evolving into plates (courtesy George Abela). The rate of change through each stage is affected by physio-chemical environmental factors. The tissues were processed for scanning electron microscopy without ethanol dehydration to avoid dissolving the CCs. Instead, tissues were dehydrated by vacuum with minimal shrinkage. (Reproduced with permission [19, 42])

structure begins to flatten into ribbons, which twist into helices, which then develop into tubules [18, 19] (Fig. 2).

Because meta-stable crystals are highly flexible and allow efficient orderly stacking of a large amount of free cholesterol in a confined compartmental space they do not impose on their surrounds. In the presence of abundant free cholesterol, meta-stable tubules eventually begin to expand, and as this occurs a myriad of microscopic flat plate CCs begin to "shed off" its end. This process is associated with the release of latent elastic energy which disperses the now solid CCs into the environment [20]. These microscopic flat plate CCs then become the platforms onto which any additional free cholesterol in the environment may attach, causing the nascent CC to grow into a macroscopic structure. The rate of CC growth may be accelerated in the presence of calcium debris [19, 20].

The transitional process described above is not unique to CC formation, as a variety of other elements and organic molecules also form flexible filaments and helices before developing into stable crystalline structures [21]. While in vivo, solid CCs appear as either flat plates or needle/rod shapes depending on their stage of development, in vitro their morphology may differ substantially depending on the solvents used during their preparation which affect the degree of hydration of cholesterol molecules [18, 22–24].

3 Intra-Cellular Cholesterol Crystals Promote the Formation of Atheroma

A unique feature of cholesterol crystals is their ability to develop and grow within cell membranes and the intra-cellular environment which stands in contrasts with other elemental crystals such as uric acid. When CCs develop in the intra-cellular environment their growth is restrained by the limited supply of free cholesterol, tight control of the physiochemical environment, and the limits imposed by cellular membranes.

Accumulation of free cholesterol and formation of CCs within the membranes of vascular endothelium predisposes to endothelial dysfunction [25] (Fig. 3). Stiffening of the endothelial membrane and damage to the underlying basement membrane enhances internalization of LDLc, and increases endothelial expression of selectins that enhance the entry of leukocytes into the subintimal space [26]. LDLc that enters the vessel wall is usually rapidly cleared by macrophages, however, if the rate of deposition of LDLc outstrips the rate of clearance, the LDLc particles begin to coalesce and form into vesicles [27]. As these vesicles enlarge, they may rupture and re-release cholesterol into the interstitial space where it is eventually cleared by macrophages that store it within their lysosomes. Further promoting the accumulation of cholesterol within macrophage is the degree of ACAT1 activity which affects reverse cholesterol transport and the release of intra-cellular lipid [28, 29].

As macrophages continue to accumulate cholesterol and store it within lysosomes, they transform into foam cells, and as the concentration of free cholesterol within the lysosomes increases, the process of cholesterol crystallization can begin. As CCs grow they disrupt the lysosomal membrane causing the release of cathepsin B, free cholesterol and CCs directly into the cytosol [30–32]. In the cytosol, CCs cannot be cleared, and in the presence of free cholesterol continue to grow and cause direct cellular trauma (Fig. 4). In addition, the surface of CCs may be recognized by complosome, which akin to complement in the interstitial space, triggers an intra-cellular cascade that together with cathepsin B leads to the activation of the pyrin domain-containing 3 (NLRP3) inflammasome that converts pro-IL-1β to an active IL-1β which in turn activates caspase-8 that eventually leads to macrophage apoptosis and release of cellular contents into the interstitial space [33, 34] (Fig. 5).

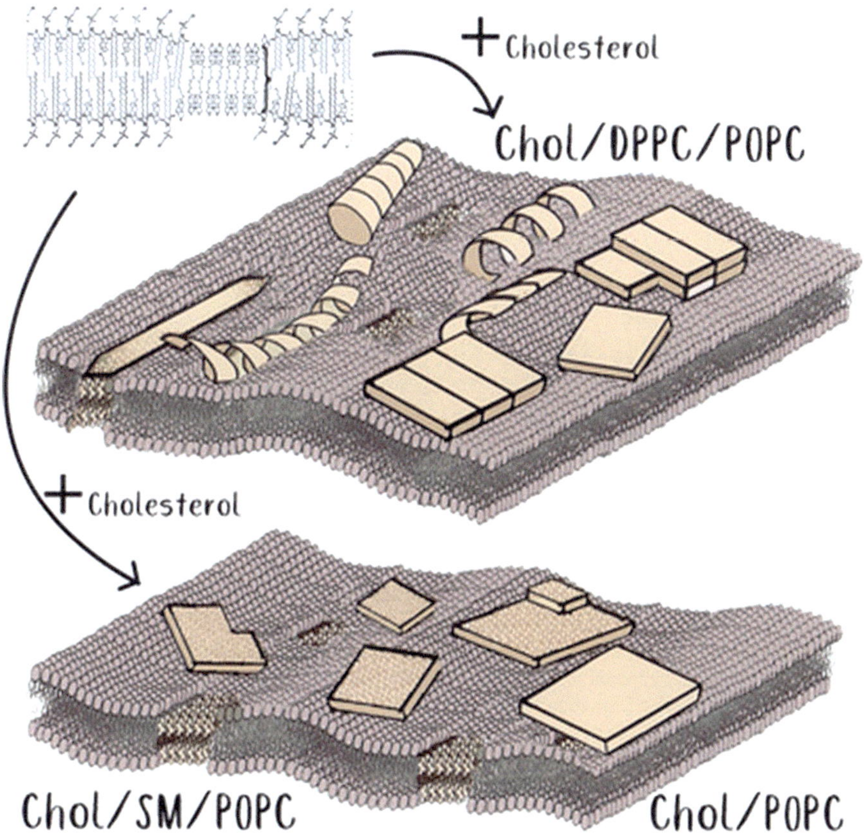

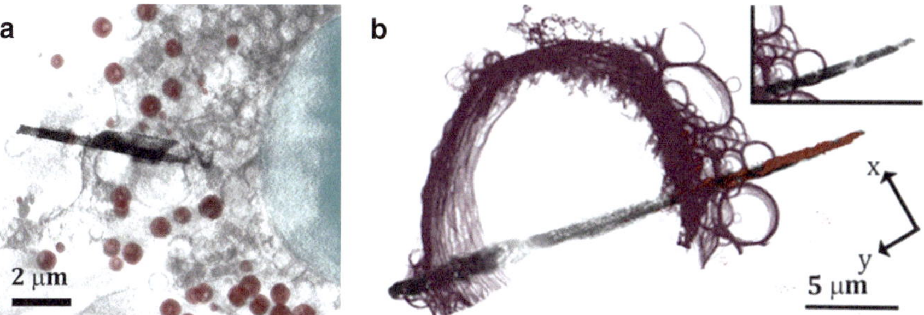

Fig. 3 The Effect of the phospholipid bilayer environment on cholesterol crystal polymorphism. The chemical environment of phospholipid bilayers affects the formation of cholesterol crystals, leading to the precipitation of different crystal morphologies. (Reproduced with permission [22])

Fig. 4 Cholesterol Crystal Interaction with macrophage. (**a**) Volume representation of a segmented cryo-soft X-ray tomograph of a helical cholesterol crystal grown by a macrophage cell in intimate contact with the cell membrane. Cell nucleus (blue), membranes and cholesterol crystal (black-grey), lipid bodies (red). (**b**) Rod-like cholesterol crystals after extended macrophage enrichment with acLDL. The 3D X-ray segmented data superimposed with the STORM signal (red) demonstrates crystal perforating the macrophage cell membrane. (Reproduced with permission [22, 25])

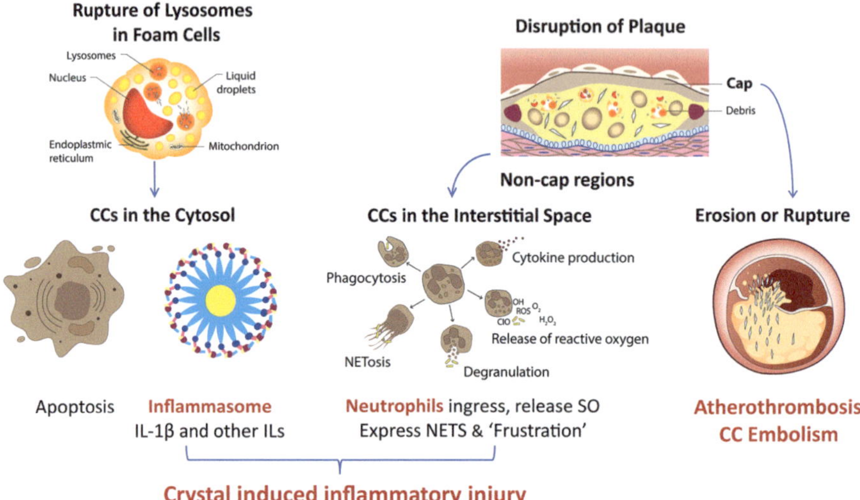

Fig. 5 Cholesterol crystal induced inflammation and plaque disruption. Schematic illustrating the rupture of lysomes by crystals in foam cells releasing cholesterol crystals (CCs) into the cytosol triggering inflammasome formation and plaque disruption with NETS formation leading to crystal induced inflammation and injury

Thus, endothelial dysfunction induced by the formation of CCs within their membrane, in concert with on-going macrophage stimulation and apoptosis driven largely by intra-cellular CCs, promotes a pro-inflammatory milieu that results in the release and sequestration of cellular debris into the interstitial space to form nascent plaques. As new foam cells become sequestered in the surrounding matrix of nascent plaque and undergo apoptosis their contents are also released and the plaque core continues to evolve [35]. Thus, the iterative process of CC induced cellular injury, apoptosis and subsequent inflammatory injury initiates and drives the development of advanced atherosclerotic plaque with a lipid rich necrotic core and a fibrous capsule fed by a neovascular network that develops from the vasa vasorum.

4 Extra-Cellular Cholesterol Crystals Promote Traumatic and Inflammatory Injury

The site in which CCs develop determines the rate at which they form, as well as their shape, size, and therefore their potential to cause injury. In contrast to the cellular environment, CCs that develop in the plaque core may grow much larger due to the size of the free cholesterol pool and the lack of cellular boundaries.

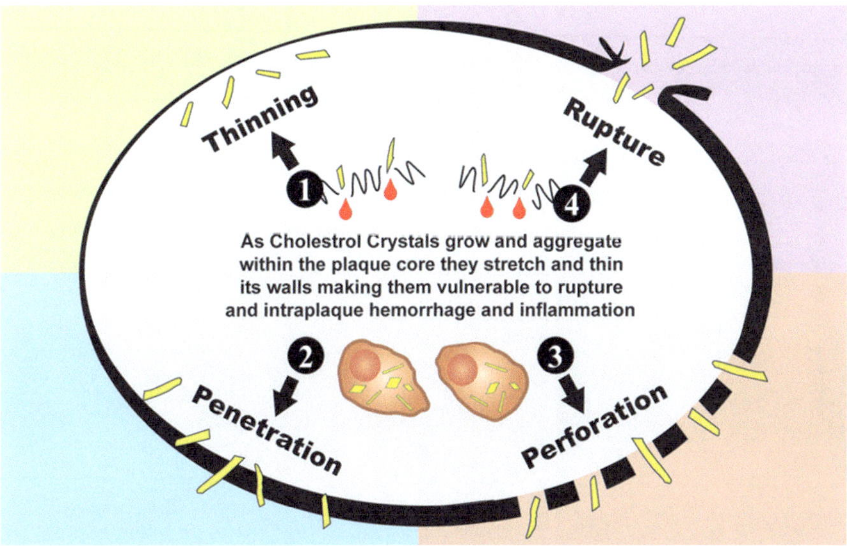

Fig. 6 Mechanical effects of cholesterol crystal growth and aggregation in the plaque core. (*1*) Increases in plaque volume and pressure thin the plaque cap leaving it more vulnerable to inflammatory and mechanical injury; (*2*) CC that penetrate the plaque cap lead to erosion and atherothrombosis; (*3*) CC that perforate the plaque corona may incite inflammation and traumatize the vasa vasorum leading to intra-plaque hemorrhage; and (*4*) Rapid CC enlargement may cause overt rupture of the plaque cap due to increased pressure or direct trauma that then leads to atherothrombosis and CC embolization

As apoptotic cells within the plaque core begin to decompose, the increased concentration of free cholesterol and the change in physiochemical composition of the plaque core may begin to favor the formation of meta-stable CCs that may, if conditions become favorable, rapidly form large solid flat plate fragments. Due to the acellular nature of the plaque core, these crystals cannot be cleared or incite an immune response. However, as they enlarge, and aggregate the increase the pressure and volume within the plaque begins to stretch and thin its walls, and their sharp leading edges may directly erode, puncture or perforate the plaque wall causing it to rupture (Fig. 6). Rupture of the plaque cap is consequential as it leads to atherothrombosis and embolization of atherosclerotic debris including CCs into the circulation where they can lead to distal ischemic and inflammatory tissue injury [5, 36].

In contrast, injury to the non-cap regions of a plaque leads to the release of CCs into the interstitial space surrounding the plaque that can damage the vasa vasorum to cause intra-plaque hemorrhage [37, 38], and incite an inflammatory response akin to gout, associated with the activation of complement and the NLRP3 inflammasome, expression of several interleukins including IL-1β and IL-6, and the ingress and expression of neutrophils which express NETs in their effort to sequester and degrade CC fragments [12, 39–41]. While most inflammatory flares induced by CCs settle, resulting in the sequestration of CCs and the larger lipid pool, and progressive sclerosis, neovascularization and calcification of the arterial wall, on occasions it may predispose to plaque rupture by weakening vulnerable portions of

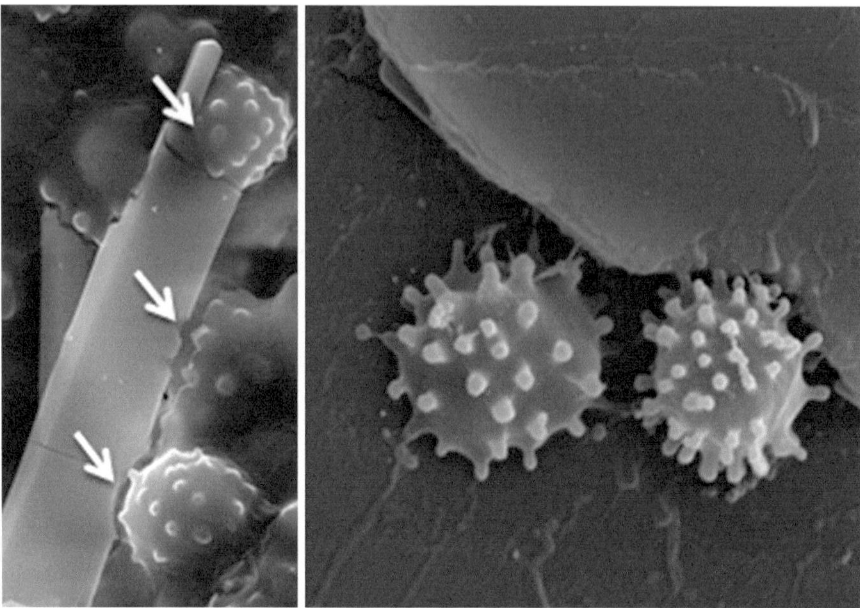

Fig. 7 Cholesterol crystals from coronary artery aspirates during myocardial infarction. Crystals are seen attached to macrophages and appear to be degrading them (arrows) as seen by the notches created at the site of macrophage and crystal contact [43]

the plaque that have been stretched and thinned due to concomitant enlargement and aggregation of CCs in its core. Large fragments of CCs that cannot be ingested by leucocytes lead to a cycle of "frustrated phagocytosis" that promotes chronic inflammatory injury and sclerosis [42, 43] (Fig. 7).

Thus, lipid rich plaques are under the constant threat of injury; from within due to enlargement and aggregation of CCs, and from without due to acute inflammatory flares triggered by the intermittent release of CCs from its core. Importantly, the intensity of the inflammatory process may be enhanced by systemic factors that prime circulating neutrophils, such as aging, smoking, hypertension, diabetes, obesity, chronic kidney disease, and chronic gout, so that they are readily activated when attracted into the site of CC deposition as they course through the atherosclerotic landscape via the neovascular network [44].

5 Hyperglycemia and Crystal Formation

In 1963, Wilkens and Krut postulated that cholesterol deposition in the artery may be caused by cholesterol crystallization, and that the process of CC formation could be enhanced by glucose [45]. Notably, recent evidence supports both contentions, which provide important insights as to why the atherosclerotic process is accelerated in diabetics. First, it has been confirmed that CCs that develop in endothelium damages them and the underlying basement membrane, enhancing the deposition of LDL and the expression of selectins that attracts circulating leukocytes to the vascular bed (Chapter "Formation of CCs in Endothelial Cells"). Second it has been demonstrated that glucose does indeed enhance the process of CC formation in vascular cell membranes in a dose-dependent manner [46]. Interestingly, however, while tight glycemic control in diabetics has been demonstrated to reduce the risk of microvascular complications of diabetcs, it has been difficult to demonstrate that it reduces the risk of macrovascular events [47]. The cause for this paradox is not known, but the observation suggests that tight glycemic control has a greater effect on the formation of CCs in endothelial membranes that drive microvascular disease than it has on the physiochemistry of the plaque core that determines the development and growth of CCs that leads to plaque trauma and macrovascular events.

6 Clinical Implications

The "cholesterol crystal paradigm" provides an understanding how and why formation of CCs in the arterial wall causes traumatic and inflammatory injury that initiates and drives the atherosclerotic process. As such it provides insights into why therapies that reduce the availability of free cholesterol, inhibit the formation of CCs, dissolve them, inhibit various aspects of crystal induced inflammation and control systemic cardiovascular risk factors will slow the progression of atherosclerosis, and potentially impact the course of other diseases in which CCs have been found.

References

1. Aschoff A. Über Entwicklungs-, Wachstums- und Altersvorgänge an den Gefäßen. Path Anat. 1909;47:1.
2. Klintworth GK. Corneal dystrophies. Orphanet J Rare Dis. 2009;4:7. https://doi.org/10.118 6/1750-1172-4-7.
3. Vijaynarayanan A, Menon MP. Cholesterol pericarditis. N Engl J Med. 2022;387:1021. https:// doi.org/10.1056/NEJMicm2118193.
4. Ettlinger RE, Hunder GG. Synovial effusions containing cholesterol crystals report in 12 patients. Mayo Clin Proc. 1979;54(6):366–74.
5. Ghanem F, Vodnala D, Kalavakunta JK, Duga S, Thormeier N, Subramaniyam P, Abela S, Abela GS. Cholesterol crystal embolization following plaque rupture: a systemic disease with unusual features. J Biomed Res. 2017;31(2):82–94.
6. Scolari F, Ravani P. Atheroembolic renal disease. Lancet. 2010;375(9726):1650–60.
7. Smith BF. Gallbladder mucin as a proucleating agent for cholesterol monohydrate crystals in bile. Hepatology. 1990;12(3):183S–6S.
8. Poloni JA. Urine sediment of the month: pathologic crystals in the urine. 2021.

9. Nair PN, Sjogren U, Sundqvist G. Cholesterol crystals as an etiological factor in non-resolving chronic inflammation: an experimental study in Guinea pigs. Eur J Oral Sci. 1998;106(2 Pt 1):644–50. https://doi.org/10.1046/j.0909-8836.1998.eos106206.x.
10. Coe JE, Aikawa JK. Cholesterol pleural effusion. Arch Intern Med. 1961;108(5):763–74. https://doi.org/10.1001/archinte.1961.03620110103014.
11. Abela GS, Aziz K. Cholesterol crystals rupture biological membranes and human plaques during acute cardiovascular events—a novel insight into plaque rupture by scanning electron microscopy. Scanning. 2006;28(1):1–10. https://doi.org/10.1002/sca.4950280101.
12. Düewell P, Kono H, Rayner KJ, et al. NLRP3 inflammasomes are required for atherogenesis and activated by cholesterol crystals. Nature. 2010;464(7293):1357–61.
13. Franklin BS, Mangan MS, Latz E. Crystal formation in inflammation. Annu Rev Immunol. 2016;34:173–202. https://doi.org/10.1146/annurev-immunol-041015-055539.
14. Loomis CR, Shipley GG, Small DM. The phase behavior of hydrated cholesterol. J Lipid Res. 1979;20(4):525–35. https://doi.org/10.1007/s00402-012-1651-z.
15. Carey MC, Small DM. The physical chemistry of cholesterol solubility in bile. J Clin Invest. 1978;61(4):998–1026. http://www.jci.org/articles/view/109025/version/1/pdf/render.
16. Holzbach RT. Cholesterol nucleation in bile. Ital J Gastroenterol. 1995;27(2):101–5.
17. Ziblat R, Fargion I, Leiserowitz L, Addadi L. Spontaneous formation of two-dimensional and three-dimensional cholesterol crystals in single hydrated lipid bilayers. Biophys J. 2012;103(2):255–64. https://doi.org/10.1016/j.bpj.2012.05.025.
18. Bajaj D, Datta SK, Lingaiah R. Needle-shaped cholesterol crystals in pleural fluid: an unusual presentation. J Appl Lab Med. 2019;3(5):899–902. https://doi.org/10.1373/jalm.2018.026211.
19. Konikoff F, Chung D, Donovan J. Filamentous, helical and tubular microstructures during cholesterol crystallization from bile. J Clin Invest. 1992;90(September):1155–60. http://academicdepartments.musc.edu/neuromodulation/epapers/horvathjcn99hypocretin.pdf%5Cn; http://scholar.google.com/scholar?hl=en&btnG=Search&q=intitle:Filamentous,+Helical,+and+Tubular+Microstructures+during+Cholesterol+Crystallization+from+Bile#0%5Cnhtt.
20. Khaykovich B, Hossain C, McManus JJ, Lomakin A, Moncton DE, Benedek GB. Structure of cholesterol helical ribbons and self-assembling biological springs. Proc Natl Acad Sci. 2007;104(23):9656–60. https://doi.org/10.1073/pnas.0702967104.
21. Reynolds NP, Adamcik J, Berryman JT, et al. Competition between crystal and fibril formation in molecular mutations of amyloidogenic peptides. Nat Commun. 2017;8(1):1338–48. https://doi.org/10.1038/s41467-017-01424-4.
22. Varsano N, Beghi F, Elad N, et al. Two polymorphic cholesterol monohydrate crystal structures form in macrophage culture models of atherosclerosis. Proc Natl Acad Sci U S A. 2018;115:7662. https://doi.org/10.1073/pnas.1803119115.
23. Portincasa P, Moschetta A, Van Erpecum KJ, et al. Pathways of cholesterol crystallization in model bile and native bile. Dig Liver Dis. 2003;35(2):118–26. https://doi.org/10.1016/S1590-8658(03)00009-4.
24. Garti N, Karpuj L, Sarig S. Correlation between crystal habit and the composition of solvated and nonsolvated cholesterol crystals. J Lipid Res. 1981;22:785. https://doi.org/10.1016/s0022-2275(20)37350-8.
25. Varsano N, Beghi F, Dadosh T, et al. The effect of the phospholipid bilayer environment on cholesterol crystal polymorphism. ChemPlusChem. 2019;84:338. https://doi.org/10.1002/cplu.201800632.
26. Baumer Y, McCurdy S, Weatherby TM, et al. Hyperlipidemia-induced cholesterol crystal production by endothelial cells promotes atherogenesis. Nat Commun. 2017;8(1):1129. https://doi.org/10.1038/s41467-017-01186-z.
27. Nordestgaard BG, Watts GF, Bruckert E, Fazio S, Ference BA, Graham I, Horton JF, Landmesser U, Laufs U, Masana L, Pasterkamp G, Raal FJ, Ray KK, Schunkert H, Taskinen M, van de Sluis B, Wiklund O, Tokgozoglu L, Catapano AL, Borén J, Chapman MJ, Krauss RM, Packard CJ, Bentzon JF, Binder CJ, Daemen MJ, Demer LL, Hegele RA. Low-density lipoproteins cause atherosclerotic cardiovascular disease: pathophysiological, genetic, and

therapeutic insights: a consensus statement from the European Atherosclerosis Society Consensus Panel. Eur Heart J. 2020;14:2313. https://doi.org/10.1093/eurheartj/ehz962.
28. Fazio S, Major AS, Swift LL, et al. Increased atherosclerosis in LDL receptor-null mice lacking ACAT1 in macrophages. J Clin Invest. 2001;107(2):163–71. https://doi.org/10.1172/JCI10310.
29. Yan RS, Dove DE, Major AS, et al. Reduced ABCA1-mediated cholesterol efflux and accelerated atherosclerosis in apolipoprotein E-deficient mice lacking macrophage-derived ACAT1. Circulation. 2005;111(18):2373–81. https://doi.org/10.1161/01.CIR.0000164236.19860.13.
30. Lima H, Jacobson LS, Goldberg MF, et al. Role of lysosome rupture in controlling Nlrp3 signaling and necrotic cell death. Cell Cycle. 2013;12(12):1868–78. https://doi.org/10.4161/cc.24903.
31. Shu F, Chen J, Ma X, et al. Cholesterol crystal-mediated inflammation is driven by plasma membrane destabilization. Front Immunol. 2018;9:1163. https://doi.org/10.3389/fimmu.2018.01163.
32. Tangirala RK, Jerome WG, Jones NL, et al. Formation of cholesterol monohydrate crystals in macrophage-derived foam cells. J Lipid Res. 1994;35(1):93–104. https://doi.org/10.1016/s0022-2275(20)40131-2.
33. Arbore G, Kemper C, Kolev M. Intracellular complement—the complosome—in immune cell regulation. Mol Immunol. 2017;89:2–9. https://doi.org/10.1016/j.molimm.2017.05.012.
34. Lappalainen J, Eklund K, Kovanen P, Välimäki E, Rajamäki EMS. Cholesterol crystals activate the NLRP3 inflammasome in human macrophages: a novel link between cholesterol metabolism and inflammation. PloS One. 2010;5(7):1–9. https://doi.org/10.1371/journal.pone.0011765.
35. Kolodgie FD, Burke AP, Nakazawa G, Cheng Q, Xu X, Virmani R. Free cholesterol in atherosclerotic plaques: where does it come from? Curr Opin Lipidol. 2007;18(5):500–7. https://doi.org/10.1097/MOL.0b013e3282efa35b.
36. Pervaiz MH, Durga S, Janoudi A, Berger K, Abela GS. PET/CT detection of muscle inflammation related to cholesterol crystal emboli without arterial obstruction. J Nucl Cardiol. 2018;25:433–40.
37. Mughal MM, Khan MK, DeMarco JK, Majid A, Shamoun F, Abela GS. Symptomatic and asymptomatic carotid artery plaque. Expert Rev Cardiovasc Ther. 2011;9:1315–30. https://doi.org/10.1586/erc.11.120.
38. Abela GS. Cholesterol crystals piercing the arterial plaque and intima trigger local and systemic inflammation. J Clin Lipidol. 2010;4:156–64. https://doi.org/10.1016/j.jacl.2010.03.003.
39. Perl-Treves D, Kessler N, Izhaky D, Addadi L. Monoclonal antibody recognition of cholesterol monohydrate crystal faces. Chem Biol. 1996;3(7):567–77. https://doi.org/10.1016/S1074-5521(96)90148-9.
40. Hasselbacher P, Hahn JL. Activation of the alternative pathway of complement by microcrystalline cholesterol. Atherosclerosis. 1980;37(2):239–45. https://doi.org/10.1016/0021-9150(80)90009-X.
41. Warnatsch A, Ioannou M, Wang QPV. Inflammation. Neutrophil extracellular traps license macrophages for cytokine production in atherosclerosis. Science (80-). 2015;349(6245):316–20.
42. Nidorf SM, Fiolet A, Abela GS. Viewing atherosclerosis through a crystal lens: how the evolving sturture of cholesterol crystals in atheroscleritc plaque alters its stability. J Clin Lipidol. 2020;14:619–30. https://doi.org/10.1016/j.jacl.2020.07.003.
43. Abela GS, Kalavakunta JK, Janoudi A, Leffler D, Dhar G, Salehi N, Cohn J, Shah I, Karve M, Kotaru VPK, Gupta V, David S, Narisetty KK, Rich M, Vanderberg A, Pathak DR, Shamoun FE. Frequency of cholesterol crystals in culprit coronary artery aspirate during acute myocardial infarction and their relation to inflammation and myocardial injury. Am J Cardiol. 2017;120:1699–707. https://doi.org/10.1016/j.amjcard.2017.07.075.
44. Nidorf SM. The challenge of reducing residual cardiovascular risk in patients with chronic kidney disease. Eur Heart J. 2022;43:4845. https://doi.org/10.1093/eurheartj/ehac531.

45. Wilkens JA, Krut LH. The effect of glucose on the crystallization of cholesterol. J Atheroscler Res. 1965;5(5):516–23. https://doi.org/10.1016/s0368-1319(65)80024-2.
46. Self-Medlin Y, Byun J, Jacob RF, Mizuno Y, Mason RP. Glucose promotes membrane cholesterol crystalline domain formation by lipid peroxidation. Biochim Biophys Acta. 2009;1788(6):1398–403. Epub 2009 Apr 17. https://doi.org/10.1016/j.bbamem.2009.04.004.
47. Giorgino F, Leonardini A, Laviola L. Cardiovascular disease and glycemic control in type 2 diabetes: now that the dust is settling from large clinical trials. Ann N Y Acad Sci. 2013;1281(1):36–50. Epub 2013 Feb 6. PMID: 23387439; PMCID: PMC3715107. https://doi.org/10.1111/nyas.12044.

Part II
Physical Properties and Imaging of Cholesterol Crystals: In Vitro

How Innovation in Tissue Preparation and Imaging Revolutionized the Understanding of the Role of Cholesterol Crystals in Atherosclerosis

Stanley Flegler, Abigail Vanderberg, Melinda Frame, Carol Flegler, Alicia Withrow, Michael Rich, Erik Shapiro, and George S. Abela

1 Background

Tissue histology using light microscopy continues to be the mainstay for the diagnosis of disease pathology. The fundamentals of tissue processing were established over two centuries ago when alcohol was introduced as a tissue dehydrating agent to facilitate trimming by a microtome and then mount thin tissue cuts on glass slides for staining and examination by a light microscope [1]. Light microscopy tissue preparation involves bathing tissues in 70% ethanol with gradual transition to 100%. This approach has persisted into the modern era because ethanol is miscible in both water of the fixative and the paraffin embedding medium. Sometimes acetone is used instead of ethanol. Although effective in stiffening the tissue for cutting, ethanol dehydration also dissolves fatty elements in the tissue including cholesterol and limits the ability to identify cholesterol crystals (CCs) when processing

S. Flegler · A. Vanderberg · M. Frame · C. Flegler · A. Withrow
Center for Advanced Microscopy, College of Natural Science, Michigan State University, East Lansing, MI, USA
e-mail: flegler@msu.edu; vandera@msu.edu; framem@msu.edu; fleglerc@msu.edu; pastorle@msu.edu

M. Rich
College of Engineering, Composite Materials and Structures Center, Michigan State University, East Lansing, MI, USA
e-mail: rich@msu.edu

E. Shapiro
Department of Radiology, Michigan State University, East Lansing, MI, USA
e-mail: shapir86@msu.edu

G. S. Abela (✉)
Department of Medicine, Division of Cardiovascular Medicine, Michigan State University, East Lansing, MI, USA
e-mail: abela@msu.edu

G. S. Abela, S. M. Nidorf (eds.), *Cholesterol Crystals in Atherosclerosis and Other Related Diseases*, Contemporary Cardiology,
https://doi.org/10.1007/978-3-031-41192-2_3

atherosclerotic plaques for light microscopy. As CCs dissolve during preparation, they leave behind empty spaces within the plaque that approximate the residual shape of crystals. Pathologists have referred to these tissue imprints as "cholesterol clefts" and understood that the clefts were the result of dissolving CCs by tissue

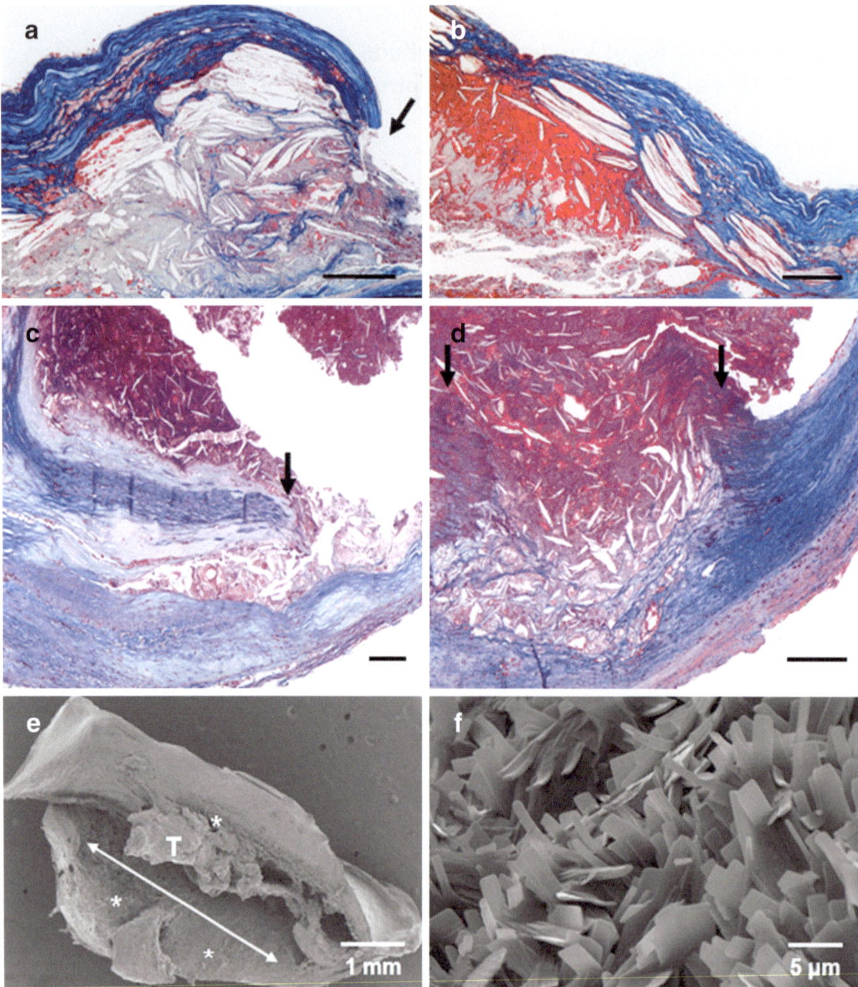

Fig. 1 Cholesterol clefts by light microscopy vs. cholesterol crystals by scanning electron microscopy. (**a–d**) Light micrographs of plaque rupture (arrows) in carotid arteries from three patients with neurologic symptoms (Masson's trichrome stain; bars = 200 µm). No crystals are seen perforating the intimal surface. (**e, f**) Low-magnification scanning electron micrography of plaque obtained on endarterectomy have extensive crystal formations (*) on the entire plaque surface (arrow) below the thrombus (T). Higher-magnification SEM shows the extensiveness and density of CCs layering the intimal surface. (Reproduced with permission [7])

preparation methods [2, 3] but they invariably dismissed their importance in the genesis and progression of atherosclerosis (Fig. 1a–d).

As microscopy evolved and developed to include scanning and transmission electron microscopy, higher tissue definition became possible [4]. However, even in the case of electron microscopy the same tissue dehydration approach is utilized [5]. Ethanol is used since it is miscible with the resin used during embedding tissue for transmission electron microscopy. It is also miscible with the liquid carbon dioxide used as the transitional fluid for critical point drying for scanning electron microscopy (SEM). In both techniques, graded ethyl alcohol is typically used at 25%, 50%, and 75% for half an hour each and then 100% for 45 min [5]. As with light microscopy, the use of solvents dissolves CCs making them undetectable by electron microscopy. Therefore, the modification of the tissue processing technique is required and critical in order to detect and quantify CCs in tissues. Specifically, with light microscopy, since CCs that are not embedded in the tissues do not leave any imprints, the amount of CCs may be vastly underestimated if they are situated at and above the tissue surface as often occurs in ruptured plaque. In contrast, when using SEM without dissolving CCs the true extent and distribution of CCs become readily visible (Fig. 1e, f).

2   Scanning Electron Microscopy Methodology

2.1   Tissue Preparation for SEM

Scanning electron microscopy provides high resolution imaging of the tissue surface by an electron beam that is discharged from an electron gun in a vacuum chamber. The electron beam interacts with atoms in a conductive sample to emit secondary electrons that form an image [5]. For optimal image quality and resolution, samples must be prepared so that they are dry and conductive. Tissues are initially prepared by fixation in buffered 4% glutaraldehyde or buffered 10% formalin and then cut into 3–5 mm long segments. In order to preserve CCs it is necessary to avoid the standard use of ethanol for tissue dehydration; hence tissue samples are dehydrated using either air drying for several days or by placing tissues in a vacuum chamber (Speed Vac SC110, Savant Instruments Inc., Farmingdale, NY) evacuated by a pump (VP110, Franklin Electric, Bluffton, IN) for up to 12 hours prior to scanning [6, 7].

Another technique developed in our laboratory is to air dry samples while placing a thin layer of silk material on them to absorb residual liquid and oily residues on the tissue so that the tissue remains stable in the in the SEM chamber. Because the samples are dry, critical point drying is not a necessary step in tissue processing. These tissue segments are then mounted on aluminum stubs and fixed with 2% osmium tetroxide vapor for at least 48 h. Vapor fixation in osmium tetroxide is used to stabilize oil/lipids on the tissue surface that could otherwise contaminate the column of the SEM. The tissue is finally coated in a gold sputter coater or osmium coater (NEOC-AT osmium CVD (chemical vapor deposition); Meiwafosis Co., Ltd., Osaka, Japan). Tissue surfaces are then examined using a JEOL SEM (model JSM-6300F, JSM-6400, or JSM-6610LV, JEOL Ltd., Tokyo, Japan).

2.2   Quantification of Cholesterol Crystals

In our Lab we developed a semi-quantification method to assess the tissue content of CCs by SEM. This includes *crystal density* defined as absent (+0), scattered few (+1), dense in a limited area (+2), or dense and widely distributed (+3). Thus, it is important to also obtain a low magnification image of the entire tissue segment surface to detect *CCs distribution* for a count of the various sites with crystal presence [7, 8]. The average CC density per specimen is then calculated by adding all the individual densities from all the sites and divided by the number of sites in a specific specimen. This approach allows for both quantification of crystal density and the area of distribution of CCs over the entire tissue segment.

2.3   Tissue Shrinkage

Tissue shrinkage is a known occurrence during tissue processing for microscopy. On an average it is expected that about 15% tissue shrinkage will occur after fixation and dehydration [8–10]. However, hardened and calcific plaques may not shrink to the same extent as soft tissues. Using standard tissue preparation by fixation and dehydration, studies have found soft arterial tissues shrink 9% in the short axis and 12% in the long axis. However, vacuum drying can result in shrinkage up to 16% in the short axis and 19% in the long axis [8]. Some reviewers have raised concern about the protocol that excludes the ethanol dehydration step claiming that air or vacuum drying will cause excessive shrinkage and create artifacts including the formation of crystals and their perforating the arterial intima seen by SEM. However, when the same tissues were examined without any tissue processing using either fluorescence, digital or cryo-transmission electron microscopy the same finding of CCs perforating the intima was confirmed on the same tissue specimens as noted with air or vacuum dried tissues by SEM (Figs. 2, and 3) [11, 12]. Moreover, other techniques using micro-optical coherence tomography (OCT), standard OCT in human coronary arteries during acute coronary syndrome, and angioscopy of spontaneous plaque rupture in human patients have all demonstrated the presence of CCs

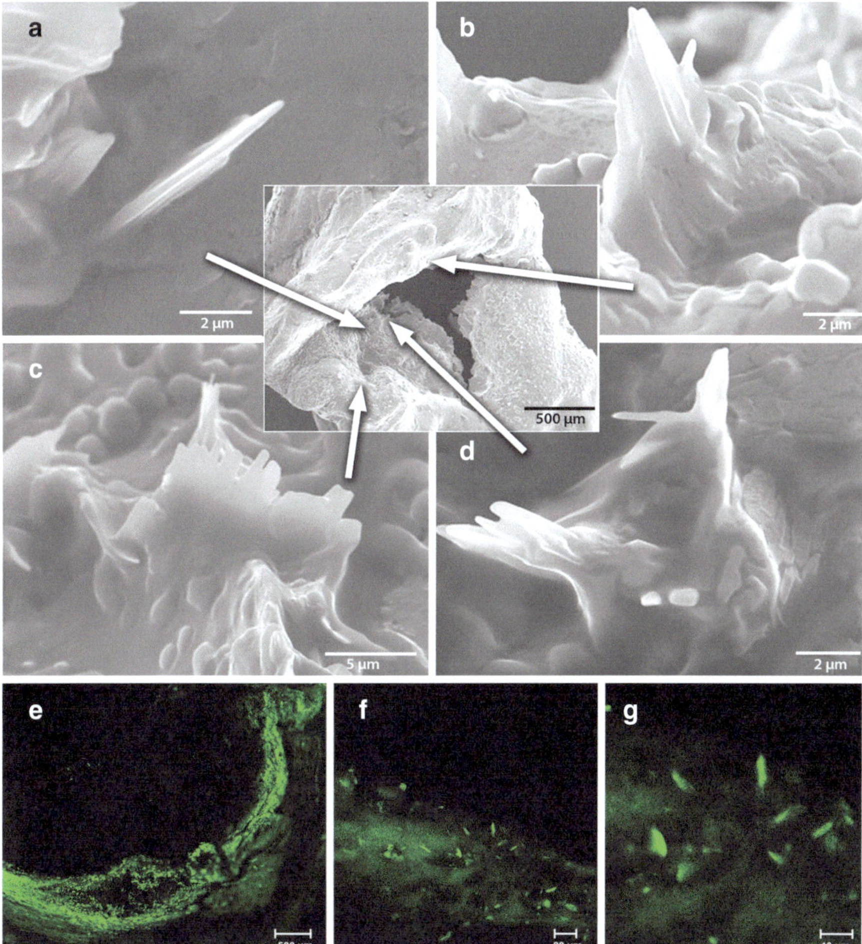

Fig. 2 Scanning electron micrographs of human coronary artery and fluorescence microscopy of carotid plaque. (**a–d**) Scanning electron micrographs of left anterior descending coronary artery from patient who died of an acute myocardial infarction. Cholesterol crystals are noted perforating the intimal surface just below the plaque rupture site. (**e–g**) Low-power image of human carotid plaque with green fluorescence. (**f, g**) Higher magnification reveals selectively stained cholesterol crystals arising from the plaque surface seen without any tissue processing. (Reproduced with permission [6, 11])

emerging from atherosclerotic plaques and penetrating the intima as seen with SEM using air or vacuum dehydration (Fig. 4) [13–15].

Detailed evaluation of the role of ethanol on tissue preparation for SEM confirmed that ethanol at the sequential concentrations used (25; 50; 75; 95 and 100%)

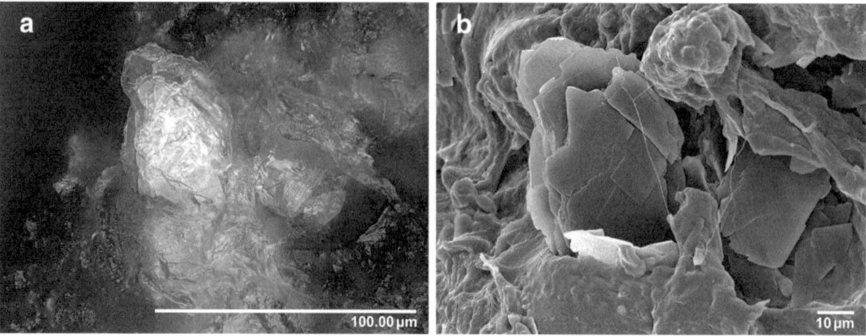

Fig. 3 Digital image of cholesterol crystal from a fresh colon cancer (**a**) with the same sample subsequently processed with air dehydration for scanning electron microscopy demonstrating almost identical crystal morphology (**b**). (Courtesy of GS Abela)

Fig. 4 Micro-optical coherence tomography of plaque. Evidence of cholesterol crystals perforating the fibrous cap and intima of human plaque. Micro-optical coherence tomography image of human carotid plaque with (**a**) dense concentration of cholesterol crystals beneath a bulging fibrous cap and (**b**) cholesterol crystals perforating the fibrous cap (arrow; *nc* necrotic core). (Courtesy of GJ Tearney and reproduced with permission [13])

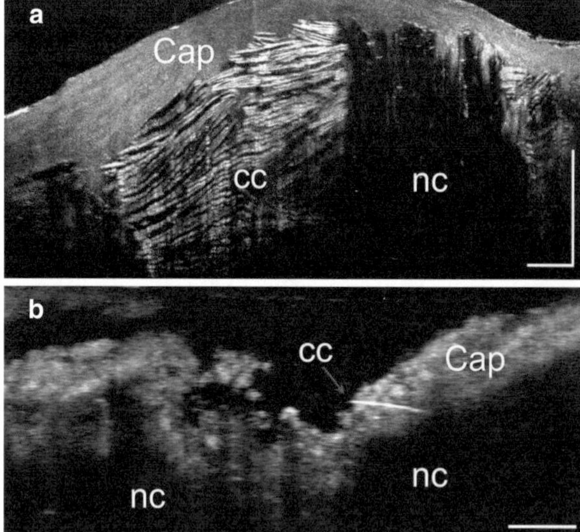

[5] causes a dose related solubilization and dissolving of the CCs, and 100% ethanol essentially eliminated all CCs present in the tissue [11]. These studies were performed by using mirror tissue segments of human carotid atherosclerotic plaque, one prepared in normal saline medium serving as control and the other matched tissue segment treated at various concentrations of ethanol (Fig. 5). Moreover, confocal microscopy with fluorescence on fresh tissues confirmed similar images obtained by SEM utilizing tissues that were dehydrated only by vacuum dehydration (Fig. 6) [7, 11]. All the microscopic techniques used confirm that the SEM modifications that were instituted with air or vacuum dehydration alleviated any concern that this approach of tissue preparation altered the tissues to create an artifact with the CCs emerging from the tissue surface and disrupting tissues.

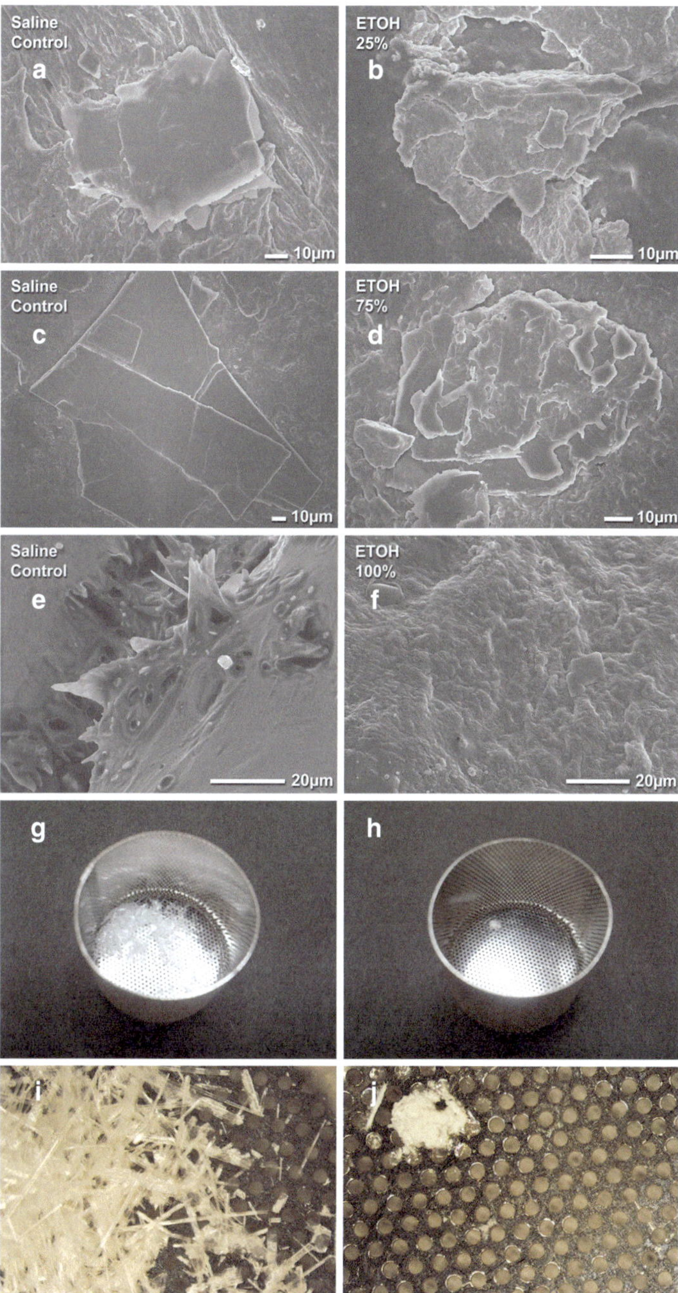

Fig. 5 Carotid artery and synthetic cholesterol crystals treated with and without ethanol preparation: scanning electron microscopy of adjacent human carotid plaque segments incubated with either saline (left column, **a–i**) or with ethanol (right column, **b–j**) at concentrations used in the standard ethanol dehydration protocol. Dissolving cholesterol crystals are noted with ethanol treatment only. (Reproduced with permission [11])

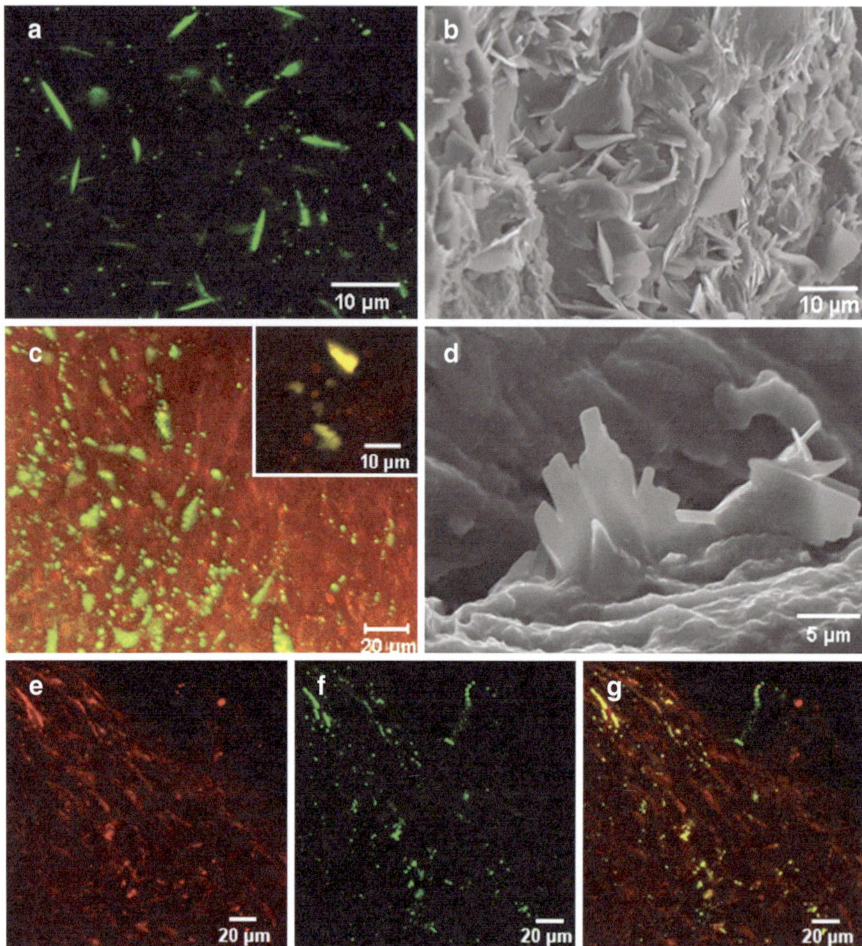

Fig. 6 Fluorescence and scanning electron microscopy of human plaques. (**a**) Fluorescence images of CCs stained with green dye at 37 °C on human plaque surface. (**c, e, f, g**) Similar findings with dual fluorescence staining, Bodipy for CCs, and eosin for intima demonstrate CCs emerging onto the intima at 37 °C. Insert at higher crystal magnification. Selective endothelial stain with acetylated low-density lipoprotein, (**e**) red fluorescence; (**f**) selective CCs stain with Bodipy, green fluorescence; and (**g**) superimposed image of both red and green fluorescence shows CCs on the surface of the endothelium. (**b, d**) SEM of same plaque shows clusters of CCs at intima. (Reproduced with permission [7])

2.4   Cholesterol Crystal Expansion

A benchtop study of the behavior of cholesterol demonstrates that cholesterol occupies a greater volume when crystalizing from a liquid to a solid state. Cholesterol is known to exist in a liquid and semiliquid state in atherosclerotic plaques [16–18]. Once crystals form, they are no longer miscible like the liquid state and spaces develop between the crystals causing them to occupy a markedly larger volume than the space occupied by the liquid phase. In vitro studies demonstrated that when pure cholesterol is melted in a test tube with a heat gun and then allowed to crystalize, the CCs expand in volume by up to 45% of the original volume forming sharp tipped crystals that cut their way into fibrous tissue placed in their path at the mouth of the test tube [6, 19]. CCs could also be seen with the naked eye and then later confirmed by SEM to be perforating fibrous tissue as was subsequently seen in human arterial plaques that had ruptured during acute myocardial infarction (Figs. 4, 5 Chapter "The Role of Cholesterol Crystals in Plaque Rupture Leading to Acute Myocardial Infarction and Stroke") (Fig. 7). Moreover, basic studies confirm that CCs have the physical structure and firmness to perforate fibrous tissues [18].

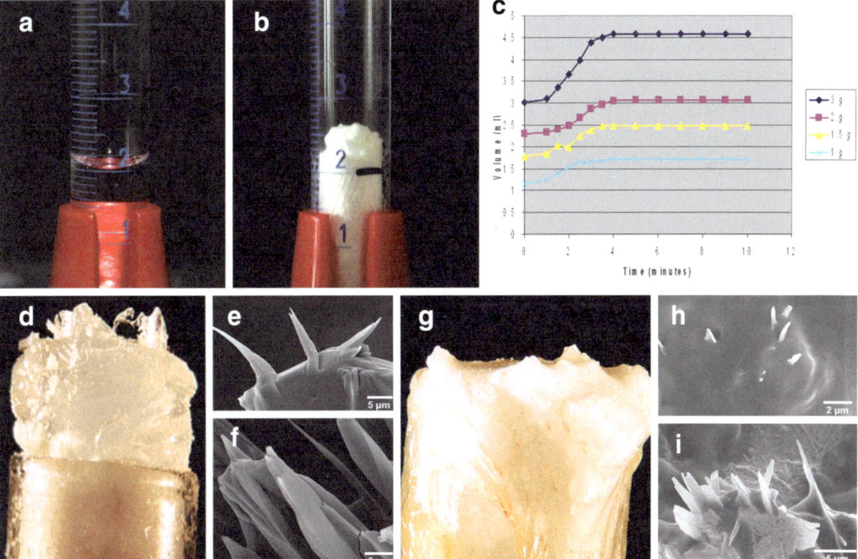

Fig. 7 Volume expansion of cholesterol during crystallization. (**a**, **b**) Melted cholesterol in a graduated cylinder expands in volume above the meniscus line. (**c**) Volume expansion is greater with increasing amounts of cholesterol (1–3 g). (**d**) Cholesterol crystals are seen growing above the edge of the test tube after crystallization. (**e**, **f**) Scanning electron micrographs demonstrate sharp-tipped crystal geometries. (**g–i**) When a fibrous membrane is placed over the mouth of the test tube, crystals perforate the membrane as noted by scanning electron microscopy (bar 5 μm). (Reproduced with permission from [6, 34])

2.5   Energy Dispersive X-Ray Spectroscopy (EDX)

EDX with SEM is very helpful in determining the composition of crystals being examined. This process detects X-rays emitted by the sample due to excitation of atoms by the incident electron beam. This interaction produces characteristic X-rays that reveal the elemental composition of the targeted SEM image. EDX measures the energy of these X-rays and utilizes the unique pattern produced by the sample to identify elements present and determine quantities of those elements [20].

CCs are primarily composed of carbon, hydrogen, and oxygen. Hydrogen cannot be detected using EDX and is therefore not included in this analysis. Calcium phosphate crystals, composed primarily of calcium, phosphorus, and oxygen, are also present in many arterial plaques. These elemental signatures found using EDX, along with morphology, contribute to the identification of the crystal type being examined. The weight percent of each element is quantified by the system [21]. It is important to note that some X-ray signal may be detected from tissue beneath the crystal (due to depth of X-ray production) so an area of tissue without crystals is also analyzed for comparison. In EDX spectra, contaminants often include gold and osmium because these are used for sample coatings (Fig. 8).

In our studies, EDX used to confirm the composition of CCs obtained from aspirates from culprit coronary arteries during acute myocardial infarction demonstrated that all crystals with needle or plate shapes were composed of carbon and oxygen as would be expected for cholesterol [21]. Furthermore, aggregates of calcium phosphate crystals were also present in the aspirates. By SEM those were seen as white nodular deposits that typically form on top of CCs and EDX confirmed they were calcium phosphate (Fig. 8). Further confirmation that these crystals were cholesterol was performed by using infrared spectroscopy (see section on spectroscopy).

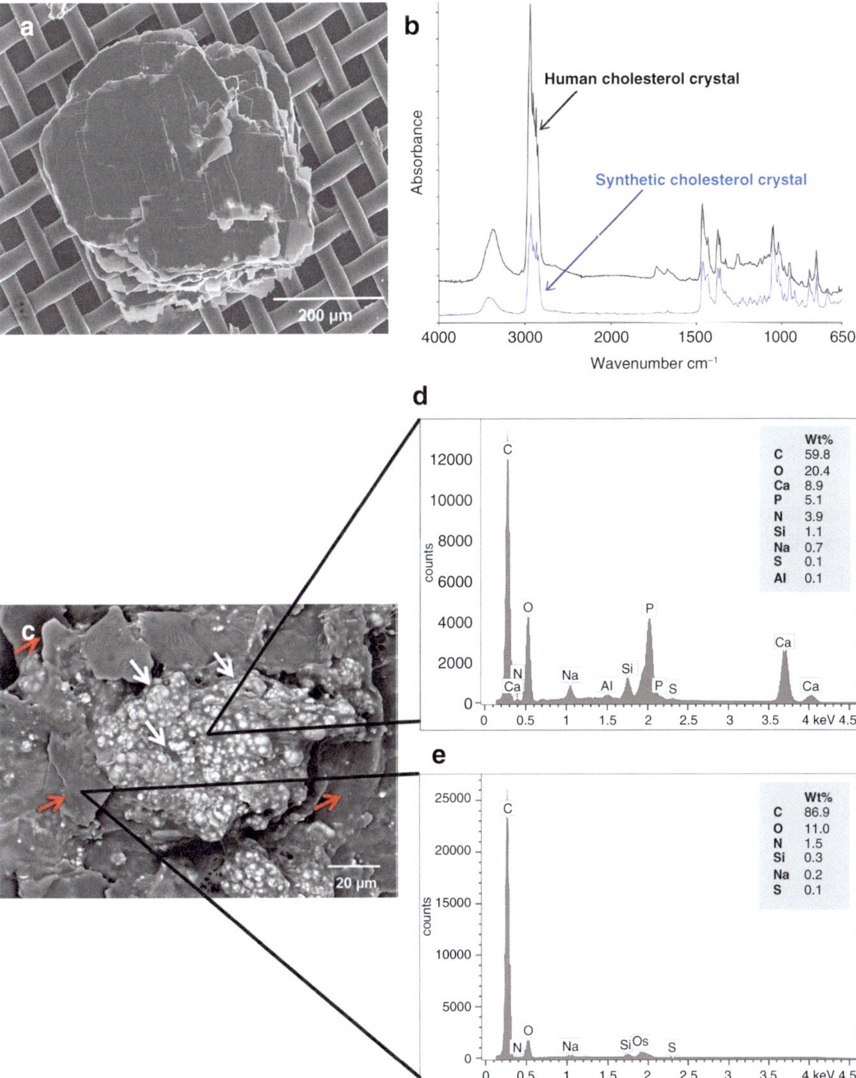

Fig. 8 Chemical composition of crystals aspirated from culprit coronary artery during acute myocardial infarction. (**a**) Scanning electron micrograph of large cholesterol crystal cluster (0.187 mm²) composed of many layers of merged individual plate crystals. (**b**) Fourier transform infrared absorption spectrum of the aspirated human cholesterol crystals is identical to synthetic cholesterol crystals. (**c**) Scanning electron micrograph of calcium crystal deposits (white arrows) overlaying cholesterol crystals (red arrows). (**d**) Calcium and phosphorus ions are detected by energy dispersive X-ray spectroscopy over the clumps of white crystal, whereas no calcium or phosphate is detected over the surrounding cholesterol crystals (**e**). *Al* aluminum, *C* carbon, *Ca* calcium, *Na* sodium, *O* oxygen, *P* phosphorus, *S* sulfur, *Si* silicon, *N* nitrogen. (Reproduced with permission from [21])

3 Transmission Electron Microscopy with Cryo-Methodology

Cryosectioning of tissue helps to preserve CCs by avoiding the use of organic compounds that dissolve CCs. Using transmission electron microscopy (TEM), the tissue is fixed in buffered 4% formaldehyde and 0.1% glutaraldehyde and then immersed in a saturated sucrose solution overnight followed by freezing and then sectioning the tissue while frozen [22]. The ultrathin sections are then transferred from the "cold" knife, thawed, and placed on a grid for examination in a transmission electron microscope (Jeol 100CX electron microscope). These tissue sections are then stained with osmium tetroxide. This approach avoids the use of uranyl acetate which is a solvent and can dissolve CCs [8]. Although this approach does not result in the usual high-quality images of tissue morphology, it does provide clear detection of CCs and their location in the tissues (Fig. 9).

Other techniques include the use of 3-dimensional electron microscopy that has demonstrated the presence of CCs in close association with intracellular lipid droplets and extracellular apolipoprotein B particles in human carotid plaques [23]. Both SEM and TEM with various combined imaging techniques including correlative

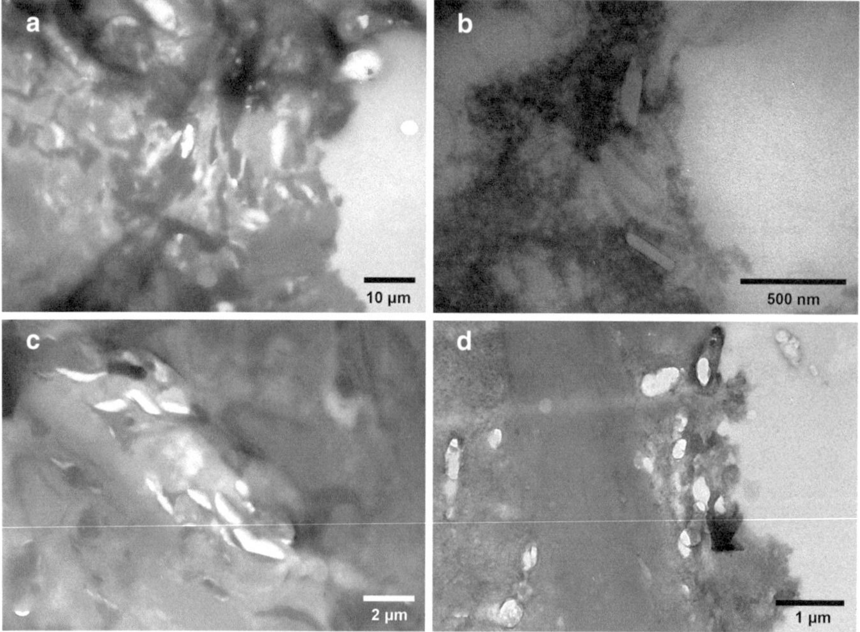

Fig. 9 Transmission electron micrographs of early crystal formation. Transmission electron microscopy of fresh frozen arterial plaques demonstrates very small cholesterol crystals forming at plaque surface of an atherosclerotic rabbit model (**a**, **b**). Also, crystals are noted infiltrating the internal elastic lamella (**c**, **d**). (Reproduced with permission from [8])

cathodoluminescence and cryo-soft X-ray tomography with stochastic reconstruction microscopy can help obtain high resolution (70 nm) and localize early crystal formation [24, 25]. These techniques have become the mainstay for the evaluation of CCs localization and where they appear to form and aggregate within the arterial wall and plaque. Electron microscopy was used to demonstrate that as LDL cholesterol accumulates in endothelial cells where it is metabolized leads to increase the intracellular cholesterol burden that eventually leads to cholesterol crystal formation [26].

4   Confocal Microscopy Methodology

Confocal microscopy can be used to complement SEM and TEM for identifying and characterizing CCs within tissue. Fluorescence light microscopy permits the use of fluorescent stains to specifically label biomolecules and organelles of interest, allowing the use of color for detection, identification, and localization of multiple intracellular targets. Specifically, confocal laser scanning microscopy (CLSM) permits the acquisition of high-contrast fluorescence images through the removal of out-of-focus background light by a pinhole aperture, providing high-resolution images even from relatively thick tissue sections [27]. In addition, CLSM methodologies typically require minimal sample preparation and can be used to image CCs in fresh unprocessed tissue, alleviating concerns that sample preparation may affect CC structure and identification [8].

Detection and localization of intracellular cholesterol by fluorescence microscopy can be performed using a variety of fluorescent molecules that can either bind to cholesterol directly or can closely mimic cholesterol [28]. BODIPY FL (Invitrogen, Waltham, MA; excitation peak 505 nm, emission peak 515 nm) is a relatively photostable fluorophore that emits a bright green fluorescence when exposed to blue excitation light. When the BODIPY moiety is bound directly to cholesterol, the BODIPY-cholesterol complex can be a useful cholesterol probe [29]. Similarly, the BODIPY FL C_{12} cholesteryl ester has been used to monitor intracellular cholesterol, including studies involving cholesterol transport and receptor-mediated endocytosis of lipoproteins [30]. In contrast, Filipin is a naturally occurring fluorescent antibiotic that binds to cholesterol that has been shown to be useful in detecting cholesterol [31]. Filipin fluorescence (excitation peak 360 nm, emission peak 480 nm) can be excited in the UV range with a blue fluorescence emission. Unfortunately, Filipin fluorescence is not appreciably photostable and can rapidly photobleach during UV excitation. Thus, when imaging Filipin care must be taken to attenuate light exposure in order to reduce photobleaching effects.

Multiple fluorescent stains can be used to identify the relationship of CCs to the arterial intima using CLSM. For endothelial staining, fresh arterial tissue is prepared by incubating tissue segments for 4 h at 37 °C in Eagle minimum essential medium with 10 µg/mL Alexa Fluor 594 acetylated-low density lipoprotein under O_2 and CO_2 (Molecular Probes, Eugene, OR). Alexa Fluor 594 acetylated-low density lipoprotein (590 nm excitation, 617 nm emission) is a red fluorescent dye that is specific for endothelium [7, 32]. After incubation, the tissue is washed with PBS and fixed with 4% glutaraldehyde. To counterstain for CCs, fixed tissue segments are placed for 3 min in a solution of cholesteryl BODIPY-C12 (Invitrogen, Eugene, OR) that had been dissolved in 75% ethanol at a 1/100 dilution. Following staining, the dual-labeled tissue segments are rapidly transferred to a slide incubator chamber filled with PBS, and the fluorescence images of the atherosclerotic plaque are acquired using a Zeiss Pascal CLSM microscope (Carl Zeiss, Inc., Jena, Germany). This approach does not allow enough time for the crystals to be dissolved by the ethanol. The cholesteryl BODIPY-C12 fluorescence is excited using the 488 nm Argon laser, and the green fluorescence emission collected using a 505–530 nm band-pass filter. The Alexa Fluor 594 fluorescence is excited using the 543 nm helium-neon laser, and the red emission is collected using a 560 nm long-pass filter. This process allows simultaneous staining of both the endothelial cells red and the CCs green demonstrating a spatial relationship that shows the crystals perforating through the arterial intima (Fig. 6).

5   Digital Microscopy Methodology

Sample preparation is not required for imaging by a VHX-6000 digital microscope because digital light microscopy uses the concept of Focus Stacking (also called Z-stacking). It combines multiple images taken at different focus distances to give a resulting image with greater depth of field. Software algorithms are used to determine which of the pixels are in sharp focus and then use these to create the final image [33]. For the study of CCs, tissue was examined using a Keyence VHX-6000 digital light microscope (Keyence Corp of America, Itasca, IL, USA). When using tissues that were fixed in formalin and air dried, CCs were visible as rectangular, iridescent plates on the arterial surface. These CCs were later confirmed by SEM on the same tissue specimen (Fig. 2).

6   Phase Contrast and Polarized Light Microscopy

Location, density, and geometries of unstained CCs, of isolated crystals as well as those located within cultured cells or thin tissue sections, can be viewed directly by several transmitted light microscopic methodologies, including bright-field microscopy, phase contrast microscopy, differential interference microscopy, and polarized light microscopy [34].

In bright-field microscopy, image contrast is often limited by the small differences in light scatter and diffraction properties of the CCs compared to the surrounding cells or tissue, limiting the usefulness of bright field microscopy in visualizing unstained specimens. Alternatively, both phase contrast and differential interference microscopy methodologies enhance contrast by taking advantage of the subtle differences in the thickness and refractive indices of structures within the specimen. In phase contrast microscopy, optics are introduced within the microscope that convert differences in phase within the sample into differences of amplitude that can be visualized through the oculars or recorded by a digital camera. Similarly, differential interference microscopy uses optics to produce shadows within the image resulting in a pseudo-3-dimensional appearance that can help resolve structures within transparent, low-contrast samples (Fig. 10).

In contrast, polarized light microscopy relies on birefringent properties produced by highly ordered structures, such as the ordered molecular arrays found within crystal structures, to create a bright image of the birefringent structure against a very dark background (Fig. 11) [28]. With a wavelength dependence that often results in highly colorized structures, polarized light microscopy provides a high-contrast imaging methodology that is highly selective for CC structure [34].

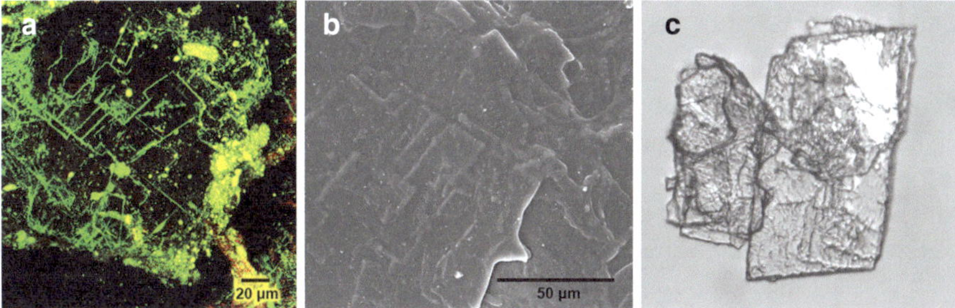

Fig. 10 Crystal images using various contrast microscopy. (**a, b**) Crystalloids are seen in atherosclerotic plaque using phase contrast microscopy (**a**) Fluorescence, (**b**) differential interference contrast, and (**c**) brightfield microscopic images demonstrating the typical features of rhomboid shaped cholesterol crystals obtained from human coronary artery during acute myocardial infarction

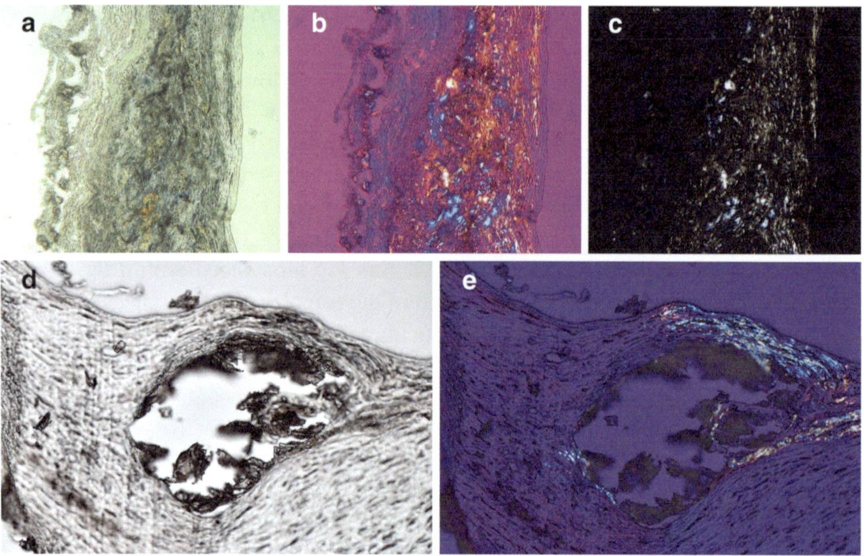

Fig. 11 Polarizing microscopy of crystals in plaque. Polarizing light microscopy of birefringent crystals in rabbit aorta (**a**, **b**, **c**) and human coronary arteries (**d**, **e**) obtained at various angles (0°, 45° and 90°). (Reproduced with permission (**d**, **e**; [42]))

7 Infrared Spectroscopy

In other studies crystals obtained from aspirates of culprit coronary arteries during myocardial infarction were collected and examined using Fourier Transform Infrared Spectroscopy (FTIR) (Perkin Elmer Spectrum One FTIR, Waltham, Massachusetts) fitted with a light microscope that permitted the FITR interrogation of the small crystals in the aspirates [22]. The spectra of crystals were compared with crystals made from a commercial synthetic cholesterol source made by dissolving cholesterol powder in methyl alcohol and allowed to evaporate leaving behind CCs. Micro-FTIR spectroscopy confirmed that the plate and needle-shaped crystals from human coronary artery aspirates and the synthetic crystals were composed of cholesterol (Fig. 8). The interferograms of aspirated crystals from patients were identical to those of synthetic CCs. To further confirm the chemical composition, EDX was also used to demonstrate that all crystals with needle or plate shapes from human coronary aspirates were composed of carbon and oxygen as would be expected for cholesterol.

Infrared spectroscopy is now being tested in the clinical setting using catheter-based technology to engage the coronary arteries during interventional procedures [35]. This approach has been able to detect the present of lipid deposits in the arterial wall during cardiac catheterization of the coronary arteries. It is hypothesized that this could allow the interventional cardiologist to identify and stent sites that may be prone to rupture.

8   Raman Spectroscopy

Coherent anti-Stokes Raman Scattering (CARS) microscopy can be used to interrogate fresh tissues by chemical imaging by molecular vibrations. It is a nonlinear optical microscopy with submicron resolution that does not require dye labeling for imaging. It is selectively effective in imaging lipids by interrogating the vibrational signatures of carbon-hydrogen bonds. It has been used to correlate the morphology and chemical composition of atherosclerotic lipids in plaques [36, 37]. Studies performed by multiplex CARS on atherosclerotic arteries from ApoE $^{-/-}$ mice using spectral ranges of Raman shift from 2650 to 3050 cm^{-1} [36] demonstrated the presence of needle shaped CCs deep in the intima (20 μm). Moreover, when mice were treated with simvastatin, the crystallized lipids detected by CARS were found to be less solidified than those seen in the non-treated group. However, both needle shaped and rhomboid shaped crystals were detected by CARS. In another study evaluating the use of hyperspectral CARS imaging/principal component analysis to image CCs in atherosclerotic arteries from LDLR$^{-/-}$ and ApoE$^{-/-}$ mice [37] a chemical map used to identify CCs within macrophages confirmed that they were composed of cholesterol. The three-dimensional feature of these systems has the potential to be applied to in vivo conditions. Since abundant CCs is a common feature of ruptured plaques, this feature may have the potential to detect plaques that are prone to rupture in real time during vascular intervention [38, 39].

9   Nuclear Magnetic Resonance Spectroscopy

Early studies on the development of the lipid core in atherosclerotic plaques suggested that CCs were important feature in plaque evolution as evidenced by their presence in fatty streaks [40]. However, this was not certain as once the tissues are fixed and processed for light and transmission electron microscopy, CCs were dissolved leaving behind empty "clefts." Furthermore, the original biochemical studies done on arterial tissue were destructive causing the loss of the specific localization of CCs.

However, NMR spectroscopy is a nondestructive approach that can be used to identify various plaque elements. As opposed to liquid-based samples, NMR of solid structures requires the use of "solid state" techniques to narrow resonance peaks, one of which is magic angle spinning (MAS NMR). Also, contrary to more commonly performed hydrogen NMR, in which the signals of metabolites or other biological materials is dwarfed by the water signal, to specifically detect cholesterol, it is possible to use ^{13}C NMR, aided by signal amplification techniques such as cross-polarization, in which magnetization is transferred from the abundant hydrogen atoms to the very nonabundant ^{13}C atoms. To detect calcium phosphate hydroxyapatite in situ, ^{31}P MAS NMR is used (no need for cross polarization as ^{31}P is the natural abundance isotope). By performing ^{13}C and ^{31}P MAS NMR it is possible to obtain quantitative measures of crystalline cholesterol and calcium phosphate, respectively, as demonstrated in ex vivo tissue specimens of human carotid plaques [41]. This method has the potential to evaluate the amount of CCs trapped within the phospholipid bilayers and determine the supersaturated state in that location and as such can help localize of the distribution of CCs in the tissue. However, these experiments cannot be performed in humans for several reasons, including resolution of the current approaches with NMR spectroscopy and the need to spin samples.

References

1. Bracegridle B. A history of microtechnique: the evolution of the microtome and the development of tissue preparation. London: Heinemann; 1978. p. 64.
2. Flory CM. Arterial occlusions produced by emboli from eroded atheromatous plaques. Am J Pathol. 1945;21:549–65.
3. Guyton JR, Klemp KF. Transitional features in human atherosclerosis: intimal thickening, cholesterol clefts, and cell loss in human aortic fatty streaks. Am J Pathol. 1993;143:1444–57.
4. Baumer Y, Mehta NN, Dey AK, Powell-Wiley TM, Boisvert WA. Cholesterol crystals and atherosclerosis. Eur Heart J. 2020;41:2236–9.
5. Flegler SL, Heckman JW Jr, Klomparens KL. Scanning and transmission electron microscopy. New York, NY: Oxford University Press; 1993. p. 240.
6. Abela GS, Aziz K. Cholesterol crystals rupture biological membranes and human plaques during acute cardiovascular events—a novel insight into plaque rupture by scanning electron microscopy. Scanning. 2006;28:1–10.
7. Abela GS, Aziz K, Vedre A, Pathak DR, Talbott JD, DeJong J. Effect of cholesterol crystals on plaques and intima in arteries of patients with acute coronary and cerebrovascular syndromes. Am J Cardiol. 2009;103:959–68.
8. Patel R, Janoudi A, Vedre A, Aziz K, Tamhane U, Rubinstein J, Abela OG, Berger K, Abela GS. Plaque rupture and thrombosis is reduced by lowering cholesterol levels and crystallization with ezetimibe and is correlated with FDG-PET. Arterioscler Thromb Vasc Biol. 2011;31:2007–14. https://doi.org/10.1161/ATVBAHA.111.226167.
9. Choy JS, Mathieu-Costello O, Kassab GS. The effect of fixation and histological preparation on coronary artery dimensions. Ann Biochem Eng. 2005;33:1027–33.
10. Dobrin PB. Effect of histologic preparation on the cross-sectional area of arterial rings. J Surg Res. 1996;61:413–5.
11. Nasiri M, Huang R, Janoudi A, Vanderberg A, Flegler C, Flegler S, Abela GS. Unraveling the role of cholesterol crystals in plaque rupture by altering the method of tissue preparation. Microsc Res Tech. 2015;78:969–74.
12. El-Khatib LA, De Feijter-Rupp H, Janoudi A, Fry L, Kehdi M, Abela GS. Cholesterol induced heart valve inflammation and injury: efficacy of cholesterol lowering treatment. Open Heart. 2020;7:e001274. https://doi.org/10.1136/openhrt-2020-001274.
13. Liu L, Gardecki JA, Nadkarni SK, Toussaint JD, Yagi Y, Bouma BE, Tearney GJ. Imaging the subcellular structure of human coronary atherosclerosis using micro–optical coherence tomography. Nat Med. 2011;17:1010–4.
14. Dai J, Tian J, Hou J, Xing L, Liu S, Ma L, Yu H, Ren X, Dong N, Yu B. Association between cholesterol crystals and culprit lesion vulnerability in patients with acute coronary syndrome: an optical coherence tomography study. Atherosclerosis. 2016;247:111–7.

15. Komatsu S, Yutani C, Ohara T, Takahashi S, Takewa M, Hirayama A, Kodama K. Angioscopic evaluation of spontaneously rupture aortic plaques. J Am Coll Cardiol. 2018;71:2893–902. https://doi.org/10.1016/j.jacc.2018.03.539.
16. Lundberg B. Atherosclerosis chemical composition and physical state of lipid deposits in atherosclerosis. Atherosclerosis. 1995;56:93–110.
17. Lang P, Insull W Jr. Lipid droplets in atherosclerotic fatty streaks of human aorta. J Clin Invest. 1970;49:1479–88.
18. Al-Handawi MB, Commins P, Karothu DP, Raj G, Li L, Naumov P. Mechanical and crystallographic analysis of cholesterol crystals puncturing biological membranes. Chem A Eur J. 2018;24:11493–7.
19. Abela GS, Vedre A, Janoudi A, Huang R, Durga S, Tamhane U. Effect of statins on cholesterol crystallization and atherosclerotic plaque stabilization. Am J Cardiol. 2011;107:1710–7.
20. Bozzola JJ, Russell LD. Electron microscopy. Burlington, MA: Jones and Bartlett; 1992.
21. Abela GS, Kalavakunta JK, Janoudi A, Leffler D, Dhar G, Salehi N, Cohn J, Shah I, Karve M, Kotaru VPK, Gupta V, David S, Narisetty KK, Rich M, Vanderberg A, Pathak DR, Shamoun FE. Frequency of cholesterol crystals in culprit coronary artery aspirate during acute myocardial infarction and their relation to inflammation and myocardial injury. Am J Cardiol. 2017;120:1699–707. https://doi.org/10.1016/j.amjcard.2017.07.075.
22. Webster P, Webster A. Cryosectioning fixed and cryoprotected biological materials. In: Kuo II J, editor. Electron microscopy: methods and protocols. Totowa, NJ: Humana Press; 2007. p. 257–89.
23. Lehti S, Nguyen SD, Belevich I, et al. Extracellular lipids accumulate in human carotid arteries as distinct three-dimensional structures and have proinflammatory properties. Am J Pathol. 2018;188:525–38.
24. Keevend K, Coenen T, Herrmann IK. Correlative cathodoluminescence electron microscopy bioimaging: towards single protein labelling with ultrastructural context. Nanoscale. 2020;12(29):15588–603.
25. Varsano N, et al. Development of correlative cryo-soft X-ray tomography andstochastic reconstruction microscopy. A study of cholesterol crystal early formation in cells. J Am Chem Soc. 2016;138(45):14931–40.
26. Baumer Y, McCurdy S, Weatherby TM, et al. Hyperlipidemia-induced cholesterol crystal production by endothelial cells promotes atherogenesis. Nat Commun. 2017;8:1129. https://doi.org/10.1038/s41467-017-01186-z.
27. Murphy DB, Davidson MW. Fundamentals of light microscopy and electronic imaging. 2nd ed. Hoboken, NJ: Wiley; 2013.
28. Maxfield FR, Wustner D. Analysis of cholesterol trafficking with fluorescent probes. Methods Cell Biol. 2012;108:367–93.
29. Hölttä-Vuori M, Uronen RL, Repakova J, Salonen E, Vattulainen I, Panula P, Li Z, Bittman R, Ikonen E. BODIPY-cholesterol: a new tool to visualize sterol trafficking in living cells and organisms. Traffic. 2008;9:1839–49.
30. https://www.thermofisher.com/us/en/home/references/molecular-probes-the-handbook/fluorophores-and-their-amine-reactive-derivatives/bodipy-dye-series.html#head1.
31. Kruth HS. Histochemical detection of esterified cholesterol within human atherosclerotic lesions using the fluorescent probe filipin. Atherosclerosis. 1984;51:281–92.
32. Voyta JC, Via DP, Butterfield CE, Zetter BR. Identification and isolation of endothelial cells based on their increased uptake of acetylated-low density lipoprotein. J Cell Biol. 1984;99:2034–40.
33. Focus Stacking. In Wikipedia. 2020. https://en.wikipedia.org/wiki/Focus_stacking.
34. Abela GS, Aziz K. Cholesterol crystals cause mechanical damage to biological membranes: a proposed mechanism of plaque rupture and erosion leading to arterial thrombosis. Clin Cardiol. 2005;28:413–20.

35. Madder RD, Goldstein JA, Madden SP, Puri R, Wolski K, Hendricks M, Sum ST, Kini A, Sharma S, Rizik D, Brilakis ES, Shunk KA, Petersen J, Weisz G, Virmani R, Nicholls SJ, Maeheara A, Mintz GS, Stone GW, Muller JE. Detection by near infrared spectroscopy of large lipid core plaques at culprit sites in patients with acute ST-segment elevation myocardial infarction. J Am Coll Cardiol Interv. 2013;6:838–46.
36. Se-H K, Lee E-S, Lee JY, Lee ES, Lee B-S, Park JE, Moon W. Multiplex coherent anti-stokes Raman spectroscopy images intact atheromatous lesions and concomitantly identifies distinct chemical profiles of atherosclerotic lipids. Circ Res. 2010;106:1332–41. https://doi.org/10.1161/CIRCRESAHA.109.208678.
37. Lim RS, Suhalim JL, Miyazaki-Anzai S, Miyazaki M, Levi M, Potma EO, Tromberg BJ. Identification of cholesterol crystals in plaques of atherosclerotic mice using hyperspectral CARS imaging. J Lipid Res. 2011;52:2177–86.
38. Virmani R, Kolodgie FD, Burke AP, Farb A, Schwartz SM. Lessons from sudden coronary death: a comprehensive morphological classification scheme for atherosclerotic lesions. Arterioscler Thromb Vasc Biol. 2000;20:1262–75.
39. Abela GS. Cholesterol crystals piercing the arterial plaque and intima trigger local and systemic inflammation. J Clin Lipidol. 2010;4:156–64.
40. Guyton JR, Klemp KF. Development of the lipid-rich core in human atherosclerosis. Arterioscler Thromb Vasc Biol. 1996;16:4–11.
41. Guo W, Morrisett JD, DeBakey ME, Lawrie GM, Hamilton JA. Quantification in situ of crystalline cholesterol and calcium phosphate hydroxyapatite in human atherosclerotic plaques by solid-state magic angle spinning NMR. Arterioscler Thromb Vasc Biol. 2000;20:1630–6.
42. Nidorf SM, Fiolet A, Abela GS. Viewing atherosclerosis through a crystal lens: how the evolving structure of cholesterol crystals in atherosclerotic plaque alters its stability. J Clin Lipidol. 2020;14:619–30. https://doi.org/10.1016/j.jacl.2020.07.003.

Crystals in Atherosclerosis: Crystal Cholesterol Structures, Morphologies, Formation and Dissolution. What Do We Know?

Jenny Capua-Shenkar, Neta Varsano, Howard Kruth, and Lia Addadi

1 Introduction

Evidence for the onset of cholesterol crystallization emerges at the initial stages of the development of an atherosclerotic lesion [1, 2]. The early events of crystallization are thought to be affected by the local lipid environment that is mostly comprised of the esterified form of cholesterol (thereafter addressed as "cholesteryl ester"), unesterified cholesterol (thereafter addressed as "cholesterol"), and phospholipids as well as by the cellular population residing in the developing lesion [1, 3]. As the lesion assumes further advanced forms, cholesterol concentration raises to super-saturation, where potential meta-stability can lead to cholesterol crystal nucleation and growth [1]. Further lesion advancement will lead to the development of an atheroma, which is characterized by an even further rise in cholesterol concentration, leading to an abundance of additional cholesterol crystal nucleation events, and the growth and thickening of pre-existent crystals. In practice, cholesterol crystals are inevitably observed in advanced atherosclerotic lesions [1, 4, 5].

J. Capua-Shenkar · L. Addadi (✉)
Department of Chemical and Structural Biology, Weizmann Institute of Science, Rehovot, Israel
e-mail: jenny.capua-shenkar@weizmann.ac.il; Lia.Addadi@weizmann.ac.il

N. Varsano
Department of Chemical Research Support, Weizmann Institute of Science, Rehovot, Israel
e-mail: Neta.Varsano@weizmann.ac.il

H. Kruth
Experimental Atherosclerosis Section, National Institutes of Health, Bethesda, MD, USA
e-mail: kruthh@nhlbi.nih.gov

© The Author(s), under exclusive license to Springer Nature Switzerland AG 2023
G. S. Abela, S. M. Nidorf (eds.), *Cholesterol Crystals in Atherosclerosis and Other Related Diseases*, Contemporary Cardiology,
https://doi.org/10.1007/978-3-031-41192-2_4

49

Examination of atherosclerotic lesions, of human or animal model origin, reveals remarkable diversity of crystalline cholesterol shapes and sizes in relation to their environment (Fig. 1). Crystal morphologies present in atherosclerotic lesions vary greatly: from slender platy morphologies seen in rabbit models, associated with lipid droplet surfaces (Fig. 1i) and with the outer surfaces of multi-lamellar bodies (Fig. 1j), to rod-like crystals extracted from human lesions (Fig. 1e), and to massive rhomboid or plate-like crystals, the classic crystalline cholesterol found in human atheromas (Fig. 1a–d, f). Not only is the morphological crystal diversity apparent in the diseased tissues, but also the association between the distinct crystalline morphologies and different tissue components. Human and rabbit advanced lesion cores are associated with large (0.2–2 μm thick, and tens of μm long) plate-like cholesterol crystals (Fig. 1d) [6, 7], whereas early stages of crystalline cholesterol are associated with lipid droplets, multi-lamellar bodies, and additional cellular components in different locations [6, 8, 9]. There is also evidence of intracellular

Fig. 1 Cholesterol crystals in atherosclerotic tissues. Images (**a–f**) concentrate specifically on the crystals, images **g–j** on the cellular context. (**a**) TEM image of human atherosclerotic lesion, cholesterol crystal clefts indicated by arrows. *E* elastic fiber. Scale bar = 1 μm. Adapted with permission from [15]. (**b**) Three-dimensional representation of extracellular lipid droplets, cholesterol crystals, and foam cells generated from SEM images. Cholesterol crystals (yellow) seem to grow out from large lipid droplets (black arrowheads and inset). Large sheet-like crystals (black arrows) can be two dimensionally as large as foam cells. The plasma membranes of the foam cells are artificially colored in transparent blue or green, the nuclei in light blue, and the intracellular lipid droplets in vermilion or maroon. Two cholesterol crystals are surrounded by the right-hand foam cell (white arrow). Reproduced with permission from [7] (**c**) SEM image of human carotid artery displaying cholesterol plate-like crystals (adapted with permission from [16]. (**d**) Cryo-SEM image of a freeze-fractured atherosclerotic lesion taken from a human carotid artery, displaying a multitude of stacked cholesterol crystals. (**e**) Light microscope image of rod-like cholesterol crystals isolated from a human atherosclerotic lesion. Adapted with permission from [17] (**f**) SEM image of a large rhomboid plate-like crystal isolated from human atherosclerotic lesion. (**g**) TEM image of intra-lysosomal cholesterol crystals found in a rabbit lesion *ly* lysosome, *D* lipid droplet. Scale bar = 1 μm. Adapted with permission from [10] (**h**) Thin intracellular cholesterol crystals (black arrows) in a single slice from cryo-focused ion beam block face serial imaging by SEM (cryo-FIB-SEM), taken from a rabbit atherosclerotic lesion. Note that the crystals are not membrane bound. (**i**) Three-dimensional representation of a lipid droplet (pink) with thin cholesterol crystals (grey) attached and merged to its outer surfaces, taken from a rabbit atherosclerotic lesion, data acquired by cryo-FIB-SEM. (**j**) Single slice from cryo-FIB-SEM of a rabbit lesion, displaying a thin cholesterol crystal (arrow) attached to the outer surface of a multi-lamellar body

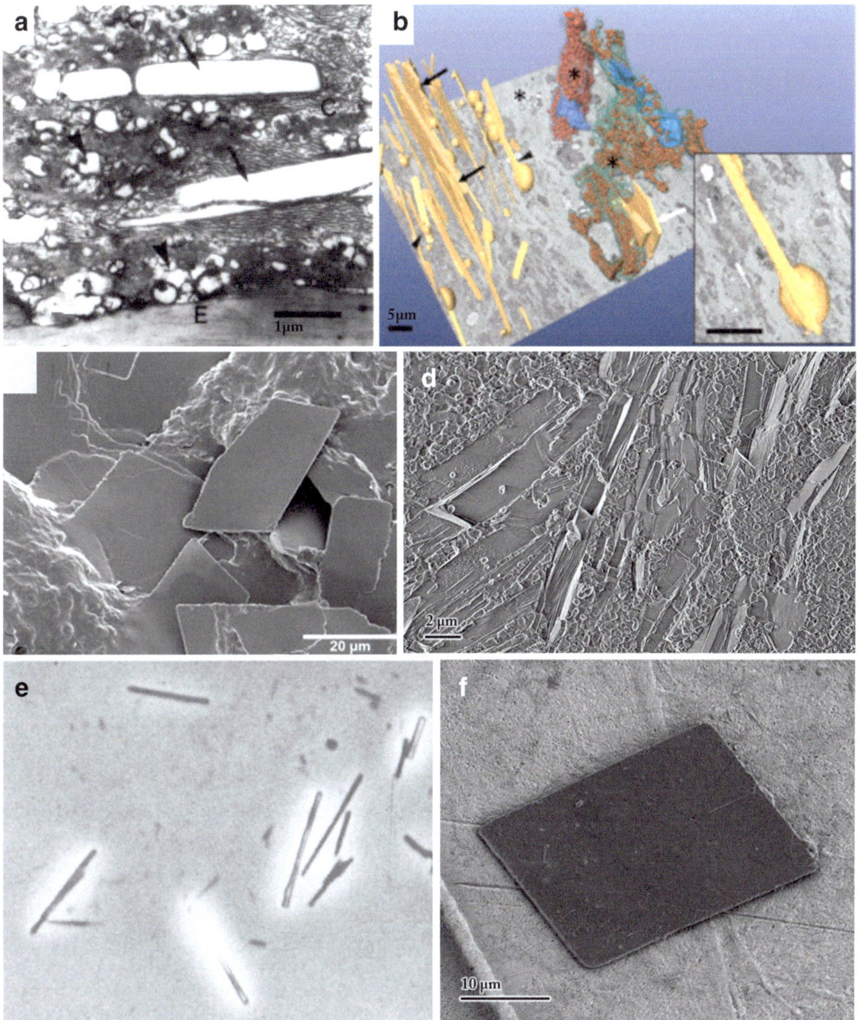

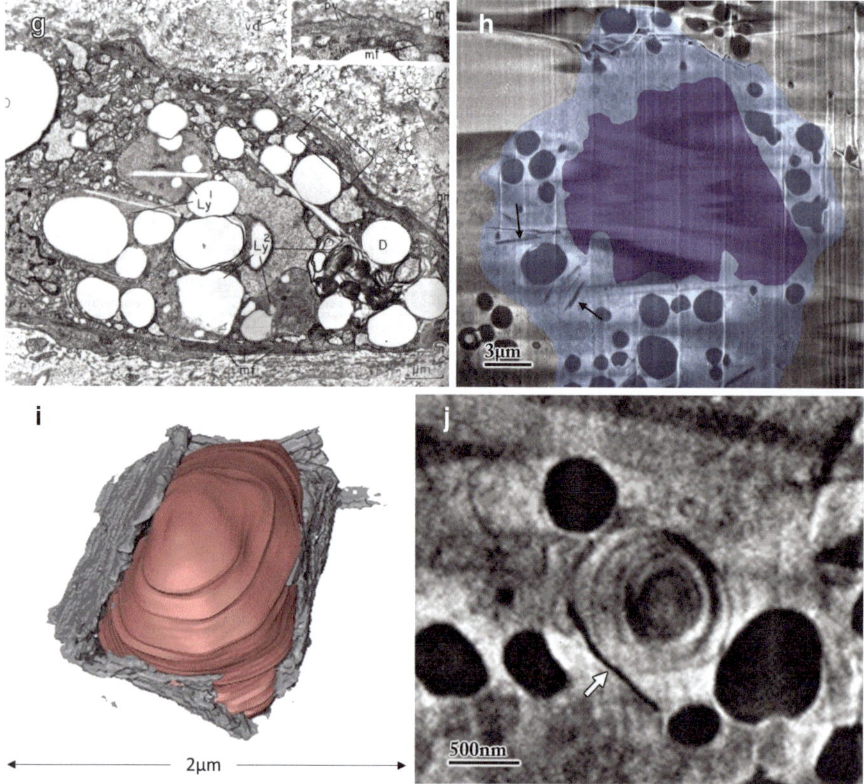

Fig. 1 (continued)

cholesterol nucleation (Fig. 1h) as well as of intra-lysosomal crystals (Fig. 1g) [6, 10]. The cholesterol molecule, from the moment it enters the diseased tissue, may take distinct routes [3, 11]. The intriguing shapes cholesterol crystals assume, while pathologically accumulating in the diseased tissue, and the interaction of these crystals with distinct tissue components give rise to some interesting questions. Is there a relation between the different cholesterol crystal morphologies and the pathway followed during crystal nucleation? Do the structures of the initial crystals remain the same with time? How do different crystal morphologies form within the same region in the lesion and what story can that tell us? Do model systems display distinct crystal characteristics similar or identical to those of the actual diseased tissue? How can environmental characteristics affect cholesterol nucleation, growth and dissolution?

We realize that we are not the first to raise these questions. We also do not claim to have definite and profound answers to all of them. We do hope that with the advent of more advanced techniques, especially in electron microscopy, more information will become accessible [12–14]. Some already available advanced techniques allow us to see the crystals in the tissue and in three dimensions at relatively high resolution, as shown in Fig. 1b (FIB-SEM) and Fig. 1i (cryo-FIB-SEM). The cryo-techniques provide direct observation of the crystals in their native hydrated environment, as shown in Fig. 1d, h–j. These techniques avoid sample preparation procedures that dissolve the crystals, leaving only an imprint of the crystal location in the form of a void, as shown in Fig. 1a, b, g, and without extracting the crystals or drying them, as they are shown in Fig. 1c, e, f.

Looking for answers requires the examination of the fundamental aspects of the processes within the context of the subject that we are examining, cholesterol crystals in atherosclerotic plaques. This we shall do in the sections below, examining first cholesterol the molecule and cholesterol crystal structures, followed by examination of what determines crystal morphologies, crystal nucleation and finally crystal dissolution.

We note that, although calcification is a prominent characteristic of human advanced atherosclerotic lesions, its deposition as well as the interaction with crystalline cholesterol will not be covered in this chapter.

2 Why Cholesterol? Cholesterol, The Molecule and Its Crystals

Cholesterol is an essentially hydrophobic molecule, with a rigid steroid backbone consisting of four fused carbon rings, one hydrocarbon tail and one hydroxyl group, the only hydrophilic group in the whole molecule (Fig. 2a). As a consequence of the molecular structure, cholesterol is almost insoluble in water but does dissolve to a

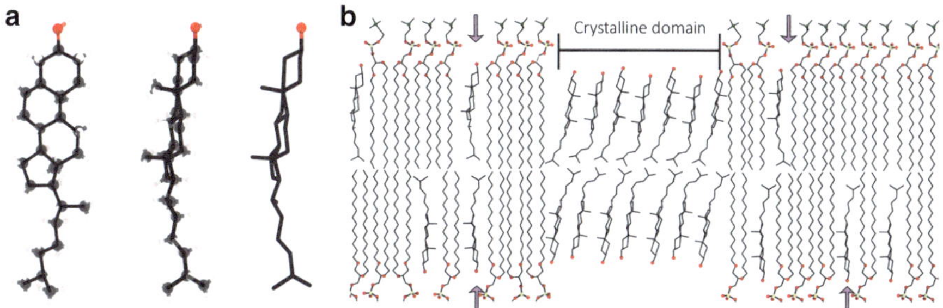

Fig. 2 Schematic representation of the cholesterol molecule and its locations in a lipid bilayer. (**a**) The cholesterol molecule in two different orientations, face-on to the carbon rings (left) and in profile (center and right). The left and center representations are in the ball and stick format, with carbon atoms in black, oxygen in red, and hydrogen in off-white. The right-hand representation of the molecule in stick format will be used all along the chapter as a model to explain the processes involving the molecule in the crystal structures, during crystal nucleation, growth, and dissolution. The molecular conformation was taken, for convenience, from one of the molecules in the monoclinic structure. (**b**) Schematic representation of a lipid bilayer composed of phosphoglycerolipids and cholesterol molecules (arrows); above a critical concentration for cholesterol, cholesterol segregates in two-dimensional crystalline domains

certain measure inside cell membranes, where it is an essential component contributing to membrane fluidity and integrity [18–21]. The hydrophobic backbone of the molecule interacts with the hydrocarbon chains of membrane phospholipids, while the hydroxyl head interacts with water in the intracellular and extracellular medium (Fig. 2b). The length of the molecule is 17 Å, about the length of palmitic acid, one of the main components of cell membrane lipids, with which cholesterol interacts particularly well [22, 23]. Inside the cell membranes, cholesterol may arrange in bilayers, with the same arrangement as the phospholipid bilayer. When its concentration in the membrane is above the solubility limit, cholesterol may separate from the phospholipids forming domains composed exclusively of cholesterol, from which crystals may nucleate [24–26] (Fig. 2b).

Two crystal structures are known to form in water-based environments, both of them containing one molecule of water per cholesterol molecule, i.e., forming crystals with molecular content of cholesterol monohydrate. The better-known structure of cholesterol monohydrate, which is also the most stable structure, is the triclinic structure that Craven determined in 1976 (Fig. 3a) [27]. The monoclinic structure,

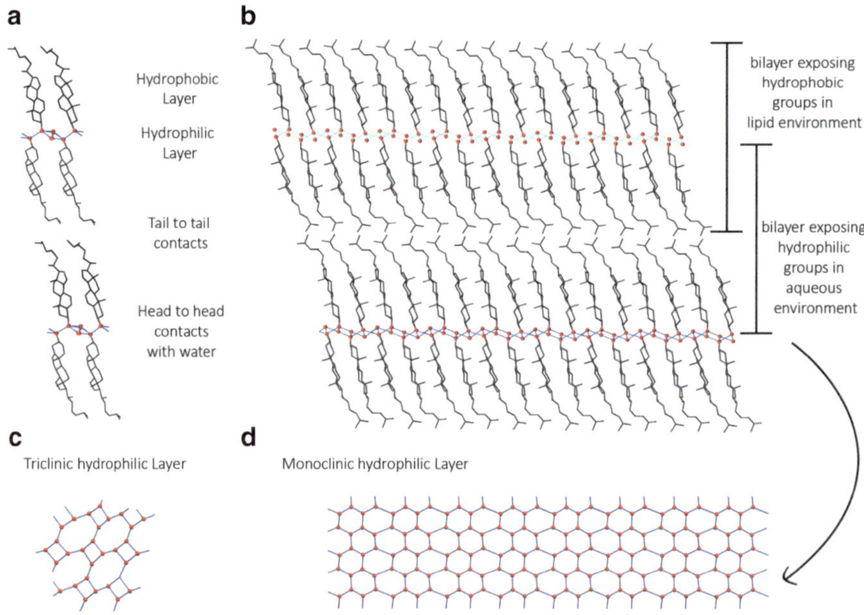

Fig. 3 Cholesterol monohydrate crystal structures. Packing arrangement of (**a**) the triclinic cholesterol.H₂O structure. (**b**) The monoclinic cholesterol.H₂O structure. Several crystallographic unit cells are represented, to make two superimposed bilayers. For convenience, we shall use the same structural arrangement of the monoclinic structure in (**b**) as a model for all the different schemes thereafter. Note that the fundamental bilayer arrangement is very similar in the monoclinic and triclinic structures. (**c**, **d**) hydrophilic layer arrangement of water and cholesterol hydroxyl moieties in the triclinic structure, and the ice-like layer in the monoclinic structure, respectively. Red: oxygen, black: carbon, blue: hydrogen bonds between water molecules and cholesterol hydroxyl groups. (Figure adapted in part from [32])

reported by Solomonov et al. [28] in 2005 and recently refined by Shepelenko et al. [29] (Fig. 3b), is metastable and preferably forms in vitro from thin layers at the air–water interface and from saturated phospholipid bilayers (Fig. 2b). Although the triclinic structure is the stable structure, cholesterol monoclinic deposits form in gallstones and in vitro in the presence of bile acids, and have unique helical and tubular superstructures (Fig. 6e) [30, 31]. Cholesterol helical superstructures growing from macrophages from the J774A.1 cell line supplemented with acetylated LDL, are also crystalline and have the monoclinic structure (Fig. 6f) [8].

Both crystal structures, triclinic and monoclinic, consist of bilayers of cholesterol molecules where the hydrophobic backbones interact laterally with each other with van der Waals forces (Fig. 3a, c), and the water molecules interact with the hydroxyl groups of the cholesterol molecule in a two-dimensional lattice (Fig. 3b, d). Within the bilayer, the molecules interact tail to tail with hydrophobic contacts (Fig. 3b), such that in an aqueous environment, as the intracellular environment or the extracellular matrix, a crystal will terminate at the surface with the hydrophilic side of the bilayer interacting with water. In a hydrophobic environment, such as might be the core of an atherosclerotic plaque, cholesterol crystals would be delimited by a surface layer exposing the hydrophobic tails of the molecules (Fig. 3).

3 Cholesterol Crystal Morphologies: What Are They, What Do They Mean, and What Do They Show Us?

The rates of growth of a crystal in the different directions, Va, Vb, and Vc, determine the crystal morphology [33, 34]. If a crystal grows very fast in one direction, say along the crystallographic axis b, relative to its rate of growth along the a and c axes, the crystal will develop as a thin rod (Fig. 4 (**1**)). The crystal will develop as a ribbon if there is also a substantial difference in the rates of growth between the other two axes (Fig. 4 (**2**)). The crystal will develop as a thin plate if its rates of growth along two directions are comparable, and much faster than in the third direction (Fig. 4 (**3**)), and will develop as a prism if the rates of growth along the three directions are in the same order of magnitude (Fig. 4 (**4**)).

The relative rates of crystal growth in the various crystallographic directions are determined, in turn, by the interactions between the molecules in the respective directions, which determine the rate at which new molecules will add up in the given orientations [35, 36]. In the case of cholesterol crystals, growth along the c axis requires the addition of new molecular layers or bilayers (Fig. 5a) [32]. The interactions between molecules in different layers are much weaker than the interactions between molecules in the same layer, and this is true for the crystals both in the stable triclinic structure and in the monoclinic structures. In agreement with this, synthetic crystals of cholesterol monohydrate in the stable triclinic structure are typically thin plates, as in case (**3**) in Fig. 4.

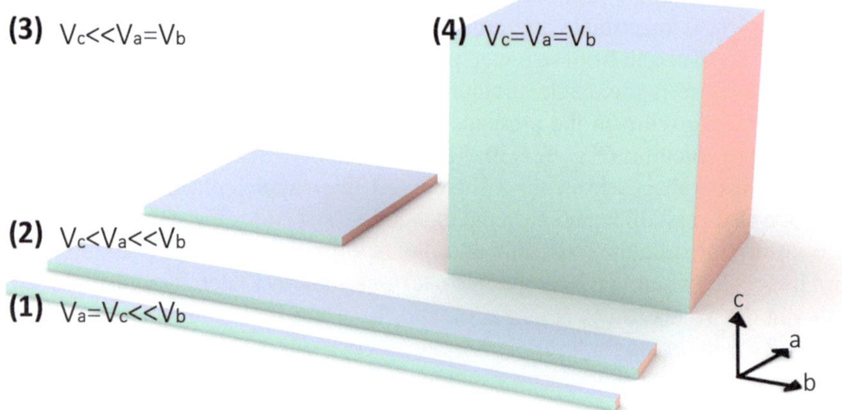

Fig. 4 Schematic representations of how crystal morphology develops depending on the relative rates of growth of the crystal in the different directions. V_a, V_b, and V_c are the rates (V = velocity) of growth of the crystal along the three crystallographic axes a, b, and c, as indicated

Crystals extracted from atherosclerotic plaques (Fig. 1f) or imaged in atherosclerotic plaques (Figs. 1a, b, d, and 6b), as well as crystals grown in macrophage cultures (Fig. 6a) are prevalently thin plates [7, 37]. There are, however, both in atherosclerotic plaques (Figs. 1e and 6d) and in macrophage cultures (Fig. 6c), crystals that assume the morphology of elongated ribbons or rods [17, 37]. If these crystals assumed the triclinic structure from their incept, it is necessary to understand why and how the crystals grew predominantly in one direction, as in the example shown in Fig. 4(1), rather than in two directions, as justified by the internal bilayer structure, resulting in thin plates as in Fig. 5c. We do not have a plausible explanation for this instance.

There exists, however, another possibility. The helical crystals that form from pathological bile or in J774A.1 macrophage cultures and assume the monoclinic structure (Fig. 6e, f) consist of very thin ribbons wrapped up around an axis [8, 38, 39]. If the ribbon is unwrapped, the morphology matches the model in Fig. 4(2), and is well justified by the crystal structure of the monoclinic polymorph.

Benedek [40] described how the diameter of the helix increases proportionally to the thickness of the ribbons, or in other words, how the helices open with the growth and thickening of the ribbons. Such process would result in a rod-like crystal with the monoclinic structure. X-ray diffraction measurements performed on crystals extracted from atherosclerotic plaques showed unambiguous presence of the triclinic cholesterol monohydrate polymorph, without any trace of any other polymorph being present [4]. This is not surprising because the stable polymorph is the triclinic one and a metastable structure would inevitably transform into the more stable triclinic structure at some stage during the long development of the plaques. The rod-like morphology might in such case preserve and manifest the metastable morphology in which it formed. In vitro crystallizations of cholesterol from lipid

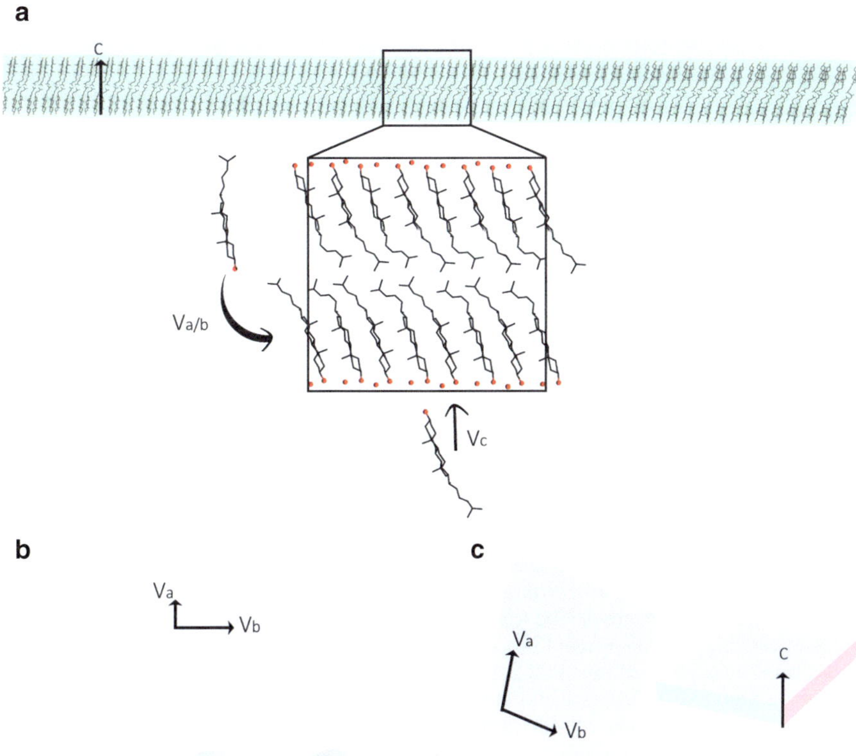

Fig. 5 Schematic representation of cholesterol crystal morphologies. (**a**) Thin cholesterol crystals develop easily parallel to the bilayer planes. The magnification of the boxed bilayer area shows how molecules added in the c direction (V_c) do not form good interactions with the existing bilayer, whereas multiple interactions develop when a molecule adds within the bilayer plane ($V_{a/b}$). (**b**) Cholesterol crystal morphologies that develop during the growth of the monoclinic polymorph: thin ribbons may grow into thin hexagonal crystals, or helical crystals because $V_b > V_a >> V_c$. (**c**) The crystal morphology of the triclinic polymorph is thin plates because $V_a \sim V_b >> V_c$

bilayers indeed showed instances in which the monoclinic polymorph deposited as helices, which subsequently underwent phase transition to the triclinic phase [30, 31, 38, 39].

Besides few thin plates and rods, the prevailing population of crystals in the atherosclerotic lesions are relatively thicker plates (Fig. 1a–d, f). These crystals presumably grew in extra-cellular locations by the addition of cholesterol present in the environment. In addition, the cholesterol crystals tend to stick one to the other forming stacks of crystals with the same orientation either because they formed from connected nuclei or because the stresses directionally imposed on the plaque reoriented them. Crystal ripening, consisting in growth of large crystals at the expense of smaller crystals that dissolve, is a well-known phenomenon (under the name of

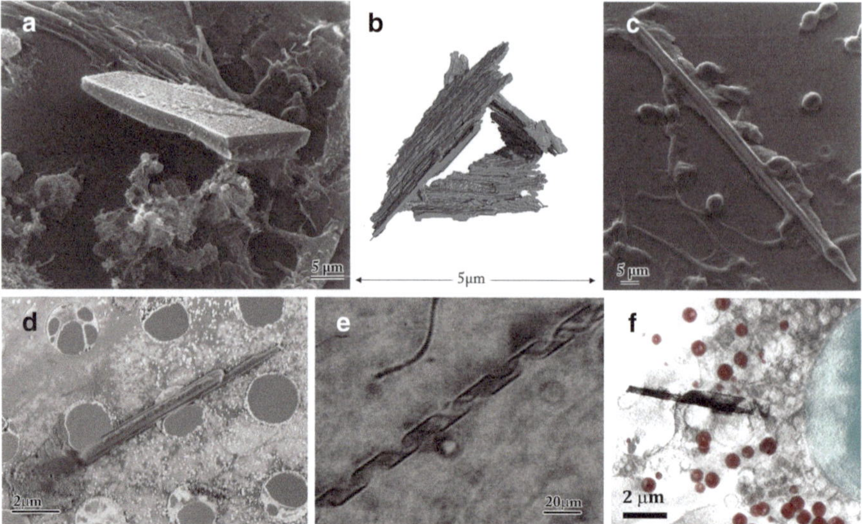

Fig. 6 Cholesterol crystal morphologies in biological context. (**a**) Crystal plate grown from macrophage culture (reproduced with permission from [37]). (**b**) 3D representation of segmented crystal plates from rabbit atherosclerotic lesion. (**c**) Crystal needle grown from macrophage culture (reproduced with permission from [37]). (**d**) rod-shaped crystal isolated from human atherosclerotic plaque. Image adapted from [32]. (**e**) Helical crystal grown from bile acids (reproduced with permission from [38]). (**f**) Helical crystal (black) grown in macrophage culture (nucleus = blue, lipid bodies = red). (Reproduced with permission from [39])

Ostwald ripening [41]) that may certainly also contribute to increase the population of larger crystals over long periods in the core of the lesions. Crystal ripening occurs because interactions with the environment at the crystal surface favor crystal dissolution whereas interaction between the molecular components in the bulk favor the crystalline phase. Because the surface-to-bulk ratio is always bigger in small crystals relative to larger ones, the big crystals are more stable relative to the small ones [42].

Specific crystal growth inhibitors may influence crystal morphology, by preferentially attaching to specific crystal faces where their molecular structure provides favorable interactions with the surface [35]. This is well exemplified in the insert shown in Fig. 5a, where any alcohol, or for what that matters water itself may inhibit growth of the crystal along the c axis, by interacting with the cholesterol molecules and the water in the ab layer, thus decreasing the rate of addition of layers along c (V_c). This would make the cholesterol plates or ribbons even thinner. On the other hand, a hydrophobic molecule that interacts well with the exposed ring system of the cholesterol molecule could be absorbed along a or b and subsequently slow down the growth (V_a and/or V_b) decreasing the rate of addition of further cholesterol molecules in these directions. The crystals in the latter case should become thicker plates. It is conceivable that they could grow as rods as consequence of preferential absorption on one of the lateral surfaces of the plate (as in Fig. 4 (2) or (1)). We deem this, however, as highly improbable because the structure along the *a* and *b* axes of the triclinic crystals is very similar [27], and so should be the molecular interactions with an external inhibitor. There are also many high-energy sites in growing crystals, especially kink sites or sites of emerging dislocations. These sites favor crystal growth, but are also target of non-specific growth inhibition [43], one example of which are the typical notches observed in cholesterol crystals extracted especially from gallstones [31].

4 Crystal Nucleation

4.1 *Cholesterol Crystal Formation: The Conceivable Routes, The Hypotheses and the Evidence*

Molecules that dissolve in a native environment favorably interact with their environment, and thus release energy. Formation of a crystal from an initially homogeneous solution requires prior organization of the molecules, and extraction of the molecules from the environment, including cutting off the associated interactions, which in turn requires an investment of energy. This is not favored in a solution that is under saturation level, where the energy associated with interaction of the molecule with its environment exceeds the energy of interaction of the molecules among themselves. However, when appropriately oriented molecules interact with each other to form a crystal in a super-saturated solution, they liberate more energy than what they need to invest to extract the molecules from the environment, such that the energy balance is in the favor of crystallization. The extra-energy that is needed to organize an initial nucleus, thus promoting the beginning of crystallization, is the activation energy, which represents a substantial barrier to crystallization from homogeneous media [44]. External surfaces may help reduce the energy of activation by providing a template to the forming crystal, both organizing the molecules in a manner that is similar to their packing in the crystal, and liberating interaction energy. In the case of cholesterol, grazing angle X-ray diffraction experiments performed on saturated phospholipid bilayers containing cholesterol showed that cholesterol molecules segregate into cholesterol domains when their concentration is above saturation level in the lipid environment (Fig. 2b) [45]. The cholesterol molecules in the segregated domains are already organized in the correct orientation to form crystal bilayers that are stabilized by interactions with water, and can give rise to three-dimensional cholesterol crystals of the monoclinic cholesterol monohydrate polymorph (Fig. 5a).

In vitro experiments showed that the crystal polymorph eventually grows either into crystal plates of the triclinic structure (Figs. 5c and 7b) or into crystal elongated plates, cylinders, or helixes in the monoclinic structures (Fig. 5b), affected by the specific lipid components of the bilayer membrane [39]. Growth of rhomboidal plate crystals occurs from the plasma membrane of macrophages supplemented with acetylated-LDL (Fig. 7c), whereas helical and cylindrical crystals of the monoclinic polymorph form from internal membranes (Fig. 6f) [8]. This type of templated nucleation is probably the mechanism responsible for the crystal nucleation from multilamellar bodies (Fig. 7e) that was observed in rabbit atherosclerotic lesions (Figs. 1j and 7d insert) [6].

Analogously, lipid droplets are delimited by a monolayer of lipid and cholesterol molecules that can provide a template to crystallization on their surface [47]. An epitaxial match exists between the cholesteryl surface of a single bilayer of the ester cholesteryl palmitate and a monoclinic cholesterol monohydrate crystal [29]. This means that a bilayer of cholesteryl palmitate or other similar cholesteryl esters, which are common components of atherosclerotic lesions, could nucleate cholesterol crystals by templating. Templated nucleation is thus most probably the mechanisms responsible for cholesterol crystal nucleation from lipid droplets (Fig. 7d) that was observed in rabbit atherosclerotic lesions (Fig. 1g, i). In agreement with this interpretation, crystals were observed to nucleate at the surface of lipid droplets close to the so-called hydrolysis pits, locations where cholesteryl ester is hydrolyzed to produce unesterified cholesterol (Fig. 7d) [48]. The crystals that were observed in rabbit atherosclerotic lesions are extremely thin plates, 20–30 nm thick. This morphology corresponds to triclinic cholesterol monohydrate crystals that just nucleated and grew rapidly in the *ab* plane (Figs. 5c and 6b). Such very thin crystals, close to the nucleation stage, were also observed in intra-cellular locations in rabbit lesions, although the cell viability at the time when the sample was withdrawn is uncertain (Fig. 1h) [6].

Fig. 7 Cholesterol crystal nucleation scenarios. (**a**) Schematic representation of a crystal (gray) nucleating at the surface of a cell membrane (green), from a domain of cholesterol molecules (red) that segregated inside the cholesterol-supersaturated bilayer. (**b**) Volume representation of a cholesterol crystal nucleated on the surface of a liposome. The data presented is reconstructed from soft X-ray tomography of a phospholipid unilamellar vesicle with attached cholesterol crystal. (**c**) Super-resolution localization map of labelled plasma membrane crystalline cholesterol on macrophage cell membranes. The crystals are labeled by an antibody that recognizes cholesterol crystals (Reproduced with permission from [8]). Inset shows high magnification of one labelled crystal (reproduced with permission from [46]). (**d**) Schematic representation of a lipid droplet, delimited by a monolayer of phospholipids and unesterified cholesterol, with dedicated proteins, and containing in the hydrophobic bulk neutral lipids, triglycerides and cholesteryl esters (reproduced with permission from [32]). Insert—cholesterol crystals nucleated on the surface of a lipid droplet (white arrow). Slice from a cryo-FIB-SEM set of images. The lipid droplet has a bright cavity (yellow arrow) consistent with what is described as a hydrolysis pit, i.e., a location where cholesteryl ester is hydrolyzed to produce cholesterol. (**e**) Schematic representation of a multilamellar body formed by onion-like arrangements of superimposed bilayer membranes. (Created with BioRender. com). Insert—multilamellar body with a cholesterol crystal attached to the outer membrane (arrow) slice from a cryo-FIB-SEM set of images

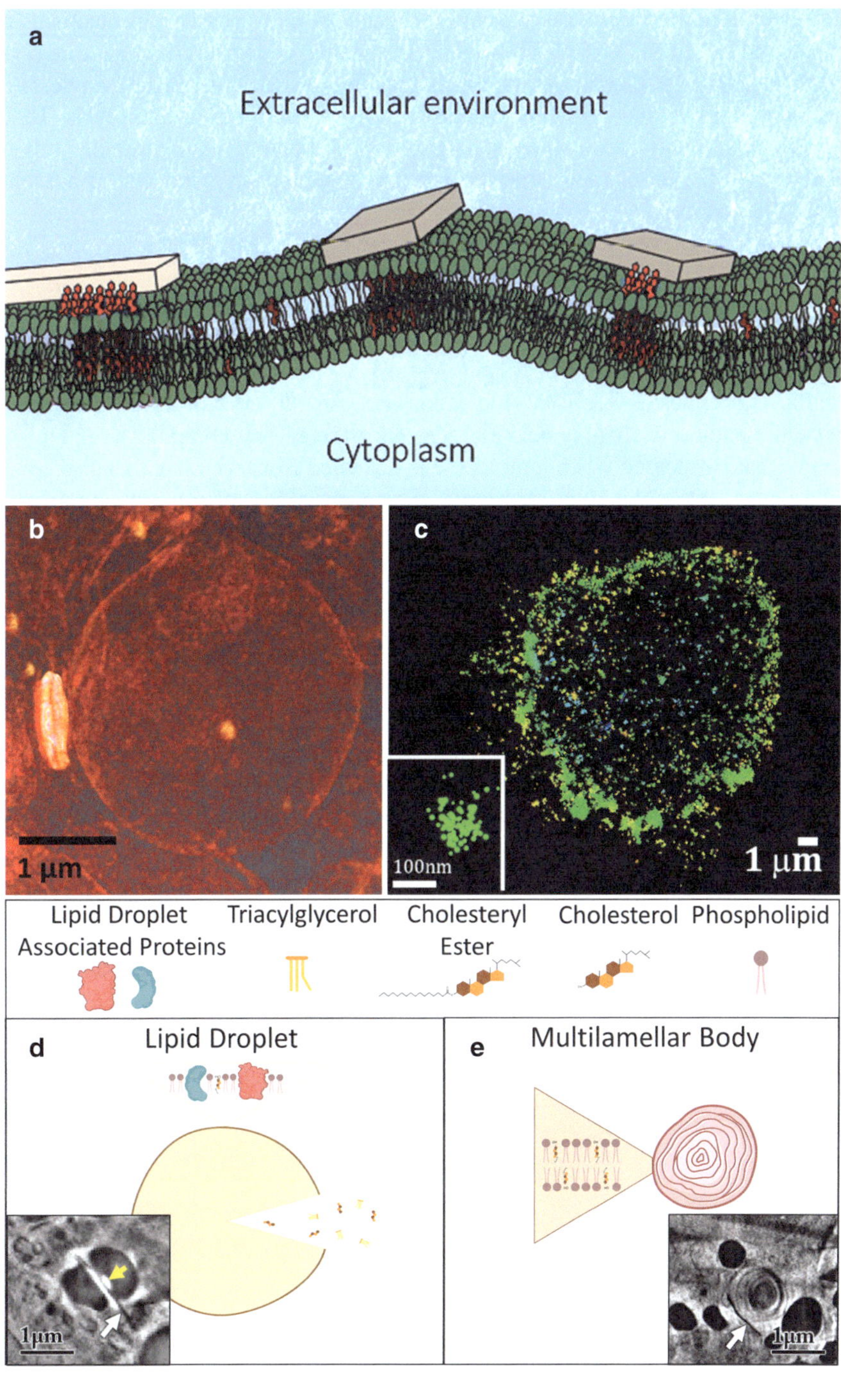

a
Extracellular environment
Cytoplasm
b
1 µm
c
100nm
1 µm
Lipid Droplet Associated Proteins
Triacylglycerol
Cholesteryl Ester
Cholesterol
Phospholipid
d
Lipid Droplet
1µm
e
Multilamellar Body
1µm

It is important to point out that these are not the only possible mechanisms of crystal nucleation and growth, as other environmental conditions can facilitate crystallization, in particular in extra-cellular locations, where unesterified cholesterol concentration may increase after cell death and cholesteryl ester hydrolysis. There are, however, plenty of membranes, particles, lipid droplets, and multilamellar bodies in extra-cellular locations, and most probably nucleation is induced, if not templated, by surfaces.

5 Crystal Dissolution

Similar and opposite to crystal nucleation and growth, crystal dissolution occurs when the environment is under-saturated with the crystal components [36]. The energy that is released when a molecule is detached from the crystal and interacts with the solvent, in this case, overcomes the energy of interaction of the molecules with their environment inside the crystal. Naturally, the molecules exposed at the crystal surface are more easily susceptible to dissolution, but there are also differences in the ease of dissolution of molecules in different positions. Thus, molecules exposed at steps or kinks on the crystal surface are more easily dissolved than molecules that are integral parts of a crystal layer, for the simple fact that they make less contact with the surrounding molecular crystal components. A molecule at a crystal step makes contact with only two other molecules on the two sides of the step, and a molecule at a crystal kink with three, instead of five contacts that a molecule makes when it is embedded in a crystal layer (Fig. 8a). For this reason, crystals dissolve more from the edges and from the corners than homogeneously from the surfaces, resulting in rounded corners and edges in dissolving crystals (Fig. 9a, b). Analogously, crystals dissolve from imperfections such as emerging screw or edge

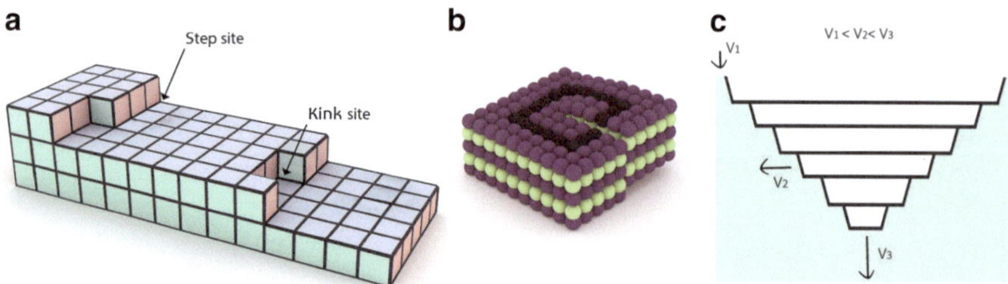

Fig. 8 Schematic representations of crystal dissolution sites. (**a**) A molecule residing in a crystal step site or in a crystal kink site is more prone to dissolution because it makes less contacts with the crystal components than a molecule residing inside the surface layer. (**b**) Screw dislocation. A molecule residing in an emerging crystal imperfection, such as a screw dislocation or an edge dislocation, is easier to remove because it makes less favorable contacts with the crystal components. (**c**) Etch pit, the result of dissolution from emerging dislocations. The etch pit sides are formed by steps along preferred crystallographic directions, dissolving with relative velocities $V_3 > V_2 >> V_1$

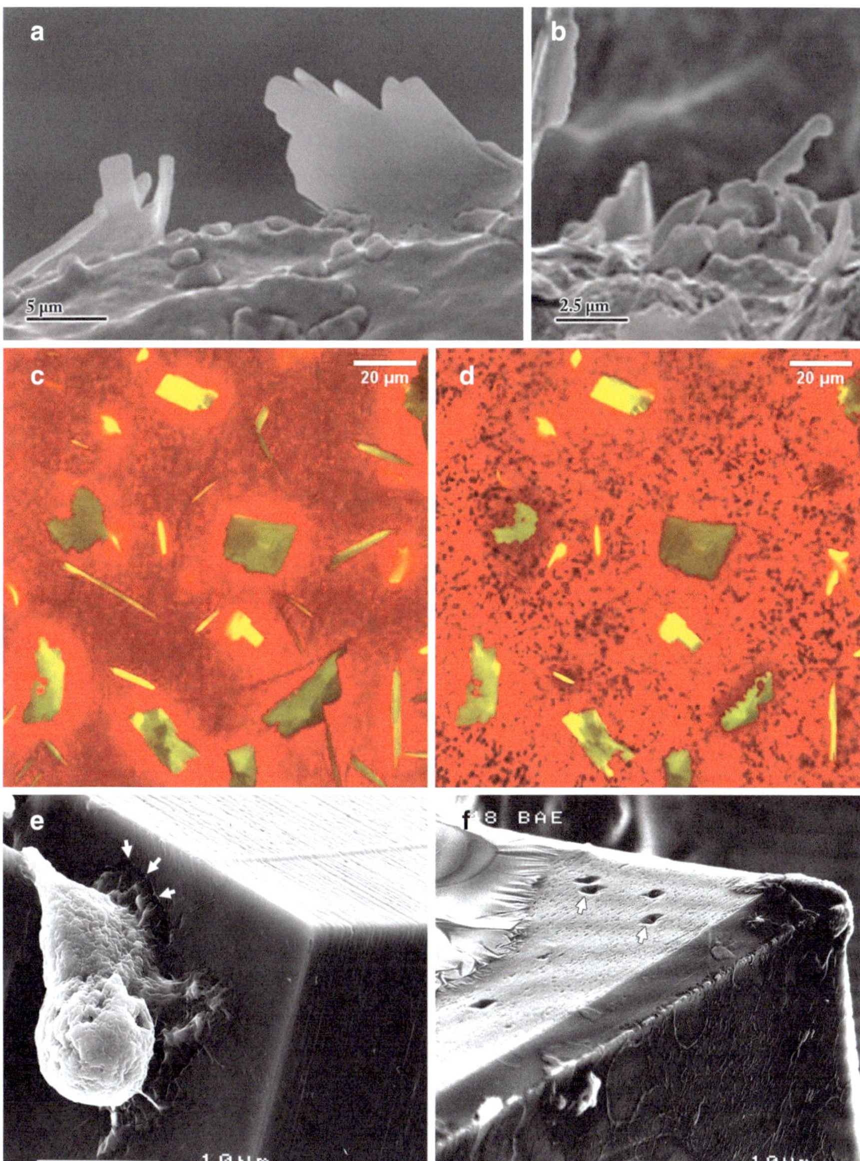

Fig. 9 Cholesterol crystal dissolution. (**a**) Scanning electron micrograph of carotid plaque from endarterectomy of a patient not on statins. (**b**) Scanning electron micrograph of carotid plaque from a patient on statins demonstrating dissolving crystals (images adapted with permission from [57]). (**c, d**) Cholesterol crystals dissolving in the presence of cyclodextrin. Frames from a movie taken during dissolution. (**c**) is the first frame of the movie, showing already dissolving crystals [50]. The rod-like crystals dissolve completely before the plates. (**e–f**) Scanning electron micrographs of cells from the epithelial cell line A6 adhering to large cholesterol crystals and locally dissolving them, forming large pits (white arrows). In (**f**) the cell moved from the location, leaving traces of its activity in the form of etch pits [58]

dislocations (Fig. 8b), simply because the molecules are easier to detach, i.e., the interactions that the solvent needs to overcome to detach them from the crystal are weaker [49]. The result of preferred dissolution from imperfections, which are very frequent in all crystals, is the formation of the so-called etch pits (Fig. 8c). A crystal that dissolves preferentially by this route will develop an irregular morphology, such as the morphology developed by cholesterol crystals dissolving in the presence of cyclodextrin (Fig. 9c, d) [50].

Cholesterol crystal dissolution can occur in several conceivable scenarios relevant to atherosclerosis, each following a different sequence of events, which we shall examine one by one below:

5.1   Lowering Cholesterol Concentration in Blood

Cholesterol solubility in water is extremely low (<2 mg in 100 mL water [18]), but there are several vehicles for cholesterol in blood. The tests of cholesterol concentration in blood take into account the total cholesterol, including but not limited to LDL and HDL with their cargo of cholesterol and cholesteryl ester. Lowering cholesterol concentration in blood led to plaque regression in nonhuman studies, including lowering the amount of crystals [1, 51–53]. The crystals in the lesion core are, however, difficult to dissolve, both because the crystals are in the most stable form of cholesterol, and because the crystals in the core are presumably more difficult to reach and act upon.

5.2   Increasing Cholesterol Solubility in Water

The solubility of cholesterol in ethanol at 37° is ~32.5 mg in 100 mL of solvent [54], more than one order of magnitude higher relative to water. It is thus to be expected that cholesterol crystals will be more easily soluble in water-ethanol mixtures than in water. Cholesterol monohydrate crystals dissolve in 10–50% ethanol-containing aqueous solutions by bilayer or multilayer step retreat and by formation of etch pits [55]. The effect is due to the mixed hydrophobic–hydrophilic character of ethanol, which induces good interactions both with water and with cholesterol and lipid molecules. When fresh human atherosclerotic plaques were exposed to ethanol/water solutions, cholesterol crystals dissolved, assuming pitted and rounded morphology [56]. Analogously, cholesterol crystals treated with cyclodextrin solutions in water dissolve forming pitted crystals with deformed morphology [50] (Fig. 9b). In the latter case, cholesterol solubility is increased in water because cyclodextrin molecules form very stable inclusion complexes with cholesterol.

Carotid plaques of patients treated with statins had cholesterol crystals showing clear evidence of dissolution in their irregular rounded morphologies [57] (Fig. 9b).

Analogously, in carotid samples treated with aspirin, "The otherwise sharp edged, dense rhomboid and needle shaped crystals appeared … significantly dissolving, … with blunted tips and altered geometry." [16]

5.3   Cell Membrane Solubilization of Cholesterol

In a process opposite to the cholesterol crystal nucleation on cell membranes mentioned above (Sect. 4), cholesterol crystals can be dissolved by adhering cells, with the cholesterol molecules becoming internalized in the cell plasma membrane itself, or in other cellular organelles. We were very surprised to see pit formation in large cholesterol crystals on which we seeded cells from the epithelial cell line A6 [58]. The cell adhered to the crystals and burrowed inside the crystals, forming large and deep etch pits, while the cells swelled assuming an appearance similar to foam cells (Fig. 9e, f). It is interesting to note that the same phenomenon did not happen with any of other crystals. The same cells adhered to several other crystals [59], but dissolution of the crystals following cell adhesion was never observed. We take this phenomenon to indicate that cholesterol may penetrate into the phospholipid bilayer membrane of the cell as separate molecules or as ordered domains, and can subsequently become internalized in the cell as cholesterol or as cholesteryl ester (see Sect. 5.4).

Adams et al. reported that liposomes form at the surface of synthetic cholesterol crystals and crystals isolated from human atherosclerotic plaques in contact with HDL. Under the reported experimental conditions this process persisted until cholesterol crystal dissolution [60, 61]. Although the mechanism of interaction responsible for crystal dissolution is not known, it is conceivable that the process involves adsorption of cholesterol molecules from the crystal onto the modified HDL particles or onto the liposomal membranes formed. Synthetic HDL particles were also reportedly involved in lowering of cholesterol crystal burden [62]. However, contrasting evidence on the role of HDL in cholesterol crystal dissolution also exists [63, 64].

5.4   Crystal Sequestration or Phagocytosis by Macrophages and Esterification or Cellular Efflux of Cholesterol

There is evidence that cholesterol crystals can be sequestrated or phagocytosed by macrophages and subsequently dissolved, with associated esterification of the dissolved molecules to cholesteryl esters [65, 66]. Kruth (1995) reported sequestration of cholesterol crystals in surface-connected (i.e., open to the extracellular space) bilayer membrane-bound compartments formed in human monocyte-derived macrophages differentiated with human serum. Some cholesterol redistributed from the surface-connected compartments into lysosomes (where the cholesterol remained unesterified) and into lipid droplets (where the cholesterol was stored as cholesteryl ester). Other cholesterol was released from the macrophages in the form of nascent HDL discoidal complexes containing cholesterol, phospholipid, and apolipoprotein E [67, 68]. The presence of apolipoprotein E within the surface-connected compartments containing the cholesterol crystals [66] suggests that the macrophage-derived nascent HDL solubilized the crystalline cholesterol within these compartments.

Human monocyte-derived macrophages differentiated with M-CSF and then enriched with cholesterol by uptake of lipoprotein- or microcrystalline-derived cholesterol, shed cholesterol into the extracellular matrix [69]. The cholesterol was contained within amorphous phospholipid deposits.

McConathy et al. examined cholesterol crystal uptake by a mouse macrophage cell line (P388Di) and observed cholesterol crystal accumulation within intracellular bilayer membrane-bound vacuoles consistent with phagocytic uptake of the crystals [65]. A small amount of the crystal-derived cholesterol became esterified within the macrophages. A similar occurrence of macrophage phagocytosing and dissolving cholesterol crystals have been advocated in human macrophages from aspirates of coronary arteries during myocardial infarction [70] (See Fig. 7, Chapter "The Cholesterol Crystal Paradigm: Overview of How Cholesterol Crystals Evolve and Induce Traumatic and Inflammatory Vascular Injury").

The above findings suggest that macrophages can function in uptake and processing of cholesterol crystals for either storage within the macrophage or excretion of crystal-derived cholesterol in a form solubilized by phospholipid.

6 Conclusions, Questions, and Suggestions

The combination of observations made on diseased tissues and model systems with structural and chemical knowledge on crystals may provide some insight into the pathways of crystal deposition during the formation of atherosclerotic lesions. The advanced electron microscope techniques nowadays available allow unprecedented observations of the tissues in conditions much closer to their original ones, relative to those that were previously available. Does all this information provide us with any additional knowledge on the pathology? Does it suggest any additional tools for the clinicians to tackle the disease? We shall sort out some considerations, thoughts, and questions below.

6.1 Cholesterol Crystal Polymorphism: Curiosity or Interesting Possibility?

We know that a metastable phase of cholesterol monohydrate crystals exists. We know that this phase forms from macrophage cell membranes and from phospholipid bilayers in vitro and is dependent on membrane composition. These same crystals, with their characteristic helical morphology, form also in artificial solutions containing cyclodextrin and in bile [38, 50], and subsequently transform into the stable triclinic crystal structure that figures conspicuously in atherosclerotic plaques [1, 17]. There is no direct evidence of a transient metastable phase during the formation of atherosclerotic lesions, although there are some observations that might suggest its existence. We note that a less stable phase, which formation is kinetically favored, may be easier to dissolve than the stable phase. In the case of cholesterol, this theoretical possibility is supported also by experiments, showing that in vitro the metastable crystals indeed dissolve faster than those of the stable phase (Fig. 9c, d) [50]. Whether these observations can have any practical value in the treatment of the pathology, we do not know.

6.2 Cholesterol Crystal Formation: The Locations. Intra-Cellular, Extra-Cellular or Both?

We know that cholesterol crystals can form in intra-cellular locations in forming rabbit lesions [6]. The observation of an intact nucleus and of a complete cell plasma membrane enclosing the area where nascent crystals appear, guarantees the intra-cellular location, and suggest that the cell is intact, although it is not possible to verify that the cell is viable at the time of crystal nucleation. The extremely thin crystal morphology, together with the absence of a lysosomal membrane envelope around them, support the notion that the crystals are in the first stages of formation, rather than undergoing dissolution, and did not undergo phagocytosis after extra-cellular nucleation. Murine macrophages from cultures supplemented with acetylated-LDL supported formation of cholesterol crystals associated with cell membranes, including the cell plasma membrane. Intracellular crystal growth can eventually lead to cell death and/or excretion in the extra-cellular space. At the same time, we do not exclude, and we actually consider most likely that crystal nucleation and growth can occur also in extra-cellular locations, supplied with cholesterol coming from external sources, or from cholesteryl ester hydrolysis after cell death.

6.3 Macrophage Activity: Crystal Formation, Dissolution or Both?

The evidence concerning macrophage activity in atherosclerotic lesions is heterogeneous and difficult to reconcile. Murine macrophages in cell culture and rabbit macrophages in atherosclerotic lesions support intra-cellular crystal deposition. In contrast, human monocyte-derived macrophages were not observed to induce cholesterol crystallization, even after accumulating considerable amounts of intracellular cholesterol. On the other hand, both murine and human monocyte-derived macrophages in cell culture are active in cholesterol crystal dissolution. It is possible that different macrophage activities exist in macrophages of different origin. It is also possible that macrophages activate different processes in different phases of lesion formation and plaque development, depending from the signals they receive from the environment. We do not know the answer to these questions, and we should wait for more information, if possible derived from the observation of human plaques rather than of model systems. These observations trigger, however, the thought that if crystal dissolution can be promoted over the crystal formation activity, potential clinical pathways could be considered.

References

1. Small DM. George Lyman Duff memorial lecture. Progression and regression of atherosclerotic lesions. Insights from lipid physical biochemistry. Arteriosclerosis. 1988;8:103–29.
2. Duewell P, Kono H, Rayner KJ, Sirois CM, Vladimer G, Bauernfeind FG, Abela GS, Franchi L, Nunez G, Schnurr M, Espevik T, Lien E, Fitzgerald KA, Rock KL, Moore KJ, Wright SD, Hornung V, Latz E. NLRP3 inflammasomes are required for atherogenesis and activated by cholesterol crystals. Nature. 2010;464:1357–61.
3. Chistiakov DA, Bobryshev YV, Orekhov AN. Macrophage-mediated cholesterol handling in atherosclerosis. J Cell Mol Med. 2016;20:17–28.
4. Katz S, Shipley GG, Small D. Physical chemistry of the lipids of human atherosclerotic lesions. Demonstration of a lesion intermediate between fatty streaks and advanced plaques. J Clin Investig. 1976;58:200–11.
5. Small DM, Shipley GG. Physical-chemical basis of Lipid deposition in atherosclerosis: the physical state of the lipids helps to explain lipid deposition and lesion reversal in atherosclerosis. Science. 1974;185:222–9.
6. Capua-Shenkar J, Varsano N, Itzhak N-R, Kaplan-Ashiri I, Rechav K, Jin X, Niimi M, Fan J, Kruth HS, Addadi L. Examining atherosclerotic lesions in three dimensions at the nanometer scale with cryo-FIB-SEM. Proc Natl Acad Sci U S A. 2022;119:e2205475119.
7. Lehti S, Nguyen SD, Belevich I, Vihinen H, Heikkilä HM, Soliymani R, Käkelä R, Saksi J, Jauhiainen M, Grabowski GA. Extracellular lipids accumulate in human carotid arteries as distinct three-dimensional structures and have proinflammatory properties. Am J Clin Pathol. 2018;188:525–38.
8. Varsano N, Beghi F, Elad N, Pereiro E, Dadosh T, Pinkas I, Perez-Berna AJ, Jin X, Kruth HS, Leiserowitz L, Addadi L. Two polymorphic cholesterol monohydrate crystal structures form in macrophage culture models of atherosclerosis. Proc Natl Acad Sci U S A. 2018;115:7662–9.
9. Tangirala RK, Jerome WG, Jones N, Small DM, Johnson W, Glick J, Mahlberg F, Rothblat G. Formation of cholesterol monohydrate crystals in macrophage-derived foam cells. J Lipid Res. 1994;35:93–104.
10. Shio H, Haley N, Fowler S. Characterization of lipid-laden aortic cells from cholesterol-fed rabbits. III. Intracellular localization of cholesterol and cholesteryl ester. Lab Invest. 1979;41:160–7.
11. Kruth HS. Macrophage foam cells and atherosclerosis. Front Biosci. 2001;6:D429–55.
12. Vidavsky N, Akiva A, Kaplan-Ashiri I, Rechav K, Addadi L, Weiner S, Schertel A. Cryo-FIB-SEM serial milling and block face imaging: large volume structural analysis of biological tissues preserved close to their native state. J Struct Biol. 2016;196:487–95.
13. Mahamid J, Tegunov D, Maiser A, Arnold J, Leonhardt H, Plitzko JM, Baumeister W. Liquid-crystalline phase transitions in lipid droplets are related to cellular states and specific organelle association. Proc Natl Acad Sci U S A. 2019;116:16866–71.

14. Spehner D, Steyer AM, Bertinetti L, Orlov I, Benoit L, Pernet-Gallay K, Schertel A, Schultz P. Cryo-FIB-SEM as a promising tool for localizing proteins in 3D. J Struct Biol. 2020;211:107528.
15. Bocan T, Schifani T, Guyton J. Ultrastructural examination of the human aortic fibrolipid lesion-formation of the atherosclerotic lipid-rich core. Am J Clin Pathol. 1985;123:413–24.
16. Fry L, Lee A, Khan S, Aziz K, Vedre A, Abela GS. Effect of aspirin on cholesterol crystallization: a potential mechanism for plaque stabilization. Am Heart J. 2022;13:100083.
17. Kruth HS. Cholesterol deposition in atherosclerotic lesions. Cholesterol. 1997;28:319–62.
18. Saad HY, Higuchi WI. Water solubility of cholesterol. J Pharm Sci. 1965;54:1205–6.
19. Haberland ME, Reynolds JA. Self-association of cholesterol in aqueous solution. Proc Natl Acad Sci U S A. 1973;70:2313–6.
20. Sackmann E. Biological membranes architecture and function. Amsterdam: Elsevier Science B.V; 1995.
21. Alberts B, Johnson A, Lewis J, Raff M, Roberts K, Walter P. Molecular biology of the cell. Scand J Rheumatol. 2003;32:125.
22. Smondyrev AM, Berkowitz ML. Structure of dipalmitoylphosphatidylcholine/cholesterol bilayer at low and high cholesterol concentrations: molecular dynamics simulation. Biophys J. 1999;77:2075–89.
23. Berg J, Tymoczko J, Stryer L. Biochemistry: international version. New York: W. H. Freeman; 2002.
24. Ziblat R, Leiserowitz L, Addadi L. Crystalline domain structure and cholesterol crystal nucleation in single hydrated DPPC: cholesterol: POPC bilayers. J Am Chem Soc. 2010;132:9920–7.
25. Ziblat R, Kjaer K, Leiserowitz L, Addadi L. Structure of cholesterol/lipid ordered domains in monolayers and single hydrated bilayers. Angew Chem Int Ed. 2009;48:8958–61.
26. Ziblat R, Fargion I, Leiserowitz L, Addadi L. Spontaneous formation of two-dimensional and three-dimensional cholesterol crystals in single hydrated lipid bilayers. Biophys J. 2012;103:255–64.
27. Craven BM. Crystal structure of cholesterol monohydrate. Nature. 1976;260:727–9.
28. Solomonov I, Weygand MJ, Kjaer K, Rapaport H, Leiserowitz L. Trapping crystal nucleation of cholesterol monohydrate: relevance to pathological crystallization. Biophys J. 2005;88:1809–17.
29. Shepelenko M, Hirsch A, Varsano N, Beghi F, Addadi L, Kronik L, Leiserowitz L. Polymorphism, structure, and nucleation of cholesterol· H2O at aqueous interfaces and in pathological media: revisited from a computational perspective. J Am Chem Soc. 2021;144:5304–14.
30. Konikoff F, Chung DS, Donovan J, Small D, Carey M. Filamentous, helical, and tubular microstructures during cholesterol crystallization from bile. Evidence that cholesterol does not nucleate classic monohydrate plates. J Clin Investig. 1992;90:1155–60.
31. Weihs D, Schmidt J, Goldiner I, Danino D, Rubin M, Talmon Y, Konikoff FM. Biliary cholesterol crystallization characterized by single-crystal cryogenic electron diffraction. J Lipid Res. 2005;46:942–8.
32. Varsano N, Capua-Shenkar J, Leiserowitz L, Addadi L. Crystalline cholesterol: the material and its assembly lines. Annu Rev Mat Res. 2022;52:52.
33. Wells A. XXV. Crystal habit and internal structure.—II. Lond Edinb Dublin Philos Mag. 1946;37:217–36.
34. Hartman P, Perdok W. On the relations between structure and morphology of crystals. I. Acta Crystallogr. 1955;8:49–52.
35. Weissbuch I, Addadi L, Lahav M, Leiserowitz L. Molecular recognition at crystal interfaces. Science. 1991;253:637–45.
36. Burton W, Cabrera N, Frank F. Role of dislocations in crystal growth. Nature. 1949;163:398–9.
37. Kellner-Weibel G, Yancey P, Jerome W, Walser T, Mason R, Phillips M, Rothblat G. Crystallization of free cholesterol in model macrophage foam cells. Arterioscler Thromb Vasc Biol. 1999;19:1891–8.

38. Chung DS, Benedek GB, Konikoff FM, Donovan JM. Elastic free energy of anisotropic helical ribbons as metastable intermediates in the crystallization of cholesterol. Proc Natl Acad Sci U S A. 1993;90:11341–5.

39. Varsano N, Beghi F, Dadosh T, Elad N, Pereiro E, Haran G, Leiserowitz L, Addadi L. The effect of the phospholipid bilayer environment on cholesterol crystal polymorphism. ChemPlusChem. 2019;84:338–44.

40. Khaykovich B, Kozlova N, Choi W, Lomakin A, Hossain C, Sung Y, Dasari RR, Feld MS, Benedek GB. Thickness–radius relationship and spring constants of cholesterol helical ribbons. Proc Natl Acad Sci U S A. 2009;106:15663–6.

41. Ostwald W. Über die vermeintliche Isomerie des roten und gelben Quecksilberoxyds und die Oberflächenspannung fester Körper. Z Phys Chem. 1900;34:495–503.

42. Ratke L, Voorhees PW. Growth and coarsening: Ostwald ripening in material processing. Berlin: Springer Science & Business Media; 2002.

43. Frank FC. The influence of dislocations on crystal growth. Discuss Faraday Soc. 1949;5:48–54.

44. Walton AG. Nucleation of crystals from solution: mechanisms of precipitation are fundamental to analytical and physiological processes. Science. 1965;148:601–7.

45. Ziblat R, Leiserowitz L, Addadi L. Crystalline Lipid domains: characterization by X-ray diffraction and their relation to biology. Angew Chem Int Ed. 2011;50:3620–9.

46. Varsano N, Dadosh T, Kapishnikov S, Pereiro E, Shimoni E, Jin X, Kruth HS, Leiserowitz L, Addadi L. Development of correlative cryo-soft X-ray tomography and stochastic reconstruction microscopy. A study of cholesterol crystal early formation in cells. J Am Chem Soc. 2016;138:14931–40.

47. Tauchi-Sato K, Ozeki S, Houjou T, Taguchi R, Fujimoto T. The surface of lipid droplets is a phospholipid monolayer with a unique fatty acid composition. J Biol Chem. 2002;277:44507–12.

48. Guyton JR, Klemp KF. The lipid-rich core region of human atherosclerotic fibrous plaques. Prevalence of small lipid droplets and vesicles by electron microscopy. Am J Clin Pathol. 1989;134:705.

49. Dove PM, Han N, De Yoreo JJ. Mechanisms of classical crystal growth theory explain quartz and silicate dissolution behavior. Proc Natl Acad Sci U S A. 2005;102:15357–62.

50. Park S, Sut TN, Ma GJ, Parikh AN, Cho N-J. Crystallization of cholesterol in phospholipid membranes follows Ostwald's rule of stages. J Am Chem Soc. 2020;142:21872–82.

51. Small DM, Bond MG, Waugh D, Prack M, Sawyer J. Physicochemical and histological changes in the arterial wall of nonhuman primates during progression and regression of atherosclerosis. J Clin Investig. 1984;73:1590–605.

52. Feig J. Regression of atherosclerosis: insights from animal and clinical studies. Ann Glob Health. 2014;80:13–23.

53. Brown B, Zhao X, Sacco D, Albers J, Lipid lowering and plaque regression. New insights into prevention of plaque disruption and clinical events in coronary disease. Circulation. 1993;87:1781–91.

54. Flynn G, Shah Y, Prakongpan S, Kwan K, Higuchi W, Hofmann A. Cholesterol solubility in organic solvents. J Pharm Sci. 1979;68:1090–7.

55. Abendan RS, Swift JA, design. Dissolution on cholesterol monohydrate single-crystal surfaces monitored by in situ atomic force microscopy. J Cryst Growth. 2005;5:2146–53.

56. Nasiri M, Janoudi A, Vanderberg A, Frame M, Flegler C, Flegler S, Abela GS, Technique. Role of cholesterol crystals in atherosclerosis is unmasked by altering tissue preparation methods. Microsc Res Tech. 2015;78:969–74.

57. Abela GS, Vedre A, Janoudi A, Huang R, Durga S, Tamhane U. Effect of statins on cholesterol crystallization and atherosclerotic plaque stabilization. Am J Cardiol. 2011;107:1710–7.

58. Zimmerman HE. Molecular mechanism of cell-substrate recognition and attachment. Feinberg Graduate School, Ph.D. Thesis; 2001.

59. Zimmerman E, Geiger B, Addadi L. Initial stages of cell-matrix adhesion can be mediated and modulated by cell-surface hyaluronan. Biophys J. 2002;82:1848–57.

60. Adams C, Abdulla Y. The action of human high density lipoprotein on cholesterol crystals. Part 1. Light-microscopic observations. Atherosclerosis. 1978;31:465–71.
61. Abdulla Y, Adams C. The action of human high density lipoprotein on cholesterol crystals. Part 2. Biochemical observations. Atherosclerosis. 1978;31:473–80.
62. Luo Y, Guo Y, Wang H, Yu M, Hong K, Li D, Li R, Wen B, Hu D, Chang L, Sun D, Shchwendeman SA, Chen YE. Phospholipid nanoparticles: therapeutic potentials against atherosclerosis via reducing cholesterol crystals and inhibiting inflammation. EBioMedicine. 2021;74:103725.
63. Niyonzima N, Samstad EO, Aune MH, Ryan L, Bakke SS, Rokstad AM, Wright SD, Damås JK, Mollnes TE, Latz E, Espevik T. Reconstituted high-density lipoprotein attenuates cholesterol crystal–induced inflammatory responses by reducing complement activation. J Immunol. 2015;195:257–64.
64. Thacker SG, Zarzour A, Chen Y, Alcicek MS, Freeman LA, Sviridov DO, Demosky SJ Jr, Remaley ATx. High-density lipoprotein reduces inflammation from cholesterol crystals by inhibiting inflammasome activation. Immunology. 2016;149:306–19.
65. McConathy WJ, Koren E, Stiers DL. Cholesterol crystal uptake and metabolism by P388D1 macrophages. Atherosclerosis. 1989;77:221–5.
66. Kruth HS, Skarlatos SI, Lilly K, Chang J, Ifrim I. Sequestration of acetylated LDL and cholesterol crystals by human monocyte-derived macrophages. J Cell Biol. 1995;129:133–45.
67. Kruth HS, Skarlatos SI, Gaynor PM, Gamble W. Production of cholesterol-enriched nascent high density lipoproteins by human monocyte-derived macrophages is a mechanism that contributes to macrophage cholesterol efflux. J Biol Chem. 1994;269:24511–8.
68. Zhang W-Y, Gaynor PM, Kruth HS. Apolipoprotein E produced by human monocyte-derived macrophages mediates cholesterol efflux that occurs in the absence of added cholesterol acceptors. J Biol Chem. 1996;271:28641–6.
69. Jin X, Dimitriadis EK, Liu Y, Combs CA, Chang J, Varsano N, Stempinski E, Flores R, Jackson SN, Muller L, Woods AS, Addadi L, Kruth HS. Macrophages shed excess cholesterol in unique extracellular structures containing cholesterol microdomains. Arterioscler Thromb Vasc Biol. 2018;38:1504–18.
70. Abela GS, Kalavakunta JK, Janoudi A, Leffler D, Dhar G, Salehi N, Cohn J, Shah I, Karve M, Kotaru VPK, Gupta V, David S, Narisetty KK, Rich M, Vanderberg A, Pathak DR, Shamoun FE. Frequency of cholesterol crystals in culprit coronary artery aspirate during acute myocardial infarction and their relation to inflammation and myocardial injury. Am J Cardiol. 2017;120:1699–707.

Part III
Physical Properties and Imaging of
Cholesterol Crystals: In Vivo

In Vivo Detection of Cholesterol Crystals in Atherosclerotic Plaque with Optical Coherence Tomography

Jinwei Tian, Xiang Peng, Yanwen Zhang, Zhifeng Qin, Peng Zhao, Yani Wang, and Bo Yu

1 Introduction

Deposition and accumulation of lipids in the arterial wall is the sine qua non of atherosclerotic plaque. Until recently the presence of cholesterol crystals (CCs) in atherosclerotic plaque had been dismissed as a post-mortem artifact and thus no consideration was given to their potential role in the evolution of atherosclerosis. In the last decade it has become increasingly clear that the development of CCs within the atherosclerotic bed are essential for the evolution of atherosclerotic plaques. Growth and aggregation of CCs within the plaque core leads to plaque trauma that precipitates atherothrombotic events, and their deposition in the plaque corona (the area surrounding the necrotic core) incites an inflammatory response that leads to the progressive sclerosis of the arterial wall [1–3]. Accordingly, the ability to detect CCs in situ in vivo provides strong support for the CC paradigm by confirming that they develop de novo in vivo, thus highlighting their role in the dynamics of plaque development, as well as plaque erosion and rupture.

Various imaging modalities have been used to assess the nature of atherosclerotic plaque in vivo, but to date, optical coherence tomography (OCT) is the only technique that has sufficient acuity to reliably detect CCs. This chapter focuses on the insights gained from OCT about the de novo appearance of CCs in stable plaques and highlights how their presence informs us about how atherosclerotic plaques evolve.

J. Tian (✉) · X. Peng · Y. Zhang · Z. Qin · P. Zhao · Y. Wang · B. Yu
Department of Cardiology, The Second Affiliated Hospital of Harbin Medical University, Harbin, China

G. S. Abela, S. M. Nidorf (eds.), *Cholesterol Crystals in Atherosclerosis and Other Related Diseases*, Contemporary Cardiology,
https://doi.org/10.1007/978-3-031-41192-2_5

2   Imaging the Atherosclerotic Landscape in Real Time

Since its introduction in 1959, coronary angiography has been employed in the diagnosis and treatment of coronary heart disease (ref). Despite its clinical utility, angiography only provides a 2-dimensional image of the vascular lumen with a resolution of >500 µm, which is insufficient to provide any specific detail about the character of individual atheromatous plaques which are mostly embedded well below the luminal surface within the arterial wall.

The first technique to obtain real-time in vivo images of atherosclerotic plaque was intravascular ultrasound (IVUS). Using a miniaturized ultrasound probe, IVUS allows the sections of coronary arteries to be analyzed using an echo signal that can differentiate tissues based upon their densities [4]. While IVUS has proven useful as an adjunct to angiography during coronary intervention, the frequency range of it transduces limit its axial resolution to 100–150 µm which is insufficient to visualize cellular structures and anything other than very large CCs within atherosclerotic plaque.

In contrast to IVUS, OCT has higher resolution that employs near-infrared light technology and computer image processing to achieve real-time tomography that provides a maximum axial resolution of 10 µm which 10× greater than the resolution of IVUS [5–8]. As a result, OCT has sufficient resolution to allow for the in vivo identification of various plaque structures and makes it possible to; distinguish a lipid rich core from thickened intima; to accurately identify and measure the thickness of the plaque cap; to visualize microvascular channels indicative of the vasa vasorum; to detect and quantify macrophages in the plaque corona, and to identify and differentiate CCs in the plaque core from the plaque corona. OCT can also be used to calculate the luminal area, the degree of stenosis of an artery, and plaque volume. Thus, in addition to what can be learned from angiography and IVUS, OCT is able to characterize many of the features of atherosclerotic plaque described by pathologists which make it the current gold standard for detecting tissue structural features in vivo [9–13] (Fig. 1).

None-the-less, OCT has limitations. While it is capable of mapping plaque features over the proximal 8–10 cm of all three coronary vessels which covers the majority of culprit lesions, it can only be performed in medium size arteries with lumen stenosis <70% [14]. Since the penetration depth is only 2–2.5 mm it may fail to detect structures including CCs located deep with the plaque and may miss those situated below overlying structures including a calcified plaque, large lipid pool, a large necrotic core or a large thrombus as these structures may attenuate the depth of penetration of the infra-red-light source. Additional factors that specifically affect the ability of OCT to detect CCs are discussed below.

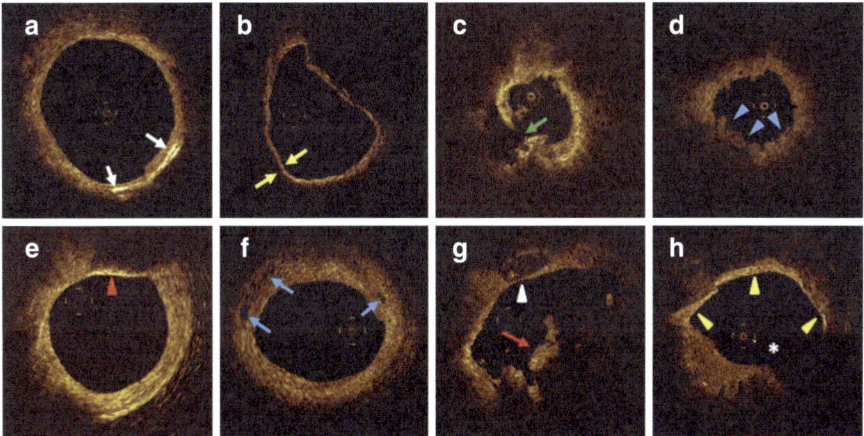

Fig. 1 Representative OCT images. (**a**) Cholesterol crystals (white arrows) defined as linear, highly backscattering structures within the plaque. (**b**) Thin Capped Fibroatheroma (yellow arrows) defined as a plaque with lipid content in two quadrants and the thinnest part of fibrous cap <65 mm. (**c**) Plaque rupture (green arrow) defined as a lipid plaque with fibrous cap discontinuity and a clear cavity formation within the plaque. (**d**) Plaque erosion (blue arrowhead) defined as the presence of attached thrombus overlying an intact and visualized plaque, luminal surface irregularity at the culprit lesion in the absence of thrombus, or attenuation of underlying plaque by thrombus without superficial lipid or calcification immediately proximal or distal to the site of thrombus. (**e**) Macrophages accumulation (red arrowhead) defined as signal-rich, distinct or confluent punctuate regions with heterogeneous backward shadows. (**f**) Microchannels (blue arrow) defined as a black hole with a diameter of 50–300 mm within a plaque that was present on at least 3 consecutive frames. (**g**) Thrombus (red arrow) defined as a mass (diameter > 250 mm) attached to the lumen surface or floating within the lumen; Spotty calcification (white arrowhead) defined a calcification within an arc <90°. (**h**) Calcification (yellow arrowhead) defined as well-delineated, low backscattering heterogeneous regions*. (Reproduced with permission [26])

3   Characterization of Atherosclerotic Plaques by OCT

Standard characterization of plaques by OCT typically involves the measurement of the lipid core arc and its length, assessment of the integrity and thickness of the plaque cap, assessment of the presence of macrophages, calcification, thrombus, microvascular channels in the plaque bed, and assessment of the presence, size and depth of CCs within the plaque. In the setting of an acute coronary syndrome, assessment can also be made of the presence and type of thrombus (white vs red) [15–17].

In comparative studies, OCT can distinguish fibrous, fibrocalcific, and lipid rich plaques with a high sensitivity (range 0.87–0.95) and specificity (range 0.94–1.0) and can identify potentially vulnerable plaques using the same criteria defined by pathologists who characterize plaque vulnerability based upon the thickness of its cap (<65 μm), the size of its lipid pool, and the presence of activated macrophages in the plaque corona [18, 19]. Consistent with the histopathology, these features have been frequently observed by OCT in the atherosclerotic segment containing the culprit lesion in patients with ST-segment elevation myocardial infarction [20].

4 Identification of Cholesterol Crystals by OCT

Animal and autopsy studies suggest that the growth and aggregation of CCs in the core of lipid rich plaques can stretch, penetrate, perforate, and rupture the plaque cap, damage embedded portions of the plaque corona to cause intra-plaque hemorrhage due to direct damage to the vasa vasorum, and trigger acute and chronic inflammation (Chapters "The Cholesterol Crystal Paradigm: Overview of How Cholesterol Crystals Evolve and Induce Traumatic and Inflammatory Vascular Injury", "How Innovation in Tissue Preparation and Imaging Revolutionized the Understanding of the Role of Cholesterol Crystals in Atherosclerosis", and "Role of CCs and Their Lipoprotein Precursors in NLRP3 and IL-1β Activation"). Studies using angioscopy to directly harvest debris from spontaneously ruptured plaques confirm that CCs within atherosclerotic plaque activate innate inflammation [21]. Similarly, aspirates from culprit lesions in patients with acute myocardial infarction have been found to contain large CCs and CC aggregates in association with elevated serum levels of IL-β [22].

Detecting CCs in vivo in culprit plaques with OCT provides strong support for the CC paradigm and has also proven useful as an independent marker of the future risk of plaque rupture, erosion, hemorrhage, and disease progression in a given segment of atheroma [23].

Importantly, despite its high-resolution OCT only has the ability to identify (large) aggregated fragments of CCs in stable atheroma and ruptured plaques. The criteria used by investigators to define CCs by OCT include the presence of a linear, high intensity signal within the plaque that has a clear border between this signal and adjacent low or intermediate density tissues. The linearity of the high intensity signal differentiates CCs from macrophages which are non-linear and lack sharp borders, and the presence of a border between the linear signal and low or intermediate intensity shadows distinguishes them from areas of calcification [17] (Fig. 1). In addition, investigators routinely describe the number and length of CCs, as well as their depth, describing them as deep, or superficial when they are seen to invade the plaque cap (Fig. 2).

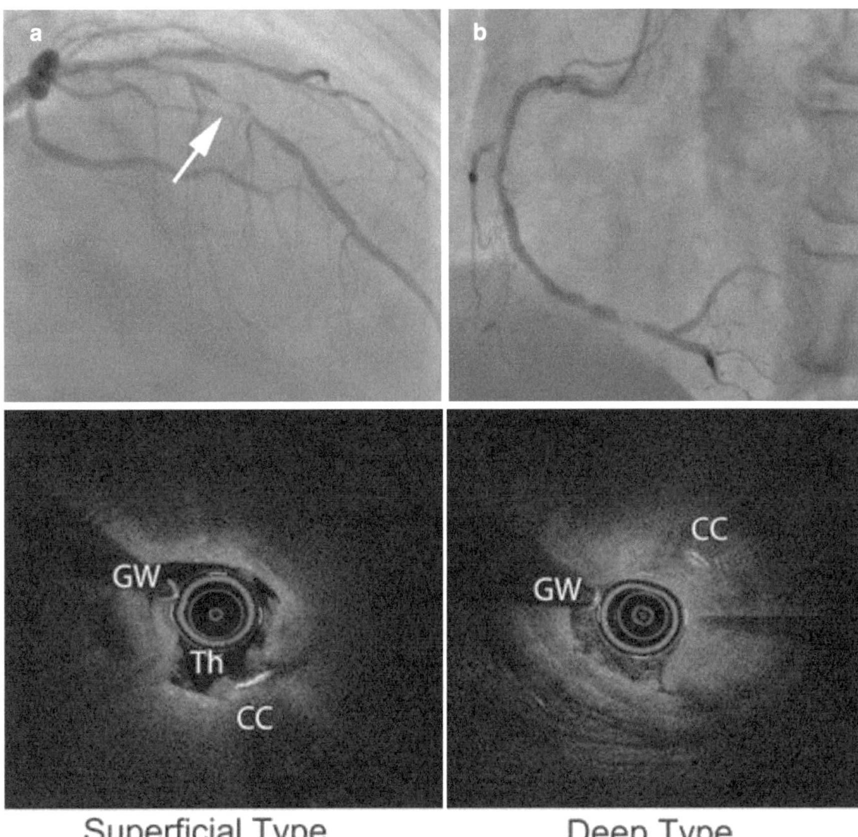

Superficial Type   Deep Type

Fig. 2 Distribution of cholesterol crystals in atherosclerotic plaque using OCT. (**a**) Superficial-type cholesterol crystals (CCs) penetrating a fibrous cap covered with a thrombus; (**b**) deep type CCs without fibrous cap invasion. *CC* indicates cholesterol crystal, *GW*, guidewire, and *Th* thrombus. (Reproduced with permission [17])

In ex vivo studies using these criteria have demonstrated that OCT has a high positive predictive value for large, aggregates of CCs and a favorable inter-observer reproducibility, but a low sensitivity when compared with histology (Fig. 3). This is not surprising as OCT can only detect large CCs and may fail to detect smaller CCs or fragments located deep in the plaque due to limited depth of imaging, as well as those adjacent calcified structures or below the necrotic core. In addition, OCT is unable to detect meta-stable CCs which lack a reflective surface and is unable to detect small and unaggregated CC fragments that may otherwise be confused with foamy macrophages. Furthermore, the ability of OCT to detect CCs may be affected by CC morphology and orientation; whereas OCT may detect the surface of flat

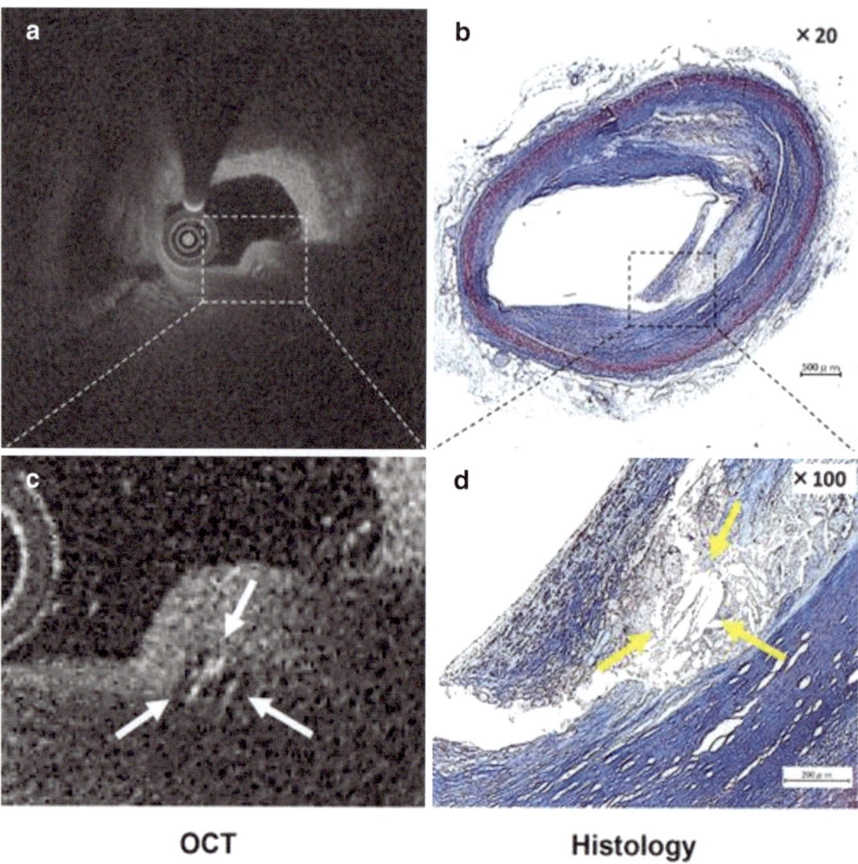

OCT   **Histology**

Fig. 3 Comparison of OCT images with histology for cholesterol crystal assessment of a human coronary artery (**a**) and a magnified version (**c**). **b** and **d**, present the corresponding histological images. OCT shows several thin, linear regions of high-signal intensity within the superficial layer of a plaque (white arrows). Several clefts can be seen (yellow arrows) at the correspondence sites in the histological image. (Reproduced with permission [17])

plate CCs that typically measure 50–100 μm, it will not be able to resolve the thin edge of a CC or appreciate needle / rod shaped CCs viewed on edge or in cross-section that typically measure 1–5 μm.

Thus, although the absence of CCs on OCT imaging does not negate their existence in a given plaque, their presence does inform us that the physiochemistry in a specific plaque core is sufficient to trigger CC development and growth in vivo. Furthermore, the detection of large CC fragments or aggregates in a large lipid and

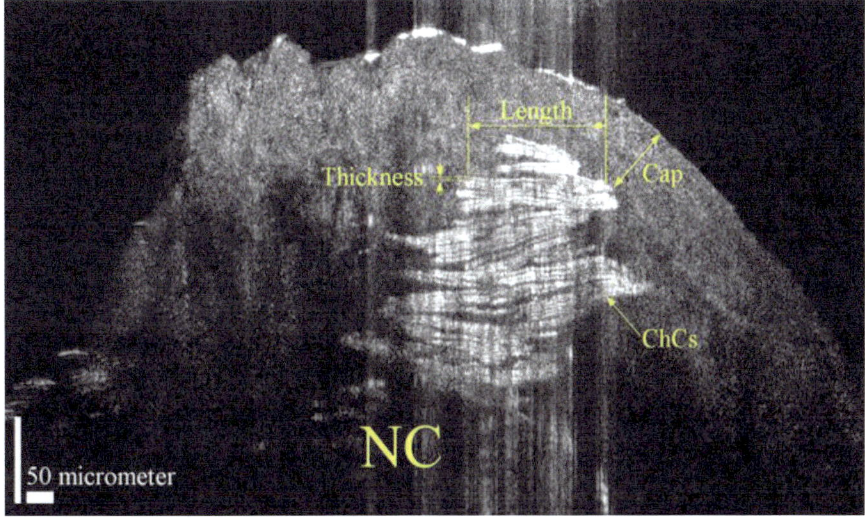

Fig. 4 A μOCT Image of a human aortic atherosclerotic plaque revealing aggregated cholesterol crystals. *ChCs* cholesterol crystals, *NC* necrotic core. Scale bar, 50 μm. (Reproduced with permission [20])

necrotic core provides potentially important independent prognostic information [18, 19]. Large CCs in the plaque corona may exert circumferential stresses on the plaque, which together with the increase in volume and pressure that CCs impose within the plaque core, increases the risk of plaque rupture [20] (Fig. 4). Moreover, OCT demonstrates lipid rich plaque and calcification with cholesterol crystallization in coronary artery stenosis, leading to plaque rupture (Fig. 5).

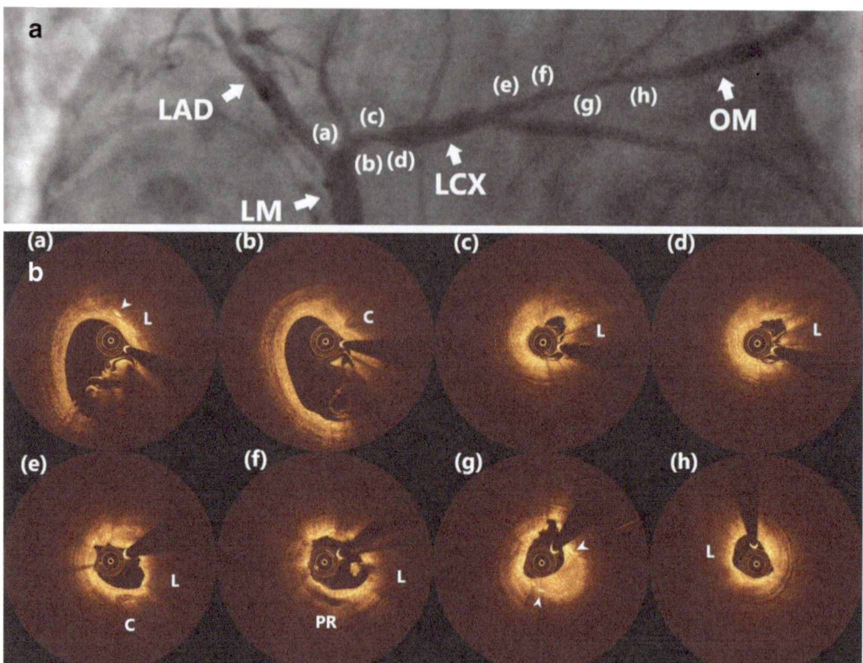

Fig. 5 Cholesterol crystals in plaque rupture (**a**) Coronary angiography prior to percutaneous coronary intervention. One stenosis (**a–d**) and another culprit lesion (**e–h**) were identified in the proximal segments of left circumflex artery (LCX) and the obtuse marginal branch (OM), respectively. *LAD* left anterior descending artery, *LM* left main. (**a–h**) corresponds to optical coherence tomography images in (**b**). (**b**) Optical coherence tomography Images prior to percutaneous coronary intervention. Non-culprit lesion (**a–d**) exhibited lipid plaque (L) or calcification (C) with cholesterol crystal (arrow head).Homogeneous high-intensity signal area at the surface of this lesion was observed. At culprit lesion (**e–h**), lipid plaque (L), multiple cholesterol crystals (arrow head), and small calcification (C) were visualized. Plaque rupture (PR) and lipid plaque (L) were visualized in (**f**). (Courtesy of the chapter authors)

5 Prevalence and Predictors of CCs in Atherosclerotic Plaque as Detected by OCT

OCT studies have reported the incidence of CCs in various settings. In stable (non-culprit) coronary plaques, CCs are more frequently found in men, in patients with chronic kidney disease and patients with peripheral vascular disease [24–28]. In addition, CCs have been associated with higher levels of glycosylated hemoglobin, LDL-c and apolipoprotein C3 [29, 30]. As in in vitro experiments where a drop in temperature of 1–2 °C has been found to be sufficient to trigger cholesterol crystallization [2], CCs are also more frequently observed in patients with slightly lower body temperature (36.1 °C vs. 36.4 °C), consistent with the belief that even slight decreases in core body temperature in vivo may be enough to trigger CC formation in stable plaques and predispose to plaque rupture.

6 Characteristic of CCs in Patients Presenting with Acute Myocardial Infarction

OCT studies have shown that a culprit (disrupted) plaque is more likely to be found in patients presenting with Type I myocardial infarction than Type 2 myocardial infarction or stable angina, and that the cap of the culprit plaque cap is eroded rather than ruptured in up to one third of patients presenting with an acute myocardial infarction [31] (Chapter "Formation of CCs in Endothelial Cells"). Consistent with angioscopy, using OCT has also found that in patients with coronary disease spontaneous asymptomatic plaque ruptures are not uncommon [21].

To determine the potential role of CCs in the evolution of plaque rupture we examined the appearance of *non-culprit* lesions in 261 patients with ST elevation myocardial infarction (STEMI) [23]. This revealed that non-culprit plaques with CCs were more likely to have other characteristics of plaque vulnerability including a greater lipid burden, more macrophages and spotty calcification than non-culprit plaque without CCs (Fig. 6). Furthermore, non-culprit lesions that contained CCs were also more likely to have a ruptured plaque cap, and the CCs within them were larger and more superficial than the CCs seen in non-ruptured plaques. Notably, longitudinal studies with OCT demonstrate that the vast majority (90–95%) of non-culprit plaques with vulnerable features including a thin cap and large lipid pool remain stable over 1–4 years, however, those containing CCs have a two to threefold higher risk of future rupture than lesions that do not contain CCs at baseline [17, 23, 26, 32–37]. Together, these observations suggest that CCs within *non-culprit* plaques had begun to form, enlarge and aggregate *prior* to plaque rupture, and that the number, size, and position of CCs within the plaque may each inform about the future risk plaque rupture. Moreover, after drug intervention, the number of CCs and corresponding parameters also changed at non-culprit plaque, demonstrating the potential of CCs for treatment evaluation (Fig. 7).

We have also observed that in patients undergoing coronary stenting, target lesions containing CCs are more prone to irregular protrusions, no-reflow, stent thrombosis, and peri-procedural myocardial injury, especially when fractional flow reserve computed tomography is <82 µm. Similarly, other investigators have found that in the setting of acute myocardial infarction, CCs in the culprit lesion are associated with an increased risk of no-reflow during angioplasty, and that the number of CCs within the plaque is a predictor of coronary no-reflow, independent of the size of the lipid arc. Finally, in keeping with the observations in non-culprit plaques,

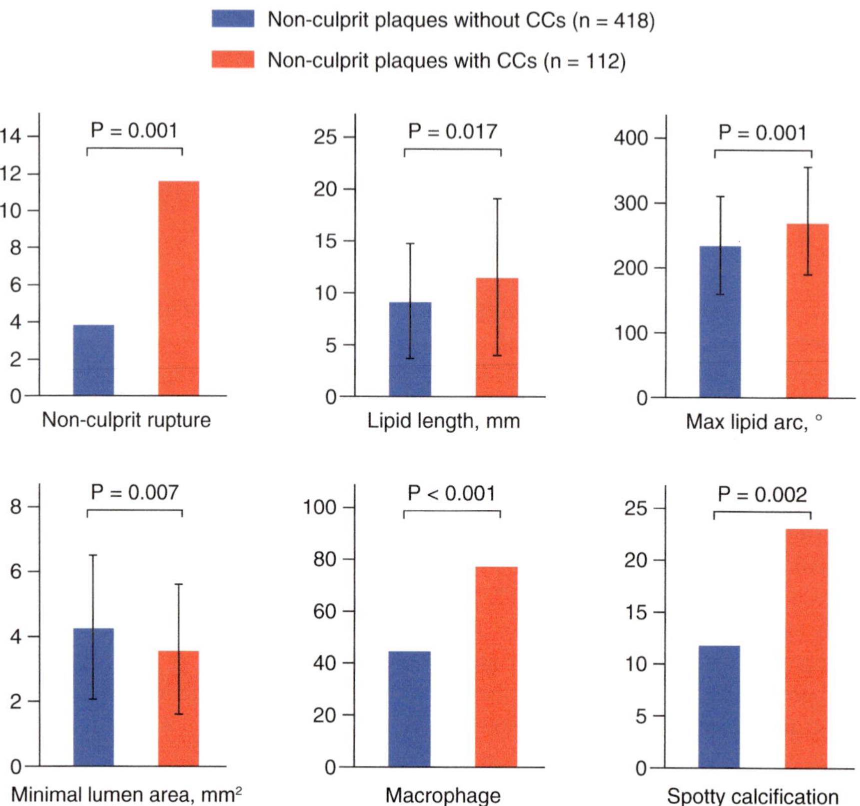

Fig. 6 Morphological characteristics of non-culprit plaques with and without CCs. Quantitative analysis revealed that non-culprit plaques with CCs had more vulnerable characteristics than those without CCs, including a greater lipid burden ($p < 0.001$), more macrophages ($p < 0.001$) and spotty calcification ($p = 0.002$) and were more likely to be associated with plaque rupture. *CC* cholesterol crystal. (Adapted from Zhifeng Qin et al. [23])

it has been found that the presence of CCs in culprit lesions that are stented in the setting of myocardial infarction are also associated with an increased risk of cardiovascular events over the subsequent 12 months [38, 39].

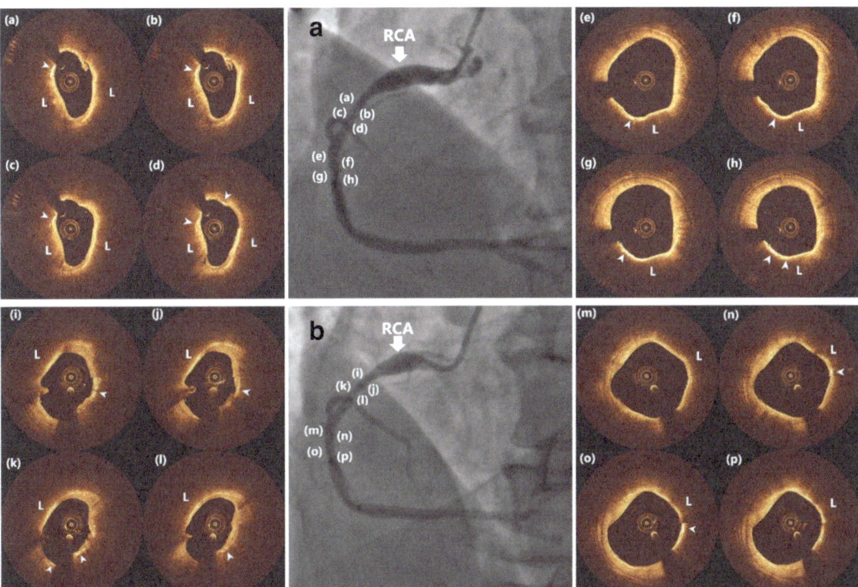

Fig. 7 Changes in cholesterol crystals after drug treatment. (**a**) Primary coronary angiography revealed two stenosis (**a–d**) and (**e–h**) in the right coronary artery (RCA). (**a–h**) corresponds to optical coherence tomography images were displayed on both sides. (**b**) Drug treatment for 1 month, Coronary angiography was reexamined. The same location was taken, and (**i–p**) corresponds to optical coherence tomography images were displayed on both sides. Lipid plaque (L), multiple cholesterol crystals (arrow head). (Courtesy of the chapter authors)

7   Conclusion

The ability of OCT to detect, locate, and quantify characteristics of CCs in vivo provides insight into their role in the progression of atherosclerosis, and erosion and rupture of the plaque cap, and provides independent prognostic information about the natural history of an atherosclerotic segment following myocardial infarction and coronary intervention.

References

1. Abela GS, Aziz K, Vedre A, et al. Effect of cholesterol crystals on plaques and intima in arteries of patients with acute coronary and cerebrovascular syndromes. Am J Cardiol. 2009;103(7):959–68.
2. Vedre A, Pathak DR, Crimp M, et al. Physical factors that trigger cholesterol crystallization leading to plaque rupture. Atherosclerosis. 2009;203(1):89–96.

3. Janoudi A, Shamoun FE, Kalavakunta JK, et al. Cholesterol crystal induced arterial inflammation and destabilization of atherosclerotic plaque. Eur Heart J. 2016;37(25):1959–67.
4. Nissen SE, Yock P. Intravascular ultrasound: novel pathophysiological insights and current clinical applications. Circulation. 2001;103(4):604–16.
5. Huang D, Swanson EA, Lin CP, et al. Optical coherence tomography. Science. 1991;254(5035):1178–81.
6. Brezinski ME, Tearney GJ, Bouma BE, et al. Optical coherence tomography for optical biopsy. Properties and demonstration of vascular pathology. Circulation. 1996;93(6):1206–13.
7. Rogowska J, Patel NA, Fujimoto JG, et al. Optical coherence tomographic elastography technique for measuring deformation and strain of atherosclerotic tissues. Heart. 2004;90(5):556–62.
8. Kawase Y, Hoshino K, Yoneyama R, et al. In vivo volumetric analysis of coronary stent using optical coherence tomography with a novel balloon occlusion-flushing catheter: a comparison with intravascular ultrasound. Ultrasound Med Biol. 2005;31(10):1343–9.
9. Boppart SA, Bouma BE, Pitris C, et al. In vivo cellular optical coherence tomography imaging. Nat Med. 1998;4(7):861–5.
10. Tearney GJ, Brezinski ME, Bouma BE, et al. In vivo endoscopic optical biopsy with optical coherence tomography. Science. 1997;276(5321):2037–9.
11. Tearney GJ, Jang IK, Bouma BE. Optical coherence tomography for imaging the vulnerable plaque. J Biomed Opt. 2006;11(2):021002.
12. Kume T, Akasaka T, Kawamoto T, et al. Assessment of coronary arterial plaque by optical coherence tomography. Am J Cardiol. 2006;97(8):1172–5.
13. Yabushita H, Bouma BE, Houser SL, et al. Characterization of human atherosclerosis by optical coherence tomography. Circulation. 2002;106(13):1640–5.
14. Prati F, Romagnoli E, Gatto L, et al. Relationship between coronary plaque morphology of the left anterior descending artery and 12 months clinical outcome: the CLIMA study. Eur Heart J. 2020;41(3):383–91.
15. Jinnouchi H, Sato Y, Torii S, et al. Detection of cholesterol crystals by optical coherence tomography. EuroIntervention. 2020;16(5):395–403.
16. Brown AJ, Obaid DR, West NE, et al. Cholesterol crystals identified using optical coherence tomography and virtual histology intravascular ultrasound. EuroIntervention. 2015;11(2):e1.
17. Katayama Y, Tanaka A, Taruya A, Kashiwagi M, Nishiguchi T, Ozaki Y, Matsuo Y, Kitabata H, Kubo T, Shimada E, Kondo T, Akasaka T. Feasibility and clinical significance of in vivo cholesterol crystal detection using optical coherence tomography. Arterioscler Thromb Vasc Biol. 2020;40(1):220–9. Epub 2019 17. https://doi.org/10.1161/ATVBAHA.119.312934.
18. Nishimura S, Ehara S, Hasegawa T, et al. Cholesterol crystal as a new feature of coronary vulnerable plaques: an optical coherence tomography study. J Cardiol. 2017;69(1):253–9.
19. Shi X, Cai H, Wang F, et al. Cholesterol crystals are associated with carotid plaque vulnerability: an optical coherence tomography study. J Stroke Cerebrovasc Dis. 2020;29(2):104579.
20. Luo Y, Cui D, Yu X, Chen S, Liu X, Tang H, Wang X, Liu L. Modeling of mechanical stress exerted by cholesterol crystallization on atherosclerotic plaques. PloS One. 2016;11(5):e0155117. PMID: 27149381; PMCID: PMC4858299. https://doi.org/10.1371/journal.pone.0155117.
21. Otsuka F, Joner M, Prati F, et al. Clinical classification of plaque morphology in coronary disease. Nat Rev Cardiol. 2014;11(7):379–89.
22. Abela GS, Kalavakunta JK, Janoudi A, Leffler D, Dhar G, Salehi N, Cohn J, Shah I, Karve M, Kotaru VPK, Gupta V, David S, Narisetty KK, Rich M, Vanderberg A, Pathak DR, Shamoun FE. Frequency of cholesterol crystals in culprit coronary artery aspirate during acute myocardial infarction and their relation to inflammation and myocardial injury. Am J Cardiol. 2017;120:1699–707. https://doi.org/10.1016/j.amjcard.2017.07.075.
23. Qin Z, Cao M, Xi X, et al. Cholesterol crystals in non-culprit plaques of STEMI patients: a 3-vessel study. Int J Cardiol. 2022;364:162–8.

24. Komatsu S, Yutani C, Takahashi S, et al. Debris collected in-situ from spontaneously ruptured atherosclerotic plaque invariably contains large cholesterol crystals and evidence of activation of innate inflammation: insights from nonobstructive general Angioscopy. Atherosclerosis. 2022;352:96. https://doi.org/10.1016/j.atherosclerosis.2022.03.010.
25. Virmani R, Kolodgie FD, Burke AP, et al. Atherosclerotic plaque progression and vulnerability to rupture: angiogenesis as a source of intraplaque hemorrhage. Arterioscler Thromb Vasc Biol. 2005;25(10):2054–61.
26. Dai J, Tian J, Hou J, et al. Association between cholesterol crystals and culprit lesion vulnerability in patients with acute coronary syndrome: an optical coherence tomography study. Atherosclerosis. 2016;247:111–7.
27. Kataoka Y, Puri R, Hammadah M, Duggal B, Uno K, Kapadia SR, Tuzcu EM, Nissen SE, King P, Nicholls SJ. Sex differences in nonculprit coronary plaque microstructures on frequency-domain optical coherence tomography in acute coronary syndromes and stable coronary artery disease. Circ Cardiovasc Imaging. 2016;9:e004506. https://doi.org/10.1161/CIRCIMAGING.116.004506.
28. Kato K, Yonetsu T, Jia H, et al. Nonculprit coronary plaque characteristics of chronic kidney disease. Circ Cardiovasc Imaging. 2013;6(3):448–56.
29. Bryniarski KL, Yamamoto E, Takumi H, et al. Differences in coronary plaque characteristics between patients with and those without peripheral arterial disease. Coron Artery Dis. 2017;28(8):658–63.
30. Fujiyoshi K, Minami Y, Ishida K, et al. Incidence, factors, and clinical significance of cholesterol crystals in coronary plaque: an optical coherence tomography study. Atherosclerosis. 2019;283:79–84.
31. Sekimoto T, Koba S, Mori H, et al. Impact of small dense low-density lipoprotein cholesterol on cholesterol crystals in patients with acute coronary syndrome: an optical coherence tomography study. J Clin Lipidol. 2022;16(4):438–46.
32. Iannaccone M, Quadri G, Taha S, et al. Prevalence and predictors of culprit plaque rupture at in patients with coronary artery disease: a meta-analysis. Eur Heart J Cardiovasc Imaging. 2016;17(10):1128–37.
33. Kataoka Y, Puri R, Hammadah M, et al. Cholesterol crystals associate with coronary plaque vulnerability in vivo. J Am Coll Cardiol. 2015;65(6):630–2.
34. Xing L, Higuma T, Wang Z, et al. Clinical significance of lipid-rich plaque detected by optical coherence tomography: a 4-year follow-up study. J Am Coll Cardiol. 2017;69(20):2502–13.
35. Tian J, Dauerman H, Toma C, et al. Prevalence and characteristics of TCFA and degree of coronary artery stenosis: an, IVUS, and angiographic study. J Am Coll Cardiol. 2014;64(7):672–80.
36. Kato K, Yonetsu T, Kim SJ, et al. Nonculprit plaques in patients with acute coronary syndromes have more vulnerable features compared with those with non-acute coronary syndromes: a 3-vessel optical coherence tomography study. Circ Cardiovasc Imaging. 2012;5(4):433–40.
37. Vergallo R, Uemura S, Soeda T, et al. Prevalence and predictors of multiple coronary plaque ruptures: in vivo 3-vessel optical coherence tomography imaging study. Arterioscler Thromb Vasc Biol. 2016;36(11):2229–38.
38. Otsuka K, Shimada K, Ishikawa H, et al. Usefulness of pre- and post-stent optical frequency domain imaging findings in the prediction of periprocedural cardiac troponin elevation in patients with coronary artery disease. Heart Vessels. 2020;35(4):451–62.
39. Katayama Y, Taruya A, Kashiwagi M, et al. No-reflow phenomenon and in vivo cholesterol crystals combined with lipid core in acute myocardial infarction. Int J Cardiol Heart Vasc. 2022;38:100953.

Detecting Cholesterol Crystals Clinically in Spontaneous Aortic Plaque Rupture

Kazuhisa Kodama, Chikao Yutani, Sei Komatsu, and Satoru Takahashi

1 History of Non-Obstructive General Angioscopy

Angioscopy was first performed in the USA in the 1980s [1], mainly for the coronary artery. As angioscopy itself cannot be demonstrated inside the vessel wall due to the abundant blood flow in the vessel, the prototype system uses a balloon to occlude coronary blood flow upstream for observation. Angioscopy was banned by the Food and Drug Administration after accidents like fatal arrhythmia secondary to coronary ischemia due to long-term occlusion of the coronary artery. Kodama et al. [2] developed the non-obstructive angioscopy (NOGA) in Japan that does not include a balloon (Fig. 1), and the visual field is obtained by removing the erythrocytes using a transparent low-molecular-weight dextran sulfate L solution (dextran 40/lactated ringer's solution; LMDS) in front of an angioscopic fiber [3]. By diluting the blood in front of a catheter with LMDS, the vessel wall can be visualized clearly, creating a safer system than those preceding because the coronary artery, aorta, and vein are not temporarily occluded. As a result, NOGA is covered by Japanese medical insurance.

By applying NOGA to the coronary artery, the number of yellow plaques (or rather the yellow color intensity of these plaques) could be a marker of coronary atherosclerosis [4]. An intensive yellow color with red thrombi may indicate a vulnerable plaque [5]. In patients with myocardial infarction, all three major coronary arteries were widely diseased and had multiple yellow, but non-disrupted plaques;

K. Kodama (✉) · S. Komatsu · S. Takahashi
Department of Cardiology, Cardiovascular Center, Osaka Gyoumeikan Hospital, Osaka, Japan

C. Yutani
Department of Pathology, Cardiovascular Center, Osaka Gyoumeikan Hospital, Osaka, Japan

G. S. Abela, S. M. Nidorf (eds.), *Cholesterol Crystals in Atherosclerosis and Other Related Diseases*, Contemporary Cardiology,
https://doi.org/10.1007/978-3-031-41192-2_6

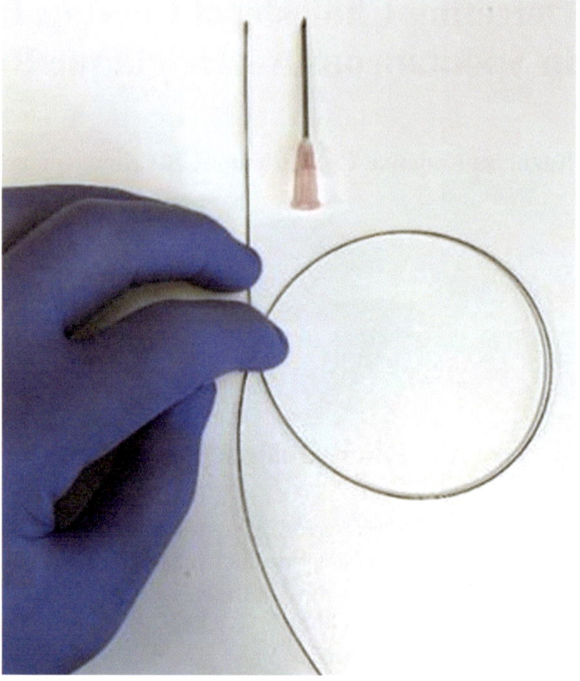

Fig. 1 A macroscopic image of the angioscopic fiber with a diameter of 0.75 mm and thinner than an 18-gauge needle

therefore, acute myocardial infarction may represent a pan-coronary process of vulnerable plaque development [6]. Patients with observed multiple yellow plaques per vessel have a higher risk of developing acute coronary syndrome (ACS) [7]. The healing process of yellow plaques at the lesions responsible for myocardial infarction was found to reduce the color grade and thrombogenicity by angioscopy [8]. In patients with coronary artery disease receiving statin treatment, serial analysis with angioscopy demonstrated an early loss of yellow color in plaques [9, 10]. In addition, the stabilization observed by NOGA, and regression observed by intravascular ultrasound of atherosclerotic plaques by statins, may differ [10]. Plaque disruption and healing occur not only at the culprit lesion but may also be a pan-coronary process in patients with acute myocardial infarction [11].

The completion of neointimal coverage of stents in human coronary arteries requires approximately 3 months [12], and in-stent atherosclerosis, which was evaluated by yellow plaque at 1 year after the implantation of a drug-eluting stent, and the absence of statin therapy were risk factors for very late stent failure [13].

The technique for NOGA requires proficiency to obtain quality images with better visual fields, and subsequently, a dual infusion system that infuses LMDS was developed to obtain a better and more effective visual field [3]. The development of this technique has allowed dynamic subintimal changes in coronary artery stenting to be detected [14]. Instant pullback, which is used in intravascular ultrasound and optical coherence tomography, cannot detect such subintimal blood flow. Moreover, new applications have opened the door to observe vessels of every size through which NOGA can pass, such as the aorta [15–17], renal artery [18], pulmonary artery [14, 19–21], and the aortic valve [22, 23]. Angioscopy-assisted interventions have also been reported [20, 24], and it is hoped that NOGA will be considered for all fields of intervention worldwide.

2 Non-Obstructive General Angioscopy

The NOGA system comprises of a fiber, probing, and guiding catheters with a standard size of 2.5-Fr, 4.2-Fr, and 6-Fr [3] that can be flexibly changed. The single infusion method, in which LMDS is infused between the fiber and probing catheter, was used initially (Fig. 2a). After dual infusion LMDS was infused between the guiding and probing catheter in addition to a single infusion, the visual field was expanded and the application for every sized vessel was established [3] (Fig. 2b). It is crucial to remove the microbubbles inside the catheter using a syringe during assembly, as these may cause a temporal air embolism and obstruct the visual field.

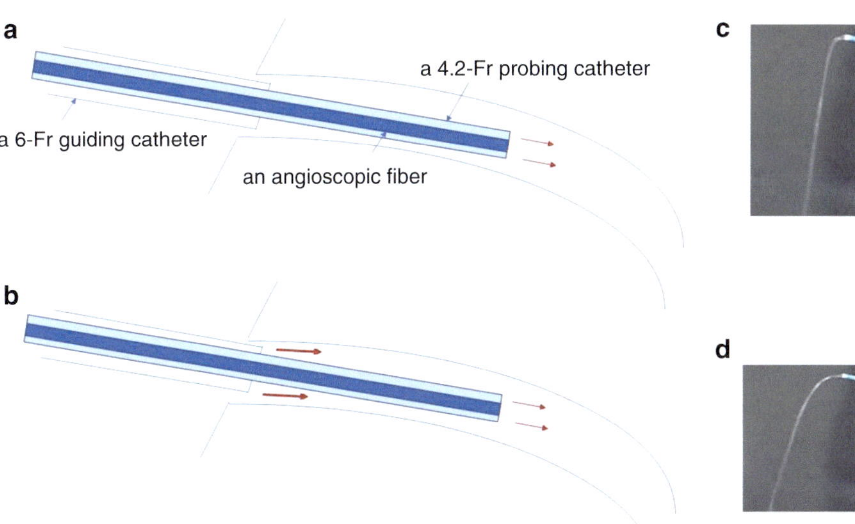

Fig. 2 A schematic image from the top of the catheters of a coronary angioscopy using non-obstructive general angioscopy and experimental models of infusion. (**a**) Single infusion method: A low-molecular-weight dextran sulfate L solution was infused between the angioscopic fiber and 4.2-Fr probing catheter. (**b**) Dual-infusion method: A low-molecular-weight dextran sulfate L solution was additionally infused between a 4.2-Fr probing catheter and 6-Fr guiding catheter. (**c**) Speed of low-molecular-weight dextran sulfate L solution from the top of catheters using a single infusion method. (**d**) Speed of low-molecular-weight dextran sulfate L solution from the top of catheters using a dual infusion method

2.1 Non-Obstructive General Angioscopy for Coronary Artery (Fig. 2)

The surgeon can select an approach from either the femoral, brachial, or radial artery. An aspiration catheter can be used in the place of the outer probing catheter. The guidewire (with a set of probing catheters) is wedged into the middle of the coronary artery, and then removed with the inner probing catheter to insert a fiber catheter. Dual infusion is then initiated to improve the visual field, and the video footage is recorded. After angioscopy of the aorta, coronary angiography was performed to check the electrocardiogram and coronary angiography without coronary slow flow or reflow.

2.2 Non-Obstructive General Angioscopy for the Aorta (Fig. 3)

Soft tip-type guiding catheters, such as the Heartrail-type, are recommended to prevent injury to the aorta and shapes such as the Ikari (IL), extra backup (EBU), super power backup(SPB), and Judkins right (JR) catheters fit well to most variations of the aorta. Specifically, the IL3.5 catheter works well because it can wedge both sides of the coronary arteries [25, 26] and allows for both coronary and aortic angioscopies to be performed. While a guiding catheter is generally 100 cm, a

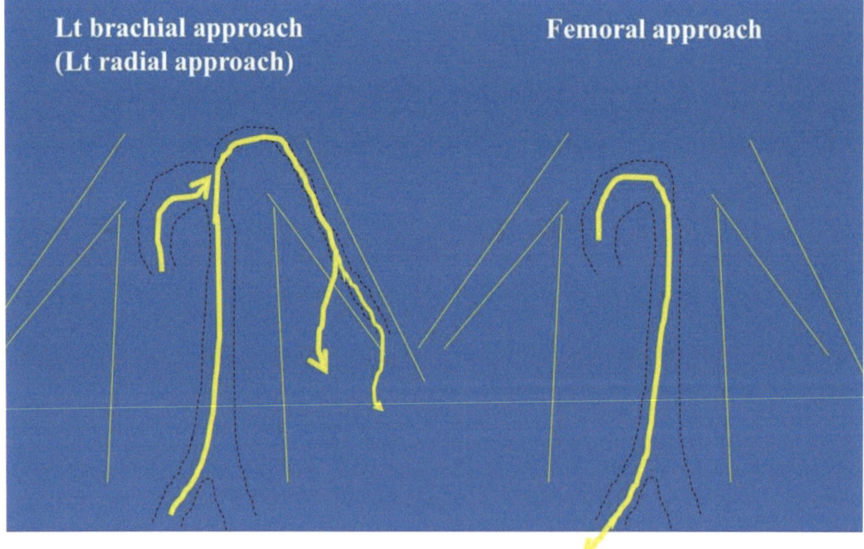

Fig. 3 A schematic image of the trajectory of a catheter performing an aortic angioscopy with left brachial approach (*left*) and femoral approach (*right*)

longer catheter with a size of 112 cm can approach longer areas of the aorta. Either the femoral, left brachial, or left radial approach can easily access the ascending aorta, aortic arch, descending aorta, abdominal aorta, and iliac arteries.

3   Detecting and Sampling Spontaneously Ruptured Aortic Plaques

There are various types of SRAPs in the aorta [17, 27]. Among SRAPs, puff rupture (Fig. 4a, b), chandelier rupture, and puff-chandelier rupture (Fig. 4c, d) are common. A puff rupture consists of white or white-yellow colored puff-like materials that are easily spontaneously blown out, while a chandelier rupture consists of

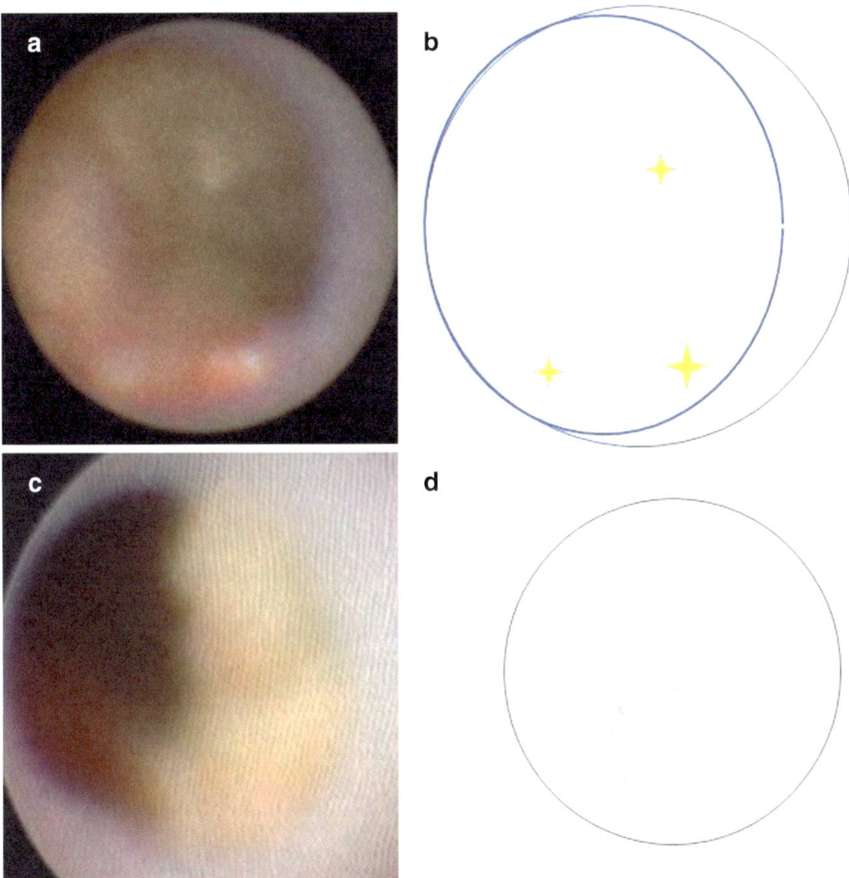

Fig. 4 An angioscopic image of puff and puff-chandelier rupture and their schema. (**a**) Puff rupture. (**b**) An illustration of (**a**). (**c**) Puff-chandelier rupture. (**d**) An illustration of (**c**)

materials that glisten against the light from the tip of the fiber catheter of a non-obstructive general angioscope that wriggle, but do not blow out. A Puff-chandelier rupture is a common ruptured plaque mixed with features of a puff and chandelier rupture. Plaque components of puff and puff-chandelier ruptures can be sampled from a guiding catheter, whereby a puff-chandelier rupture consists of atheromatous materials (including cholesterol crystals), fibrin, calcification, and macrophages [16], and a puff rupture predominantly contains fibrin. Cholesterol crystals sometimes are associated with a puff rupture, although they are not visually reflected in the light of NOGA.

After removing the guiding catheter from the coronary artery, a fiber catheter with an outer probing catheter is inserted at the top of the guiding catheter (Fig. 5a). Dual infusion to gain the visual field is then initiated, and a set of catheters is rotationally pulled back from the ascending aorta to the iliac artery. The video feed, along with comments, are recorded. If SRAPs are detected, a weak infusion is recommended. To sample the SRAPs, a fiber catheter with an outer probing catheter is removed, and the syringe is gently pulled from the guiding catheter (Fig. 5b).

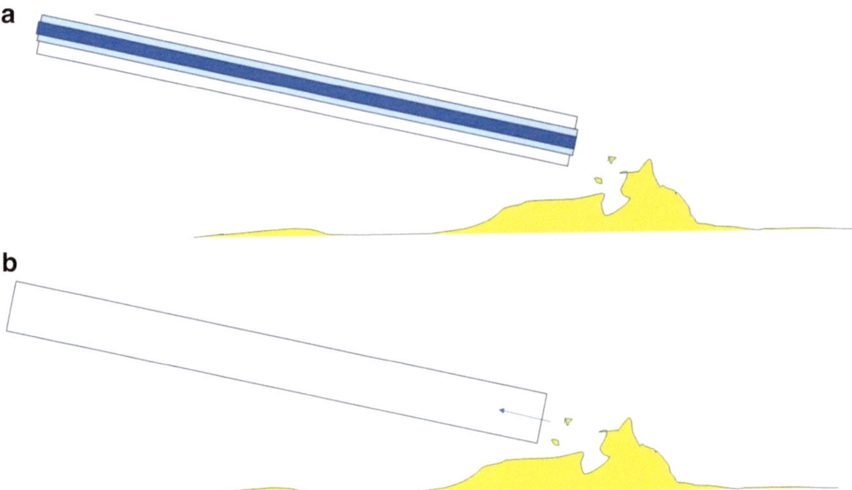

Fig. 5 Sampling for spontaneously ruptured aortic plaques using a non-obstructive general angioscopic system. (**a**) Detecting spontaneously ruptured aortic plaques by non-obstructive general angioscopic system. (**b**) Both an angioscopic fiber and a 4.2-Fr probing catheter are gently removed, then blood is gently sampled from a 6-Fr guiding catheter

4 Detecting Cholesterol Crystals from Human Blood Samples

If a blood sample with SRAPs is observed by light microscopy, a multilayer of erythrocytes around the cholesterol crystals (CCs) may interfere with their detection (Fig. 6) and therefore need to be removed by chemical or mechanical preparation for an effective observation. Denaturization of erythrocytes can be performed using solvents, although CCs are also soluble in solvents. The size of the CCs are generally 40×30 µm, and the diameter of a erythrocytes are approximately 5 µm. To mechanically sift particles of this size may be expensive, and if CCs are broken, their size may be similar to that of erythrocytes. Alternatively, diluting samples with distilled water may induce hemolysis, although the concentration of CCs would decrease. The melting point of the CCs is 148 °C, and heat shock may distinguish erythrocytes from CCs, although it is difficult to remove denatured proteins. Qualitative and quantitative analyses of CCs from SRAPs can be performed.

Fig. 6 Cholesterol crystals surrounded multi-layered erythrocytes

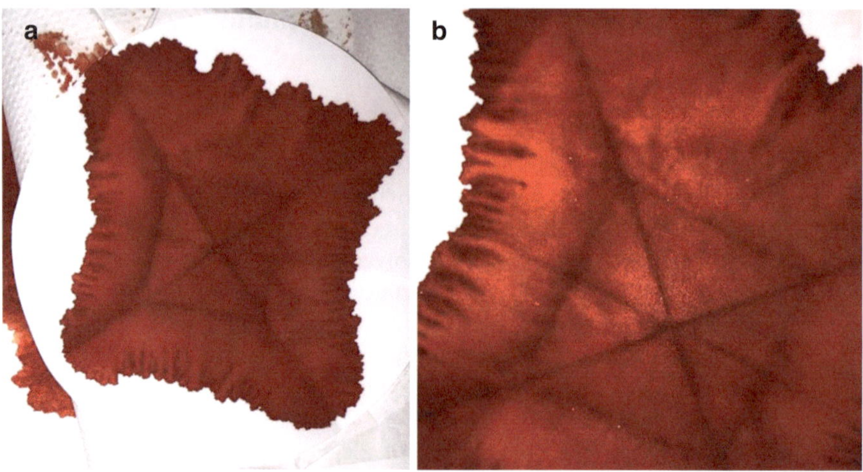

Fig. 7 Sampled spontaneously ruptured aortic plaques on a 15-cm filter paper. (**a**) Filter the paper under wet conditions. (**b**) Filter paper under dried conditions

4.1 Qualitative Analysis of CCs from Blood Samples

When blood sampled from SRAPs was spread onto fine-pore cellulose filter paper (pore size 7 μm, diameter 15 cm, spherical type No. 5A, Advantech Co., Tokyo, Japan; Fig. 7a), the filter paper glitters under light conditions of at least 500 lx after drying (Fig. 7b). The filter paper is then rinsed with 3 mL of distilled water and the rinsed water placed on a glass slide [28]. This sample is then observed by a polarized light microscopy, and if CCs are present, the parallelepipeds reflect blue or orange (Fig. 8a, b). There are two kinds of CCs observed, namely free and atheroma that may be multilayered.

4.2 Quantitative Analysis of CCs from Blood Samples

The sampled blood is placed on a glass slide and covered with a coverslip with its edges sealed with resin and hardened for approximately 30 min in an ultraviolet light-irradiated box. If a sample is observed by polarized light microscopy, multi-layered erythrocytes can be used to quantitatively detect and analyze the CCs. Specimens can be instantly frozen at −20 °C using a freezing solvent and gently thawed to 25 °C to destroy erythrocytes [28], and quantitative analysis of CCs and their approximate lengths can be measured by treating erythrocytes as size markers (Fig. 8c, d).

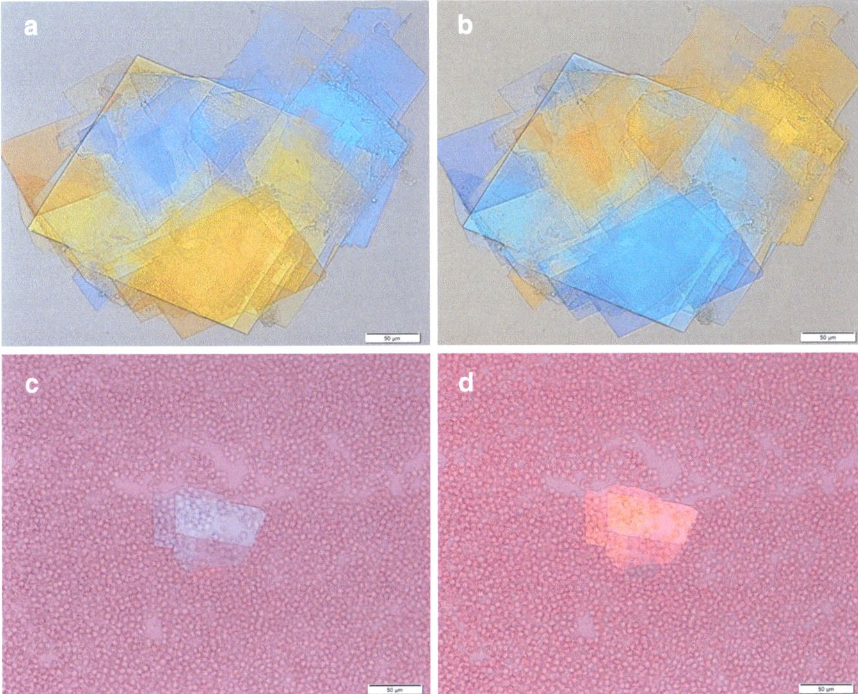

Fig. 8 Examples of multi-layered cholesterol crystals in spontaneously ruptured aortic plaques obtained by a filter-paper rinse method (**a** and **b**) and a freeze-thaw method for sampled blood (**c** and **d**). Each crystal is expressed blue or orange alternatively by a polarized light microscopy without background (**a** and **b**) and with fewer erythrocytes compared to that of Fig. 6

5 Clinical Significance of Detecting SRAPs and Cholesterol Crystals: Is Aortic Plaque Really Innocent?

Cholesterol crystals perforating the cap and intimal surface are thought to be formed in plaques [29]. SRAPs are thought to cause organ dysfunction through ischemia and inflammation [30, 31] by mechanical obstruction and the NLRP3 inflammasome. Furthermore, the incidence of thromboembolism in the aorta is estimated to be up to 5%, and the limitation of the detection of large aortic plaques by CT or echocardiography suggests that arterial thromboembolism is mainly iatrogenic [32]. Large plaques, such as complex aortic plaques defined as ≥4-mm-thick, ulcerated, or containing mobile thrombi, are considered a major source of stroke [33], and whether aortic atherosclerotic plaques are associated with potential cardiac or cerebrovascular events remains controversial [34].

A total of 324 consecutive patients diagnosed with or suspected of having coronary artery disease were subjected to intra-aortic scans with NOGA [16]. SRAPs were detected in 262 patients (80.9%). SRAPs were commonly scattered, and their dimensions were smaller than those previously reported. Atheromatous materials, including CCs (median length × width, 650 × 313 μm), fibrin, macrophages, calcification, and their mixture may be blown out from SRAPs. The free form of the monolayer (median length × width, 40 μm × 30 μm) and multilayer CCs may scatter. Interestingly, sampling CCs from SRAPs in live patients has revealed a difference between human and commercially available CCs made from animals [26], whereby those from humans were more diverse in size and form than experimental CCs.

This might be key to determining the unknown pathogenesis of systemic organ dysfunction [35], such as that of the brain [36, 37], heart [38–40], kidney, peripheral arteries [41], and muscles [42] to cholesterol embolization syndrome [32, 43]. After detecting either puff or puff-chandelier rupture scattering by NOGA, there was no significantly high record of embolic complications [16, 17, 35, 44]. Thus, most SRAPs are asymptomatic, silent, and have been present for several years [45]. The accumulation of asymptomatic injuries caused by silent embolism may rather be related to aging and chronic inflammation [16, 17].

In future, a multicenter prospective study of patients with SRAPs and cerebrovascular events should be performed [35]. Furthermore, the free forms of CCs and CCs in atheromatous materials have not been distinguished from each other, and as the free form of CCs without atheromatous material or fibrin is responsible for embolism, the term 'cholesterol embolization' may not be appropriate [17].

6 Future Perspectives

Using CCs from live patients instead of experimental CCs, implies that concepts in the various fields of CC embolism and CC induced inflammation may need to be updated or revised. Ziltivekimab, a human monoclonal antibody directed against the IL-6 ligand, markedly reduces the biomarkers of inflammation and thrombosis, which are important in the development of atherosclerosis [46]. Analyzing SRAPs might reveal when anti-inflammatory drugs are effective in the aorta and coronary artery. Furthermore, continuous organ dysfunction can lead to aging, and the SRAPs detected by NOGA may contribute to clarifying the mechanism of aging [17].

References

1. Spears JR, Marais HJ, Serur J, et al. In vivo coronary angioscopy. J Am Coll Cardiol. 1983;1:1311–4. https://doi.org/10.1016/s0735-1097(83)80145-4.
2. Nanto S, Ohara T, Mishima M, et al. Coronary angioscopy: a monorail angioscope with movable guide wire. Am J Card Imaging. 1991;5:1–5.
3. Komatsu S, Ohara T, Takahashi S, et al. Improving the visual field in coronary artery by with non-obstructive angioscopy: dual infusion method. Int J Cardiovasc Imaging. 2017;33:789–96. https://doi.org/10.1007/s10554-017-1079-1.

4. Ueda Y, Hirayama A, Kodama K. Plaque characterization and atherosclerosis evaluation by coronary angioscopy. Herz. 2003;28:501–4. https://doi.org/10.1007/s00059-003-2486-8.

5. Ueda Y, Ohtani T, Shimizu M, et al. Assessment of plaque vulnerability by angioscopic classification of plaque color. Am Heart J. 2004;148:333–5. https://doi.org/10.1016/j.ahj.2004.03.047.

6. Asakura M, Ueda Y, Yamaguchi O, et al. Extensive development of vulnerable plaques as a pan-coronary process in patients with myocardial infarction: an angioscopic study. J Am Coll Cardiol. 2001;37:1284–8. https://doi.org/10.1016/s0735-1097(01)01135-4.

7. Ohtani T, Ueda Y, Mizote I, et al. Number of yellow plaques detected in a coronary artery is associated with future risk of acute coronary syndrome: detection of vulnerable patients by angioscopy. J Am Coll Cardiol. 2006;47:2194–200. https://doi.org/10.1016/j.jacc.2006.01.064.

8. Ueda Y, Asakura M, Yamaguchi O, et al. The healing process of infarct-related plaques. Insights from 18 months of serial angioscopic follow-up. J Am Coll Cardiol. 2001;38:1916–22. https://doi.org/10.1016/s0735-1097(01)01673-4.

9. Hirayama A, Saito S, Ueda Y, et al. Qualitative and quantitative changes in coronary plaque associated with atorvastatin therapy. Circ J. 2009;73:718–25. https://doi.org/10.1253/circj.cj-08-0755.

10. Kodama K, Komatsu S, Ueda Y, et al. Stabilization and regression of coronary plaques treated with pitavastatin proven by angioscopy and intravascular ultrasound—the TOGETHAR trial. Circ J. 2010;74:1922–8. https://doi.org/10.1253/circj.cj-10-0038.

11. Okada K, Ueda Y, Matsuo K, et al. Frequency and healing of nonculprit coronary artery plaque disruptions in patients with acute myocardial infarction. Am J Cardiol. 2011;107:1426–9. https://doi.org/10.1016/j.amjcard.2011.01.016.

12. Ueda Y, Nanto S, Komamura K, et al. Neointimal coverage of stents in human coronary arteries observed by angioscopy. J Am Coll Cardiol. 1994;23:341–6. https://doi.org/10.1016/0735-1097(94)90417-0.

13. Ueda Y, Matsuo K, Nishimoto Y, et al. In-stent yellow plaque at 1 year after implantation is associated with future event of very late stent failure: the DESNOTE study (detect the event of very late stent failure from the drug-eluting stent not well covered by Neointima determined by Angioscopy). JACC Cardiovasc Interv. 2015;8:814–21. https://doi.org/10.1016/j.jcin.2014.12.239.

14. Komatsu S, Ohara T, Takahashi S, et al. Extraordinary subintimal bleeding after coronary stenting. JACC Cardiovasc Interv. 2016;9:e207–9. https://doi.org/10.1016/j.jcin.2016.07.043.

15. Komatsu S, Ohara T, Takahashi S, et al. Early detection of vulnerable atherosclerotic plaque for risk reduction of acute aortic rupture and thromboemboli and atheroemboli using non-obstructive angioscopy. Circ J. 2015;79:742–50. https://doi.org/10.1253/circj.CJ-15-0126.

16. Komatsu S, Yutani C, Ohara T, et al. Angioscopic evaluation of spontaneously ruptured aortic plaques. J Am Coll Cardiol. 2018;71:2893–902. https://doi.org/10.1016/j.jacc.2018.03.539.

17. Komatsu S, Takahashi S, Yutani C, et al. Spontaneous ruptured aortic plaque and injuries: insights for aging and acute aortic syndrome from non-obstructive general angioscopy. J Cardiol. 2020;75:344–51. https://doi.org/10.1016/j.jjcc.2019.12.004.

18. Komatsu S, Ohara T, Takewa M, et al. Nonobstructive angioscopy in patient with atherosclerotic renal artery stenosis. J Cardiol Cases. 2013;9:18–21. https://doi.org/10.1016/j.jccase.2013.08.014.

19. Nakanishi N, Nakamura T, Yamano T, et al. Angioscopic observation in chronic thromboembolic pulmonary hypertension before and after balloon pulmonary angioplasty. J Cardiovasc Med (Hagerstown). 2016;17 Suppl 2:e129–31. https://doi.org/10.2459/JCM.0000000000000166.

20. Komatsu S, Takahashi S, Toyama Y, et al. Angioscopy-guided selective aspiration thrombectomy for acute pulmonary thromboembolism. BMJ Case Rep. 2017;2017:bcr2017220059. https://doi.org/10.1136/bcr-2017-220059.

21. Nakanishi N, Fukai K, Tsubata H, et al. Angioscopic evaluation during balloon pulmonary angioplasty in chronic thromboembolic pulmonary hypertension. Heart Lung Circ. 2019;28:655–9. https://doi.org/10.1016/j.hlc.2018.08.008.

22. Komatsu S, Takahashi S, Ohara T, et al. Aortic valve stenosis and atheromatous ascending aorta. Intern Med. 2017;56:2685–6. https://doi.org/10.2169/internalmedicine.8486-16.

23. Kojima K, Fukamachi D, Hirayama A, et al. Clinical insights of non-obstructive general angioscopy for assessing atherosclerotic pathology of aortic valve in vivo. Int J Cardiovasc Imaging. 2021;37:1839. https://doi.org/10.1007/s10554-021-02183-6.

24. Nishi H, Higuchi Y, Takahashi T, et al. Aortic angioscopy assisted thoracic endovascular repair for chronic type B aortic dissection. J Cardiol. 2020;76:60–5. https://doi.org/10.1016/j.jjcc.2020.02.011.

25. Ikari Y, Nagaoka M, Kim JY, et al. The physics of guiding catheters for the left coronary artery in transfemoral and transradial interventions. J Invasive Cardiol. 2005;17:636–41.

26. Ikari Y, Masuda N, Matsukage T, et al. Backup force of guiding catheters for the right coronary artery in transfemoral and transradial interventions. J Invasive Cardiol. 2009;21:570–4.

27. Hiro T, Komatsu S, Fujii H, et al. Consensus standards for acquisition, measurement, and reporting of non-obstructive aortic Angioscopy studies: a report from the working Group of Japan Vascular Imaging Research Organization for standardization of non-obstructive aortic Angioscopy (version 2017). Angioscopy. 2018;4:1–11.

28. Iwa N, Yutani C, Komatsu S, et al. Novel methods for detecting human cholesterol crystals from sampled blood. Lab Med. 2021;53:255. https://doi.org/10.1093/labmed/lmab078.

29. Abela GS. Cholesterol crystals piercing the arterial plaque and intima trigger local and systemic inflammation. J Clin Lipidol. 2010;4:156–64. https://doi.org/10.1016/j.jacl.2010.03.003.

30. Duewell P, Kono H, Rayner KJ, et al. NLRP3 inflammasomes are required for atherogenesis and activated by cholesterol crystals. Nature. 2010;464:1357–61. https://doi.org/10.1038/nature08938.

31. Janoudi A, Shamoun FE, Kalavakunta JK, et al. Cholesterol crystal induced arterial inflammation and destabilization of atherosclerotic plaque. Eur Heart J. 2016;37:1959–67. https://doi.org/10.1093/eurheartj/ehv653.

32. Kronzon I, Saric M. Cholesterol embolization syndrome. Circulation. 2010;122:631–3.

33. Harloff A, Simon J, Brendecke S, et al. Complex plaques in the proximal descending aorta: an underestimated embolic source of stroke. Stroke. 2010;41:1145–50. https://doi.org/10.1161/STROKEAHA.109.577775.

34. Meissner I, Khandheria BK, Sheps SG, et al. Atherosclerosis of the aorta: risk factor, risk marker, or innocent bystander? A prospective population-based transesophageal echocardiography study. J Am Coll Cardiol. 2004;44:1018–24. https://doi.org/10.1016/j.jacc.2004.05.075.

35. Kojima K, Komatsu S, Kakuta T, et al. Aortic plaque burden predicts vascular events in patients with cardiovascular disease: the EAST-NOGA study. J Cardiol. 2022;79:144–52. https://doi.org/10.1016/j.jjcc.2021.08.028.

36. Higuchi Y, Hirayama A, Komatsu S, et al. Embolic stroke caused by aortic ruptured plaque and thrombus visualized by Angioscopy. JACC Case Rep. 2020;2:705–6. https://doi.org/10.1016/j.jaccas.2020.02.023.

37. Matsumoto N, Takahashi M, Katano T, et al. Cholesterol crystal in thrombus removed by mechanical thrombectomy should be a strong marker for Aortogenic embolic stroke. J Stroke Cerebrovasc Dis. 2020;29:105178. https://doi.org/10.1016/j.jstrokecerebrovasdis.2020.105178.

38. Yutani C, Nagano T, Komatsu S, et al. Visible-free cholesterol crystal emboli adjacent to microinfarcts in myocardial capillaries and arterioles on H&E-stained frozen sections of an autopsied patient. BMJ Case Rep. 2018;2018:bcr2018225558. https://doi.org/10.1136/bcr-2018-225558.

39. Komatsu S, Yutani C, Takahashi S, et al. Acute myocardial infarction caused by distal embolization from a proximal ruptured plaque. JACC Case Rep. 2020;2:33–4. https://doi.org/10.1016/j.jaccas.2019.11.042.

40. Abela GS, Kalavakunta JK, Janoudi A, et al. Frequency of cholesterol crystals in culprit coronary artery aspirate during acute myocardial infarction and their relation to inflammation and myocardial injury. Am J Cardiol. 2017;120:1699–707. https://doi.org/10.1016/j.amjcard.2017.07.075.

41. Narula N, Dannenberg AJ, Olin JW, et al. Pathology of peripheral artery disease in patients with critical limb ischemia. J Am Coll Cardiol. 2018;72:2152–63. https://doi.org/10.1016/j.jacc.2018.08.002.
42. Pervaiz MH, Durga S, Janoudi A, et al. PET/CTA detection of muscle inflammation relate to cholesterol crystal emboli without arterial obstruction. J Nucl Cardiol. 2018;25:433–40. https://doi.org/10.1007/s12350-017-0826-y.
43. Komatsu S, Yutani C, Takewa M, et al. Detecting free cholesterol crystals in a patient with spontaneous cholesterol embolization syndrome. JACC Case Rep. 2020;2:615–8. https://doi.org/10.1016/j.jaccas.2019.12.022.
44. Kojima K, Kimura S, Hayasaka K, et al. Aortic plaque distribution, and association between aortic plaque and atherosclerotic risk factors: an aortic Angioscopy study. J Atheroscler Thromb. 2019;26(11):997–1006. https://doi.org/10.5551/jat.48181.
45. Takahashi S, Komatsu S, Yutani C, et al. Serial observation of aortic puff-chandelier rupture for 2 years by non-obstructive general Angioscopy. Circ J. 2021;86:476. Epub ahead of print. https://doi.org/10.1253/circj.CJ-21-0767.
46. Ridker PM, Devalaraja M, Baeres FMM, et al. IL-6 inhibition with ziltivekimab in patients at high atherosclerotic risk (RESCUE): a double-blind, randomised, placebo-controlled, phase 2 trial. Lancet. 2021;10289:2060–9.

Part IV
Lipidology of Atherosclerosis

Disorders of Cholesterol Trafficking and the Formation of Cholesterol Crystals in Atherosclerotic Plaque

Sean P. Gaine, Steven R. Jones, and Peter P. Toth

1 Introduction

Atherosclerosis is a highly prevalent disease and a major cause of morbidity and mortality worldwide [1]. The role of cholesterol in the development of atherosclerosis is one of the most intensively studied issues in the history of medicine and its causal role is well established [2, 3].

The pathogenesis of atherosclerosis begins early in life with the formation of fatty streaks, decades before it manifests as clinically overt disease [4]. Inflammation associated with lipid-rich atherosclerotic plaques, and crystallization of cholesterol within their core can lead to plaque erosion, ulceration, or rupture, causing athero-thrombosis that in turn leads to tissue ischemia and infarction.

Cholesterol crystals (CCs) have been implicated in these processes because they can activate the production of pro-inflammatory mediators, increase vascular permeability, and cause direct trauma to cell membranes as well as the fibrous cap of atherosclerotic plaque [5]. The rate and extent to which CCs form is a result of a complex interplay of local physical factors involving cholesterol saturation, pH, and hydration status of the cholesterol molecule [6]. Thus, understanding how abnormal

S. P. Gaine · S. R. Jones
Ciccarone Center for the Prevention of Cardiovascular Disease, Johns Hopkins University School of Medicine, Baltimore, MD, USA

P. P. Toth (✉)
Ciccarone Center for the Prevention of Cardiovascular Disease, Johns Hopkins University School of Medicine, Baltimore, MD, USA

CGH Medical Center, Sterling, IL, USA
e-mail: Peter.toth@cghmc.com

G. S. Abela, S. M. Nidorf (eds.), *Cholesterol Crystals in Atherosclerosis and Other Related Diseases*, Contemporary Cardiology, https://doi.org/10.1007/978-3-031-41192-2_7

105

cholesterol trafficked in the arterial wall can lead to accumulation of free cholesterol and the development of CCs is important as it provides insight into how to target atherogenesis in order to prevent its clinical sequelae.

2 Genetic Factors Associated with Elevated Serum Levels of Low-Density Lipoprotein (LDL-c)

By far the most common genetic disorders that influence the risk of developing atherosclerosis relate to variants of the genes responsible for the regulation of serum levels of LDL-c. The prototypic example is autosomal dominant familial hypercholesterolemia (FH) which results in life-long elevations of LDL-c. It is estimated that 5% of patients who have had a myocardial infarction (MI) before 60 years of age have heterozygous FH, and around 50% of untreated FH heterozygotes will have an MI by age 60 [7].

FH is most commonly associated with the loss of the function variant in the low-density lipoprotein receptor (LDLR) gene that leads to reduced systemic clearance of LDL-c [8]. Other genetic abnormalities that give rise to phenotypic FH include the loss-of-function variants in the genes for apoprotein B100 (*apo-B*) [9], and the LDLR adaptor protein-1 [9, 10], as can gain of function variants in the gene for proprotein convertase subtilisin kexin 9 (PCSK9) [11]. Conversely, loss-of-function variants in the *PCSK9* gene has been associated with a 40% reduction in circulating LDL-C and significant reduction in the incidence of coronary events, even in populations with a high prevalence of non-lipid-related cardiovascular risk factors [12, 13].

Other proteins which regulate LDL-c have been identified including angiopoietin-like protein 3 (ANGPTL3), a hepatic protein which plays a key role in regulating circulating triglycerides and cholesterol levels through reversible inhibition of lipoprotein lipase and endothelial lipase. Loss-of-function variants of the *ANGPTL3* gene have been identified in many persons with familial combined hypolipidemia [14]. Similarly, lower levels of triglycerides and LDL-c have been observed with loss-of-function mutations in the angiopoietin-like 4 (ANGPTL4) gene corresponding to lower risk of atherosclerosis in these individuals [15].

3 Transcytosis of LDL-c into the Arterial Subendothelial Space

Atherosclerosis is characterized by thickening of the intimal layer of arteries over the course of decades. It is generally understood that the process begins with endothelial dysfunction and accumulation of LDL-C within the subendothelial space. The deposition of LDL-C compromises the protective endothelial monolayer [16]. Damage to the endothelium and basement membrane can elicit the production of vasoactive mediators including histamine and thrombin that can enhance endothelial permeability by acting on intercellular gap junctions [17]. Similarly, shear stresses can promote endothelial permeability especially in the areas of low shear stress to enhance plaque progression [18, 19]. When the vascular endothelium is exposed to elevated levels of LDL-c and other atherogenic lipoproteins in addition to these factors, it becomes increasingly dysfunctional. This leads to reduced endothelial production of nitric oxide and increased elaboration of adhesion molecules, including intercellular adhesion molecule-1 (ICAM-1), vascular cell adhesion molecule-1 (VCAM-1), and selectin P, among others. These adhesion molecules promote the binding, rolling, and transmigration of circulating leukocytes including neutrophils, monocytes, T helper cells, and mast cells into the subendothelial space where they establish an inflammatory nidus [20, 21]. Concentration dependent uptake is one mechanism by which LDL-c accumulates in the subendothelial space and higher plasma circulating LDL-c levels are associated with the progression of atherosclerosis [2] (Fig. 1).

Cell membrane transport proteins such as LDL-R, scavenger receptor B1 (SR-B1), caveolin, and activin receptor-like kinase 1 (ALK-1) receptors play a significant role in the process by assisting LDL-c transcytosis across the endothelium [22–24]. Under normal circumstances healthy endothelium transports many molecules including lipoproteins across the cell membrane [25]. The size of circulating lipoprotein particles determines their ability to translocate into the subendothelial space. Whereas normal sized LDL-c (25–30 nm) is readily translocated, larger lipoproteins (>70 nm) do not translocate due to the size and volume limitations of transcytotic vesicles [26]. In contrast, smaller LDL-c particles are readily translocated. This is important as small dense LDL-c and lipoprotein(a) (Lp(a)) have been associated with increased CC formation in atherosclerotic plaque and a significantly increased risk of plaque rupture as detected by optical coherence tomography during acute coronary syndrome [27].

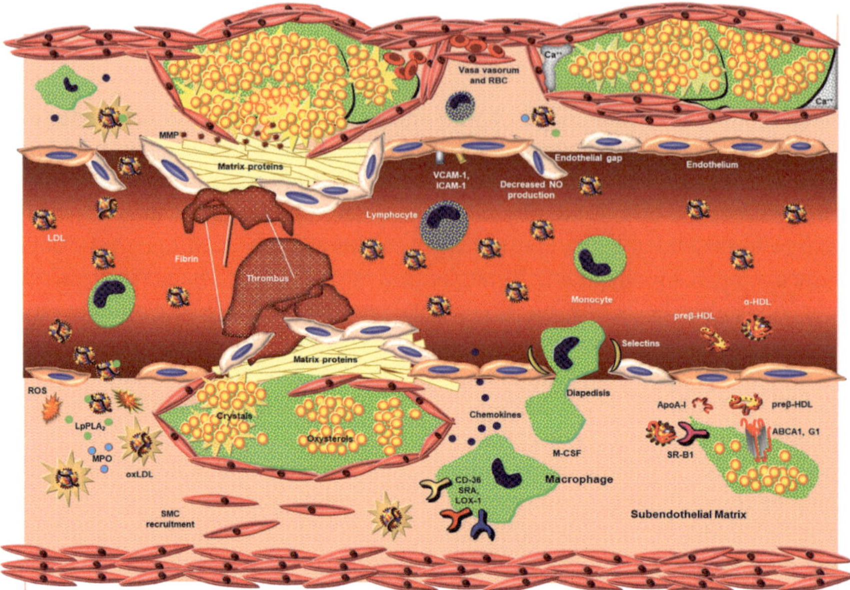

Fig. 1 This figure shows processes involved in atherogenesis and plaque rupture. Top left quadrant shows an advanced atherosclerotic plaque with intra-plaque hemorrhage from ruptured vasa vasora. The sudden increase in plaque volume and cholesterol load from erythrocyte membranes increases intra-plaque pressure and may precipitate cholesterol crystal formation. Plaque rupture ensues, exposing underlying collagen and release of factors which promote platelet aggregation and thrombus formation. Matrix metalloproteinases (MMP) can degrade the fibrous cap resulting in increased susceptibility to rupture. (Figure reproduced with permission from Dr. Thomas Dayspring.) Centre/top right quadrant shows LDL entry into the subendothelial space via dysfunctional endothelium. Fatty streak development results from the accumulation of cholesterol-rich foam cells. As lipid and cellular debris increases an atheromatous lesion is formed with a large lipid core. Macrophages are unable able to clear the lipid and cellular debris efficiently and a necrotic core develops. Lymphocytes are present, these may bind to cell surface adhesion molecules and function as antigen presenting cells (APC) which induce inflammatory mediator production. Bottom right quadrant shows a monocyte binding to adhesion molecules (ICAM-1, VCAM-1, selectin-P) expressed on dysfunctional endothelium. Chemokines promote monocyte entry through loosened gap junctions between cells. Within the subendothelial space it secretes inflammatory interleukins and cytokines. Monocytes subsequently convert to macrophages and express surface receptors such as CD36, scavenger receptor A (SRA), and lectin-like oxidized low-density lipoprotein receptor (LOX-1). These allow macrophages to scavenge oxidized low-density lipoproteins (LDL) and remnant lipoproteins. Intracellular cholesterol content progressively increases, and the macrophage becomes a lipid-laden foam cell. In order to remove cholesterol, macrophages express the transmembrane cholesterol transport proteins ATP-binding membrane cassette transport proteins (ABC) A1 and G1 which assist with the process of efferocytosis. Bottom left quadrant shows LDL particles which have become oxidized by various reactive oxygen species (ROS) including superoxide anion, peroxynitrite, and hydrogen peroxide which are produced by MPO and lipoxygenases. These oxidized LDL particles (OxLDL) are scavenged by macrophages. Lipoprotein-associated phospholipase A2 (LpPLA2) hydrolyzes phospholipids into lecithin and a free fatty acid, which promote inflammation. Macrophages may store scavenged OxLDL as pools of oxysterol or cholesterol crystals. These cholesterol crystals form sharp-rigid edges which may promote inflammasome activation, cell death or pierce through the plaque cap resulting in platelet activation and thrombosis

4 Trapping of LDL-c and Remnant Particle in the Subendothelial Space

Mucopolysaccharides, known as glycosaminoglycans (GAGs), and arterial proteoglycans composed of GAGs with a core protein, form the intercellular and extracellular matrix around cells along with collagens, elastin, and proteins such as fibronectin, laminin, and tenascin [28]. The main GAGs are heparan sulfate (HS), dermatan sulfate (DS), and chondroitin sulfate (CS) which form the GAG component of proteoglycans versican (CS-based), decorin and biglycan (DS-based), and perlecan (HS-based). The proteoglycans of the extracellular matrix are thought to play an important part in the binding and retention of LDL-C and remnant particle trapping within the subendothelial space [3, 29, 30].

Transgenic mice with proteoglycan-defective-binding LDL-c have been shown to develop significantly less atherosclerosis than their wild-type counterparts [31]. The composition of proteoglycans synthesized by local cells changes depending on a variety of factors, such as exposure to transforming growth factor-β1 (TGF-B1) and platelet derived growth factor (PDGF) which can enhance proteoglycan-LDL binding [32, 33].

5 Transport of Lipoproteins into Plaque Via the Adventitia, and Deposition of Cholesterol from Erythrocyte Membranes into the Plaque Core Following Plaque Hemorrhage

The adventitial layer may contribute to atherosclerosis through lipoprotein transport and inflammation. Advanced atherosclerotic lesions have been shown to contain dense predominantly B-cell adventitial infiltrates which may resemble lymphoid follicles [34]. The humoral response generated by these cells may contribute to further reactice oxygen species generation, inflammation, and oxidation of LDL-c [35].

Yet another mechanism by which cholesterol may become deposited into atherosclerotic lesions is through intraplaque hemorrhage. Increasing intimal thickness due to atherosclerosis may exceed the capacity of oxygen diffusion. The resultant cellular hypoxia triggers the activation of hypoxia-inducible factor-1 (HIF-1) pathway which in turn increases vascular endothelial growth factor (VEGF) production, thereby promoting angiogenesis [36]. Growing evidence suggests that neovascularization occurs early in the development of atherosclerotic plaque [37]. Neo-vascular networks are inherently fragile, leaky, and particularly vulnerable to damage that may lead to plaque hemorrhage [38]. Since the free cholesterol content of erythrocyte membranes is larger than any other cell type, it is thought that they may contribute to the plaque's lipid pool following (non-fatal) plaque hemorrhage thus forming a large the lipid pool, which is a hallmark of plaque instability [39, 40].

6 Oxidation and Scavenging of LDL-c in the Arterial Wall

As LDL-c is deposited in the subendothelial space it can become oxidized by oxygen free radicals (superoxide anion, peroxynitrite, and hydrogen peroxide) produced by smooth muscle cells, endothelial cells, or macrophages into oxidized LDL (ox-LDL). Some of the enzymes involved in these reactions include NAD:NADH oxidase, xanthine oxidase, myeloperoxidase, and a variety of lipoxygenases [41]. This results in changes to the protein, phospholipids, and lipids carried by the LDL-C particle such that it is no longer recognized by the LDL-R and there occurs a shift towards recognition by the scavenger family of receptors such as scavenger receptor-BI (SR-BI) and scavenger receptor A (SR-A) [42]. Macrophages and endothelial cells express these scavenger receptors. The SR-BI receptor also regulates the delivery of HDL cholesterol (HDL-C) to the liver and steroidogenic tissues (adrenal glands, ovaries, testis, and placenta). SR-BI is highly expressed by macrophages and can decrease atherosclerosis by reducing foam cell formation as it is one of a number of cell surface translocase proteins that mediates cholesterol removal from macrophages [43]. The SR-A receptors are thought to play a role in the formation of foam cells by ox-LDL uptake into macrophages, a key driver of atherogenesis [44], however, subsequent knockout mouse models have provided discrepant results regarding its role in the development of atherosclerosis. The SR-A receptor may also be protective against MI-induced cardiomyocyte necrosis and may exhibit different effects at various stages of atherosclerosis [45–47] (Fig. 2).

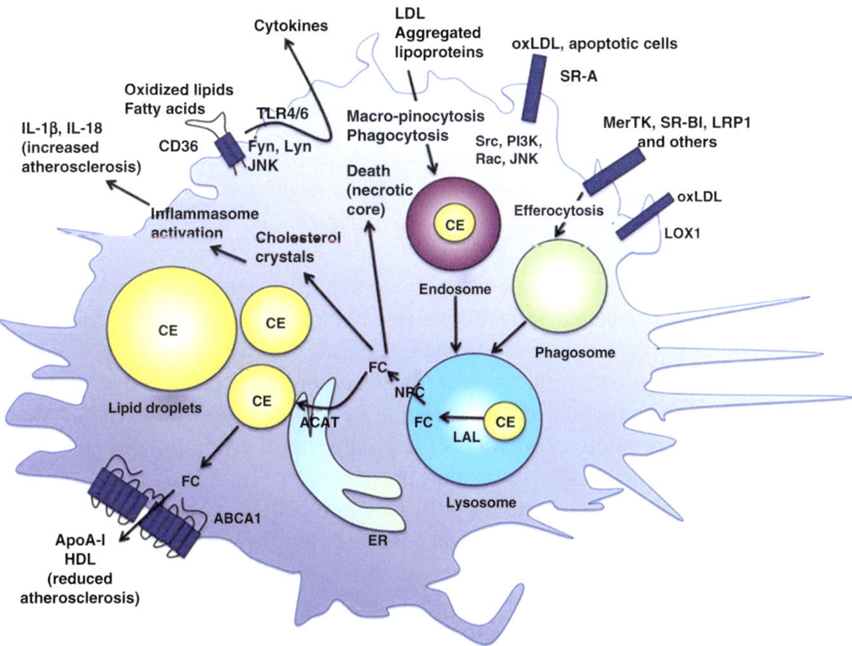

Fig. 2 This figure depicts the process of lipoprotein uptake by macrophages through micropino-cytosis, phagocytosis, and via scavenger receptors (SRs) such as SR-A, CD36, SR-BI, and LOX1. These lipoproteins are subsequently degraded in endosomes-lysosomes. CE is converted to FC by lysosomal acid lipase (LAL) and distributed to various cellular compartments via Niemann–Pick disease, type C (NPC) proteins. FC can then be converted back to CE by acyl-CoA cholesterol acyltransferase (ACAT) in the endoplasmic reticulum (ER). CE can be hydrolyzed back to FC by cholesteryl ester hydrolase (CEH) (not pictured) before it is effluxed from the cell through the cholesterol exporters ATP-binding cassette, sub-family A, member 1 (ABCA1) and ATP-binding cassette, sub-family G, member 1 (ABCG1) to apolipoprotein A-I (ApoA-I) or high-density lipo-protein. Excess FC not effluxed or converted to CE may accumulate and form cholesterol crystals or exert detrimental effects including ER stress and cell death which may promote atherogenesis and necrotic core expansion. (Reproduced with permission [47])

7   Cellular Cholesterol Efflux Via Transporters

High-density lipoprotein cholesterol (HDL-c) is a key component of reverse cholesterol transport that moves cholesterol out of cells (including foam cells in atherosclerotic plaque) and is excreted or delivered to hepatocytes where it is metabolized
to bile salts via 7α-hydroxylase. Although HDL-c levels are inversely related with
cardiovascular risk, efforts to raise HDL-c have not resulted in a reduction in cardiovascular risk [48, 49].

Excess free cellular cholesterol can be toxic to macrophages and adaptive mechanisms are present to manage intracellular free cholesterol. Free cholesterol may be
stored as cholesterol esters in cytoplasmic inclusions by acyl-CoA:cholesterol acyltransferase (ACAT). In addition, nuclear transcription factors such as liver X receptor (LXRs) may be upregulated in the setting of elevated intracellular cholesterol
levels which then promote expression of key cholesterol efflux proteins including
ATP binding membrane cassette transport proteins A1 (ABCA1) and G1 (ABCG1)
[50]. These transporters facilitate the efflux of intracellular cholesterol to nascent
discoidal HDL and spherical HDL, respectively. After cholesterol transfer to HDL
particles, a variety of receptors can mediate HDL holoparticle uptake by hepatocytes, including SR-BI, scavenger receptor CD36, and the ecto-F_1-ATPase/P2Y13R
pathway [50–53]. In the liver, free cholesterol can then be repackaged for secretion
in VLDL particles, converted to bile acids via 7-α-hydroxylase, or transported by
biliary tract ABCG5 and ABCG8 proteins into bile for fecal excretion [54].

8   Polymorphisms in Macrophage Transport Proteins and Impairment in Reverse Cholesterol

While the role of genetic polymorphisms in LDL-R and other regulators of cholesterol in atherosclerosis is well established, the contribution of polymorphisms in
macrophage transport proteins is less clear.

Tangier disease, for instance, is an autosomal codominant disorder caused by
loss-of-function mutations in the ABCA1 transport protein. Manifestations of this
disease include hepatosplenomegaly, neuropathy, cholesterol accumulation in macrophages, and extremely low levels of HDL. While these patients are at elevated risk
for atherosclerosis with around sixfold higher incidence of coronary artery over
30 years, the risk is not as profound as one might expect given that they have an
almost complete absence of HDL [55].

Heterozygotic loss-of-function mutations in ABCA1 similarly have reduced
HDL levels but the relationship with cardiovascular risk is not been consistently
demonstrated [56, 57]. Homozygous loss-of-function ABCG1 mutations by contrast are not described in humans; however, knockout models in mice have been
associated with excess cholesterol accumulation in macrophages [58]. Furthermore,

certain single nucleotide polymorphisms in the ABCG1 promoter region have indeed been associated with reduced cholesterol efflux from macrophages and increased incidence of atherosclerosis in humans [59]. SR-B1 polymorphisms have also been described which are characterized by high levels of both HDL and Lp(a); however, the implications these polymorphisms have for risk of developing athero-sclerosis are not known [60].

Sitosterolemia is an autosomal recessive disease caused by mutations in ABCG5 or ABCG8 characterized by increased intestinal absorption and decreased biliary excretion of cholesterol. These patients demonstrate substantial phenotypic hetero-geneity with some developing premature coronary disease in life while others remain asymptomatic even in the same family of symptomatic patients [61]. Heterozygous carriers of loss-of-function mutations in ABCG5 have been demon-strated to have significant increased circulating LDL levels and a twofold increase in risk of coronary artery disease [62].

9 Toxicity of Cholesterol and Oxysterols with Macrophages

Excess free cholesterol and oxysterols are known to be toxic to macrophages and are associated with macrophage apoptosis and necrosis by several mechanisms. The oxysterols 7β-hydroxycholesterol and keto-cholesterol contained within ox-LDL trigger apoptosis by inducing lysosomal destabilization and activating the caspase pathway [63]. One way by which free cholesterol causes toxicity in macrophages and other cells is through alterations in cell membrane fluidity. Excess free choles-terol can alter the physiological membrane free cholesterol to phospholipid ratio which in turn may inhibit or alter the function of one or more integral membrane proteins important for normal cellular function [64].

Other mechanisms of cell toxicity associated with cholesterol accumulation include intracellular CC formation. Although mostly observed extracellularly, cho-lesterols crystals have been visualized in foam cells from coronary atherosclerotic lesions [65]. These intracellular needle-shaped CCs may cause direct damage to cells by disrupting intracellular structure and organization (see Chapter "In Vivo Detection of Cholesterol Crystals in Atherosclerotic Plaque with Optical Coherence Tomography"). Excess cholesterol may also increase cholesterol oxidation to oxys-terols such as 7α-hydroxycholesterol, 7β-hydroxycholesterol, 7-ketocholesterol, 25-hydroxycholesterol, and 26-hydroxycholesterol, all of which are associated with cellular toxicity [66]. The oxysterols can form via both nonenzymatic and enzy-matic (e.g., CYT P450 isozymes) means [67].

Free cholesterol accumulation can also result in mitochondrial dysfunction and subsequent cytochrome-c release and caspase-9 activation leading to cellular apop-tosis [68]. In addition, cell necrosis where plasma membrane become leaky, and organelles swell result in cell death and leakage of cell contents into the extracel-lular environment that can induce a strong inflammatory response. Necrotic cell death is to be differentiated from apoptosis in which is a programmed form of cell death where cells retain intact membranes and condensed organelles and does not usually induce an inflammatory response unless the cells are not cleared by phagocytes [69].

10 Impairment of Macrophage Efferocytosis Leading to Formation of Fatty Streaks

Efferocytosis is the process by which phagocytes such as macrophages clear apoptotic cells and cellular debris efficiently and without promoting inflammation. These functions prevent cellular necrosis by clearing apoptotic cells when the cellular and organelle membranes are still intact. Preventing necrosis is important as this reduces the risk of the release of intracellular pro-inflammatory mediators into the extracellular milieu.

In addition, efferocytosis can result in the secretion of anti-inflammatory mediators such as transforming growth factor-β (TGF-β), IL-10, and prostaglandin E2 (PGE2) by efferocytes to apoptotic cells [70]. The efficiency of this process is critical, and the ability of healthy phagocytes to ingest apoptotic cells is typically very high. Thus, while apoptosis is increased in regions of plaque, the accumulation of uncleared apoptotic cells, as is seen in advanced atherosclerotic lesions, primarily reflects the dysfunction of phagocyte efferocytosis as the process is overwhelmed secondary to a rate of plaque progression that exceeds the capacity of macrophages to control [71].

Impaired efferocytosis occurs by several mechanisms. The production of reactive oxygen species within plaque has been shown to impair macrophage capacity to phagocytose apoptotic cells [72]. Furthermore, the production of cytokines such as tumor necrosis-α (TNF-a) within plaque promotes upregulation of anti-phagocytic surface ligands such as CD47 on vascular smooth muscle and the suppression of pro-efferocytic ligands such as MFG-E8 (milk fat globule epidermal growth factor 8, aka lactadherin) contribute to the defective clearance of apoptotic cells [73, 74]. Oxidized LDL present in plaque is also thought to contribute by competing with apoptotic cells for scavenger receptors and preventing recognition of pro-efferocytic ligands on apoptotic cells [75]. Reduced clearance of these apoptotic cells means that dying cells are allowed time to undergo breakdown of their cell membranes and promote inflammation and angiogenesis. The lack of anti-inflammatory mediator (TGF-B, IL-10) release from normal macrophages to apoptotic cells also contributes to this process [76] (Fig. 3).

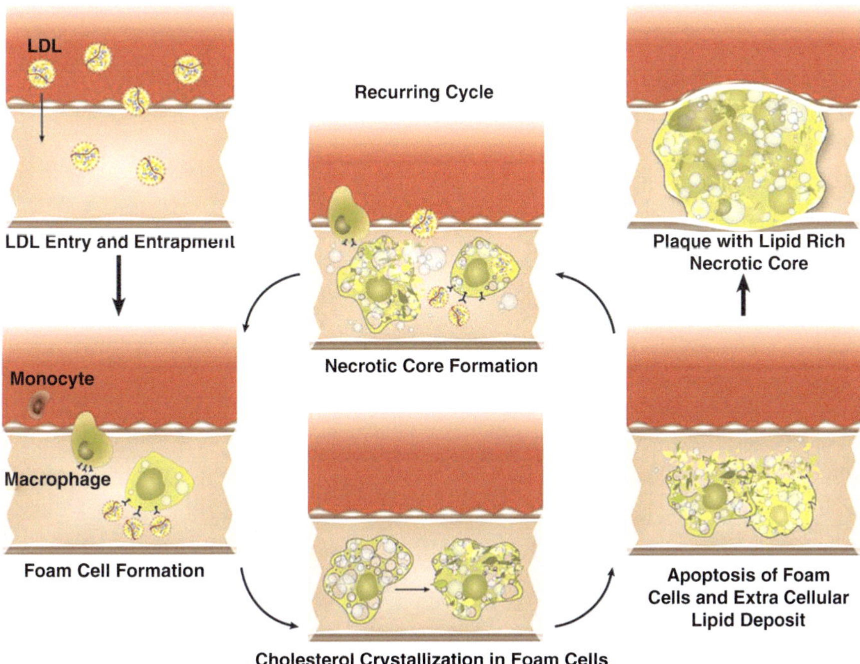

Fig. 3 Necrotic core formation within advanced atherosclerotic plaque. The first step is LDL entry through dysfunctional endothelium and entrapment within the subendothelial space. Monocytes enter and differentiate into macrophages which then become lipid-laden foam cells from uptake of surrounding lipoproteins. A cycle of inflammation and cholesterol crystal formation ensues resulting in macrophage apoptosis and accumulation of lipid and cellular debris. The cycle continues and a vulnerable plaque with a lipid-rich necrotic core is formed. (Reproduced with permission [94])

11 Expansion of the Lipid Core in Atherosclerotic Plaque Correlates with Inflammation and Architectural Instability

Culprit plaque morphology in acute coronary syndromes typically demonstrates evidence of plaque rupture or erosion with resultant atherothrombosis [77, 78]. Ruptured plaques are usually characterized by an expansive remodeling with a large necrotic core and thin, disrupted fibrous cap infiltrated by foamy macrophages. Plaque erosions, on the other hand, often show evidence of negative remodeling, and are rich in proteoglycans and smooth muscle cells with minimal inflammation [79] (Fig. 4).

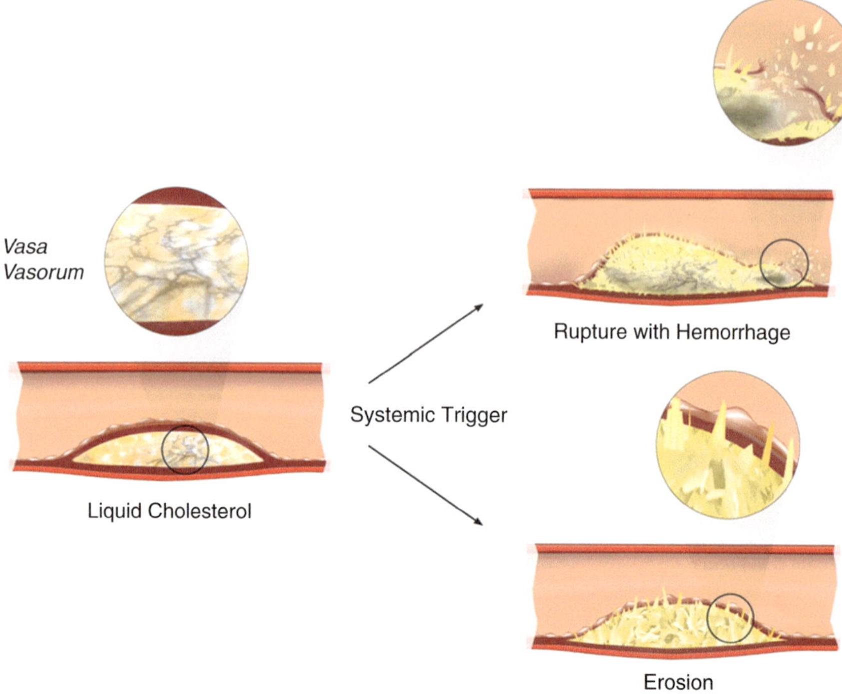

Fig. 4 Cartoon image of plaque rupture or erosion induced by cholesterol crystal formation within a lipid-rich plaque. Disruption of the vasa vasorum by cholesterol crystals and intra-plaque hemorrhage may increase intra-plaque volume and pressure. In the setting of a large necrotic core the fibrous cap may become torn and rupture, whereas a smaller necrotic core may result in erosion. (Reproduced with permission [94])

Architectural instability is an important feature of unstable plaque [80]. These plaques tend to have large lipid cores with increased density of macrophages and inflammatory mediator expression with reduced smooth muscle cells [81]. The thin fibrous cap seen in these lesions provides vulnerability to fissuring in response to stressors such as increasing cholesterol deposition and inflammatory debris deposition, coronary vasospasm or intraplaque hemorrhage. Intraplaque hemorrhage resulting in plaque expansion may be caused by perforation and leakage from at risk plaque microvessels formed by neovascularization [82]. In contrast to stable plaque, vulnerable plaque tends to show features such as rapid plaque progression and luminal obstruction ay angiography [83].

12   Cholesterol Ester Accumulation and Cholesterol Crystal Formation in Atherosclerosis

Cholesterol crystals have long been demonstrated in advanced and ruptured atherosclerotic plaque [84]. The lipid in atheromatous lesions exists mainly as cholesterol which may be free or esterified cholesterol or phospholipid. Free cholesterol can be associated with phospholipid and cholesterol esters or form condensed CCs. In the process of fatty streak development macrophages take up more cholesterol than they can excrete into the extracellular milieu. Some of this cholesterol may be organized as cholesterol ester droplets within cells which can subsequently be hydrolyzed back into free cholesterol by cholesteryl ester hydrolase (CEH) and effluxed during reverse cholesterol transport [85]. The conversion of cholesterol into cholesterol esters is a relatively rapid process and is not the rate-limiting step in the reversal of atherosclerotic plaque; rather, the hydrolysis of cholesterol esters into free cholesterol may limit its removal [86]. Intracellular cholesterol esters are maintained in a dynamic equilibrium with free cholesterol by the activities of ACAT1 and CEH. Free cholesterol released by CEH can be either re-esterified by ACAT or effluxed to extracellular cholesterol acceptors (Fig. 5).

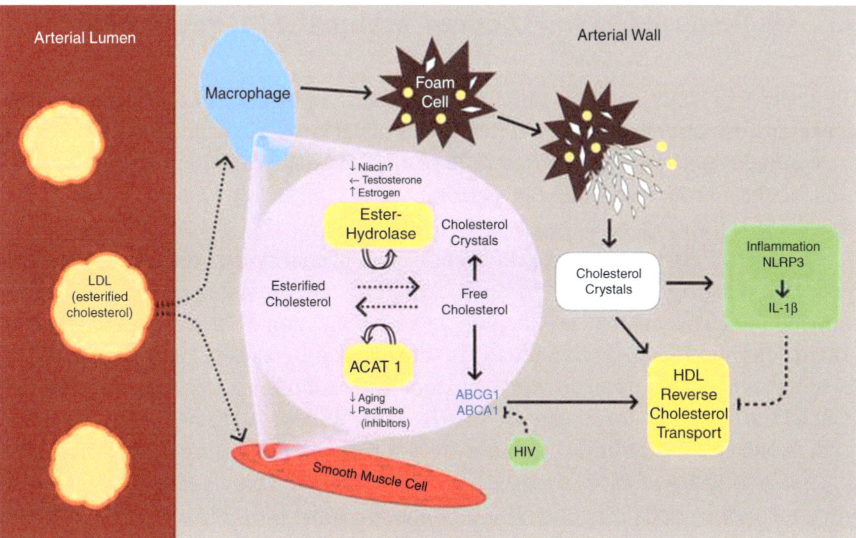

Fig. 5 Cholesterol transport within cells and extracellular space. Equilibrium between esterified and free cholesterol is noted with membrane transporters driving free cholesterol into the extracellular space where it is taken up by high-density lipoprotein. Dying foam cells overloaded with esterified cholesterol and crystals release their content into the extracellular space. Free cholesterol build-up in the extracellular space leads to crystallization. *ABCA1, ABCG1* ATP-binding cassette A-1, G-1, *ACAT 1* acyl-coenzyme A cholesterol acyltransferase 1, *HDL* high-density lipoprotein, *HIV* human immunodeficiency virus, *IL-1b* interleukin-1b, *LDL* low-density lipoprotein, *NLRP3* NLRP3 inflammasome. (Reproduced with permission [87])

Several factors trigger CC precipitation from free cholesterol in cells. Free cholesterol saturation (exceeding the solubility constant of cholesterol) is an important factor in this process. It is recognized that a large lipid pool is an important feature of ruptured plaques; moreover, it has been demonstrated ex vivo that the size of the lipid pool is a critical factor in the rate of cholesterol crystallization. Cholesterol pools can form in the necrotic core, and in the membranes of endothelium and macrophages where they may function as sources of free cholesterol that lead to CC formation [87].

In addition, disrupting normal cholesterol homeostasis by ACAT inhibition may result in accumulation of free cholesterol with resultant cell toxicity and cholesterol crystallization [64]. In the setting of heightened systemic inflammation, HDL can become dysfunctional [88, 89]. Under these circumstances, ABCA1 and ABCG1 may translocate unesterified cholesterol out of macrophages without functional HDL to serve as an acceptor. As free cholesterol accumulates and reaches its saturation point, it crystallizes [87]. In addition, CC formation may be precipitated by a drop in temperature, as well as shifts in local calcium concentration, pH, and hydration. Alteration in these physiochemical factors may explain the increased risk of plaque rupture associated with winter and acute febrile [90, 91].

13 Cholesterol Crystal Induced Traumatic Plaque Rupture

Cholesterol crystals are frequently seen in ruptured plaques. As cholesterol undergoes transformation from a liquid to a solid crystal state it expands [92, 93]. Within the confined space of an atherosclerotic plaque, crystal expansion can lead to thinning of the fibrous cap, and cap perforation, rupture or erosion by sharp tipped crystals [87, 94] (Fig. 6).

Cholesterol crystals can take different forms; primarily triclinic CCs are associated with plasma membrane and monoclinic CCs are more commonly seen in the intracellular environment (see Chapter "In Vivo Detection of Cholesterol Crystals in Atherosclerotic Plaque with Optical Coherence Tomography") [95]. Expansion of CCs in the plaque core can disrupt the plaque cap resulting in exposure of serum and platelets to tissue factor, collagen, Ca (II), von Willebrand factor, and adenosine 5′-diphosphate. In addition, inflammatory mediators including IL-6, CRP, and platelet aggregation factors such as TxA2 are released. CCs can further exacerbate inflammation by activating the NLRP3 inflammasome [96]. Platelet activation and aggregation ensues with concomitant triggering of the coagulation cascade causing thrombosis [97].

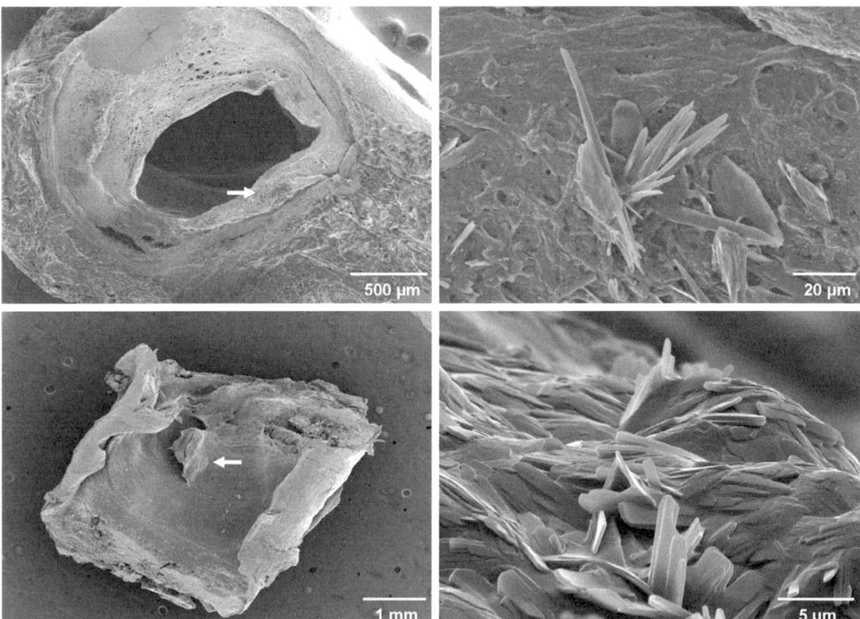

Fig. 6 Image of coronary artery at plaque rupture site. (Top left) scanning electron micrograph of diagonal coronary artery just below plaque rupture site from a 57-year-old male patient who died with acute coronary syndrome. (Top right; arrow) At higher magnification extensive crystals perforating the intimal surface are visible. (Bottom left) SEM of carotid artery plaque from a patient after endarterectomy showing plaque with a thin thrombus layer. (Bottom right; arrow) At higher magnification many cholesterol crystals are noted over the carotid intima. (Reproduced with permission [90])

14 Agents That Affect Cholesterol Crystal Formation and Morphology

The role of CCs in cell necrosis, plaque inflammation, erosion, and rupture, suggests that therapies that prevent CC formation, alter CC morphology or dissolve them should reduce the progression of atherosclerosis and plaque trauma. To date, several medications have been demonstrated to have such actions [98] (Fig. 7).

14.1 Lipid Lowering Agents

Statins, the most prescribed class of LDL-c lowering medication, have been demonstrated to prevent the formation of CCs and to dissolve them in both in vitro, and in in vivo animal models and humans [93]. While reducing LDL-c reduces the

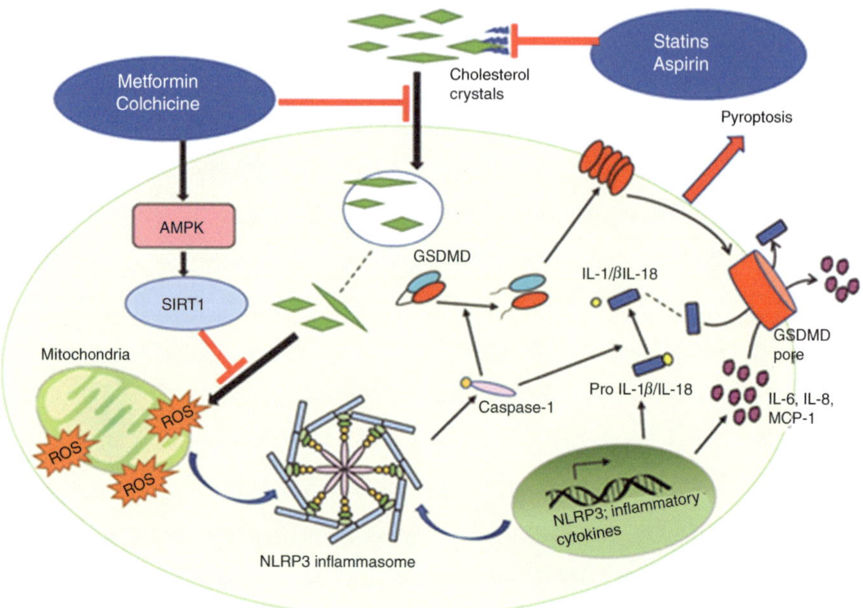

Fig. 7 Agents with known effects on cholesterol crystallization. *Metformin and colchicine* induce activation of AMPK/SIRT1 and prevent downstream expression of NLRP3 inflammasome, reactive oxygen species, and related pro-inflammatory proteins. *Metformin* also promotes cholesterol efflux from cells by enhancing ABCA1 and ABCG1 expression. *Statins, ezetimibe, aspirin metformin, and colchicine* have been shown to interact with cholesterol molecules and preventing the formation of crystals or alter their morphology. *Statins and ezetimibe* reduce the total cholesterol pool, the saturation of which is an important factor in cholesterol crystallization. (Reproduced with permission [98])

availability of free cholesterol [99, 100], statins have also been found to interfere with the CC lattice through hydrophobic interactions that alter CC morphology and thereby reduce the risk of direct CC induced plaque trauma.

14.2 Metformin

It has been shown to reduce CC formation within coronary plaques in a study performed on patients with diabetes and coronary artery disease. Also, in vitro experiments with metformin were effective in inhibiting crystal growth [101]. Metformin activates AMP-activated protein kinase (AMPK) which inhibits NLRP3 inflammasome activation and downstream inflammatory mediator production [102]. The lower prevalence of CCs in atherosclerotic plaques may relate to its ability to promote cholesterol efflux into HDL particles by enhancing expression of ABCA1 and ABCG1, thereby reducing intracellular cholesterol concentrations [102–104].

14.3   Aspirin

In vitro studies have demonstrated that aspirin can reduce cholesterol crystallization and dissolve CCs in a dose-dependent manner. This likely relates to the fact that aspirin contains alcohol and lipid domains that can interact with cholesterol to increase its solubility when incorporated in lipid membranes [105, 106]. Although the cardioprotective effects of aspirin have traditionally been attributed to its anti-platelet properties which reduces the risk of atherothrombosis following plaque erosion or rupture, the effect of aspirin on CC formation provides a mechanism by which it may reduce the risk of plaque rupture [106].

14.4   Colchicine

Traditionally used to treat and prevent gout flares caused by the precipitation of uric acid crystals within joints, colchicine has recently been shown to also reduce the risk of myocardial infarction and ischemic stroke in patients with coronary disease [107]. It is well recognized that colchicine suppresses expression of the gene for familial Mediterranean fever (MEFV gene encodes pyrin) within macrophages and impairs the production and assembly of the NLRP3 inflammasome. This in turn reduces the production of various pro-inflammatory cytokines such as IL-1β. IL-18, IL-6, and CRP [108]. Colchicine also promotes signaling via AMP-activated protein kinase and the histone/protein deacetylase sirtuin1 (AMPK/SIRT1) which plays a key role in enhancing the expression of antioxidant enzymes such as heme oxygenase 1 (HO-1) as well superoxide dismutase 1 and 2 (SOD-) and (SOD-2) within cells (see Chapters "The Cholesterol Crystal Paradigm: Overview of How Cholesterol Crystals Evolve and Induce Traumatic and Inflammatory Vascular Injury" and "Interaction Between Crystals, Inflammation, and Cancer"). Interestingly, recent studies in animal models have demonstrated that colchicine also decreases cellular uptake of CCs and alters their morphology by blunting their sharp edges akin to the changes seen with statin therapy (see Chapter "The Potential Role of Cholesterol Crystals in Preeclampsia"). Thus colchicine likely has benefits in atherosclerosis beyond its inflammatory effects [98].

15   Conclusions

Atherosclerosis is a complex disease that results from abnormal cholesterol trafficking in the arterial wall that leads to accumulation of free cholesterol within atherosclerotic plaque. As free cholesterol accumulates in intracellular and extracellular compartments, it predisposes to the formation of CCs that can cause direct cellular and tissue trauma and promote inflammation that can lead to plaque growth followed by erosion or rupture. Aside lipid lowering therapies, several other medications can alter CC morphology which may in part explain their ability to reduce cardiovascular risk.

References

1. Arnett DK, Blumenthal RS, Albert MA, et al. ACC/AHA guideline on the primary prevention of cardiovascular disease: a report of the American College of Cardiology/American Heart Association task force on clinical practice guidelines. Circulation. 2019;2019:140.
2. Boren J, Chapman MJ, Krauss RM, et al. Low-density lipoproteins cause atherosclerotic cardiovascular disease: pathophysiological, genetic, and therapeutic insights: a consensus statement from the European atherosclerosis society consensus panel. Eur Heart J. 2020;41:2313–30.
3. Borén J, Chapman MJ, Krauss RM, et al. Low-density lipoproteins cause atherosclerotic cardiovascular disease: pathophysiological, genetic, and therapeutic insights: a consensus statement from the European atherosclerosis society consensus panel. Eur Heart J. 2020;41:2313–30.
4. Joseph A, Ackerman D, Talley JD, Johnstone J, Kupersmith J. Manifestations of coronary atherosclerosis in young trauma victims—an autopsy study. J Am Coll Cardiol. 1993;22:459–67.
5. Abela GS, Aziz K, Vedre A, Pathak DR, Talbott JD, Dejong J. Effect of cholesterol crystals on plaques and intima in arteries of patients with acute coronary and cerebrovascular syndromes. Am J Cardiol. 2009;103:959–68.
6. Nidorf SM, Fiolet A, Abela GS. Viewing atherosclerosis through a crystal lens: how the evolving structure of cholesterol crystals in atherosclerotic plaque alters its stability. J Clin Lipidol. 2020;14:619–30.
7. McGowan MP, Hosseini Dehkordi SH, Moriarty PM, Duell PB. Diagnosis and treatment of heterozygous familial hypercholesterolemia. J Am Heart Assoc. 2019;8:e013225.
8. Watts GF, Gidding S, Wierzbicki AS, et al. Integrated guidance on the care of familial hypercholesterolaemia from the international FH foundation. Eur J Prev Cardiol. 2015;22:849–54.
9. Batais MA, Almigbal TH, Shaik NA, Alharbi FK, Alharbi KK, Ali KI. Screening of common genetic variants in the APOB gene related to familial hypercholesterolemia in a Saudi population: a case–control study. Medicine. 2019;98:e14247.
10. Vaverkova H, Tichy L, Karasek D, Freiberger T. A case of autosomal recessive hypercholesterolemia caused by a new variant in the LDL receptor adaptor protein 1 gene. J Clin Lipidol. 2019;13:405–10.
11. Benjannet S, Hamelin J, Chrétien M, Seidah NG. Loss- and gain-of-function PCSK9 variants: cleavage specificity, dominant negative effects, and low density lipoprotein receptor (LDLR) degradation. J Biol Chem. 2012;287:33745–55.
12. Cohen J, Pertsemlidis A, Kotowski IK, Graham R, Garcia CK, Hobbs HH. Low LDL cholesterol in individuals of African descent resulting from frequent nonsense mutations in PCSK9. Nat Genet. 2005;37:161–5.
13. Cohen JC, Boerwinkle E, Mosley TH, Hobbs HH. Sequence variations in PCSK9, low LDL, and protection against coronary heart disease. N Engl J Med. 2006;354:1264–72.
14. Gusarova V, Alexa CA, Wang Y, et al. ANGPTL3 blockade with a human monoclonal antibody reduces plasma lipids in dyslipidemic mice and monkeys. J Lipid Res. 2015;56:1308–17.
15. Folsom AR, Peacock JM, Demerath E, Boerwinkle E. Variation in ANGPTL4 and risk of coronary heart disease: the atherosclerosis risk in communities study. Metabolism. 2008;57:1591–6.

16. Cahill PA, Redmond EM. Vascular endothelium—gatekeeper of vessel health. Atherosclerosis. 2016;248:97–109.
17. Lum H, Malik AB. Mechanisms of increased endothelial permeability. Can J Physiol Pharmacol. 1996;74:787–800.
18. LaMack JA, Himburg HA, Li X-M, Friedman MH. Interaction of wall shear stress magnitude and gradient in the prediction of arterial macromolecular permeability. Ann Biomed Eng. 2005;33:457–64.
19. Hartman EMJ, De Nisco G, Gijsen FJH, et al. The definition of low wall shear stress and its effect on plaque progression estimation in human coronary arteries. Sci Rep. 2021;11:11.
20. Libby P, Ridker PM, Hansson GK. Inflammation in atherosclerosis: from pathophysiology to practice. J Am Coll Cardiol. 2009;54:2129–38.
21. Libby P, Nahrendorf M, Swirski FK. Leukocytes link local and systemic inflammation in ischemic cardiovascular disease: an expanded "cardiovascular continuum". J Am Coll Cardiol. 2016;67:1091–103.
22. Zhang X, Sessa WC, Fernández-Hernando C. Endothelial transcytosis of lipoproteins in atherosclerosis. Front Cardiovasc Med. 2018;5:130.
23. Armstrong SM, Sugiyama MG, Fung KYY, et al. A novel assay uncovers an unexpected role for SR-BI in LDL transcytosis. Cardiovasc Res. 2015;108:268–77.
24. Jang E, Robert J, Rohrer L, von Eckardstein A, Lee WL. Transendothelial transport of lipoproteins. Atherosclerosis. 2020;315:111–25.
25. Nordestgaard BG, Nielsen LB. Atherosclerosis and arterial influx of lipoproteins. Curr Opin Lipidol. 1994;5:252–7.
26. Khalil MF, Wagner WD, Goldberg IJ. Molecular interactions leading to lipoprotein retention and the initiation of atherosclerosis. Arterioscler Thromb Vasc Biol. 2004;24:2211–8.
27. Sekimoto T, Shinji K, Mori H, et al. Impact of small dense low-density lipoprotein cholesterol on cholesterol crystals in patients with acute coronary syndrome: an optical coherence tomography study. J Clin Lipidol. 2022;16:438–46.
28. Mattson JM, Turcotte R, Zhang Y. Glycosaminoglycans contribute to extracellular matrix fiber recruitment and arterial wall mechanics. Biomech Model Mechanobiol. 2017;16:213–25.
29. Wight TN, Merrilees MJ. Proteoglycans in atherosclerosis and restenosis. Circ Res. 2004;94:1158–67.
30. Borén J, Williams KJ. The central role of arterial retention of cholesterol-rich apolipoprotein-B-containing lipoproteins in the pathogenesis of atherosclerosis: a triumph of simplicity. Curr Opin Lipidol. 2016;27:473–83.
31. Skålén K, Gustafsson M, Rydberg EK, et al. Subendothelial retention of atherogenic lipoproteins in early atherosclerosis. Nature. 2002;417:750–4.
32. Schönherr E, Järveläinen HT, Sandell LJ, Wight TN. Effects of platelet-derived growth factor and transforming growth factor-beta 1 on the synthesis of a large versican-like chondroitin sulfate proteoglycan by arterial smooth muscle cells. J Biol Chem. 1991;266:17640–7.
33. Little PJ, Tannock L, Olin KL, Chait A, Wight TN. Proteoglycans synthesized by arterial smooth muscle cells in the presence of transforming growth factor-β1 exhibit increased binding to LDLs. Arterioscler Thromb Vasc Biol. 2002;22:55–60.
34. Schwartz CJ, Mitchell JRA. Cellular infiltration of the human arterial adventitia associated with atheromatous plaques. Circulation. 1962;26:73–8.
35. Srikakulapu P, McNamara CA. B cells and atherosclerosis. Am J Physiol Heart Circ Physiol. 2017;312:H1060–7.
36. Forsythe JA, Jiang BH, Iyer NV, et al. Activation of vascular endothelial growth factor gene transcription by hypoxia-inducible factor 1. Mol Cell Biol. 1996;16:4604–13.
37. Jeziorska M, Woolley DE. Neovascularization in early atherosclerotic lesions of human carotid arteries: its potential contribution to plaque development. Hum Pathol. 1999;30:919–25.
38. Parma L, Baganha F, Quax PHA, De Vries MR. Plaque angiogenesis and intraplaque hemorrhage in atherosclerosis. Eur J Pharmacol. 2017;816:107–15.

39. Kolodgie FD, Gold HK, Burke AP, et al. Intraplaque hemorrhage and progression of coronary atheroma. N Engl J Med. 2003;349:2316–25.
40. Madder RD, Husaini M, Davis AT, et al. Large lipid-rich coronary plaques detected by near-infrared spectroscopy at non-stented sites in the target artery identify patients likely to experience future major adverse cardiovascular events. Eur Heart J CV Imag. 2016;17:393–9.
41. Leopold JA, Loscalzo J. Oxidative enzymopathies and vascular disease. Arterioscler Thromb Vasc Biol. 2005;25:1332–40.
42. Yoshida H, Kisugi R. Mechanisms of LDL oxidation. Clin Chim Acta. 2010;411:1875–82.
43. Vergeer M, Korporaal SJA, Franssen R, et al. Genetic variant of the scavenger receptor BI in humans. N Engl J Med. 2011;364:136–45.
44. Goldstein JL, Ho YK, Basu SK, Brown MS. Binding site on macrophages that mediates uptake and degradation of acetylated low density lipoprotein, producing massive cholesterol deposition. Proc Natl Acad Sci. 1979;76:333–7.
45. Robbins CS, Hilgendorf I, Weber GF, et al. Local proliferation dominates lesional macrophage accumulation in atherosclerosis. Nat Med. 2013;19:1166–72.
46. Ben J, Zhu X, Zhang H, Chen Q. Class A1 scavenger receptors in cardiovascular diseases. Br J Pharmacol. 2015;172:5523–30.
47. Tabas I, Bornfeldt KE. Macrophage function and cholesterol crystal formation. Circ Res. 2016;118:653–67.
48. Navab M, Reddy ST, Van Lenten BJ, Fogelman AM. HDL and cardiovascular disease: atherogenic and atheroprotective mechanisms. Nat Rev Cardiol. 2011;8:222–32.
49. Singh K, Rohatgi A. Examining the paradox of high high-density lipoprotein and elevated cardiovascular risk. J Thorac Dis. 2018;10:109–12.
50. Kellner-Weibel G, Jerome WG, Small DM, et al. Effects of intracellular free cholesterol accumulation on macrophage viability. Arterioscler Thromb Vasc Biol. 1998;18:423–31.
51. Röhrl C, Stangl H. HDL endocytosis and resecretion. Biochim Biophys Acta. 2013;1831:1626–33.
52. Brundert M, Heeren J, Merkel M, et al. Scavenger receptor CD36 mediates uptake of high density lipoproteins in mice and by cultured cells[S]. J Lipid Res. 2011;52:745–58.
53. Goffinet M, Tardy C, Boubekeur N, et al. P2Y13 receptor regulates HDL metabolism and atherosclerosis in vivo. PloS One. 2014;9:e95807.
54. Ouimet M, Barrett TJ, Fisher EA. HDL and reverse cholesterol transport. Circ Res. 2019;124:1505–18.
55. Oram J. Tangier disease and ABCA1. Biochim Biophys Acta Mol Cell Biol Lipids. 2000;1529:321–30.
56. Strong A, Rader DJ. Clinical implications of lipid genetics for cardiovascular disease. Curr Cardiovasc Risk Rep. 2010;4:461–8.
57. Frikke-Schmidt R. Association of loss-of-function mutations in the ABCA1 gene with high-density lipoprotein cholesterol levels and risk of ischemic heart disease. JAMA. 2008;299:2524.
58. Kennedy MA, Barrera GC, Nakamura K, et al. ABCG1 has a critical role in mediating cholesterol efflux to HDL and preventing cellular lipid accumulation. Cell Metab. 2005;1:121–31.
59. Liu F, Wang W, Xu Y, et al. ABCG1 rs57137919G<A polymorphism is functionally associated with varying gene expression and apoptosis of macrophages. PloS One. 2014;9:e97044.
60. Yang X, Sethi A, Yanek LR, et al. *SCARB1* gene variants are associated with the phenotype of combined high high-density lipoprotein cholesterol and high lipoprotein (a). Circ Cardiovasc Genet. 2016;9:408–18.
61. Yoo E-G. Sitosterolemia: a review and update of pathophysiology, clinical spectrum, diagnosis, and management. Ann Pediatr Endocrinol Metab. 2016;21:7.
62. Nomura A, Emdin CA, Won HH, et al. Heterozygous ABCG5 gene deficiency and risk of coronary artery disease. Circ Genom Precis Med. 2020;13:417–23.
63. Evans TD, Sergin I, Zhang X, Razani B. Modulating oxysterol sensing to control macrophage apoptosis and atherosclerosis. Circ Res. 2016;119:1258–61.
64. Yeagle PL. Modulation of membrane function by cholesterol. Biochimie. 1991;73:1303–10.

65. Kellner-Weibel G, Yancey PG, Jerome WG, et al. Crystallization of free cholesterol in model macrophage foam cells. Arterioscler Thromb Vasc Biol. 1999;19:1891–8.
66. Clare K, Hardwick SJ, Carpenter KLH, Weeratunge N, Mitchinson MJ. Toxicity of oxysterols to human monocyte-macrophages. Atherosclerosis. 1995;118:67–75.
67. Crick PJ, Yutuc E, Abdel-Khalik J, et al. Formation and metabolism of oxysterols and cholestenoic acids found in the mouse circulation: lessons learnt from deuterium-enrichment experiments and the CYP46A1 transgenic mouse. J Steroid Biochem Mol Biol. 2019;195:105475.
68. Yao PM, Tabas I. Free cholesterol loading of macrophages is associated with widespread mitochondrial dysfunction and activation of the mitochondrial apoptosis pathway. J Biol Chem. 2001;276:42468–76.
69. Edinger AL, Thompson CB. Death by design: apoptosis, necrosis and autophagy. Curr Opin Cell Biol. 2004;16:663–9.
70. Fadok VA, Bratton DL, Konowal A, Freed PW, Westcott JY, Henson PM. Macrophages that have ingested apoptotic cells in vitro inhibit proinflammatory cytokine production through autocrine/paracrine mechanisms involving TGF-beta, PGE2, and PAF. J Clin Investig. 1998;101:890–8.
71. Thorp E, Tabas I. Mechanisms and consequences of efferocytosis in advanced atherosclerosis. J Leukoc Biol. 2009;86:1089–95.
72. Schrijvers DM, De Meyer GRY, Kockx MM, Herman AG, Martinet W. Phagocytosis of apoptotic cells by macrophages is impaired in atherosclerosis. Arterioscler Thromb Vasc Biol. 2005;25:1256–61.
73. Kojima Y, Volkmer J-P, McKenna K, et al. CD47-blocking antibodies restore phagocytosis and prevent atherosclerosis. Nature. 2016;536:86–90.
74. Komura H, Miksa M, Wu R, Goyert SM, Wang P. Milk fat globule epidermal growth factor-factor VIII is Down-regulated in sepsis via the lipopolysaccharide-CD14 pathway. J Immunol. 2009;182:581–7.
75. Schrijvers D, Demeyer G, Herman A, Martinet W. Phagocytosis in atherosclerosis: molecular mechanisms and implications for plaque progression and stability. Cardiovasc Res. 2007;73:470–80.
76. Kojima Y, Weissman IL, Leeper NJ. The role of Efferocytosis in atherosclerosis. Circulation. 2017;135:476–89.
77. Libby P. Act local, act global: inflammation and the multiplicity of "vulnerable" coronary plaques. J Am Coll Cardiol. 2005;45:1600–2.
78. Hansson GK, Libby P, Tabas I. Inflammation and plaque vulnerability. J Intern Med. 2015;278:483–93.
79. Luo X, Lv Y, Bai X, et al. Plaque erosion: a distinctive pathological mechanism of acute coronary syndrome. Front Cardiovasc Med. 2021;8:8.
80. Silvestre-Roig C, Winther MP, Weber C, Daemen MJ, Lutgens E, Soehnlein O. Atherosclerotic plaque destabilization. Circ Res. 2014;114:214–26.
81. Davies MJ, Richardson PD, Woolf N, Katz DR, Mann J. Risk of thrombosis in human atherosclerotic plaques: role of extracellular lipid, macrophage, and smooth muscle cell content. Heart. 1993;69:377–81.
82. Falk E, Nakano M, Bentzon JF, Finn AV, Virmani R. Update on acute coronary syndromes: the pathologists' view. Eur Heart J. 2013;34:719–28.
83. Ahmadi A, Leipsic J, Blankstein R, et al. Do plaques rapidly Progress prior to myocardial infarction? Circ Res. 2015;117:99–104.
84. Stewart GT. Liquid crystals of lipid in normal and atheromatous tissue. Nature. 1959;183:873–5.
85. Ghosh S, Zhao B, Bie J, Song J. Macrophage cholesteryl ester mobilization and atherosclerosis. Vascul Pharmacol. 2010;52:1–10.
86. North BE, Katz SS, Small DM. The dissolution of cholesterol monohydrate crystals in atherosclerotic plaque lipids. Atherosclerosis. 1978;30:211–7.
87. Janoudi A, Shamoun FE, Kalavakunta JK, Abela GS. Cholesterol crystal induced arterial inflammation and destabilization of atherosclerotic plaque. Eur Heart J. 2016;37:1959–67.

88. Pirillo A, Catapano AL, Norata GD. Biological consequences of dysfunctional HDL. Curr Med Chem. 2019;26:1644–64.
89. Kosmas CE, Silverio D, Sourlas A, Montan PD, Guzman E. Dysfunctional high-density lipoprotein and atherogenesis. Vessel Plus. 2019;3:2.
90. Vedre A, Pathak DR, Crimp M, Lum C, Koochesfahani M, Abela GS. Physical factors that trigger cholesterol crystallization leading to plaque rupture. Atherosclerosis. 2009;203:89–96.
91. Konikoff FM, De La Porte PL, Laufer H, Domingo N, Lafont H, Gilat T. Calcium and the anionic polypeptide fraction (APF) have opposing effects on cholesterol crystallization in model bile. J Hepatol. 1997;27:707–15.
92. Abela GS, Aziz K. Cholesterol crystals rupture biological membranes and human plaques during acute cardiovascular events—a novel insight into plaque rupture by scanning electron microscopy. Scanning. 2006;28:1–10.
93. Abela GS, Vedre A, Janoudi A, Huang R, Durga S, Tamhane U. Effect of statins on cholesterol crystallization and atherosclerotic plaque stabilization. Am J Cardiol. 2011;107:1710–7.
94. Abela GS. Cholesterol crystals piercing the arterial plaque and intima triggers local and systemic inflammation. J Clin Lipidol. 2010;4:156–64.
95. Varsano N, Beghi F, Elad N, et al. Two polymorphic cholesterol monohydrate crystal structures form in macrophage culture models of atherosclerosis. Proc Natl Acad Sci U S A. 2018;115:7662–9.
96. Duewell P, Kono H, Rayner KJ, et al. NLRP3 inflammasomes are required for atherogenesis and activated by cholesterol crystals. Nature. 2010;464:1357–61.
97. Badimon L, Padró T, Vilahur G. Atherosclerosis, platelets and thrombosis in acute ischaemic heart disease. Eur Heart J Acute Cardiovasc Care. 2012;1:60–74.
98. Yang M, Lv H, Liu Q, et al. Colchicine alleviates cholesterol crystal-induced endothelial cell Pyroptosis through activating AMPK/SIRT1 pathway. Oxid Med Cell Longev. 2020;2020:9173530.
99. Patel R, Janoudi A, Vedre A, Aziz K, Tamhane U, Rubinstein J, Abela O, Berger K, Abela GS. Plaque rupture and thrombosis is reduced by lowering cholesterol levels and crystallization with ezetimibe and is correlated with FDG-PET. Arterioscler Thromb Vasc Biol. 2011;31:2007–14.
100. Lettiero B, Inasu M, Kimbung S, Borgquist S. Insensitivity to atorvastatin is associated with increased accumulation of intracellular lipid droplets and fatty acid metabolism in breast cancer cells. Sci Rep. 2018;8:5462.
101. Boumegouas M, Grondal B, Fry L, De Feijter-Rupp H, Janoudi A, Abela GS. Metformin inhibition of volume expansion with cholesterol crystallization may contribute to reducing plaque rupture and improved cardiac outcomes. J Clin Lipidol. 2020;579(171):14.
102. Tang G, Duan F, Li W, et al. Metformin inhibited nod-like receptor protein 3 inflammasomes activation and suppressed diabetes-accelerated atherosclerosis in apoE−/− mice. Biomed Pharmacother. 2019;119:109410.
103. Kataoka Y, Nicholls SJ, Andrews J, et al. Plaque microstructures during metformin therapy in type 2 diabetic subjects with coronary artery disease: optical coherence tomography analysis. Cardiovasc Diag Therapy. 2022;12:77–87.
104. Luo F, Guo Y, Ruan G-Y, et al. Combined use of metformin and atorvastatin attenuates atherosclerosis in rabbits fed a high-cholesterol diet. Sci Rep. 2017;7:2169.
105. Alsop RJ, Barrett MA, Zheng S, Dies H, Rheinstädter MC. Acetylsalicylic acid (ASA) increases the solubility of cholesterol when incorporated in lipid membranes. Soft Matter. 2014;10:4275–86.
106. Fry L, Lee A, Khan S, Aziz K, Vedre A, Abela GS. Effect of aspirin on cholesterol crystallization: a potential mechanism for plaque stabilization. Am Heart J Plus Cardiol Res Pract. 2022;13:100083.
107. Nidorf SM, Fiolet ATL. Mosterd a, et al for the LoDoCo2 trail investigators. Colchicine in patients with chronic coronary disease. N Engl J Med. 2020;383:1838–47.
108. Nidorf SM, Eikelboom JW, Thompson PL. Targeting cholesterol crystal-induced inflammation for the secondary prevention of cardiovascular disease. J Cardiovasc Pharmacol Ther. 2014;19:45–52.

Formation of CCs in Endothelial Cells

Yvonne Baumer, Lola R. Ortiz-Whittingham, Andrew S. Baez,
Tiffany M. Powell-Wiley, and William A. Boisvert

1 Endothelial Cells and Atherogenesis

Currently, cardiovascular diseases (CVD) are the leading cause of death in the
United States (US), with an economic burden of about \$219 billion in the US each
year (www.CDC.gov) [1]. Research over the past several decades has revealed that
atherosclerosis is a major underlying cause for CVD, and the processes initiating
and accelerating atherogenesis are tightly linked to chronic inflammation and dyslipidemia [2–4]. Atherosclerosis is considered a chronic disease, develops over
decades, and often goes undetected until a major cardiovascular event occurs. It is
characterized by the build-up of lipids and immune cell-filled plaques within the
tunica intima immediately beneath the endothelial lining of the vessel wall which
was recently visualized in detail utilizing cryo-focused ion beam (FIB) scanning
electron microscopy (SEM) [5]. Atherogenesis is a complex process and is still not
fully understood, with scientists globally aiming to determine the underlying mechanisms and investigating potential treatments against atherosclerosis and CVD.

One cell type of major importance at all stages of atherogenesis—from first initiation to plaque rupture—are endothelial cells (ECs) [6–8]. The vascular endothelium is the innermost layer of blood vessels, facing the bloodstream and forming the
barrier between blood and the surrounding tissue (Fig. 1a). However, the role of
ECs is more than just barrier formation; ECs also regulate blood pressure,

Y. Baumer (✉) · L. R. Ortiz-Whittingham · A. S. Baez · T. M. Powell-Wiley
Social Determinants of Obesity and Cardiovascular Risk Laboratory, National Heart, Lung,
and Blood Institute, Bethesda, MD, USA
e-mail: yvonne.baumer@nih.gov

W. A. Boisvert
Center for Cardiovascular Research, University of Hawaii, Honolulu, HI, USA

G. S. Abela, S. M. Nidorf (eds.), *Cholesterol Crystals in Atherosclerosis and
Other Related Diseases*, Contemporary Cardiology,
https://doi.org/10.1007/978-3-031-41192-2_8

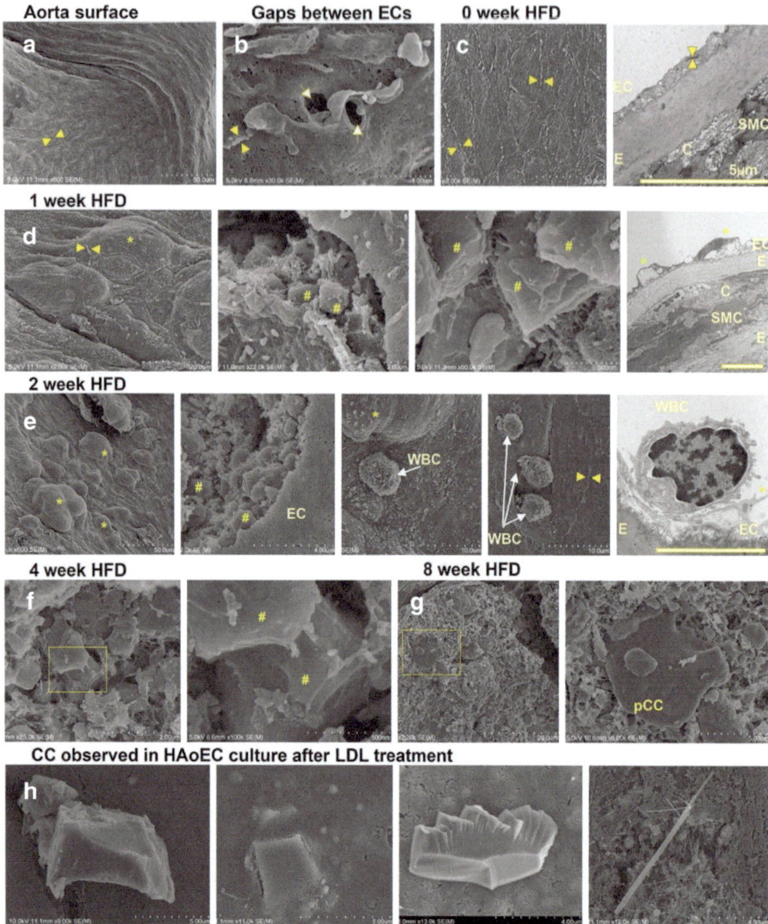

Fig. 1 The endothelium and cholesterol crystals. (**a–g**) Scanning and transmission electron microscopy images of *Ldlr*$^{-/-}$ mouse aortas on various stages of atherogenesis after being fed a high fat diet (HFD). (**a**) Image of the aorta surface displaying the continuous endothelial layer with interendothelial junction clearly visible (arrow heads). (**b**) Within 1 week of HFD gap formation (arrows) at the interendothelial junctions (arrow heads) can be seen. (**c**) At baseline the endothelium is a continuous layer (left panel) with almost not subendothelial space (right panel; space between EC and E) to be detected. The TEM on the right panel also shows intact junctions between two adjacent ECs (arrow heads). (**d**) Within 1 week of HFD aorta surface displaying subendothelial deposition (*) covered by the endothelial layer. Crack in the aorta due to preparation allow a view in the subendothelial depositions which are filled with lipids and early CC (#). In TEM (right panel) formation of the subendothelial space between the ECs and the internal elastic lamina (E) can be observed. (**e**) Within 2 weeks of HFD the subendothelial deposits are increasing in frequency and size. Additionally, an increasing amount of adherent and seemingly transmigrating white blood cells can be seen adherent to the endothelial layer often in close proximity to areas with subendothelial deposits. (**f/g**) Within the following weeks of HFD complex atherosclerotic plaques are formed with various sizes and shapes of CCs present. (**h**) Human aortic endothelial cells treated with LDL for various timepoints in vitro and examined by SEM display deposition or outlines of solid smooth objects from plate to needle shapes likely to represent CCs. (Samples utilized in this Figure were prepared as described previously by our laboratory with ethanol-based dehydration)

coagulation, angiogenesis, and inflammation. ECs are also crucially important for the controlled and well-regulated transport of nutrients, hormones, proteins, and immune cells across the vascular beds [9, 10]. Considering that the endothelium is a thin monolayer of cells collectively spanning the size of 4000–7000 m^2 and weighing approximately 1 kg within a human body, its proper function is vital for maintaining cardiovascular health [11]. Endothelial dysfunction, or the loss of adequate EC function, is a hallmark for various diseases including CVD and CVD risk factors, such as diabetes, obesity, and hypertension [8].

In the early stages of atherogenesis a dysfunctional endothelial lining facilitates pathogenic steps towards atherosclerotic plaque formation. Two of the major pathophysiological functions are described as follows: first, dysfunctional ECs display upregulated surface expression of various cellular adhesion molecules such as intercellular adhesion molecule 1 (ICAM-1), vascular cell adhesion molecule 1 (VCAM-1), or E-selectin. This allows for circulating immune cells to roll, adhere, and transmigrate through the endothelium into the subendothelial space, which can happen along inter-endothelial junctions and, in some cases, across the endothelial cell itself (transcellular migration) (Fig. 1) [12]. Second, in the very early stages of atherogenesis, the vascular endothelium allows for disturbed transport of contents from the serum—including lipoproteins such as low-density lipoproteins (LDL)—into the subendothelial space. Since the endothelial barrier does not allow for macromolecules to pass freely, transport of lipid particles involves tightly controlled transcytosis [13]. This process of LDL transcytosis was clearly demonstrated using transmission electron microscopy (TEM) in 1983 by Dr. Simionescu's laboratory whose early studies demonstrated that within minutes of treating ECs with high concentrations of LDL particles (80–200 mg/dL), the LDL can be taken up and transcytosed by the ECs to the subendothelial space [14]. The process of LDL transcytosis and its various facets, receptors, and organelles involved (e.g., caveolae) are summarized in a recent review by Zhang et al. [13] while aspects of endothelial lipid uptake, metabolism, as well as transcytosis have been extensively been summarized in a review from Dr. Goldberg's laboratory [15]. Additionally, endothelial barrier disruption during atherogenesis is also characterized by the formation of intercellular gaps (Fig. 1b) and transcellular pores [16] potentially allowing for deposition and accumulation of lipids and unesterified cholesterol [17] in an alternative secondary pathway.

In 2017, our laboratory highlighted another effect of hyperlipidemia on the endothelium in the early stages of atherogenesis. By using various microscopy techniques, we demonstrated that after only 1 week of high fat diet (HFD) feeding the so-called subendothelial space was formed and enlarged in aortas of $Ldlr^{-/-}$ mice. Within this subendothelial space, we observed the presence of lipoprotein/lipid-like structures as well as early cholesterol crystals (CCs) (Fig. 1d). The presence of such early CC deposition was corroborated by another study published in 2010 by Duewell et al. [18]. In support of our data Park et al. mention in their recent publication that CCs could also be detected in ECs during atherogenesis in SIV-infected macaques [19]. In our studies [20–23] we were able to demonstrate first CC deposits directly underneath the endothelial lining within only 1 week of HFD in

Ldlr^{-/-} mice. Within 2 weeks of HFD we were able to detect increases in size and frequency of CC/lipid filled deposits as well as the subendothelial space itself (Fig. 1e). Furthermore, after 2 weeks of HFD adherence and potential transmigration of immune cells could be observed (Fig. 1e). With increasing period of HFD feeding complexity of plaque composition as well as plaque size increased and was always accompanied by CC presence and deposition in various regions of the atherosclerotic plaque (Fig. 1f, g). This phenomenon was very recently visualized using cryo-FIB/SEM atherosclerotic lesions of HFD fed rabbits [5]. Additionally, our lab was able to demonstrate that human aortic endothelial cells (HAoECs, Fig. 1h) are capable of CC production and deposition upon LDL treatment [21] which was further exacerbated under pro-inflammatory conditions [24]. Interestingly, our lab was not able to demonstrate CC formation in human umbilical vein endothelial cells (HUVECs), suggesting that different endothelial cell types derived from various vascular beds process lipids, and in particular LDL, differently [21].

The deposition and presence of CCs has widely been recognized as an important hallmark during atherosclerosis initiation and progression [18, 20, 23, 25–28]. Since about 2010, there has been a plethora of research highlighting the importance of CCs, which, to our knowledge, was first described in atherosclerotic plaques more than 100 years ago in 1909 [29]. Most studies addressing the impact of CCs in atherogenesis focus on macrophages, with little being known about the impact of CCs on EC function. Additionally, most studies investigating CCs address the importance of CC uptake or treatment-initiated cellular behavior rather than the formation of CCs within cells. Hence, in this book chapter we will highlight the need for further research understanding the formation of CCs in various cell types, aiming to identify potential common pathways of CC formation and allowing for the development of future innovative therapies. Furthermore, we will highlight, based on past literature, potential pathways of investigation from various diseases shown to be of importance for CC formation and presence in various cells and organs.

1.1 The Impact of Acute CC Treatment on Endothelial Cells

As mentioned above, past CC research has focused on other cell types especially monocyte/macrophages and has often involved the determination of pathways activated by acute CC treatment; our team and others have highlighted pathways initiated by acute CC treatment in various cell types [22, 23]. However, there are very few publications addressing the impact of CC treatment on endothelial cells, and we would like to emphasize the importance of further understanding the impact of CCs on endothelial dysfunction in future research as a crucial step in atherogenesis. Several studies, including our own, have shown that ECs can uptake CCs [21, 30]. One of the first studies linking CC treatment with enhanced endothelial adhesion molecule expression was to our knowledge conducted in 2014 by Nymo et al. This team demonstrated that treatment of ECs with CCs induced E-selectin and ICAM-1 expression in a dose-dependent manner [31]. Jin et al. [30] demonstrated that decreased endothelial nitric oxide (NO) levels, lower eNOS activity and expression, and upregulation of endothelial adhesion molecules all associated with increased monocyte adhesion. Interestingly, these observed effects were mitigated when SIRT6 (sirtuin 6) was overexpressed involving Nrf2, a molecule previously implicated in CC-induced effects in macrophages [32]. In a follow-up study, the authors further determined that ACE2 (angiotensin-converting enzyme 2) is also heavily involved in CC-induced Sirt6-dependent endothelial barrier dysfunction [33]. Jin et al., in accordance with a previous study by Richawaram ct al. [34], also found an increase of intercellular adhesion molecules. These molecules facilitated enhanced monocyte adhesion to and transmigration through the endothelium, a process of absolute importance for the pathogenesis of atherosclerosis. In this study, CC-induced upregulation of ICAM-1 and VCAM-1 was dependent on NF|B signaling mediated by H_2O_2 production [34]. Interestingly, the authors showed that resolving D1—an agent shown to have anti-inflammatory properties—prevented CC-induced effect, which could provide a future therapeutic avenue [35, 36]. This thought, while provoking, could be plausible as resolving D1 in mice was utilized in a recent study to prevent doxorubicin-mediated cardiotoxicity involving several pathways including Nfr-2 [36], which as mentioned above was shown to be impacted by CCs in ECs. CCs have been found to disrupt the endothelial barrier by disrupting adherens junctions by phosphorylation of VE-cadherin through SHP2 signaling [37] and xanthine oxidase-mediated H_2O_2 production. Again, these effects were completely prevented when ECs were co-incubated with resolvin D1, further highlighting the potential protective effect of resolving D1 on the endothelium.

A second sirtuin (Sirt1) was implicated in the protective effects exhibited by colchicine on CC-induced damage to ECs. The authors of this study showed that colchicine decreased the amount of CC uptake by ECs, reduced intracellular ROS levels, and enhanced cell survival by inhibiting NLRP3 inflammasome activation [38]. The importance of endothelial NLRP3 inflammasome in CC-induced damage has been previously highlighted [39, 40].

In summary, relatively little is known about the impact of acute CC treatment on the endothelium and its subsequent effects on CVD development and progression, thus highlighting the importance of further research examining the pathways involved in CC-induced endothelial dysfunction and the potential of common pathways amongst various cell types (Fig. 2).

1.2 CC Formation by EC and the Potential Impact of Its Subendothelial Accumulation

CCs have been demonstrated to be generated by various cell types including endothelial cells [21, 24, 41]. Besides the impact of CCs on ECs as described above, we have postulated that EC-derived CCs are released into the subendothelial space [20, 24]. Once there, various migrating immune cells—especially monocytes—will encounter the accumulated CCs and lipoproteins and take up CCs to initiate various

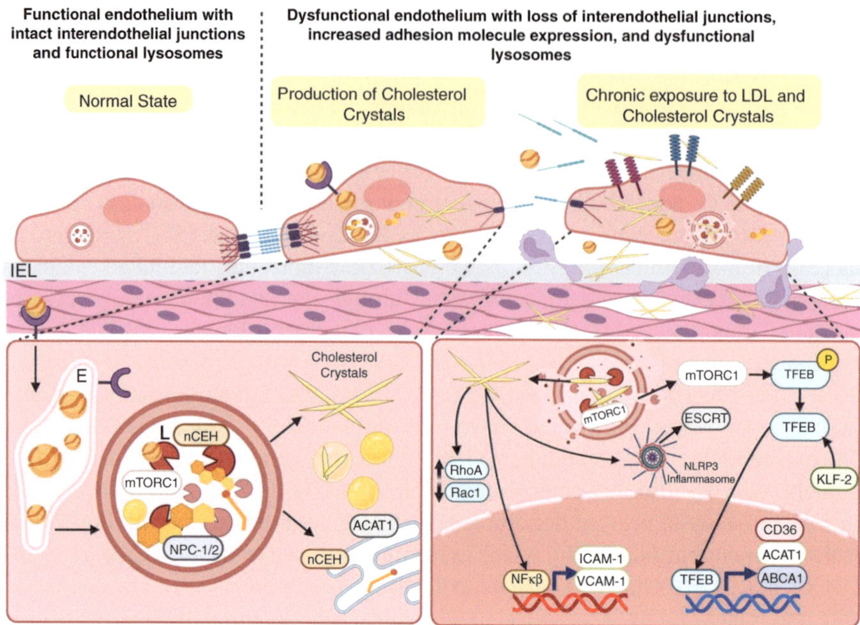

Fig. 2 Graphical summary of processes involved the formation of cholesterol crystals and the effects of its presence during atherogenesis

pro-atherosclerotic pathways, as we and others have described previously [22, 23, 27, 42–44].

We postulate an additional pathway by which CCs accumulated in the subendo-thelial space could impact endothelial function. The maintenance of endothelial barrier integrity is dependent on the mechanical microenvironment and the sur-rounding extracellular matrix stiffness [45]. To our knowledge, no study has been published connecting the presence of CCs with matrix stiffness and endothelial bar-rier dysfunction. This is of key importance, as one of the major mechanisms involved in stiffness-related endothelial dysfunction and recovery involves the reorganization of the actin cytoskeleton. For example, the presence of actin stress fibers due to thrombin treatment in cultured ECs is the highest when cultured on high stiffness substrates, as mediated by Rho/Rac signaling [45]. Interestingly, in our own study, we showed that human aortic endothelial cells cultured on CC-coated surface dis-played reduced barrier integrity (increased permeability) and decreased regenera-tive potential. These changes are accompanied by increased monocyte transmigration, increased RhoA, and decreased Rac1 activity [21]. While we were not able to con-nect substrate stiffness to the observed effect of CC-coated surface on EC dysfunc-tion, we postulate that the observed effects are at least partially due to CC-induced changes in matrix stiffness.

Other pathways which have been associated with substrate stiffness-related EC dysfunction involve autophagy, a process of potential importance in CC-induced damage to various cell types and postulated to be impaired in the presence of CCs in macrophages [46]. The importance of intact endothelial autophagy during atherogenesis, especially in ECs, has been summarized recently by Hua et al. [47]. Hu et al. published that increasing substrate stiffness in ECs reduced endothelial autophagy levels by altering a variety of genes associated with endothelial dysfunction [48]. Interestingly, in this study the impact of stiffness on vascular smooth muscle cells was the opposite when compared to the ECs, highlighting the importance of cell-specific research and the need for more endothelial-specific research as the impact of CCs might vary between different cell types. Additional pathways activated by substrate stiffness in ECs are: (1) the YAP-DII4-Notch signaling ultimately determining cellular function [49] or (2) VE-cadherin specific signaling [50] ultimately facilitating pro-atherosclerotic processes such as neutrophil transmigration [51], endothelial cytokine and chemokine secretion [52], trans-endothelial migration of lymphocytes or natural killer cells [53], or proliferation of ECs [54]. To summarize we want to highlight the importance of future research addressing the potential impact of CC accumulation in the subendothelial space on ECM stiffness and composition, and its potential impact on the endothelial function that affect atherogenesis (Fig. 2).

1.3 Cellular Lipid Metabolism and Homeostasis Possibly Linked to CC Formation

Cellular lipid metabolism and homeostasis is a tightly regulated process that is crucial for a healthy, living organism. Undoubtedly, CVD development and progression is intimately connected to both inflammation and altered lipid metabolism or lipid profile [2, 4, 55]. Several key enzymes involved in lipid uptake, efflux or homeostasis have been brought in connection with CC presence and/or formation, a few of which are highlighted below (Fig. 2).

Cholesterol is essential for the survival and function of all cells, as it is the basis for cellular as well as vesicular membranes, hormones, steroids, and bile synthesis. As cholesterol itself is insoluble in water, it is transported through the body as cholesterol esters stored in spherical lipoprotein particles, LDL in particular. LDL is taken up by cells through receptor-mediated endocytosis [56] or macropinocytosis [57–59]. Once taken up into cells, LDL is delivered to lysosomes where cholesterol esters are hydrolyzed to free cholesterol, and lysosomal transmembrane proteins transfer the free cholesterol to the endoplasmic reticulum (ER). Two important enzymes located at the ER are responsible for sensing and regulating cellular levels of free cholesterol, namely acyl coenzyme A cholesterol acyltransferases (ACATs) and neutral cholesterol ester hydrolase (nCEH).

Interestingly, alterations of intracellular lipid balance by either inhibiting nCEH activity or ACAT1 activity in human aortic endothelial cells impacted CC shape after LDL treatment [21]. In ECs, treatment with LDL in the presence of a nCEH inhibitor increased lipid droplet formation; the presence of needle shaped elongated CC was also observed. On the other hand, in the presence of an ACAT1 inhibitor, plate-shaped CCs were detected [26]. In both human as well as mouse atherosclerotic plaques, the presence of both CC shapes has been described [60]. Utilizing Coherent Anti-Stokes Raman Scattering (CARS) imaging, it has been shown that both types of CCs have similar composition [61], which could potentially indicate that the origin of the observed CCs could determine CC shape rather than chemical composition, a notion supported by a study using cryo-TEM techniques [62].

Decreasing levels of free cholesterol within cells are controlled by nCEH, which hydrolyzes cholesterol esters stored in lipid droplets to unesterified cholesterol and unesterified fatty acid molecules. In patients with fibrosing nonalcoholic steatohepatitis (NASH), presence of CCs within hepatocyte lipid droplets was observed in almost all patients as well as in HepG2 liver cells *in vitro* under hyperlipidemic conditions [63]. Similarly, livers of patients with cholesterol ester storage diseases (CESD) show the presence of CCs in lipid droplets of macrophages and foam cells [64, 65]. A very recent study performed in hyperlipidemic rabbits utilizing innovative cryo-FIB/SEM techniques indicates that thin CCs are often found in very close proximity to CCs in various regions of the atherosclerotic plaque [5], further highlighting the potential of lipid droplets to impact CC presence in advancing atherosclerotic lesions.

Certainly, the process of intracellular cholesterol homeostasis involves several other key regulators, some of which have been connected with CC formation or presence. For example, 3-hydroxy-3-methylglutaryl-coenzyme A (HMG-CoA) reductase inhibitors (statins) can reduce the presence and formation of CCs within the atherosclerotic plaque [66], potentially via alteration of cellular lipid metabolism, anti-oxidative effects, and/or altering of cell membrane composition [67]. Familial hypercholesteremia (FH) is a disorder affecting lipid metabolism and often arises due to mutations in the *LDLR* gene; individuals with FH display increased presence of CCs in their vessel walls [68]. Additionally, a recent study investigating the conversion from brown to "white-like" adipose tissue, reported that a lack of adipose triglyceride lipase (Atgl), a key enzyme in lipolysis, resulted in deposition of CCs as examined by TEM [69]. While this study lacks proof of CC presence by polarized light microscopy, it provides evidence of a potential role of Atgl and disturbed lipolysis in CC formation in adipose tissue. As the processes of lipid metabolism and cellular cholesterol homeostasis are relatively well understood, it seems clear that alteration of each of the regulators of cholesterol homeostasis discussed above have the potential to impact CC formation and subsequent CC-related pathologies (Fig. 2). It is therefore crucial to further elucidate the factors and signaling pathways impacting CC formation.

2   Cholesterol Crystals, Lysosomes, and Lysosomal Damage

The exact underlying mechanism and the location of CC formation are not fully understood. Lysosomes have been postulated to be a potential place of CC formation within cells [22]. One of the first indications suggesting lysosomes as a potential place for CC nucleation utilized TEM was published by Tangirala et al. in 1994, in which the authors observed CC in lysosomes of J477 cells loaded with cholesteryl oleate droplets [70]. Almost 20 years later, oxLDL-induced CC formation was observed in lysosomes of macrophages in a study by Sheedy et al. [71]. In regard to ECs, we were able to demonstrate that increases in lysosomal pH were linked to increased endothelial CC formation under pro-inflammatory conditions [24]. Several studies ultimately linked CC formation to inefficient lysosomal function under hyperlipidemic conditions in various cell types. We have highlighted a few potentially important pathways linking lysosomal proteins and CC formation/presence in a recent review [22], including lysosomal acid lipase (LAL, *LIPA* gene) [64, 72, 73] and Niemann-Pick C1 and C2 (NPC1/2) [74].

Second, independent of CC formation, it has been shown that cholesterol overload impacts lysosomal function in macrophages likely due to altered pH [75, 76]. Third and very importantly, *in vitro* treatment of various cell types—especially macrophages—with CCs demonstrated that uptake of CCs induce lysosomal dysfunction likely due to disruption of lysosomal membranes [77, 78], alterations of lysosomal pH and proteolytic activity. It is clear that lysosomal dysfunction is linked to the presence of CCs and subsequently atherogenesis [78, 79].

As CC formation as well as hyperlipidemia and lipid uptake have been linked to lysosomal dysfunction and lysosomal damage, it is important to highlight the cellular response mechanisms known to clear or repair damaged lysosomes. Damaged lysosomes are known to leak their contents—including protons, reactive oxygen species, cathepsins and many more—into the cytosol. There, these contents result in NLRP3 activation, an excessive inflammatory response, and ultimately cell death [80]. As a first line of action, cells likely attempt to repair damaged lysosome membranes [81] via various mechanism and signaling molecules, including ESCRT (endosomal sorting complexes required for transport) [82] and enhanced activity of sphingolipase as well as binding to lipid bisphosphonates in a Hsp70-dependent manner [83, 84]. A potential for ESCRT-dependent lysosomal repair in CC treated cells should be explored in the future, as it could provide another avenue for therapeutical intervention (Fig. 2).

If a cell is unable to repair damages, a selective subprocess of autophagy called lysophagy will be initiated [80, 81]. The driving factor of initiation of lysophagy is ubiquitination of damaged lysosomes involving, among others, galectin-regulated pathways [81, 85, 86]. To our knowledge, it has yet to be determined if formation or uptake of CC results in activation of lysophagy. From our own data, one might speculate that this is not the case, however, more detailed studies are needed to provide clear evidence that induction of autophagy with subsequent replacement of lysosomes could provide a path to prevent the detrimental impact of CCs on lysosomes and cells.

The third path a cell might initiate if lysosomal damage is detected is the activation of lysosomal biogenesis. During lysosomal damage, mTORC1 is dissociated from the lysosome. Under normal circumstances, mTOR phosphorylates transcription factor EB (TFEB) keeping it inactive. After dissociation, TFEB is dephosphorylated and translocates to the nucleus where it will lead to induction of a set of genes initiating lysosome biogenesis and autophagy [87].

2.1 A Potential Role for TFEB as a Master Regulator of Cell-Derived CC Formation

Interestingly, it has been shown for macrophages [78] and ECs [88] as well as other major cell types involved in atherogenesis [89], that induction of lysosome biogenesis due to overexpression of TFEB inhibits atherosclerosis progression [90–92]. Furthermore, TFEB has gained heightened interest in CVD-related research as it was also demonstrated to regulate lipid homeostasis beyond lysosomal function or autophagy. For example, it was shown that TFEB also regulates lipolysis and lipophagy, lipid oxidation, uptake, efflux, and degradation, all of which point to preventing excessive lipid accumulation within cells and potentially CC formation and deposition (summarized in [93]).

Interestingly, regulation of TFEB activity and action has been linked to various signaling pathways known to be dysregulated and altered during atherogenesis, highlighting its potential therapeutic importance as a target to treat CVD in the future. For example, TFEB promoter activity is controlled by Janus kinase 2 (JAK2) presence, regulating nuclear localization and expression of TFEB leading to the inhibition of lysosomal function and autophagy. JAK2 deficiency in macrophages has just recently been shown to lead to defective cholesterol efflux and subsequently worsen atherosclerosis [94]. Taken together, a potential role for TFEB in atherosclerosis could be postulated. Another important regulator of endothelial function as well as atherogenesis is Krüppel-like factor 2 (KLF-2). KLF-2 was shown to increase TFEB in endothelial cells of diabetic mice [95] and atherosclerosis (recently summarized in [96]). Furthermore, TFEB transcriptional activity has also been linked to ACAT1 by enhancement of TFEB posttranslational modification ultimately affecting TFEB localization and activity [93]. Increasing levels of cholesterol derived from LDL ultimately activates ACATs, converting free cholesterol to cholesterol esters, with subsequent storage within lipid droplets. The role of ACAT in CC formation and subsequent disease development and progression, however, has yet to be determined, with the literature containing conflicting results, especially for the ACAT1 isoform. Utilizing an atherosclerosis mouse model on high fat diet (HFD), depletion of ACAT1 induced changes in atherosclerotic plaque composition and additionally resulted in the development of skin xanthomas filled with CCs [97], a finding supported by another study demonstrating the presence of CC-filled skin xanthomas in bone marrow-specific ACAT1 knockout mice [98]. In contrast, in a study by Melton et al. myeloid depletion of ACAT1 decreased presence of CC in atherosclerotic lesion and reduced early as well as late-stage atherosclerotic plaque size [99]. A potential downfall for either of these studies might be that no techniques—such as a combination of laser reflection and fluorescence confocal microscopy or polarized light microscopy—were used that are capable of identifying small CCs in atherosclerotic plaques [18, 21].

As mentioned above, lipid droplets have been speculated to be another place of origin for CC within cells. Lipophagy is the process by which lipid droplets are degraded utilizing a specific autophagy-related process [100, 101] and has been linked to metabolic disorders [102]. Interestingly, TFEB in nonalcoholic fatty liver disease has been connected in a recent review by Yu et al. to be beneficial in regulating lipophagy and lipolysis [103]. TFEB activation or overexpression could hence have therapeutical benefit on cell-derived CC formation by its impact of diminishing lipid droplets as a potential source for intracellular CC formation.

TFEB has additionally been linked to the regulation of the expression of various lipid metabolism/homeostasis regulating receptors like ATP-binding cassette transporter A1 (ABCA1) [93]. Cholesterol efflux is an active process transporting free cholesterol out of a cell mainly via two transporters, ABCA1 and ABCG1. Various diseases have been linked to dysfunctional cholesterol efflux. Psoriasis, a chronic inflammatory skin disease, is accompanied by increased risk for CVD [104–106]. Psoriasis has been demonstrated to impair macrophage cholesterol efflux upon lipid loading and accelerate CC formation *in vitro* as well as *in vivo* [107]. Also, the ABCA1 gene is affected in Tangier disease leading to the accumulation of cholesterol esters within cells [108–110]. Needle-shaped birefringent CCs were shown to be present in foam cells of patients with Tangier disease. However, from the present literature, one can only speculate that deficiency in cholesterol efflux does indeed result in enhanced foam cell CC formation, indicating the need to further understand mechanisms and pathways involved in this process.

TFEB has also been shown to impact CD36 mRNA expression [93], a receptor on phagocytes and ECs able to function as a scavenger receptor for lipoproteins and oxidized phospholipids [111]. Interestingly, CD36 has been described to be crucial for oxLDL-derived lysosomal CC formation in macrophages [71] and endothelial CD36 has recently been demonstrated to reduce atherosclerosis [112], implying its potential importance for the vascular endothelium.

The most well-studied signaling pathway involving CCs is the activation of the NLRP3 inflammasome in various cell types, particularly macrophages [18, 25, 32]. Very recently, in the setting of severe asthma, Theofani et al. [113] demonstrated that the activation of the NLRP3 inflammasome was accompanied by impaired autophagy which could be attenuated by TFEB activation, ultimately linking the two major pathways involved in CC-induced cell damage and laying important groundwork for a potential future therapy.

In summary, TFEB has been implicated in most major processes known to be important in CC formation or for CC-induced signaling. However, its role specifically in ECs is still unknown, especially in the setting of hyperlipidemia, CC formation, or CVD development and progression. It will be of crucial importance to enhance our knowledge on TFEB signaling in CC-related processes to potentially develop new and innovative therapies.

Acknowledgments The authors would like to thank Tina M. Weatherby and Dr. Christopher K.E. Bleck, two excellent electron microscopists, for their support and help over all these years.

Funding This work was partly supported by a grant 19TPA34850150 from the American Heart Association to WAB.

Conflict of Interest None.

References

1. Tsao CW, et al. Heart disease and stroke statistics; 2022 update: a report from the American Heart Association. Circulation. 2022;145(8):e153–639.
2. Libby P, Aikawa M, Schonbeck U. Cholesterol and atherosclerosis. Biochim Biophys Acta. 2000;1529(1-3):299–309.
3. Libby P. Inflammation in atherosclerosis. Arterioscler Thromb Vasc Biol. 2012;32(9):2045–51.
4. Libby P, Hansson GK. From focal lipid storage to systemic inflammation: JACC review topic of the week. J Am Coll Cardiol. 2019;74(12):1594–607.
5. Capua-Shenkar J, et al. Examining atherosclerotic lesions in three dimensions at the nanometer scale with cryo-FIB-SEM. Proc Natl Acad Sci U S A. 2022;119(34):e2205475119.
6. Howe KL, Cybulsky M, Fish JE. The endothelium as a hub for cellular communication in Atherogenesis: is there directionality to the message? Front Cardiovasc Med. 2022;9:888390.
7. Mussbacher M, et al. More than just a monolayer: the multifaceted role of endothelial cells in the pathophysiology of atherosclerosis. Curr Atheroscler Rep. 2022;24(6):483–92.
8. Botts SR, Fish JE, Howe KL. Dysfunctional vascular endothelium as a driver of atherosclerosis: emerging insights into pathogenesis and treatment. Front Pharmacol. 2021;12:787541.
9. Kolka CM, Bergman RN. The barrier within: endothelial transport of hormones. Phys Ther. 2012;27(4):237–47.
10. Al-Soudi A, Kaaij MH, Tas SW. Endothelial cells: from innocent bystanders to active participants in immune responses. Autoimmun Rev. 2017;16(9):951–62.
11. Aird WC. 3—Endothelium. In: Kitchens CS, Kessler CM, Konkle BA, editors. Consultative hemostasis and thrombosis. 3rd ed. Philadelphia: W.B. Saunders; 2013. p. 33–41.
12. Muller WA. How endothelial cells regulate transmigration of leukocytes in the inflammatory response. Am J Pathol. 2014;184(4):886–96.
13. Zhang X, Sessa WC, Fernández-Hernando C. Endothelial transcytosis of lipoproteins in atherosclerosis. Front Cardiovasc Med. 2018;5:130.
14. Vasile E, Simionescu M, Simionescu N. Visualization of the binding, endocytosis, and transcytosis of low-density lipoprotein in the arterial endothelium in situ. J Cell Biol. 1983;96(6):1677–89.
15. Abumrad NA, et al. Endothelial cell receptors in tissue lipid uptake and metabolism. Circ Res. 2021;128(3):433–50.
16. Kluza E, et al. Diverse ultrastructural landscape of atherosclerotic endothelium. Atherosclerosis. 2021;339:35–45.
17. Kruth HS. Subendothelial accumulation of unesterified cholesterol. An early event in atherosclerotic lesion development. Atherosclerosis. 1985;57(2–3):337–41.
18. Duewell P, et al. NLRP3 inflammasomes are required for atherogenesis and activated by cholesterol crystals. Nature. 2010;464(7293):1357–61.

19. Park MH, et al. Non-linear optical imaging of atherosclerotic plaques in the context of SIV and HIV infection prominently detects crystalline cholesterol esters. PloS One. 2021;16(5):e0251599.
20. Baumer Y, et al. Ultramorphological analysis of plaque advancement and cholesterol crystal formation in Ldlr knockout mouse atherosclerosis. Atherosclerosis. 2019;287:100–11.
21. Baumer Y, et al. Hyperlipidemia-induced cholesterol crystal production by endothelial cells promotes atherogenesis. Nat Commun. 2017;8(1):1129.
22. Baumer Y, McCurdy SG, Boisvert WA. Formation and cellular impact of cholesterol crystals in health and disease. Adv Biol (Weinh). 2021;5(11):e2100638.
23. Baumer Y, et al. Cholesterol crystals and atherosclerosis. Eur Heart J. 2020;41(24): 2236–9.
24. Baumer Y, et al. Hyperlipidaemia and IFNgamma/TNFalpha synergism are associated with cholesterol crystal formation in endothelial cells partly through modulation of lysosomal pH and cholesterol homeostasis. EBioMedicine. 2020;59:102876.
25. Rajamaki K, et al. Cholesterol crystals activate the NLRP3 inflammasome in human macrophages: a novel link between cholesterol metabolism and inflammation. PloS One. 2010;5(7):e11765.
26. Abela GS. Cholesterol crystals piercing the arterial plaque and intima trigger local and systemic inflammation. J Clin Lipidol. 2010;4(3):156–64.
27. Grebe A, Latz E. Cholesterol crystals and inflammation. Curr Rheumatol Rep. 2013;15(3):313.
28. Kataoka Y, et al. Cholesterol crystals associate with coronary plaque vulnerability in vivo. J Am Coll Cardiol. 2015;65(6):630–2.
29. Aschoff A. Zur Morphologie der lipoiden Substanzen. Über Entwicklungs-, Wachstums- und Altersvorgänge an den Gefäßen. Path Anat. 1909;47:1.
30. Jin Z, et al. SIRT6 inhibits cholesterol crystal-induced vascular endothelial dysfunction via Nrf2 activation. Exp Cell Res. 2020;387(1):111744.
31. Nymo S, et al. Cholesterol crystal-induced endothelial cell activation is complement-dependent and mediated by TNF. Immunobiology. 2014;219(10):786–92.
32. Freigang S, et al. Nrf2 is essential for cholesterol crystal-induced inflammasome activation and exacerbation of atherosclerosis. Eur J Immunol. 2011;41(7):2040–51.
33. Zheng Z, et al. Protective effect of SIRT6 on cholesterol crystal-induced endothelial dysfunction via regulating ACE2 expression. Exp Cell Res. 2021;402(1):112526.
34. Pichavaram P, et al. Cholesterol crystals promote endothelial cell and monocyte interactions via H2O2-mediated PP2A inhibition, NFkappaB activation and ICAM1 and VCAM1 expression. Redox Biol. 2019;24:101180.
35. Hiram R, et al. The inflammation-resolution promoting molecule resolvin-D1 prevents atrial proarrhythmic remodelling in experimental right heart disease. Cardiovasc Res. 2021;117(7):1776–89.
36. Wang M, et al. Resolvin D1 attenuates doxorubicin-induced cardiotoxicity by inhibiting inflammation, oxidative and endoplasmic reticulum stress. Front Pharmacol. 2022;12:749899.
37. Mani AM, et al. Cholesterol crystals increase vascular permeability by inactivating SHP2 and disrupting adherens junctions. Free Radic Biol Med. 2018;123:72–84.
38. Yang M, et al. Colchicine alleviates cholesterol crystal-induced endothelial cell Pyroptosis through activating AMPK/SIRT1 pathway. Oxid Med Cell Longev. 2020;2020:9173530.
39. Zhang Y, et al. Coronary endothelial dysfunction induced by nucleotide oligomerization domain-like receptor protein with pyrin domain containing 3 inflammasome activation during hypercholesterolemia: beyond inflammation. Antioxid Redox Signal. 2015;22(13):1084–96.
40. Samstad EO, et al. Cholesterol crystals induce complement-dependent inflammasome activation and cytokine release. J Immunol. 2014;192(6):2837–45.
41. Hawi SR, et al. Raman microspectroscopy of intracellular cholesterol crystals in cultured bovine coronary artery endothelial cells. J Lipid Res. 1997;38(8):1591–7.
42. Abela GS, et al. Effect of cholesterol crystals on plaques and intima in arteries of patients with acute coronary and cerebrovascular syndromes. Am J Cardiol. 2009;103(7):959–68.

43. Geng YJ, et al. Cholesterol crystallization and macrophage apoptosis: implication for atherosclerotic plaque instability and rupture. Biochem Pharmacol. 2003;66(8):1485–92.
44. Ho-Tin-Noe B, et al. Cholesterol crystallization in human atherosclerosis is triggered in smooth muscle cells during the transition from fatty streak to fibroatheroma. J Pathol. 2017;241(5):671–82.
45. Birukova AA, et al. Endothelial barrier disruption and recovery is controlled by substrate stiffness. Microvasc Res. 2013;87:50–7.
46. Sergin I, Razani B. Self-eating in the plaque: what macrophage autophagy reveals about atherosclerosis. Trends Endocrinol Metab. 2014;25(5):225–34.
47. Hua Y, et al. The induction of endothelial autophagy and its role in the development of atherosclerosis. Front Cardiovasc Med. 2022;9:831847.
48. Hu M, et al. Substrate stiffness differentially impacts autophagy of endothelial cells and smooth muscle cells. Bioact Mater. 2021;6(5):1413–22.
49. Matsuo E, et al. Substrate stiffness modulates endothelial cell function via the YAP-Dll4-Notch1 pathway. Exp Cell Res. 2021;408(1):112835.
50. Andresen Eguiluz RC, et al. Substrate stiffness and VE-cadherin mechano-transduction coordinate to regulate endothelial monolayer integrity. Biomaterials. 2017;140:45–57.
51. Stroka KM, Aranda-Espinoza H. Endothelial cell substrate stiffness influences neutrophil transmigration via myosin light chain kinase-dependent cell contraction. Blood. 2011;118(6):1632–40.
52. Jeon H, et al. Combined effects of substrate topography and stiffness on endothelial cytokine and chemokine secretion. ACS Appl Mater Interfaces. 2015;7(8):4525–32.
53. Onken MD, et al. Endothelial monolayers and transendothelial migration depend on mechanical properties of the substrate. Cytoskeleton. 2014;71(12):695–706.
54. LaValley DJ, et al. Matrix stiffness enhances VEGFR-2 internalization, signaling, and proliferation in endothelial cells. Converg Sci Phys Oncol. 2017;3:3.
55. Aikawa M, Libby P. Lipid lowering therapy in atherosclerosis. Semin Vasc Med. 2004;4(4):357–66.
56. Goldstein JL, Anderson RG, Brown MS. Receptor-mediated endocytosis and the cellular uptake of low density lipoprotein. Ciba Found Symp. 1982;92:77–95.
57. Kruth HS. Fluid-phase pinocytosis of LDL by macrophages: a novel target to reduce macrophage cholesterol accumulation in atherosclerotic lesions. Curr Pharm Des. 2013;19(33):5865–72.
58. Anzinger JJ, et al. Native low-density lipoprotein uptake by macrophage colony-stimulating factor-differentiated human macrophages is mediated by macropinocytosis and micropinocytosis. Arterioscler Thromb Vasc Biol. 2010;30(10):2022–31.
59. Kruth HS, et al. Macropinocytosis is the endocytic pathway that mediates macrophage foam cell formation with native low density lipoprotein. J Biol Chem. 2005;280(3):2352–60.
60. Abela GS, et al. Frequency of cholesterol crystals in culprit coronary artery aspirate during acute myocardial infarction and their relation to inflammation and myocardial injury. Am J Cardiol. 2017;120(10):1699–707.
61. Lim RS, et al. Identification of cholesterol crystals in plaques of atherosclerotic mice using hyperspectral CARS imaging. J Lipid Res. 2011;52(12):2177–86.
62. Varsano N, et al. Two polymorphic cholesterol monohydrate crystal structures form in macrophage culture models of atherosclerosis. Proc Natl Acad Sci U S A. 2018;115(30):7662–9.
63. Ioannou GN, et al. Cholesterol crystallization within hepatocyte lipid droplets and its role in murine NASH. J Lipid Res. 2017;58(6):1067–79.
64. Thompson RJ, Portmann BC, Roberts EA. Genetic and metabolic liver disease. In: Burt AD, Portmann BC, Ferrell LD, editors. MacSween's pathology of the liver. Edinburgh: Churchill Livingstone; 2012. p. 157–259.
65. Di Bisceglie AM, et al. Cholesteryl ester storage disease: hepatopathology and effects of therapy with lovastatin. Hepatology. 1990;11(5):764–72.
66. Abela GS, et al. Effect of statins on cholesterol crystallization and atherosclerotic plaque stabilization. Am J Cardiol. 2011;107(12):1710–7.

67. Mason RP, Walter MF, Jacob RF. Effects of HMG-CoA reductase inhibitors on endothelial function: role of microdomains and oxidative stress. Circulation. 2004;109(21 Suppl 1):II34–41.
68. Taghizadeh E, et al. The atherogenic role of immune cells in familial hypercholesterolemia. IUBMB Life. 2020;72(4):782–9.
69. Kotzbeck P, et al. Brown adipose tissue whitening leads to brown adipocyte death and adipose tissue inflammation. J Lipid Res. 2018;59(5):784–94.
70. Tangirala RK, et al. Formation of cholesterol monohydrate crystals in macrophage-derived foam cells. J Lipid Res. 1994;35(1):93–104.
71. Sheedy FJ, et al. CD36 coordinates NLRP3 inflammasome activation by facilitating intracellular nucleation of soluble ligands into particulate ligands in sterile inflammation. Nat Immunol. 2013;14(8):812–20.
72. Fasano T, et al. Lysosomal lipase deficiency: molecular characterization of eleven patients with Wolman or cholesteryl ester storage disease. Mol Genet Metab. 2012;105(3):450–6.
73. Valayannopoulos V, et al. Lysosomal acid lipase deficiency: expanding differential diagnosis. Mol Genet Metab. 2017;120(1):62–6.
74. Afzali M, et al. Association between the rs1805081 polymorphism of Niemann-pick type C1 gene and cardiovascular disease in a sample of an Iranian population. Biomed Rep. 2017;6(1):83–8.
75. Cox BE, et al. Effects of cellular cholesterol loading on macrophage foam cell lysosome acidification. J Lipid Res. 2007;48(5):1012–21.
76. Jerome WG, et al. Lysosomal cholesterol accumulation inhibits subsequent hydrolysis of lipoprotein cholesteryl ester. Microsc Microanal. 2008;14(2):138–49.
77. Sergin I, Evans TD, Razani B. Degradation and beyond: the macrophage lysosome as a nexus for nutrient sensing and processing in atherosclerosis. Curr Opin Lipidol. 2015;26(5):394–404.
78. Emanuel R, et al. Induction of lysosomal biogenesis in atherosclerotic macrophages can rescue lipid-induced lysosomal dysfunction and downstream sequelae. Arterioscler Thromb Vasc Biol. 2014;34(9):1942–52.
79. Marques ARA, et al. Lysosome (Dys)function in atherosclerosis—a big weight on the shoulders of a small organelle. Front Cell Dev Biol. 2021;9:658995.
80. Papadopoulos C, Kravic B, Meyer H. Repair or Lysophagy: dealing with damaged lysosomes. J Mol Biol. 2020;432(1):231–9.
81. Zhu SY, et al. Lysosomal quality control of cell fate: a novel therapeutic target for human diseases. Cell Death Dis. 2020;11(9):817.
82. Skowyra ML, et al. Triggered recruitment of ESCRT machinery promotes endolysosomal repair. Science. 2018;360(6384):eaar5078.
83. Kirkegaard T, et al. Hsp70 stabilizes lysosomes and reverts Niemann-Pick disease-associated lysosomal pathology. Nature. 2010;463(7280):549–53.
84. Petersen NH, et al. Connecting Hsp70, sphingolipid metabolism and lysosomal stability. Cell Cycle. 2010;9(12):2305–9.
85. Yao RQ, et al. Organelle-specific autophagy in inflammatory diseases: a potential therapeutic target underlying the quality control of multiple organelles. Autophagy. 2021;17(2):385–401.
86. Kravic B, Behrends C, Meyer H. Regulation of lysosome integrity and lysophagy by the ubiquitin-conjugating enzyme UBE2QL1. Autophagy. 2020;16(1):179–80.
87. Bala S, Szabo G. TFEB, a master regulator of lysosome biogenesis and autophagy, is a new player in alcoholic liver disease. Digest Med Res. 2018;1:16.
88. Lu H, et al. TFEB inhibits endothelial cell inflammation and reduces atherosclerosis. Sci Signal. 2017;10(464):eaah4214.
89. Wang Y-T, et al. Activation of TFEB ameliorates dedifferentiation of arterial smooth muscle cells and neointima formation in mice with high-fat diet. Cell Death Dis. 2019;10(9):676.
90. Lu H, et al. Transcription factor EB regulates cardiovascular homeostasis. EBioMedicine. 2021;63:103207.
91. Di Malta C, Cinque L, Settembre C. Transcriptional regulation of autophagy: mechanisms and diseases. Front Cell Dev Biol. 2019;7:114.

92. Settembre C, et al. TFEB links autophagy to lysosomal biogenesis. Science. 2011;332(6036):1429–33.
93. Li M, et al. TFEB: a emerging regulator in lipid homeostasis for atherosclerosis. Front Physiol. 2021;12:639920.
94. Dotan I, et al. Macrophage Jak2 deficiency accelerates atherosclerosis through defects in cholesterol efflux. Commun Biol. 2022;5(1):132.
95. Song W, et al. Endothelial TFEB (Transcription Factor EB) restrains IKK (IkB Kinase)-p65 pathway to attenuate vascular inflammation in diabetic db/db mice. Arterioscler Thromb Vasc Biol. 2019;39(4):719–30.
96. Dabravolski SA, et al. The role of KLF2 in the regulation of atherosclerosis development and potential use of KLF2-targeted therapy. Biomedicine. 2022;10(2):254.
97. Accad M, et al. Massive xanthomatosis and altered composition of atherosclerotic lesions in hyperlipidemic mice lacking acyl CoA:cholesterol acyltransferase 1. J Clin Invest. 2000;105(6):711–9.
98. Wakabayashi T, et al. Inflammasome activation aggravates cutaneous Xanthomatosis and atherosclerosis in ACAT1 (acyl-CoA cholesterol acyltransferase 1) deficiency in bone marrow. Arterioscler Thromb Vasc Biol. 2018;38(11):2576–89.
99. Melton EM, et al. Myeloid Acat1/Soat1 KO attenuates pro-inflammatory responses in macrophages and protects against atherosclerosis in a model of advanced lesions. J Biol Chem. 2019;294(43):15836–49.
100. Kounakis K, et al. Emerging roles of Lipophagy in health and disease. Front Cell Dev Biol. 2019;7:185.
101. Schott MB, et al. Lipophagy at a glance. J Cell Sci. 2022;135(5):jcs259402.
102. Shin DW. Lipophagy: molecular mechanisms and implications in metabolic disorders. Mol Cells. 2020;43(8):686–93.
103. Yu S, et al. The regulation of TFEB in lipid homeostasis of non-alcoholic fatty liver disease: molecular mechanism and promising therapeutic targets. Life Sci. 2020;246:117418.
104. Dey AK, et al. Association between skin and aortic vascular inflammation in patients with psoriasis: a case-cohort study using positron emission tomography/computed tomography. JAMA Cardiol. 2017;2(9):1013–8.
105. Gelfand JM, Mehta NN, Langan SM. Psoriasis and cardiovascular risk: strength in numbers, part II. J Invest Dermatol. 2011;131(5):1007–10.
106. Lerman JB, et al. Coronary plaque characterization in psoriasis reveals high-risk features that improve after treatment in a prospective observational study. Circulation. 2017;136(3):263–76.
107. Baumer Y, et al. Chronic skin inflammation accelerates macrophage cholesterol crystal formation and atherosclerosis. JCI Insight. 2018;3(1):e97179.
108. Bodzioch M, et al. The gene encoding ATP-binding cassette transporter 1 is mutated in Tangier disease. Nat Genet. 1999;22(4):347–51.
109. Brooks-Wilson A, et al. Mutations in ABC1 in Tangier disease and familial high-density lipoprotein deficiency. Nat Genet. 1999;22(4):336–45.
110. Rust S, et al. Tangier disease is caused by mutations in the gene encoding ATP-binding cassette transporter 1. Nat Genet. 1999;22(4):352–5.
111. Silverstein RL, Febbraio M. CD36, a scavenger receptor involved in immunity, metabolism, angiogenesis, and behavior. Sci Signal. 2009;2(72):re3.
112. Rekhi UR, et al. Endothelial cell CD36 reduces atherosclerosis and controls systemic metabolism. Front Cardiovasc Med. 2021;8:768481.
113. Theofani E, et al. TFEB signaling attenuates NLRP3-driven inflammatory responses in severe asthma. Allergy. 2022;77(7):2131–46.

Part V

Cholesterol Crystals and Tissue Injury

Atherosclerotic Plaque Morphology and the Conundrum of the Vulnerable Plaque

Stefan Mark Nidorf, Ryan Madder, Ahmed Elshafie, and George S. Abela

1   Introduction

Any theory as to why atherosclerotic plaques become vulnerable to atherothrombosis must explain both the processes that occur within the plaque prior to erosion or rupture and provide insight as to why the incidence of atherothrombotic events is affected by circadian rhythm, the seasons, social upheaval, and moments of intense emotional stress [1, 2]. Although it is recognized that the risk of plaque rupture is higher in patients with more extensive coronary disease, there is no consensus as to why individual plaques become vulnerable to atherothrombosis at a given point in time.

This chapter summarizes factors that make patients vulnerable to cardiovascular events and provides insight into the dynamic nature of plaque vulnerability related

S. M. Nidorf (✉)
Heart and Cardiovascular Research Institute, Perkins Research Institute, Perth, WA, Australia
e-mail: smnidorf@gmail.com

R. Madder
Interventional Cardiology, Corewell Health and Michigan State University,
Grand Rapids, MI, USA
e-mail: ryan.madder@corewellhealth.org

A. Elshafie
Division of Cardiovascular Medicine, Department of Medicine, College of Human Medicine,
East Lansing and Sparrow Hospital, Michigan State University, Lansing, MI, USA
e-mail: elshafie@msu.edu

G. S. Abela
Department of Medicine, Division of Cardiovascular Medicine, Michigan State University,
East Lansing, MI, USA
e-mail: abela@msu.edu

G. S. Abela, S. M. Nidorf (eds.), *Cholesterol Crystals in Atherosclerosis and Other Related Diseases*, Contemporary Cardiology,
https://doi.org/10.1007/978-3-031-41192-2_9

to changes in the physiochemistry of the lipid core that can lead to intermittent development of cholesterol crystals (CCs) that make plaques vulnerable to erosion and rupture that leads to atherothrombosis.

2   Historical Understanding of the Nature of Atherosclerosis

Atherosclerosis is a chronic disease that begins in early life and presents decades later most often as a sudden catastrophic atherothrombotic event [3]. Although considered a disease of modern times, yet it has been found in 3000-year-old Egyptian mummies suggests it is largely driven by genetic factors [4].

Over 600 years ago, during the Renaissance, Leonardo da Vinci (1452–1519) illustrated luminal narrowing of atherosclerotic vessels, and Antonio Scarpa (1752–1832) commented that "ulceration and rupture are likewise common in the arteries" [5]. It took another 500 years before the term "Atherosclerosis" was coined by Jean-Fredrick Lobstein to describe the disease and popularized by Felix Marchand in 1904 [5, 6]. In the nineteenth century Virchow opined that inflammation played a primary role in the development of atherosclerosis while Rokitansky postulated that thrombi on the arterial wall were the nidus for plaque [7–9]. In 1913, Anitschkow and Chalatov induced atherosclerosis in rabbits by feeding them pure cholesterol, providing the first evidence that atherosclerosis was a cholesterol-induced disease [10]. Thus, for over a century it has been evident that atherosclerosis is a "cholesterol-induced" inflammatory disease. Despite this, skepticism about the primary role of cholesterol in atherosclerosis persisted for decades because it was not possible to invariably induce the disease with cholesterol rich diets in other animals most especially canines [11, 12].

Over the last 50 years, increasing research based upon epidemiology, specialized imaging techniques as well as the improved understanding of immunology has led to a vastly more sophisticated understanding of atherosclerosis. This has also led to the development of two broad concepts, the first related to identifying patients vulnerable to cardiovascular events and the second related to identifying the reasons why individual atherosclerotic plaques become vulnerable to injury and atherothrombosis [13–16].

3   The Vulnerable Patient

Clinicians have always been concerned about how to accurately identify patients at high risk of cardiovascular events because it leads to appropriate use of diagnostic resources and treatments [16]. Aside identification of atherosclerosis by coronary imaging with CT scanning and angiography, several systemic factors have been associated with an increased risk of cardiovascular events.

3.1 Serum Cholesterol, Hypertension, Smoking, Diabetes

The Framingham Study was the first to confirm that serum cholesterol, together with blood pressure, smoking, sex, and diabetes as well as age and family history were independent risk factors for cardiovascular events [17]. Even though the mechanistic link between these factors and atherothrombosis was not known, this work paved the way for the development of highly effective strategies to reduce cardiovascular risk.

3.2 Circadian and Seasonal Factors

Although the seemingly random occurrence of acute cardiovascular events remains puzzling, population studies demonstrated that the risk of atherothrombosis changes with circadian and seasonal rhythms, with the risk of an event peaking in the early morning hours especially in winter months [1, 18]. This has led to speculation that the risk of atherothrombosis relates to circadian and seasonal changes in blood pressure, LDLc, and circulating levels and function of leukocytes and platelets.

3.3 Emotional and Physical Stress

The risk of cardiovascular events has been shown to increase following acute social upheaval, natural disasters, and even the final game of seasonal sports, as well as strenuous exercise, anger, and sexual activity [19–21]. Each of these scenarios was believed to cause a sudden rise in blood pressure sufficient to disrupt plaques. However, this explanation seems insufficient as studies using finite element analysis have failed to demonstrate that atherosclerotic plaques rupture when exposed to pressures that are physiologically attainable [22].

3.4 Systemic Inflammation

In the past few decades serum markers of inflammation including high-sensitivity C-reactive protein, serum amyloid A, elevated white blood cell count, and fibrinogen have been found to add to the assessment of cardiovascular risk over and above traditional risk factors even in patients with proven coronary disease [23]. This has strengthened the belief that systemic inflammation related to infection or chronic inflammatory disease may play a role in the development of plaque instability [24, 25].

4 The "Vulnerable Plaque"

While it is now relatively easy to identify patients with coronary atherosclerosis most at risk of a cardiovascular event by simple clinical and laboratory means, identifying individual plaques at risk of atherothrombosis remains a major challenge, in part because plaques become unstable for seemingly disparate reasons [13] (Fig. 1).

Autopsy studies in patients who died after myocardial infarction have long revealed that plaque rupture is the most common cause of atherothrombosis and is often associated with plaques with a thin fibrous cap, a large lipid pool and inflammatory infiltration in its shoulder regions that were thought to have made them "vulnerable" to rupture. However, subsequent longitudinal studies using intravascular imaging that made it possible to identify some of these characteristics in coronary artery lesions in vivo, found that these morphologic features were poorly predictive of future cardiovascular events [14–16]. Thus, it has become clear that plaque morphology at a point in time does not provide insight into the evolving processes within the plaque prior to rupture that ultimately determined its fate. Although innovations in imaging have allowed serial non-invasive assessment of

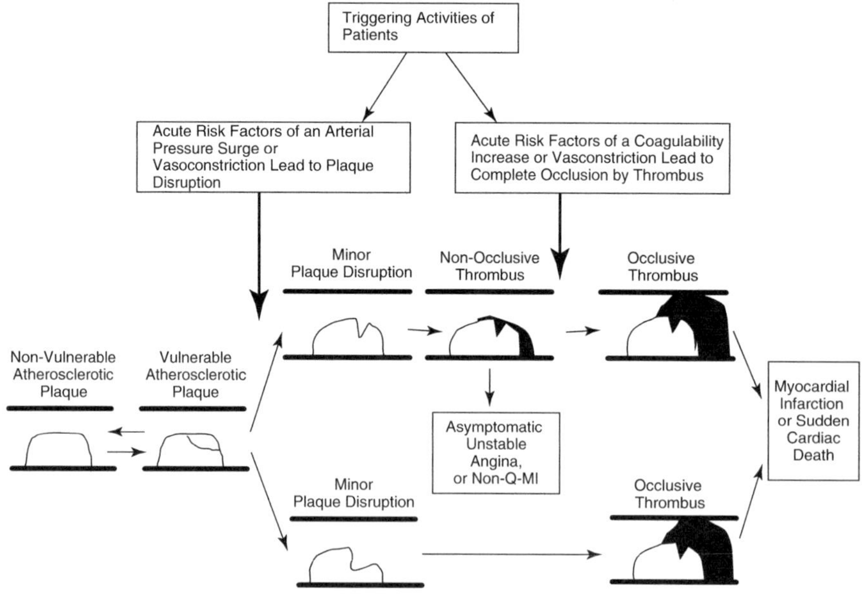

Fig. 1 Illustration of a hypothetical method by which daily activities may trigger coronary thrombosis. Three triggering mechanisms are presented: (1) physical or mental stress producing hemodynamic changes leading to plaque rupture, (2) activities causing an increase in coagulability, and (3) stimuli leading to vasoconstriction. The scheme depicting the role of coronary thrombosis in unstable angina, myocardial infarction, and sudden cardiac death has been well described by numerous investigators. The novel portion of this figure is the additional of triggers. (Reproduced with permission [13])

other features of coronary plaques including the presence of CCs and inflammation that identify vulnerable patients, all have had difficulty in identifying specific vulnerable plaques with high specificity.

5   Plaque Injuries That Lead to Atherothrombosis

5.1   *Plaque Rupture*

By definition rupture of the plaque cap exposes the highly thrombogenic contents of its core including necrotic gruel and CCs to tissue factor that attracts platelets which then aggregate to form a platelet rich thrombus followed by a fibrin rich thrombus that may occlude the artery [1, 13–15, 25–28] (Fig. 2). Although it is believed that thin cap fibroatheroma (<65 μm) are the precursor lesions of ruptured plaques [15,

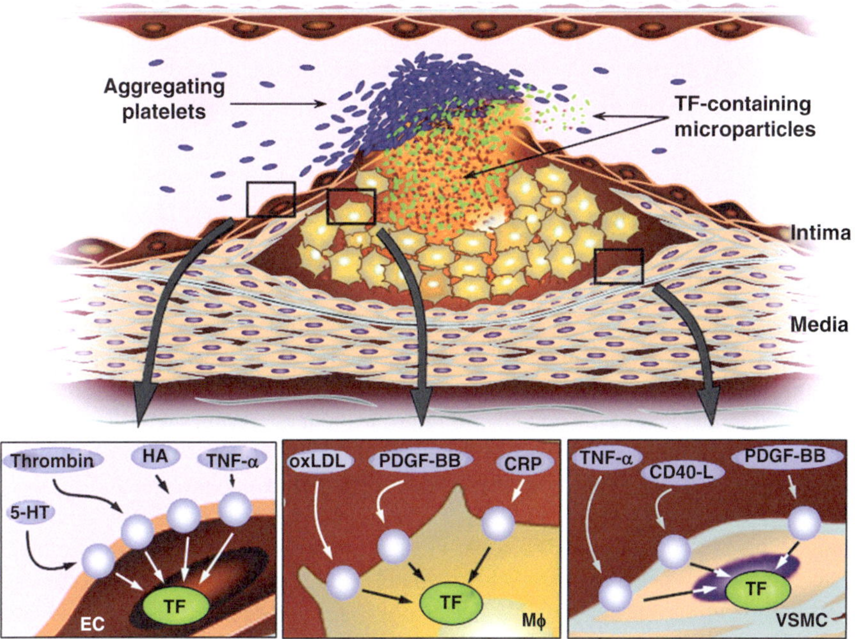

Fig. 2 Tissue factor in the atherosclerotic plaque. In the inflammatory environment of atherosclerotic plaques, tissue factor (TF) is present at high levels in endothelial cells, vascular smooth muscle cells, macrophages/foam cells, and in the necrotic core. TF induction is exemplified by selected mediators in endothelial cells (EC, left panel), macrophages (Mç, middle panel), and vascular smooth muscle cells (VSMC, right panel). On plaque rupture, highly procoagulant material including TF-containing microparticles is released into the blood, leading to rapid initiation of coagulation, platelet aggregation, and, ultimately, thrombus formation with vessel occlusion. (Reproduced with permission [28])

29, 30] it is now understood that atherothrombosis may also occur in plaques with thick caps that undergo erosion [15, 16]. Furthermore, while a relatively large necrotic core is a common feature of ruptured plaques at post-mortem pathology, the detection of lipid cores in vivo has proved to be a poor predictor of future cardiovascular events [31–36].

The cause of plaque rupture remained elusive until imaging with scanning electron microscopy in specimens untreated with ethanol revealed that CCs actually pierced the cap of ruptured plaques, thus providing a mechanical means for plaque rupture [37, 38]. While this did not explain how or why CCs developed, it was confirmed that CCs were more likely to develop in lipid rich plaques and the process of crystallization was driven by the size of the cholesterol pool, ambient temperature, high pH, and hydration of the cholesterol molecule [39]. Furthermore, CCs were found to be capable of triggering inflammation, and thus had the potential to enhance the risk of inflammatory injury that could lead to plaque rupture [40–42].

These late observations fit with more recent studies using intracoronary near-infrared spectroscopy to assess the lipid content of the plaques core in vivo which have confirmed that culprit plaques are typically rich in cholesterol compared to non-culprit plaques, and that non-culprit non-obstructive plaques with a high lipid content are also at higher risk of triggering future events over subsequent years [34] (Fig. 3). Thus, the size of the lipid core may be an important factor that determines the risk of developing CCs which in turn may determine their fate [35, 36].

5.2 Plaque Erosion

In up to one third of patients presenting with an acute coronary syndrome the underlying plaque injury relates to erosion rather than rupture of the plaque cap [43–45] (Fig. 4). The occurrence of plaque erosion has been well documented at autopsy and can now be detected in vivo with optical coherence tomography (OCT). Erosion it is typified by the loss of the endothelial lining without overt rupture of the cap overlying non-obstructive plaques with relatively small lipid cores and more fibrous caps that are rich in smooth muscle cells and extracellular matrix including hyaluronic acid and proteoglycan [43–45]. These plaques are also less likely to be infiltrated with macrophages and T cells. Furthermore, the composition of thrombus associated with erosion appears richer in platelets compared to the thrombus associated with plaque rupture, possibly because it is free of debris from the lipid core [46, 47].

Although the exact pathophysiology of plaque erosion is uncertain, electron microscopic studies have revealed that in some instances CCs can pierce the plaque cap without causing overt rupture [48, 49]. This may be important, as CCs have the ability to attract and activate neutrophils and cause the expression NETs that may lead to erosion of the plaques surface [50]. In addition, in vitro studies have

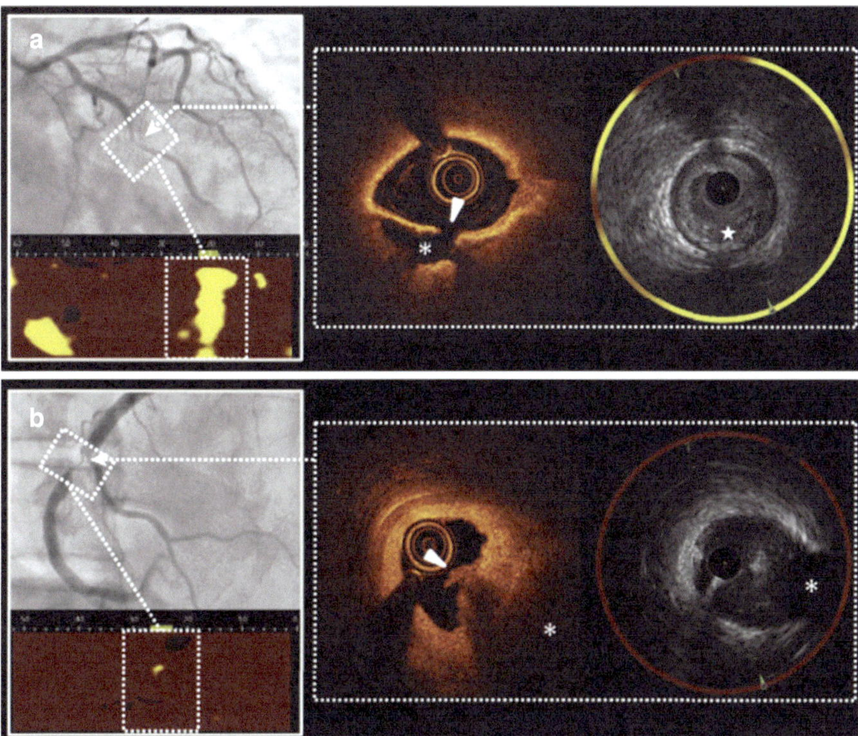

Fig. 3 (**a**) A STEMI case with a culprit lesion in the mid-left circumflex artery. OCT demonstrates PR characterized by a fibrous-cap disruption (arrowhead) and a cavity (asterisk) formation inside the plaque. IVUS reveals a cavity (star) inside the plaque. NIRS identifies a large lipid content (maxLCBI4mm 1/4 881) in the culprit lesion. (**b**) An STEMI case with a culprit lesion in the mid-right coronary artery. OCT demonstrates PE characterized by the presence of attached thrombus (arrowhead) overlying an intact fibrotic plaque. IVUS reveals the absence of plaque cavity. NIRS identifies a small lipid content (maxLCBI4mm 1/4 93) in the culprit lesion. Asterisks indicate signal attenuation behind the plaque. (Reproduced with permission [34])

demonstrated that accumulation of hyaluronic acid at the border of the plaque/thrombus interface is a prominent feature. Although it is not known if this is a secondary phenomenon, it is notable that hyaluronic acid can bind to a variety of receptors, including CD44 and hyaluronic acid-mediated motility receptors that promote smooth muscle cell proliferation and migration, raise inflammatory cells and trigger the coagulation cascade which can exacerbate erosion [51, 52]. Hyaluronic acid can also promote cellular stress and apoptosis, aggravating endothelial activation, and impairing endothelial cell adherence via the toll-like receptor 2 (TLR2) dependent pathway that may further promote plaque erosion [53]. Because plaque erosion tends to occur at vessel bifurcations, it has been postulated that local hemodynamics factors also contribute in some way to endothelial injury [54–56].

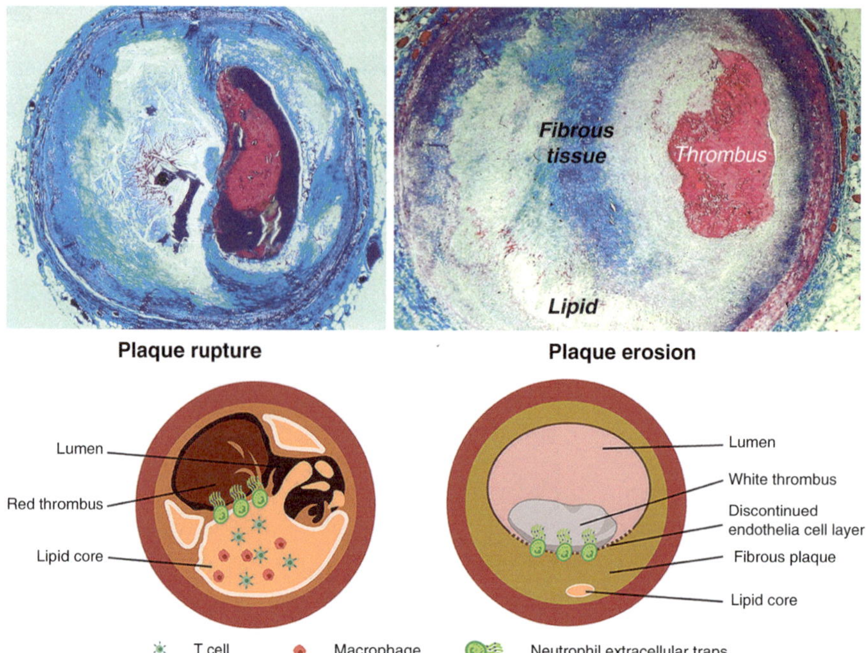

Fig. 4 Histology of Plaque rupture vs. Plaque erosions. (Top left image) Histology of a cross-sectioned coronary artery containing a ruptured plaque with a non-occlusive platelet-rich thrombus superimposed. The actual defect in the fibrous cap is not seen in this section but is located nearby. Note the cholesterol crystals in the plaque core (Trichrome stain, rendering thrombus red, collagen blue, and lipid colorless). Adapted with permission from Falk E and Fuster V. Atherogenesis and its determinants. In: Hursts the Heart. tenth edition. Fuster V, et al., editors. McGraw-Hill, 2001:1065–94. (Top right image). Plaque erosion. Cross section of a coronary artery containing a stenotic atherosclerotic plaque with an occlusive thrombosis superimposed. The endothelium is missing at the plaque–thrombus interface, but the plaque surface is otherwise intact. Note the cholesterol crystal crypts in the fibrous zone. (Trichrome stain, rendering thrombus red, collagen blue, and lipid colorless). (Courtesy of Dr. Erling Falk, Aarhus, Denmar). *Cartoon of the characteristics of plaque rupture and plaque erosion.* Pathological characteristics of plaque rupture and plaque erosion. Ruptured plaque (left image) is featured with a larger lipid core containing abundant macrophages and T cells. Red thrombus is observed in the small lumen. Eroded plaque (right image) has a large lumen with white thrombus and fibrous plaque tissue characterized by little or no lipid deposition. In particularly, there is discontinuous endothelial cell layer in eroded plaque. Neutrophil extracellular traps was found at the junction of plaque tissue and thrombus in both eroded and ruptured plaque. (Reproduced with permission [68])

6 The Dynamic Nature of Plaque Morphology

Longitudinal studies using OCT to assess plaque morphology, and PET scanning to identify inflammation in the atherosclerotic arterial bed, confirm that over time most plaques with features thought to make them vulnerable to rupture remain stable or show signs of healing [16]. Thus, despite their appearance, a "picture in time" is poorly predictive of future atherothrombotic events, and inflammatory activity in the plaque bed is more often associated with healing rather than rupture [57].

Today there is little doubt that inflammation occurs in response to vascular injury and is a driving force in the development and progression of atherosclerosis and destabilization of plaques; Histopathology and angioscopic studies confirm the presence of inflammatory infiltrates in the shoulders of culprit plaques and in the exudates of ruptured plaques [57, 58]; Studies using PET imaging suggest that "hot" atherosclerotic plaque identify patients at high risks of future coronary events [59–61] (Fig. 5). Additionally, clinical trials confirming that inhibition of the NLRP3 inflammasome is effective in reducing the risk of atherosclerotic events in patients with chronic coronary disease [62, 63]. Furthermore, the circadian and seasonal variation of atherothrombosis can possibly be explained by changes in leukocytes and platelet activity that occur with these rhythms [1, 2], and risk factors associated with atherothrombotic risk such as smoking, diabetes, chronic renal disease, gout, and ongoing inflammatory disease that can be linked to an increase in systemic inflammation, could plausibly affect the inflammatory milieu in the plaque bed as primed leukocytes transit through the vasa vasorum [64].

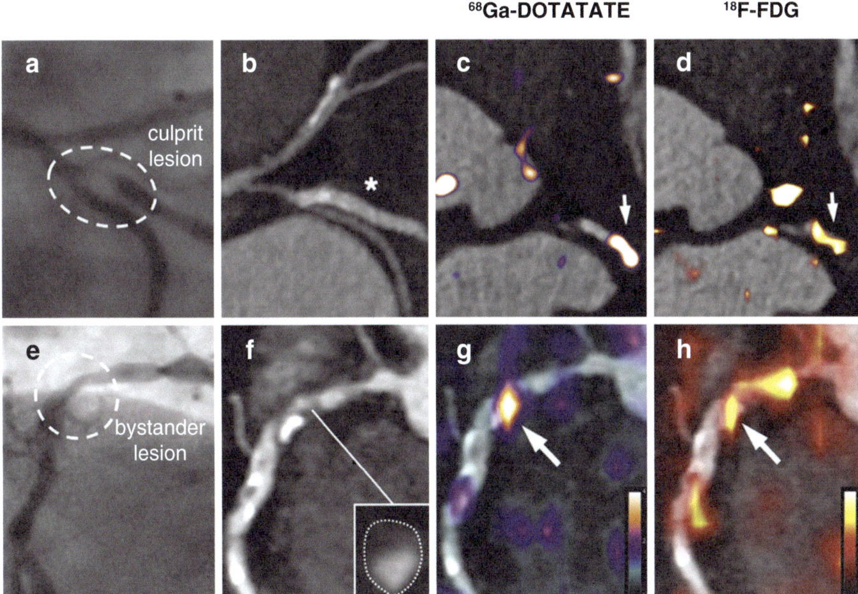

Fig. 5 PET Images of the coronary arteries. X-ray angiography images from a 59-year-old man with ACS, showing a culprit first obtuse marginal lesion ([**a**] hatched oval) and non-culprit (bystander) right coronary artery disease ([**e**] circle). Identification of a culprit artery was aided by electrocardiographic findings of lateral T-wave inversion. Corresponding CT angiography images (**b, f**) show stented culprit lesion (*) and native bystander lesion with high-risk plaque morphology ([inset] low attenuation, cross-section of artery with outer wall boundary marked by dotted outline). In both lesions, intense inflammation (arrows) detected by 68Ga-DOTATATE PET (**c, g**) is reproduced by [18F]FDG PET (**d, h**). (Reproduced with permission [61])

Despite all of the data on the role of inflammation, the outstanding issue related to the inflammatory theory of plaque rupture is uncertainty as to the injurious trigger that acutely potentiates the inflammatory process in stable plaques. Thus, it is still not clear why the decades-long inflammatory process that generally leads to sequestration of extracellular deposits of cholesterol and cellular debris should appear "to suddenly go awry" and disrupt a stable plaque. Furthermore, the inflammatory theory does not make it clear as to whether cholesterol in the plaque core is passive or plays a more active role in the atherosclerotic process, or how or why the lipid core can appear to suddenly expand, or how inflammation alone can explain the range of appearances of atherosclerotic plaque, or cause plaque erosion or plaque hemorrhage.

These remaining conundrums raise the possibility that while *chronic inflammation in the atherosclerotic bed* leads to sequestration of extracellular debris, sclerosis, and calcification of the arterial wall, *dynamic changes in the physiochemistry of the lipid core that intermittently favors the formation of cholesterol crystals may be the trigger that changes the fate of an individual plaque.*

7   The Dynamic Nature of Plaque Vulnerability

As atherosclerotic plaques evolve the nature of their core changes. As senescent cells become trapped in the surrounding fibrin-collogen matrix they are incorporated into the core, and as they degenerate their contents dissociate into their elemental forms. Thus, the core becomes rich in both necrotic gruel and cholesterol that is both esterified (bound) and unesterified (free) [37, 38, 65, 66]. These changes also alter the physiochemical environment of the core, which may begin to favor the spontaneous self-assembly of free cholesterol molecules into stable crystalline structures.

This is illustrated in Fig. 6, which is a conceptual diagram designed to show *the dynamic nature of plaque vulnerability* [67]. Specifically, it shows how changes in the size of the free (unesterified) cholesterol pool, its physiochemistry, and the state of inflammation surrounding the core may affect the stability of a plaque. Thus, plaques with a small lipid pool that is none-the-less rich in free cholesterol may become vulnerable to erosion if the physiochemical environment favors CC formation, and may become vulnerable to rupture if in addition the surrounding inflammatory milieu is already primed. In contrast, plaques rich in lipid may remain stable if the amount of free cholesterol is limited or the physiochemical environment is not conducive to CC formation.

Thus, understanding how changes in the plaque core affect the development of CCs addresses several conundrums related to the dynamics of plaque vulnerability.

1. It explains the disconnect between plaque morphology and the risk of atherothrombosis, as it explains why CCs can form and disrupt plaque independent of the size of the lipid pool as long as the conditions that promote CC formation are present.

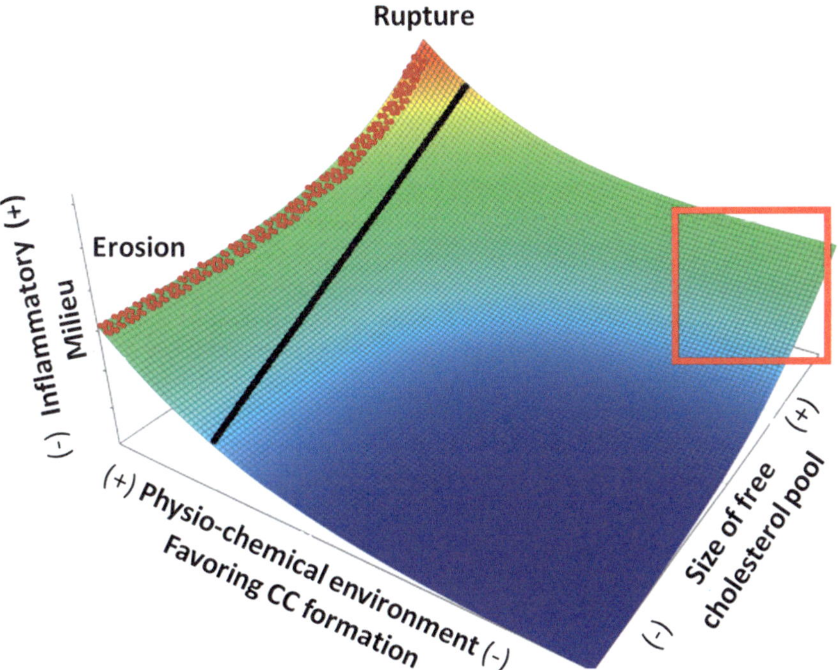

Fig. 6 The dynamic nature of plaque vulnerability. Conceptual graphic with arbitrary units demonstrating that the vulnerability of a plaque to rupture or erosion varies in relation to the size of the pool of free cholesterol, its physiochemical environment and the inflammatory milieu surrounding the lipid core. The blue regions represent quiescent plaque, the green regions represent potentially vulnerable plaques, and the red region represent eroded and rupture plaques. Plaques with a small lipid pool rich in free cholesterol may become vulnerable to erosion if the physiochemical environment is sufficient to initiate CC formation, and rupture if the surrounding inflammatory milieu is already primed (Black line). In contrast, plaques rich in lipid may remain stable (red square) if the amount of free cholesterol is limited or the physiochemical environment is not conducive to CCs formation. Erosion can occur independent of the inflammatory milieu in the plaque bed. Rupture is more likely to occur if the inflammatory milieu around the lipid core is primed by prior release of CCs or other colloids in the plaque bed, or modified by systemic factors including diabetes, renal dysfunction, sepsis or smoking and affected by circadian rhythm, seasonal change and major societal events or disasters or acute emotional stress. (Adapted with permission [67])

2. It highlights why thinning of the cap is not a prerequisite feature of vulnerability, as CCs are strong enough to pierce pericardium and can therefore readily pierce thick capped plaques. Furthermore, it highlights that it is likely that the cap of a lipid rich culprit plaque thins prior to rupture because it is stretched when CC form and aggregate and expand the lipid core.

3. It explains why even lipid rich plaques that contain CCs may stabilize if CC growth cannot be sustained before the plaque is injured. Thus, plaque vulnerability is dynamic and under circumstances when CCs cannot continue to grow healing around the plaque can continue unabated and maintain its stability.

4. It offers a mechanism by which plaque erosion can occur regardless of the inflammatory milieu of the plaque, as CCs that pierce rather than rupture the plaque cap can attract and activate circulating neutrophils [50].
5. It provides a mechanism for plaque hemorrhage, as CCs released into the plaque bed can pierce the vasa-vasorum.
6. It provides a mechanism by which cholesterol in the plaque core can change the trajectory of the inflammatory milieu in the plaque bed, as cholesterol in its crystalline form can incite acute destructive inflammatory injury to promote plaque rupture.
7. It provides an understanding as to why the incidence of cardiovascular events peaks in the early hours of the night and in winter months, because a fall in core body temperature of a few degrees centigrade may be sufficient to trigger cholesterol crystallization [37].
8. It offers a paradigm as to how to reduce the risk of cardiovascular events, by either reducing CC formation, with statins, aspirin, metformin, and colchicine, or by dampening CC induced inflammation with canakinumab or low-dose colchicine.

8 Summary

The cholesterol crystal paradigm can explain the "conundrum of the vulnerable plaque" as it highlights how the dynamic nature of plaque vulnerability may relate to the changes in the physiochemistry of the lipid core that can intermittently favor the formation of CCs that can cause plaque trauma and alter the trajectory of the inflammatory milieu in the atherosclerotic bed from one that favors healing to one that promotes inflammatory injury.

References

1. Marchant B, Ranjadayalan K, Stevenson R, Wilkinson P, Timmis AD. Circadian and seasonal factors in the pathogenesis of acute myocardial infarction: the influence of environmental temperature. Br Heart J. 1993;69(5):385–7. https://doi.org/10.1136/hrt.69.5.385.
2. Xin M, Zhang S, Zhao L, Jin X, Kim W, Cheng XW. Circadian and seasonal variation in onset of acute myocardial infarction. Medicine (Baltimore). 2022;101(28):e29839. https://doi.org/10.1097/MD.0000000000029839.
3. Mehta D, Curwin J, Gomes A, Fuster V. Sudden death in coronary artery disease: acute ischemia versus myocardial substrate. Circulation. 1997;96:3215–23. https://doi.org/10.1161/01.cir.96.9.3215.
4. Ruffer MA. On arterial lesions found in Egyptian mummies (1580 BC-525 AD). J Pathol Bacteriol. 1911;15:453–62.
5. Gotto AM. Some reflections on arteriosclerosis: past, present, and future. Circulation. 1985;72:8–17. https://doi.org/10.1161/01.CIR.72.1.8.
6. Capron L. Évolution des théories sur Íathérosclérosis. Rev Prat. 1996;46:533–7.

7. Virchow R. Cellular pathology as based upon physiological and pathlogical histoly (translated by Frank Chance from 2nd German Edition). London: John Churchill; 1860. p. 360.

8. Abela GS. Atherosclerosis as an inflammatory arterial disease "Déjà vu"? ACC Curr J Rev. 2003;12:23–5. https://doi.org/10.1016/S1062-1458(03)00337-4.

9. Rokitansky C. A manual of pathological anatomy (translated by William Swaine from German), vol. 1. London: Sydenham Society; 1854. p. 97.

10. Anitschkow NN, Chalatow S. Ueber experimentelle Cholesterinsteatose und ihre Bedeutung fur die Entstehung eini-ger pathologischer Prozesse. Zentralbl Allg Pathol. 1913;24:1–9.

11. Shull KH, Mann GV, Andrus SB, Stare FJ. Response of dogs to cholesterol feeding. Am J Physiol. 1954;176:475–82. https://doi.org/10.1152/ajplegacy.1954.176.3.475.

12. Roberts WC. We think we are one, we act as if we are one, but we are not one. Am J Cardiol. 1990;66:896.

13. Muller JE, Abela GS, Nesto RW, Tofler GH. Triggers, acute risk factors and vulnerable plaques: the lexicon of a new frontier. J Am Coll Cardiol. 1994;23:809–13. https://doi.org/10.1016/0735-1097(94)90772-2.

14. Stone GW, Maehara A, Lansky AJ, et al. A prospective natural-history study of coronary atherosclerosis. N Engl J Med. 2011;364:226–35. https://doi.org/10.1056/NEJMoa1002358.

15. Naghavi M, Libby P, Falk E, et al. From vulnerable plaque to vulnerable patient: a call for new definitions and risk assessment strategies: part I. Circulation. 2003;108:1664–72. https://doi.org/10.1161/01.CIR.0000087480.94275.97.

16. Arbab-Zadeh A, Fuster V. The myth of the "vulnerable plaque": transitioning from a focus on individual lesions to atherosclerotic disease burden for coronary artery disease risk assessment. J Am Coll Cardiol. 2015;65:846–55. https://doi.org/10.1016/j.jacc.2014.11.041.

17. Castelli WP, Anderson K, Wilson PWF, Levy D. Lipids and risk of coronary heart disease. The Framingham Study. Ann Epidemiol. 1992;2:23–8. https://doi.org/10.1016/1047-2797(92)90033-m.

18. Muller JE, Stone PH, Turi ZG, et al. Circadian variation in the frequency of onset of acute myocardial infarction. N Engl J Med. 1985;313:11315–22. https://doi.org/10.1056/NEJM198511213132103.

19. Mittleman MA, Maclure M, Tofler GH, Sherwood JB, Goldberg RJ, Muller JE. Triggering of acute myocardial infarction by heavy physical exertion. Protection against triggering by regular exertion. Determinants of myocardial infarction onset study investigators. N Engl J Med. 1993;329:1677–83. https://doi.org/10.1056/NEJM199312023292301.

20. Mittleman MA, Maclure M, Sherwood JB, Mulry RP, Tofler GH, Jacobs SC, Friedman R, Benson H, Muller JE. Circulation. 1985;92:1720–5. https://doi.org/10.1161/01.cir.92.7.1720.

21. Muller JE, Mittleman MA, Maclure M, Sherwood JB, Tofler GH. Triggering myocardial infarction by sexual activity. Low absolute risk and prevention by regular physical exertion. Determinants of myocardial infarction onset study investigators. JAMA. 1996;275:1405–9. https://doi.org/10.1001/jama.275.18.1405.

22. Chen GC, Loree HM, Kamm RD, Fishbein MC, Lee RT. Distribution of circumferential stress in rutptured and stable atherosclerotic lesions. A structural analysis with histopatholgical correlation. Circulation. 1993;87:1179–87. https://doi.org/10.1161/01.cir.87.4.1179.

23. Pearson TA, Mensah GA, Alexander RW, Anderson JL, Cannon RO 3rd, Criqui M, et al. Centers for Disease Control and Prevention; American Heart Association. Markers of inflammation and cardiovascular disease: application to clinical and public health practice: a statement for healthcare professionals from the Centers for Disease Control and Prevention and the American Heart Association. Circulation. 2003;107:499–511. https://doi.org/10.1161/01.CIR.0000052939.59093.45.

24. Libby P, Nahrendorf M, Swirski FK. Leukocytes link local and systemic inflammation in ischemic cardiovascular disease: an expanded "cardiovascular continuum". J Am Coll Cardiol. 2017;67:1091–103. https://doi.org/10.1016/j.jacc.2015.12.048.

25. Mason JC, Libby P. Cardiovascular disease in patients with chronic inflammation: mechanisms underlying premature cardiovascular events in rheumatologic conditions. Eur Heart J. 2015;36:482–9. https://doi.org/10.1093/eurheartj/ehu403.

26. Moreno PR. Vulnerable plaque: definition, diagnosis, and treatment. Cardiol Clin. 2010;28:1–30. https://doi.org/10.1016/j.ccl.2009.09.008.

27. Davies MJ. The pathophysiology of acute coronary syndromes. Heart. 2000;83:361–6. https://doi.org/10.1136/heart.83.3.361.

28. Steffel J, Luscher TF, Tanner F. Tissue factor in cardiovascular diseases. Circulation. 2006;113:722–31. https://doi.org/10.1161/CIRCULATIONAHA.105.567297.

29. Fayad ZA, Fuster V. Clinical imaging of the high-risk or vulnerable atherosclerotic plaque. Circ Res. 2001;89:305–16. https://doi.org/10.1161/hh1601.095596.

30. de Feyter PJ, Nieman K. New coronary imaging techniques: what to expect? Heart. 2002;87:195–7. https://doi.org/10.1136/heart.87.3.195.

31. Sosnovsk DE, Muiler JE, Kathiresan S, Brady TJ. Non-invasive imaging of plaque vulnerability: an important tool for the assessment of agents to stabilise atherosclerotic plaques. Expert Opin Investig Drugs. 2002;11:693–704. https://doi.org/10.1517/13543784.11.5.693.

32. Arampatzis CA, Ligthart JM, Schaar JA, Nieman K, Serruys PW, de Feyter PJ. Images in cardiovascular medicine. Detection of a vulnerable coronary plaque: a treatment dilemma. Circulation. 2003;108:e34–5. https://doi.org/10.1161/01.CIR.0000075303.04340.EF.

33. MacNeill BD, Lowe HC, Takano M, Fuster V, Jang IK. Intravascular modalities for detection of vulnerable plaque: current status. Arterioscler Thromb Vasc Biol. 2003;23:1333–42. https://doi.org/10.1161/01.ATV.0000080948.08888.BF.

34. Terada K, Kubo T, Kameyama T, et al. NIRS-IVUS for differentiating coronary plaque rupture, erosion, and calcified nodule in acute myocardial infarction. J Am Coll Cardiol Cardiovasc Imag. 2021;14:1440–50. https://doi.org/10.1016/j.jcmg.2020.08.030.

35. Madder RD, Puri R, Muller JE, et al. Confirmation of the intracoronary near-infrared spectroscopy threshold of lipid-rich plaques that underlie ST-segment-elevation myocardial infarction. Athero Thromb Vasc Biol. 2016;36:1010–5. https://doi.org/10.1161/ATVBAHA.115.306849.

36. Karlsson S, Anesäter E, Fransson K, Andell P, Persson J, Erlinge D. Intracoronary near-infrared spectroscopy and the risk of future cardiovascular events. Open Heart. 2019;6:e000917. https://doi.org/10.1136/openhrt-2018-000917.

37. Abela GS, Aziz K. Cholesterol crystals rupture biological membranes and human plaques during acute cardiovascular events—a novel insight into plaque rupture by scanning electron microscopy. Scanning. 2006;28:1–10. https://doi.org/10.1002/sca.4950280101.

38. Al-Handawi MB, Commins P, Prasad Karothu D, Raj G, Li L, Naumov P. Mechanical and crystallographic analysis of cholesterol crystals puncturing biological membranes. Chem A Eur J. 2018;24:11493–7. https://doi.org/10.1002/chem.201802251.

39. Vedre A, Pathak DR, Crimp M, Lum C, Koochesfahani M, Abela GS. Physical factors that trigger cholesterol crystallization leading to plaque rupture. Atherosclerosis. 2008;203:89–96. https://doi.org/10.1016/j.atherosclerosis.2008.06.027.

40. Janoudi A, Shamoun FE, Kalavakunta JK, Abela GS. Cholesterol crystal induced arterial inflammation and destabilization of atherosclerotic plaque. Eur Heart J. 2016;37:1959–67. https://doi.org/10.1093/eurheartj/ehv653.

41. Nidorf SM, Fiolet A, Abela GS. Viewing atherosclerosis through a crystal lens: how the evolving sturture of cholesterol crystals in atheroscleritc plaque alters its stability. J Clin Lipidol. 2020;14:619–30. https://doi.org/10.1016/j.jacl.2020.07.003.

42. Düewell P, Kono H, Rayner KJ, Sirois CM, Vladimer G, Bauernfeind F, Abela GS, Franchi L, Nunez G, Schnurr M, Espevik T, Lien G, Fitzgerald KA, Rock KL, Moore KJ, Wright SD, Hornung V, Latz E. NLRP3 inflammasomes are required for atherogenesis and activated by cholesterol crystals. Nature. 2010;464:1357–61. https://doi.org/10.1038/nature08938.

43. Jia H, Abtahian F, Aguirre AD, Lee S, Chia S, Lowe H, et al. In vivo diagnosis of plaque erosion and calcified nodule in patients with acute coronary syndrome by intravascular optical

coherence tomography. J Am Coll Cardiol. 2013;62:1748–58. https://doi.org/10.1016/j.jacc.2013.05.071.

44. Yamamoto E, Yonetsu T, Kakuta T, Soeda T, Saito Y, Yan BP, et al. Clinical and laboratory predictors for plaque erosion in patients with acute coronary syndromes. J Am Heart Assoc. 2019;8:e012322. https://doi.org/10.1161/JAHA.119.012322.

45. Grégory F. Role of mechanical stress and neutrophils in the pathogenesis of plaque erosion. Atherosclerosis. 2021;318:60–9. https://doi.org/10.1016/j.atherosclerosis.2020.11.002.

46. Fang C, Lu J, Zhang S, Wang J, Wang Y, Li L, et al. Morphological characteristics of eroded plaques with noncritical coronary stenosis: an optical coherence tomography study. J Atheroscler Thromb. 2021;29:126. https://doi.org/10.5551/jat.60301.

47. Sato Y, Hatakeyama K, Yamashita A, Marutsuka K, Sumiyoshi A, Asada Y. Proportion of fibrin and platelets differs in thrombi on ruptured and eroded coronary atherosclerotic plaques in humans. Heart. 2005;91:526–30. https://doi.org/10.1136/hrt.2004.034058.

48. Abela GS. Cholesterol crystals piercing the arterial plaque and intima trigger local and systemic inflammation. J Clin Lipidol. 2010;4:156–64. https://doi.org/10.1016/j.jacl.2010.03.003.

49. Mughal MM, Khan MK, DeMarco JK, Majid A, Shamoun F, Abela GS. Symptomatic and asymptomatic carotid artery plaque. Expert Rev Cardiovasc Ther. 2011;2011(9):1315–30. https://doi.org/10.1586/erc.11.120.

50. Singh P, Kumar N, Singh M, Kaur M, Singh G, Narang A, Kanwal A, Sharma K, Singh B, Napoli MD, Mastana S. Neutrophil extracellular traps and NLRP3 Inflammasome: a disturbing duo in atherosclerosis, inflammation and atherothrombosis. Vaccine. 2023;11(2):261. PMID: 36851139; PMCID: PMC9966193. https://doi.org/10.3390/vaccines11020261.

51. Tavianatou AG, Caon I, Franchi M, Piperigkou Z, Galesso D, Karamanos NK. Hyaluronan: molecular size-dependent signaling and biological functions in inflammation and cancer. FEBS J. 2019;286:2883–908. https://doi.org/10.1111/febs.14777.

52. Wilkinson TS, Bressler SL, Evanko SP, Braun KR, Wight TN. Overexpression of hyaluronan synthases alters vascular smooth muscle cell phenotype and promotes monocyte adhesion. J Cell Physiol. 2006;206:378–85. https://doi.org/10.1002/jcp.20468.

53. Yamamoto E, Thondapu V, Poon E, Sugiyama T, Fracassi F, Dijkstra J, et al. Endothelial shear stress and plaque erosion: a computational fluid dynamics and optical coherence tomography study. JACC Cardiovasc Imag. 2019;12:374–5. https://doi.org/10.1016/j.jcmg.2018.07.024.

54. McElroy M, Kim Y, Niccoli G, Vergallo R, Langford-Smith A, Crea F, et al. Identification of the haemodynamic environment permissive for plaque erosion. Sci Rep. 2021;11:7253. https://doi.org/10.1038/s41598-021-86501-x.

55. Vergallo R, Papafaklis MI, D'Amario D, Michalis LK, Crea F, Porto I. Coronary plaque erosion developing in an area of high endothelial shear stress: insights from serial optical coherence tomography imaging. Coron Artery Dis. 2019;30:74–5. https://doi.org/10.1097/MCA.0000000000000673.

56. Vergallo R, Crea F. Atherosclerotic plaque healing. N Engl J Med. 2020;383(9):846–57. https://doi.org/10.1056/NEJMra2000317.

57. Virmani R, Burke A, Farb A, Kolodgie FD. Pathology of the vulnerable plaque. J Am Coll Cardiol. 2006;47(8_Supplement):C13–8. https://doi.org/10.1016/j.jacc.2005.10.065.

58. Komatsu S, Yutani C, Takahashi S, Takewa M, Ohara T, Hirayama A, Kodama K. Debris collected in-situ from spontaneously ruptured atherosclerotic plaque invariably contains large cholesterol crystals and evidence of activation of innate inflammation: insights from non-obstructive general angioscopy. Atherosclerosis. 2022;352:96–102. https://doi.org/10.1016/j.atherosclerosis.2022.03.010.

59. McCubrey RO, Mason SM, Le VT, Bride DL, Horne BD, Meredith KG, Sekaran NK, Anderson JL, Knowlton KU, Min DB, Knight S. A highly predictive cardiac positron emission tomography (PET) risk score for 90-day and one-year major adverse cardiac events and revascularization. J Nucl Cardiol. 2023;30(1):46–58. https://doi.org/10.1007/s12350-022-03028-y.

60. Aziz K, Berger K, Claycombe K, Huang R, Patel R, Abela GS. Noninvasive detection and localization of vulnerable plaque and arterial thrombosis with computed tomography angiography/

positron emission tomography. Circulation. 2008;117:2061–70. https://doi.org/10.1161/CIRCULATIONAHA.106.652313.

61. Tarkin JM, Joshi FR, Evans NR, et al. Detection of atherosclerotic inflammation by 68Ga-DOTATATE PET compared to [18F]FDG PET imaging. J Am Coll Cardiol. 2017;11:1774–91. https://doi.org/10.1016/j.jacc.2017.01.060.

62. Ridker PM, Everett BM, Thuren T, MacFadyen JG, Chang WH, Ballantyne C, Fonseca F, Nicolau J, Koenig W, Anker SD, JJP K, Cornel JH, Pais P, Pella D, Genest J, Cifkova R, Lorenzatti A, Forster T, Kobalava Z, Vida-Simiti L, Flather M, Shimokawa H, Ogawa H, Dellborg M, PRF R, RPT T, Libby P, Glynn RJ, CANTOS Trial Group. Antiinflammatory therapy with Canakinumab for atherosclerotic disease. N Engl J Med. 2017;377(12):1119–31. https://doi.org/10.1056/NEJMoa1707914.

63. Nidorf SM, Fiolet ATL, Mosterd A, Eikelboom JW, Schut A, Opstal TSJ, The SHK, Xu XF, Ireland MA, Lenderink T, Latchem D, Hoogslag P, Jerzewski A, Nierop P, Whelan A, Hendriks R, Swart H, Schaap J, Kuijper AFM, van Hessen MWJ, Saklani P, Tan I, Thompson AG, Morton A, Judkins C, Bax WA, Dirksen M, Alings M, Hankey GJ, Budgeon CA, Tijssen JGP, Cornel JH, Thompson PL. LoDoCo2 trial investigators. Colchicine in patients with chronic coronary disease. N Engl J Med. 2020;383(19):1838–47. https://doi.org/10.1056/NEJMoa2021372.

64. Maiellaro K, Taylor WR. The role of the adventitia in vascular inflammation. Cardiovasc Res. 2007;75(4):640–8. https://doi.org/10.1016/j.cardiores.2007.06.023.

65. Kruth HS. Localization of unesterified cholesterol in human atherosclerotic lesions. Demonstration of filipin-positive, oil-red-O-negative particles. Am J Pathol. 1984;114(2):201–8. PMID: 6198918; PMCID: PMC1900338.

66. Small DM, Bond MG, Waugh D, Prack M, Sawyer JK. Physicochemical and histological changes in the arterial wall of nonhuman primates during progression and regression of atherosclerosis. J Clin Invest. 1984;73:1590–605. https://doi.org/10.1172/JCI111366.

67. Stefanadis C, Antoniou C-K, Tsiachris D, Pietri P. Coronary atherosclerotic vulnerable plaque: current perspectives. J Am Heart Assoc. 2017;6:e005543. https://doi.org/10.1161/JAHA.117.005543.

68. Luo X, Lv Y, Bai X, Qi J, Weng X, Liu S, Bao X, Jia H, Yu B. Plaque erosion: a distinctive pathological mechanism of acute coronary syndrome. Front Cardiovasc Med. 2021;8:711453. https://doi.org/10.3389/fcvm.2021.711453.

The Role of Cholesterol Crystals in Plaque Rupture Leading to Acute Myocardial Infarction and Stroke

George S. Abela and Kusai Aziz

1 Background

Crystals are abundant in nature. They form when matter undergoes a phase change from a liquid to a solid state that has a highly organized stable lattice structure with a geometric shape related to its specific chemical composition. Examples are conversion of water to ice, magma to rubies, and the formation of diamonds. Crystals are also present though out the universe as evidence by their presence in some meteorites. When crystals form within the body, they are invariably associated with pathological states. As they form and aggregate into stones within the urinary or biliary track they can act as a nidus for infection or cause obstruction. Moreover, their presence in contact with tissues can trigger an inflammatory response.

The cardiovascular system is no exception, and a variety of crystals can form in the arterial wall, cardiac valves, and skeleton. The foremost example is the formation of cholesterol crystals (CCs) starting in the early atheroma and up to advanced atherosclerosis. Their primary process in plaque development, growth, inflammation, and rupture has only recently been recognized. Since the authors of this chapter published the initial bench model demonstrating that CCs expand during crystallization that perforates and tears biological membranes including the arterial intima in 2005 and 2006 [1, 2], the role of CCs has gained increased attention and has led to a vast range of reports demonstrating their role in plaque rupture and other conditions (i.e., diabetic retinopathy, valvulopathy, cancer) [3–5]. In this chapter we

G. S. Abela (✉)
Department of Medicine, Division of Cardiovascular Medicine, Michigan State University, East Lansing, MI, USA
e-mail: abela@msu.edu

K. Aziz
Visalia Cardiovascular and Medical Center, Visalia, CA, USA

G. S. Abela, S. M. Nidorf (eds.), *Cholesterol Crystals in Atherosclerosis and Other Related Diseases*, Contemporary Cardiology,
https://doi.org/10.1007/978-3-031-41192-2_10

review the different aspects of CCs formation and their role in triggering inflammation and plaque rupture that leads to myocardial infarction and stroke. We also address the challenges and future research frontiers.

2 Plaque Formation and Rupture

When LDL cholesterol enters and is deposited in the arterial wall it accumulates to form atheromatous plaques. As plaques grow within the arterial wall the artery undergoes a process of positive remodeling that accommodates the plaque without encroaching on the arterial lumen. However, as the plaque continues to grow, the plaque begins to encroach on the arterial lumen to eventually impinge on the arterial blood flow through the vessel (Fig. 1) [6, 7]. The arterial remodeling phase is a

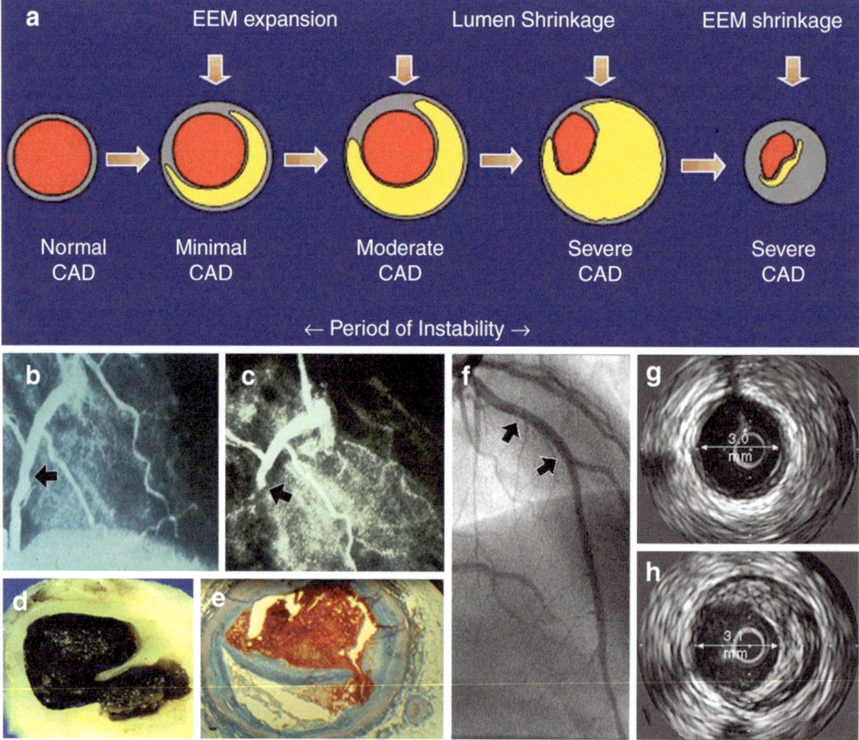

Fig. 1 Positive Remodeling of Plaque. (**a**) Description of positive remodeling where the plaque buildup is accommodated in the arterial wall. After about 40% of deposition of plaque the atherosclerosis begins to encroach on the arterial lumen. (**b, c, d, e**) These evolving lesions are the ones at increased risk for rupture. (**f, g, h**) The angiogram does not detect the presence of plaque since the lumen is not compromised yet the intravascular ultrasound demonstrates the presence of extensive plaque. (Reproduced with permission [6, 7, 11, 17])

relatively unstable state where tissues primarily collagen are being broken down by matrix metalloproteinases to accommodate the growth of the plaque in the arterial wall. Consequently, plaque rupture becomes more likely under those conditions and these lesions are the ones most frequently associated with acute cardiovascular events [8, 9]. However, that alone does not seem to explain the rupture process since the large lipid pool which is a major driver and the substrate leading to crystal formation that can physically damage the surrounding tissues including the fibrous cap [10].

2.1 Coronary Artery Angiographic Limitations in the Assessment of Atheroma

Many atheromas, including those that are do not obstruct the arterial lumen may have a large lipid pool that has the potential of rapidly expanding to rupture the plaque cap due to changing local physico-chemical conditions. Little et al. observed by angiography that even mildly non-stenotic arterial lesions (<50% stenosis) could lead to arterial thrombosis at the same site causing a myocardial infarction [11]. Nobuyoshi et al. also reported that most myocardial infarctions occurred in coronary arteries with lesions that were previously found to have mild stenosis by angiography [12–15] (Fig. 2). Studies with intravascular ultrasound subsequently confirmed that angiography often failed to appreciate the extent of plaque buildup of in these non-stenotic intramural lesions that were embedded within the arterial wall. In the PROSPECT (Prospective Natural-History Study of Coronary Atherosclerosis) trial, patients who underwent percutaneous coronary intervention for an acute cardiovascular event had gray-scale intravascular ultrasound with radiofrequency assessment of the non-infract related arteries. In this study 20% of the subsequent coronary events proved to be related to lesions that were initially assessed to being mild by angiography [16].

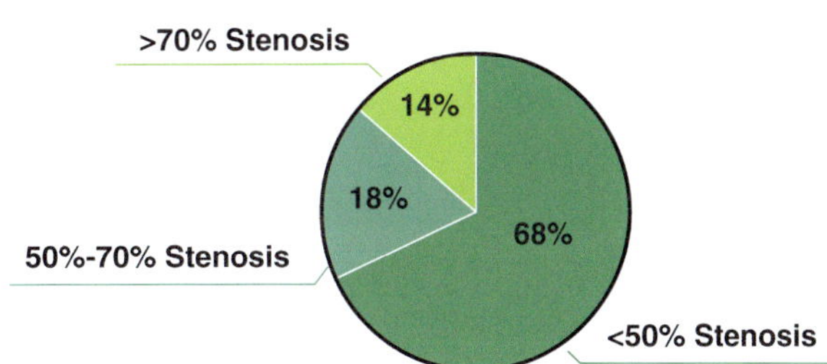

Fig. 2 Pie Graph of Arterial Stenosis by Angiography and % Myocardial Infarction. Most myocardial infarctions occur with less than 50% stenosis by angiography. (Reproduced with permission [13])

2.2   *Plaque Rupture Leading to Thrombosis Is the Dominant Cause of Myocardial Infarction*

Plaque rupture as the underlying cause for most acute myocardial infarctions was only recognized in the last few decades [17, 18]. These landmark reports demonstrated by histology that plaques at sites of arterial thrombosis were frequently "torn" and were the nidus for thrombus formation. These observations fit well with angiographic studies that indicated myocardial infarctions may be related to disruption of non-occlusive intramural lesions with positive remodeling features [11, 12].

The clinical outcome following plaque rupture is also dependent on the coagulability of the circulating blood, the amount of particulate material released from the plaque core and exposure to tissue thromboplastin [19]. Thus, not all plaque ruptures lead to the formation of a thrombus large enough to totally occlude the artery and cause a myocardial infarction. Although thrombus was often seen at the site of a ruptured plaque at autopsy, it was not known exactly how this thrombus formed. As a consequence, the development of arterial thrombosis following plaque rupture was only recognized as the occlusive mechanism during acute events by angiographic and subsequent angioscopic studies [20, 21] (Fig. 3). In the early 1980s DeWood et al. performed coronary angiography on 322 patients within 24 h of myocardial infarction. Total coronary occlusion was found in 110 of 126 patients (87%) within 4 h of symptom onset. Moreover, at bypass surgery 55 of 59 patients (88%) had thrombus that was retrieved by a balloon embolectomy catheter. These insights initiated the search for the underlying mechanism of plaque rupture and imaging techniques that could identify the "vulnerable plaques" prone to rupture.

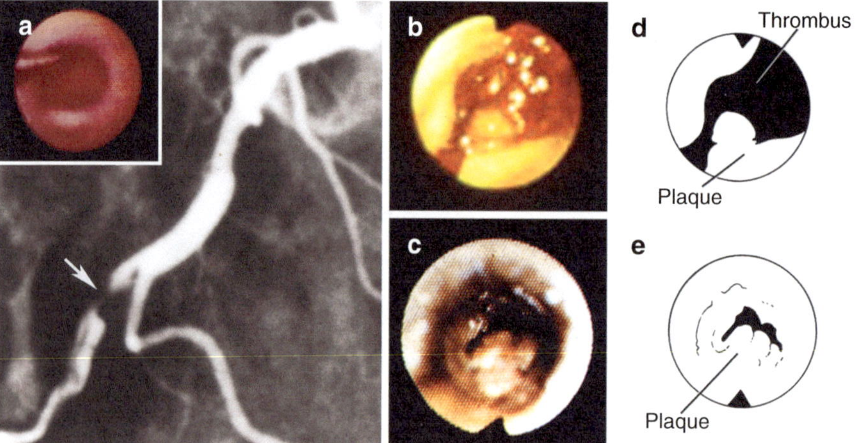

Fig. 3 Angioscopy of Arterial Stenosis. (**a**) Angiogram of right coronary artery with a 1-cm filling defect and trace amount of contrast agent crossing the obstruction (arrow). (insert) Angioscopic view of bulging red thrombus occluding the arterial lumen with guide wire crossing in the left upper quadrant. (**b**, **c**) Angioscopic images of a ruptured plaques with thrombus and (**d**, **e**) diagrams illustrating the angioscopic sites of ruptured plaque and thrombus. (Reproduced with permission [100, 101])

3   Morphology of the Vulnerable Plaque

The lexicon of the "vulnerable plaque" was defined by the group at the Institute for Prevention of Cardiovascular Disease at Harvard Medical School and became the buzz word for the plaque that was primed to disrupt and rupture [22]. Histopathologic features of the "vulnerable plaque" that ruptured were described based on a limited number of samples obtained at postmortem. Perhaps the most critical feature of ruptured plaques was the relatively large lipid pool underlying a thin fibrous cap [10, 23]. This lipid pool also known as the "gruel" in the older pathology literature is typically surrounded by an active sterile inflammation at its perimeter or shoulder. It is recognized that as inflammatory cells undergo apoptosis their cellular content is "sloughed" into the plaque core contributing to cellular debris that includes membranes from degrading red blood cells extruded from vasa vasorum supplying the plaque [24, 25] (Fig. 4). This mix of necrotic materials within the core alters its physico-chemical environment and increases free cholesterol to reach a saturation level that leads to CCs formation and subsequent growth.

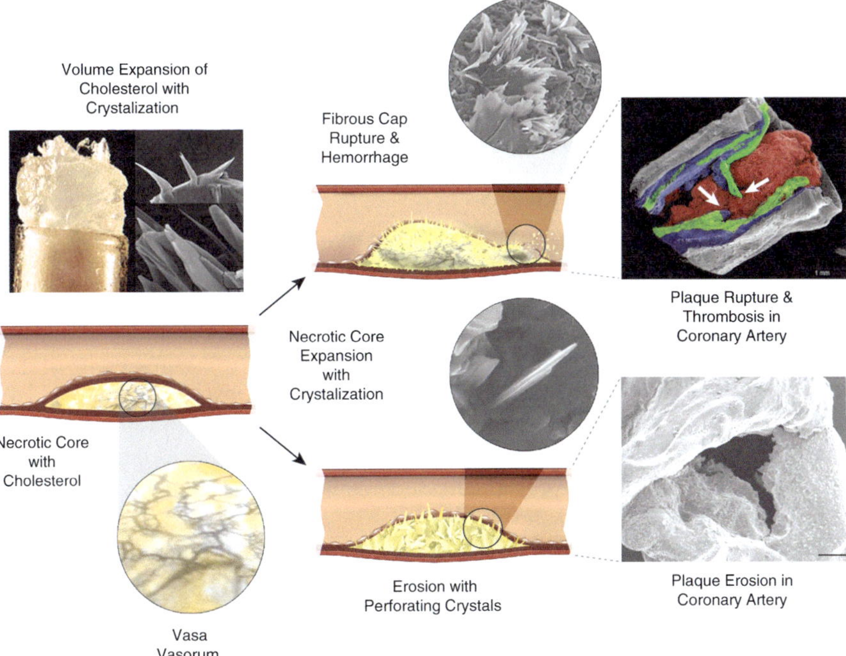

Fig. 4 Mechanism of Plaque Hemorrhage, Rupture, and/or Erosion Induced by Cholesterol Crystallization with Volume Expansion of the Plaque Necrotic Core. In the case of a large necrotic core (top), the plaque cap is torn, leading to rupture, whereas in the case of a small necrotic core (bottom), it leads to erosion. Human plaques with rupture and erosion are shown with corresponding scanning images. Also, trauma to the vasa vasorum caused by expanding cholesterol crystals within the plaque causes intra-plaque hemorrhage. (Modified with permission from [2, 30, 56])

For many years, CCs seen within atheroma and ruptured plaques were considered to be innocent bystanders that developed postmortem rather than active participants in plaque development or rupture [26]. However, few reports suggested that CCs were a marker for plaque evolution from fatty streaks into lipid rich cores [27] and that they were present in ruptured plaques [28]. However, failure to fully appreciate the potential for CCs to induce plaque trauma is understandable given the use of ethanol in tissue preparation that often eliminated their role and extent of their presence in ruptured plaques [29]. The limitation of histology is that it only provides a static image of the end stage of a complex physico-chemical process making it difficult to appreciate how the evolution of CCs in vivo might have actually led to a clinical event being evaluated at postmortem. However, by avoiding the use of ethanol in evaluating plaque rupture using scanning electron microscopy, CCs could be detected perforating the fibrous cap and their extensive amounts became visible surrounding the rupture site during acute cardiovascular events [30].

4 Understanding the Mechanism of Plaque Rupture

The search for the underlying mechanism of plaque rupture and imaging to identify the "vulnerable plaque" prone to rupture became the "Holy Grail" for cardiovascular medicine. Autopsy studies evaluating plaque morphology at ruptured sites revealed that plaques associated with acute cardiovascular events often had certain characteristic histologic features including a large lipid core, a thin fibrous cap, inflammatory cell infiltrates, and loss of myocyte content [23]. However, these histologic features represent a late phase in the evolution of the plaque and do not provide insight into the evolutionary process occurring within the plaque that led to rupture.

Initial thoughts considered that plaque might relate to factors that varied with the circadian rhythm since most heart attacks occur in the early morning hours [31]. It was proposed that elevation in blood pressure at the time of awakening increased the strain on the arterial wall and plaque, thereby acting as a trigger for rupture but testing this hypothesis using finite element analysis of arterial plaques did not support this theory because the level of blood pressure required to cause rupture far exceeded the physiologically attainable levels [10].

The search for the potential trigger of plaque rupture then shifted focus towards the role of inflammation [32]. Recognition of the inflammatory process in atherosclerosis dates back to Rudolf Virchow in 1860 who first suggested that atherosclerosis was an inflammatory condition and coined the term "endarteritis deformans" as an indication of reactive fibrosis following injury [33]. In more recent decades, there has been a resurgence in the understanding of the central role of inflammation in atherosclerosis. Russell Ross proposed that vascular injury was the cause for atherosclerosis and Peter Libby focused on various cytokines as markers of inflammation associated with atherosclerosis [34, 35].

Extension of the inflammatory hypothesis suggested that inflammation mediated by macrophages and lymphocyte infiltration in the subintimal space associated with the release of metalloproteinases could erode the fibrous cap and lead to rupture [8, 36, 37]. However, while inflammation is an integral part of plaque growth and destabilization, alone it is probably not sufficient to explain most of the rupture events that require a force to disrupt the fibrous cap architecture. Thus, the inflammation theory alone does not identify the trigger for the event.

As the search for the mechanism of plaque rupture continued the potential role of systemic inflammation as a trigger of plaque rupture was also considered [38]. In fact, patient examination using intravascular ultrasound and angioscopy revealed that during acute cardiovascular events several arterial sites besides the culprit vessel were involved with plaque rupture [39, 40]. This included not only other coronary arteries but also other vascular beds such as carotid arteries that had evidence of concurrent plaque ruptures. This aspect made it more challenging to understand the rupture process as a localized event but rather a broader systemic process suggesting that there may not only be a "vulnerable plaque" but a "vulnerable patient" as well. However, this systemic concept, however, still did not explain the mechanism of plaque rupture and failed to appreciate that the evolution of atherosclerotic plaque in one vascular bed could also be driven simultaneously by the same (local) factors in other vascular beds.

5 Cholesterol Crystals as a Cause of Plaque Rupture and Thrombosis

Thus far, each of the models proposed to explain the rupture of a vulnerable plaque have not been fully supported by investigation and failed to provide a clear link between ongoing pathophysiologic changes in the plaque core and acute rupture. This includes chemical-enzymatic injury that results from inflammation [8, 36]; intra-plaque hemorrhage induced by leaking vasa vasorum [41]; increasing shear stress on the plaque cap [10, 42], and other physical factors including changes in ambient temperature which may affect blood pressure [43].

In 2005, we first proposed that crystallization of cholesterol with volume expansion within atherosclerotic plaques is the integral link that connects all the various models (Fig. 4) [1, 2]. As cholesterol crystalizes from its liquid state in foamy macrophages it leads to cell death that releases lytic enzymes [44, 45]. When CCs form, continue to grow and aggregate in the necrotic core, they expand the plaque causing Its fibrous cap to stretch, thin, and eventually rupture or become damaged due to the ability of CCs to directly perforate it by virtue of their sharp leading edges. In addition, by these same mechanisms, CCs can cut the vasa vasorum causing intra-plaque hemorrhage. Moreover, CCs present in the arterial lumen after rupture may injure platelets promoting the release their prothrombotic contents to further promote athero-thrombosis [46].

5.1 Localization of Cholesterol Crystals in Atheromatous Plaque

CCs are a prominent component of many atherosclerotic plaques and are usually found in the advanced stage of cholesterol evolution within the plaque. They have been recognized in association with plaque lipids since the early 1900s [47]. Studies had also demonstrated that LDL cholesterol has a great affinity to the glycoproteins in the elastic tissues of the artery, leading to free cholesterol deposition and formation of CCs within the elastic lamina that in turn have the potential to destroy the arterial architecture (Chapter "Atherosclerosis as a Crystalloid Disease: The Discovery of the Role of Cholesterol Crystals in the Formation and Rupture of Atherosclerotic Plaques", Figs. 3 and 4). This assessment has been made from microscopic observations and the accumulation of cholesterol in the glycoprotein within the arterial wall [48, 49]. In a similar way, CCs accumulation in tendons forming xanthomas and corneal arcus have also been described, in patients with familial hypercholesterolemia (Chapter "Atherosclerosis as a Crystalloid Disease: The Discovery of the Role of Cholesterol Crystals in the Formation and Rupture of Atherosclerotic Plaques", Fig. 2) [50].

Cholesterol crystals can form in the lipid bilayers of endothelial cell membranes which act to stiffen the intima and activate surface adhesion molecules that attract monocytes to enter the subintimal space [51–54]. Subsequent uptake of cholesterol by monocytes eventually leads to their transforming into macrophages that transition further into foam cells as they continue to accumulate lipid within their lysosomes. CCs that form within the lysosomes can lead to lysosomal rupture that results in their release into the cytoplasm where they can trigger inflammatory processes and lead to either traumatic cell death or apoptosis. This causes the release of cellular contents into the interstitial space or into the plaque core as described above (Chapters "Atherosclerotic Plaque Morphology and the Conundrum of the Vulnerable Plaque" and "The Role of Cholesterol Crystals in the Development and Progression of Degenerative Valve Disease"). Also, this contributes further to the amount of CCs in the lipid pool and aggravates the inflammatory response while releasing free cholesterol from membranes of dying cells that are very rich in cholesterol [25]. Eventually, CCs begin to form and aggregate in the lipid pool of the plaque core due to increasing saturation of free cholesterol, pH shifts and possibly pressure elevation [55]. As CCs form, they occupy a greater space from the liquid phase that can occur relatively suddenly causing the lipid pool to expand and thin down the overlying fibrous cap by stretching that can lead to either rupture and/or erosion [30].

6 Cholesterol Crystals Perforate the Fibrous Plaque Cap and Vasa Vasorum

Evidence supporting the fact that CCs perforate the fibrous cap in humans has been demonstrated in patients who died following acute myocardial infarction where CCs were found perforating the fibrous cap at the site of the ruptured plaque [56] (Fig. 5). Moreover, the edges of these ruptured plaques were seen to be tethered as if rented in a violent manner. These findings were not present in coronary arteries with advanced atherosclerotic plaques taken from patients who died of non-acute cardiovascular events. Furthermore, extensive amounts of CCs were found in the aspirates of the occlusive athero-thrombotic material obtained from patients during acute myocardial infarction [57] (Fig. 6). Also, arteries from an atherosclerotic rabbit model had similar findings of CCs perforating the intima as seen in the human coronary arteries [58]. These observations were made possible by avoiding ethanol as a dehydrating agent during tissue preparation for scanning electron microscopy [29] (Chapter "How Innovation in Tissue Preparation and Imaging Revolutionized the Understanding of the Role of Cholesterol Crystals in Atherosclerosis"). Moreover, similar findings of crystals perforating the intima above atheromatous plaques were observed by confocal and digital microscopy without tissue processing.

6.1 CCs Can Disrupt the Vasa Vasorum

Since intra-plaque hemorrhage is often seen especially in plaque rupture, it was hypothesized that trauma to the vasa vasorum an important mechanism responsible for plaque rupture in some circumstances [41, 59]. The blood supply to the arterial wall and atherosclerotic plaques is provided by small, tortuous, and often fragile vessels known as vasa vasorum that usually originate from the adventitial side of the artery. These vessels have reduced smooth muscle cells and often leak red blood cells into the plaque matrix [60]. Previously recognized potential sources of vasa vasorum injury have included the presence of oxidized iron released from red blood cell hemoglobin; protease activity [61] and hypoxia that may affect the release of vascular endothelial growth factor (VEGF) and E26 transformation-specific-1 (Ets-1) [62]. While these factors may be important, the potential of growing CCs within the plaque to perforate any portion of the plaque, including the vasa vasorum to cause intra-plaque hemorrhage is also apparent.

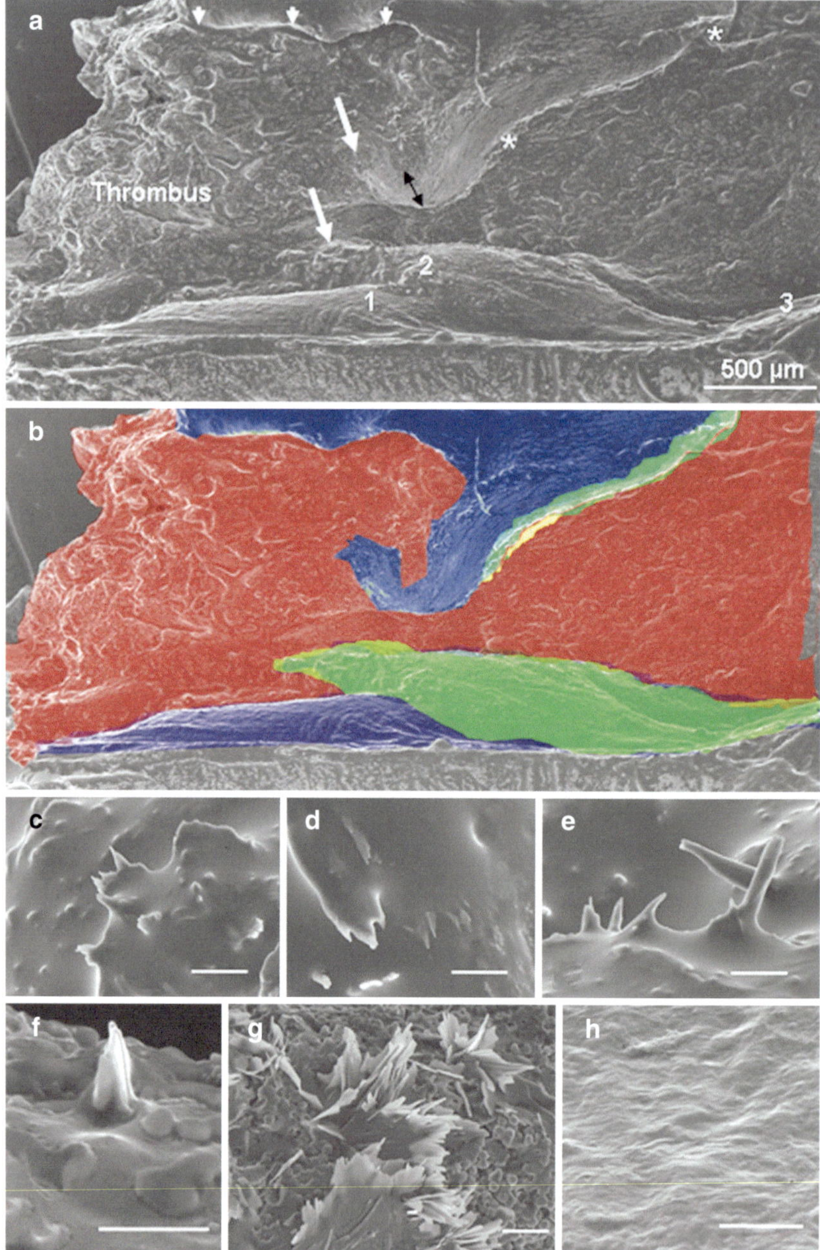

Fig. 5 Cholesterol Crystals Perforating the Fibrous Cap. (**a**) Scanning electron micrograph of right coronary artery from a 57-year-old female cut longitudinally demonstrates the site of plaque rupture with frayed plaque cap edges (long white arrows). Cap thickness was 131 μm (dual black arrows). The plaque basin (small white arrows) and arterial lumen are filled with thrombus. (**b**) A color-coded image at low magnification defines the thrombus (red); ruptured plaque (blue), and sites of crystals perforating the intima (green-yellow). (**c**, **d**, **e**) Examples of CC perforating the intimal surface at the plaque shoulders 1 (bar = 20 μm); 2 (bar = 10 μm); 3 (bar = 10 μm) and *. (**f**, **g**, **h**). Additional examples of crystals perforating the intima without and with thrombus (**f**, bar = 5 μm; **g**, bar = 10 μm) and normal endothelium (**h**, bar = 25 μm). (Reproduced with permission [56])

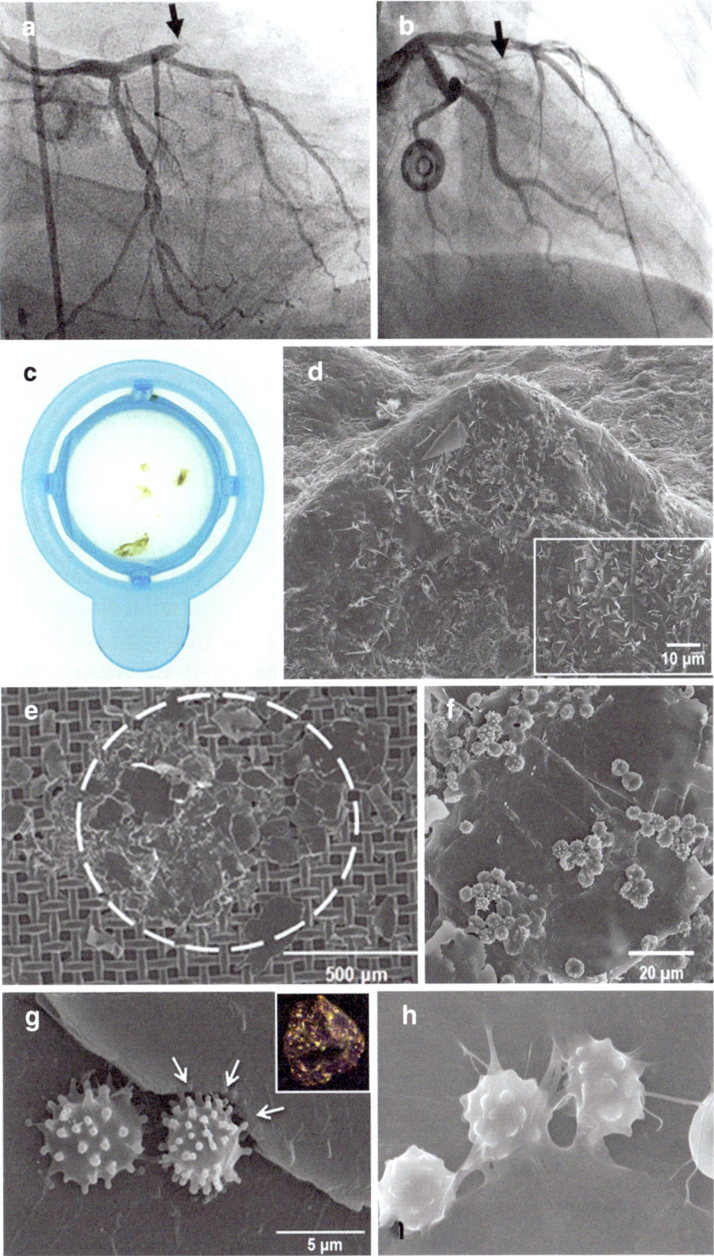

Fig. 6 Aspirated cholesterol crystals during an acute myocardial infarction. (**a**, **b**) angiograms of occluded left anterior descending artery before and after aspiration. (**c**) Gross view of aspirates (**d**) low power scanning electron micrograph of aspirate with insert demonstrating extensive cholesterol crystals (**e**) Clusters of cholesterol crystals aspirated (**f**) macrophages attached to the crystals (**g**) macrophages engaging and breaking down the crystals with crystalline material stained in the macrophage cytoplasm (insert). (**h**) Macrophages attached to crystals and disrupting them. (Reproduced with permission [57])

7 Factors That Trigger Cholesterol Crystallization and Increase the Risk of Plaque Rupture

Crystallization is a dynamic process. As with other forms of material crystallization, the process of cholesterol crystallization is dependent on several factors that affect the local milieu of the plaque.

7.1 Size of the Lipid Pool

Under the appropriate ambient conditions, cholesterol undergoes rapid crystallization within a few minutes that leads to sudden expansion of the plaque's lipid core resulting in a disruptive process that leads to rupture. This process is driven primarily by the size of the lipid pool. A large pool would be expected to have a greater and more rapid volume expansion. This has been demonstrated in vitro experiments where a greater amount of cholesterol placed in a test tube and dissolved or melted will crystallize more rapidly and expand at a greater rate (Chapter "How Innovation in Tissue Preparation and Imaging Revolutionized the Understanding of the Role of Cholesterol Crystals in Atherosclerosis", Fig. 7) [1, 2]. Moreover, if a fibrous membrane (i.e., rabbit pericardium) is placed over the mouth of the test tube during crystallization, the crystals will perforate and tear the membrane [1, 2]. A basic study that evaluated the mechanical features of CCs formed during crystallization revealed that CCs similar to those typically present in human plaques (cholesterol monohydrate) have the physical capacity to perforate fibrous membranes [63].

7.2 Physio-Chemical Factors

Cholesterol is abundant in both liquid and semi-liquid states in atherosclerotic plaques, [64] and CC formation is dependent on the local saturation of cholesterol, the ambient temperature, hydration of the cholesterol molecule, and pH [55]. Furthermore, a dynamic interaction between these factors is conducive for crystallization.

A study to evaluate the physical conditions on cholesterol crystallization was conducted at a controlled temperature of 37 °C to mimic stable in vivo conditions. The role of cholesterol saturation was then evaluated by dissolving cholesterol in a mixture of corn oil and water as described by Jandacek et al. [65]. The water oil interphase is a site for crystallization. These in vitro experiments using dissolved cholesterol at 37 °C demonstrated that as cholesterol saturation is increased the crystal volume expansion increased and crystallization occurred at a faster rate (Fig. 7). In separate experiments, as ambient temperature was dropped even by a

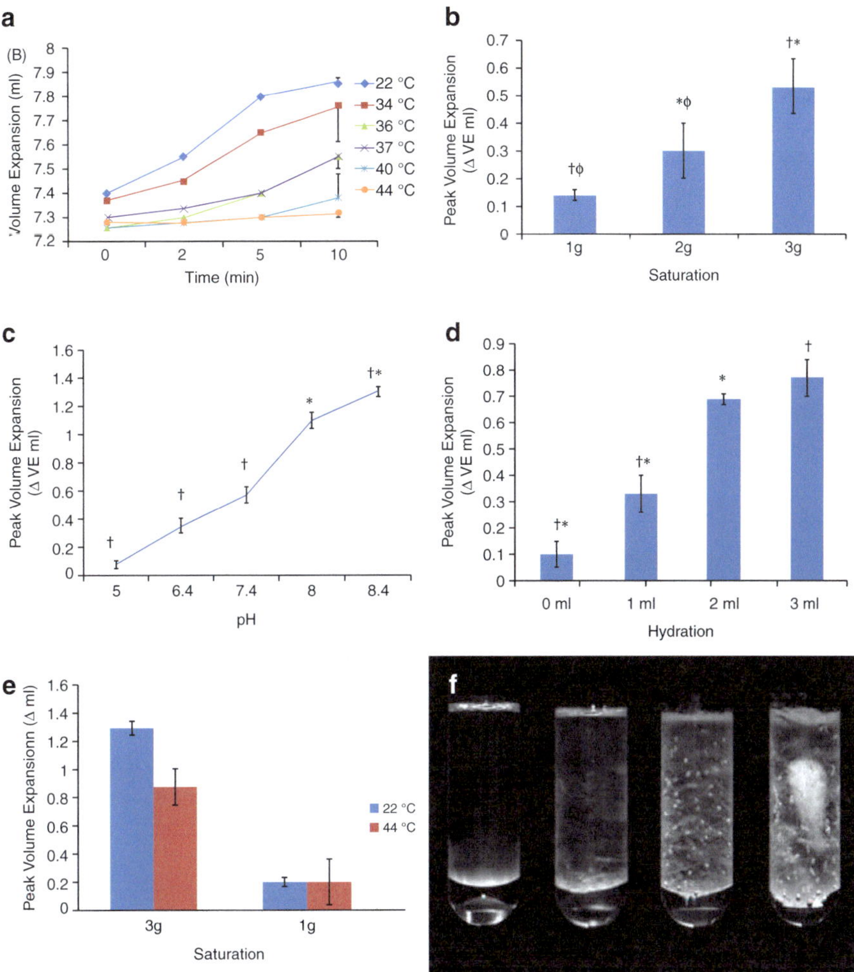

Fig. 7 Physical Factors Affecting Cholesterol Crystal Formation. (**a**) Ambient temperature drop; (**b**) increased saturation; (**c**) pH shift to basic; and (**d**) hydration of the cholesterol molecule all increase cholesterol crystallization. (**e**) Combined effects of saturation and temperature demonstrates lower temperature and saturation is synergistic. (**f**) Test tubes with greater cholesterol saturation have greater crystallization at 37 °C. (Modified and reproduced with permission [55])

few degrees centigrade and within normal physiological levels (36–40 °C), crystallization was enhanced, and volume expansion was increased. The same effects on crystallization were also seen with both a rise in pH and hydration of the cholesterol molecule to the monohydrate moiety. More impressively, a combination of some of these physical factors, primarily saturation and a drop in temperature, was found to enhance the crystallization process in a synergistic manner.

7.3   The Location of CCs Within the Plaque Core

There is evidence that the location of CC in the plaque core may also influence their effect on plaque instability and rupture. Using finite element analysis Luo et al. demonstrated that circumferential stress was directly proportional to crystal growth and accumulation of CCs in the plaque shoulders has a great impact on the peak circumferential stress [66] (Fig. 8). This is also the site where ruptures tend to occur, and macrophages seem to aggregate [67, 68]. Moreover, Frink et al. reported that parallel arrangement of CCs within the plaque matrix was an index of their association with rupture [69] (Fig. 9). A more recent study using optical coherence tomography of plaques in all three coronary arteries during ST-elevation myocardial infarction demonstrated that plaques with CCs were found to have more vulnerable features including a larger lipid burden, more macrophages, and more spotty calcification [70].

7.4   Environmental Temperature

Many reports have confirmed heart attacks and strokes cluster in the early morning hours [31]. Some of this effect was attributable to more "sticky" platelets in the early morning hours [71]. However, the model of plaque rupture by cholesterol crystallization may also help to explain the clustering of plaque rupture in the early morning hours as core temperature is usually a few degrees lower in the early morning hours. It has been shown in that even a small drop in ambient temperature can lead to rapid crystallization in vitro, especially in a saturated solution of cholesterol [55] (Fig. 7). Moreover, many heart attacks cluster in the fall season in the Northern Hemisphere and spring season in the Southern Hemisphere when the ambient temperature drops [72]. Reports have noted similar effects on triggering cardiovascular events with snow shoveling [73]. It is the change in the temperature rather that the baseline levels that seems to be the trigger for crystallization. Therefore, it would be reasonable to suggest that the circadian effect noted with both early morning and seasonal changes may also be related to a temperature variation that influences cholesterol crystallization.

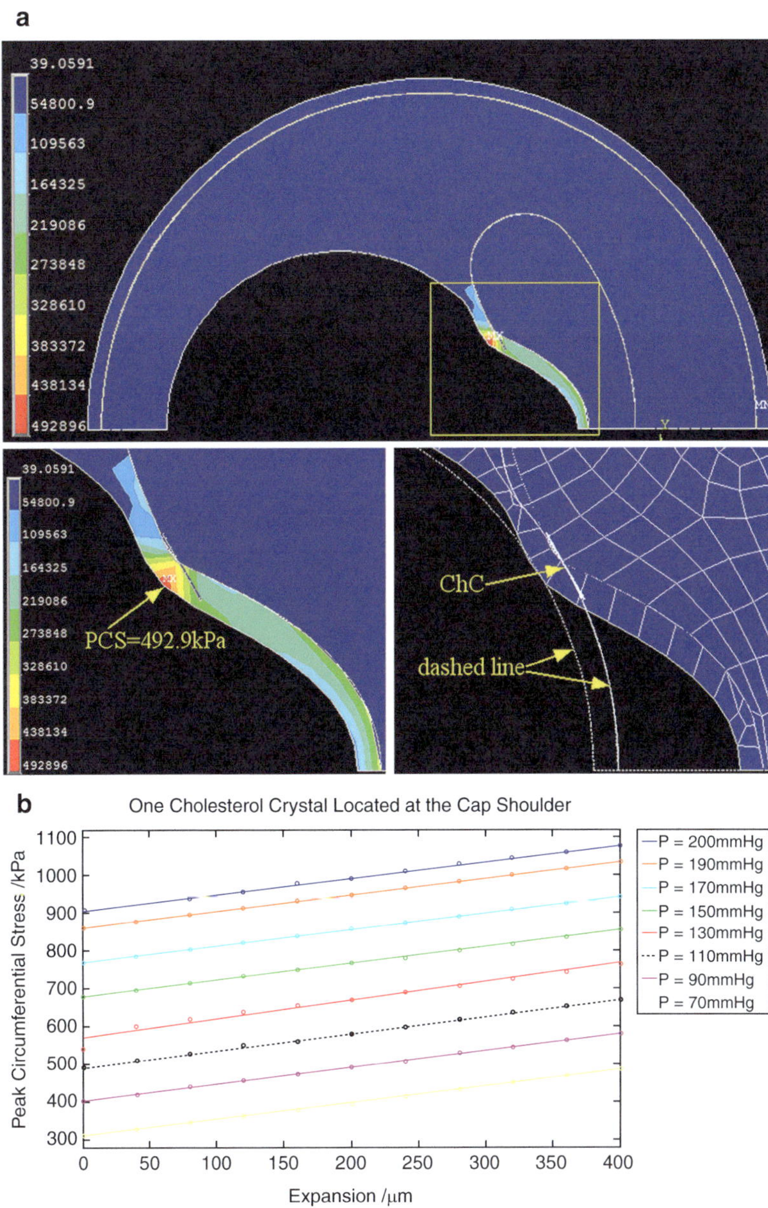

Fig. 8 Stress and Strain of the Artery with One Cholesterol Crystal at the Cap Shoulder. (**a**) Stress distribution of the overall coronary artery with a contour plot of the stress on the fibrous cap (yellow dashed box). Contour plot of the strain on the fibrous cap. The dashed line is the original contour before loading, and the meshed section is the deformed cap after loading (PCS: peak circumferential stress. ChC: cholesterol crystal). (**b**) Graphic demonstrating the effect of crystal expansion at the cap shoulder on peak circumferential stress with varying blood pressure. (P = intracoronary blood pressure). (Reproduced with permission [66])

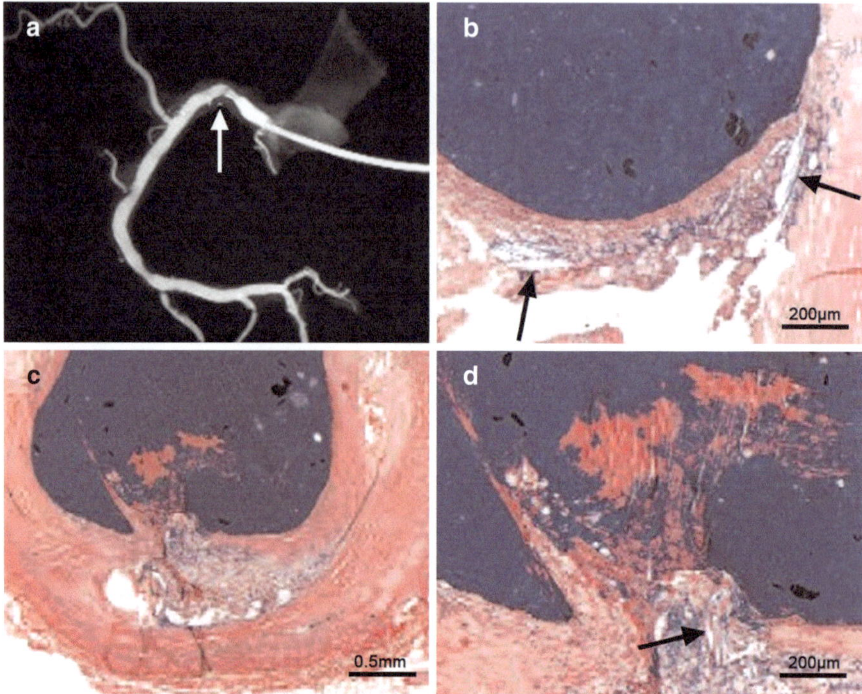

Fig. 9 Plaque rupture with parallel crystal formations. (**a**) Postmortem angiogram of right coronary artery from with plaque rupture (arrow) from a man who died suddenly. (**b**) Cholesterol crystals noted in the fibrous cap upstream from the rupture and (**c, d**) at the site of plaque rupture with an "explosive-like" ejection of cholesterol crystals. (Modified and reproduced with permission [69])

8 Crystal Induced Inflammation

Various inflammatory cells have been found in atherosclerotic plaques, the most prominent are monocytes and macrophages that eventually transform into foam cells as described earlier. Other inflammatory cells include lymphocytes and those have a role in activating an inflammatory response especially in plaque erosion [74, 75].

George Abela suggested that CCs could be acting as a source of inflammation similar to uric acid crystals in gout [76, 77] and in collaboration with Eike Latz, they demonstrated that CCs trigger the innate immune system causing an inflammation via the NLRP3 inflammasome similar to what has been described for uric acid crystals [5, 78–81]. This process involves the activation of caspase-1 that converts the stable precursor pro-IL-1β to active IL-1β and then leads to formation of IL6 that signals the liver to produce C-reactive protein. In fact, this inflammation by CCs can also be triggered via the compliment system as well [82] (Chapters "Atherosclerotic Plaque Morphology and the Conundrum of the Vulnerable Plaque" and "Infarction

Without Plaque Rupture"). In fact, a meta-analysis of patients with gout flares demonstrated that this was associated with subsequent cardiovascular events, suggesting a potentially similar mechanism for uric acid crystals in triggering inflammation and possible plaque injury with rupture as with cholesterol crystals [83].

9   Cholesterol Crystals Can Cause Distal Intimal Injury

Once an atherosclerotic plaque ruptures CCs are released into the arterial circulation where their sharp edges can cause direct endothelial damage. The risk of damage may be exaggerated by systemic blood pressure and rapid flow that together force the crystals to the margins of the lumen where they can scrape the endothelium and eventually become deposited [84]. Endothelial injury leading to arterial spasm may further promote distal ischemia [85–87] and increase the extent of end organ tissue injury.

In an earlier report the effect of CCs on the endothelium was tested in a dual vascular perfusion chamber using carotid and femoral arteries obtained from normal rabbits [84]. Vascular reactivity was monitored by an overhead digital camera attached to a computer system that measured vascular diameter of the arteries using an edge detection software. One chamber contained an artery exposed to circulating CCs while the second chamber had circulating microspheres in physiological normal saline solution or normal saline solution alone as controls. Arteries were pre-constricted with nor-epinephrine and then exposed to CCs, microspheres or physiologic buffered saline. Only the CCs exposed arteries remained significantly constricted after exposure to acetylcholine. Treatment with nitroprusside dilated all vessels to their original baseline demonstrating normal muscular function. Thus, only the arteries exposed to CCs had a significantly reduced response to acetyl choline indicating a loss of normal endothelial function and remained vasoconstricted while the controls responded normally and remained dilated (Chapter "Omega-3 Fatty Acids Influence Membrane Cholesterol Distribution and Crystal Formation in Models of Atherosclerosis", Fig. 2).

Scanning electron microscopy has also been used to examine arteries exposed to circulating CCs. These studies have demonstrated that CCs can become embedded in the intima and cause scraping injury as evidenced by tearing of the endothelial lining. In these studies, atomic microscopy of the arterial surface also demonstrated a significant increase in the roughness index of the crystal treated arteries [84]. Altogether, these findings suggest that the release of CCs during plaque rupture can cause direct endothelial injury and induce endothelial dysfunction and arterial vasospasm which together may lead to the no-reflow phenomenon often found following percutaneous coronary interventions and during myocardial infarction. A recent study in patients who had no-reflow following coronary intervention, CCs were found to be present in those culprit plaques by optical coherence tomography [87] (Chapter "In Vivo Detection of Cholesterol Crystals in Atherosclerotic Plaque with Optical Coherence Tomography").

10 Cholesterol Crystals Can Incite Inflammatory Muscle Injury

Release of large quantities of CCs into the arterial circulation can cause obstruction to the distal microvascular circulation leading to ischemic injury, and CCs that lodge in the tissues can trigger an inflammatory response that can cause further tissue damage (Chapter "Omega-3 Fatty Acids Influence Membrane Cholesterol Distribution and Crystal Formation in Models of Atherosclerosis"). In a study using a rabbit model, as well as a case report in a human heart at postmortem, it has been demonstrated that the release of CCs into the distal circulation resulted in muscle injury due to a crystal induced inflammatory response as evidenced by the presence of CCs in macrophages and by loss of striations in the myocytes consistent with muscle death [88, 89].

11 Gender Differences in Crystallization

The model of plaque rupture by expanding CCs during the crystallization may help explain some of the gender differences with symptomatology noted between men and women during acute cardiovascular events [30]. Specifically, women often have more generalized malaise and protracted symptom course while men have a more abrupt and severe onset of symptoms [90]. As mentioned earlier the larger the lipid core, the more rapid and greater the volume expansion [1, 2]. Studies using magnetic resonance angiography have demonstrated that men typically have a larger lipid pool in atherosclerotic plaques than women [91, 92]. This is probably related to a larger arterial space that accommodates a greater build up over time in men while women have the protective effect of estrogens that defers this process over time, at least by 10 years regarding acute cardiovascular events [93]. Therefore, the volume expansion is greater in men than in women leading to an acute rupture versus erosion that is more often seen in women [94]. This may translate to different symptomatology between the sexes because if the expansion is not large enough the crystals do not rupture the plaque but can perforate the intimal surface causing a slower thrombotic process and more protracted symptomatology. Thus, this could also explain why women have a higher mortality given that many may go unrecognized to having an acute cardiovascular event or do not seek medical attention (Fig. 10). Moreover, estrogens have been found to suppress cholesterol crystal volume expansion while testosterone did not [95].

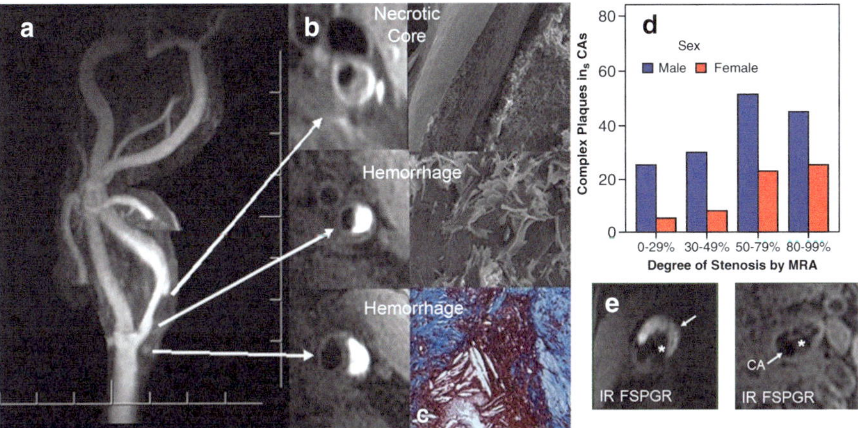

Fig. 10 Left carotid artery confirming intra-plaque hemorrhage by black-blood T1-weighted cross sectional images using 3D magnetization-prepared rapid acquisition gradient echo sequence, where the intra-plaque hemorrhage is bright. (**a**, **b**) Along the inferior aspect of the intra-plaque hemorrhage there is a 1 mm thick fibrous cap between the dark lumen and the bright deep intra-plaque hemorrhage. Superiorly there is a well-defined fibrous cap (<500 μm) between the lumen and lipid core. (**c**) Following endarterectomy, light and scanning electron microscopy demonstrate extensive cholesterol crystals with intra-plaque hemorrhage and thin fibrous cap. (**d**) Graphic demonstrates that for the same degree of stenosis on magnetic resonance angiography (MRA) males had more complex plaques (thin fibrous caps and larger lipid cores) than females. (**e**) A representative case of large hemorrhagic lipid rich necrotic core with a ruptured fibrous cap obtained from a male patient (left). A representative case of calcified plaque from a female patient (right). Area with hypointensity on contrast-enhanced T1-weighted and hyperintensity on inversion recovery fast spoiled gradient recalled indicates a hemorrhagic lipid-rich/necrotic core (arrows). *Lumen. (Modified and reproduced with permission [91, 92])

12 The Future

Appreciation and understanding how CC develop and act in the different stages of plaque development, inflammation, rupture, and thrombus formation may lead to the development of new diagnostic and therapeutic targets in patients with atherosclerosis. One of the many challenges is that CCs are small, and the process of crystallization is dynamic. Thus, understanding the potential role of CCs in the development and disruption of atherosclerotic plaque provides a new paradigm that provides an explanation for both direct mechanical and inflammatory injury of atherosclerotic plaque.

Currently there is no PET radioligand for imaging CCs [96], nuclear tracers specific to inflammation or other processes associated with cholesterol crystallization, however, radioactive labeled cholesterol has been used to track free cholesterol in plaque [97] and may be an approach to evaluate the crystallization process in vivo.

In addition, there is evidence that nano technology may also hold promise in the study of the evolving pathophysiology with the plaques to reduce CCs and inhibit inflammation [98, 99]. Therefore, further studies will likely be needed to understand crystal behavior in vivo under different circumstances.

13 Summary

Although CCs in atherosclerotic plaque were once viewed as inert bystanders, they are now recognized as central players in plaque development, growth, inflammation, and rupture. From this perspective atherosclerosis can be viewed as a disease driven by crystalloid formation that if left unchecked may lead to complications related to "death by crystallization." Efforts to reduce the development of CC formation and attenuate the inflammatory process they trigger have shown promise in retarding the progression of atherosclerosis, however, a significant treatment gap still exists and is the focus on ongoing research.

References

1. Abela GS, Aziz K. Cholesterol crystals cause mechanical damage to biological membranes: a proposed mechanism of plaque rupture and erosion leading to arterial thrombosis. Clin Cardiol. 2005;28:413–20.
2. Abela GS, Aziz K. Cholesterol crystals rupture biological membranes and human plaques during acute cardiovascular events: a novel inghight into plaque rupture by scanning electron microscopy. Scanning. 2006;28:1–10.
3. Hammer SS, Dorweiler TF, McFarland D, et al. Cholesterol crystal formation is a unifying pathogenic mechanism in the development of diabetic retinopathy. Diabetologia. 2023;66(9):1705–18.
4. El-Khatib LA, de Feijter-Rupp H, Janoudi A, Fry L, Kehdi M, Abela GS. Cholesterol induced heart valve inflammation and injury: efficacy of cholesterol lowering treatment. Open Heart. 2020;7:e001274.
5. Abela GS, Leja M, Janoudi A, Perry D, Richard J, De Feijter-Rupp H, Vanderberg A. Relationship between atherosclerosis and certain solid cancer tumors. J Am Coll Cardiol. 2019;73(9 Suppl 1):156.
6. Glagov S, Weisenberg E, Zarins CK, Stankunavicius R, Kolettis GJ. Compensatory enlargement of human atherosclerotic coronary arteries. N Engl J Med. 1987;316:1371–5.
7. Nissen SE, Yock P. Intravascular ultrasound: novel pathophysiological insights and current clinical applications. Circulation. 2001;103:604–16.
8. Henney AM, Wakeley PR, Davies MJ, Foster K, Hembry R, Murphy G, Humphries S. Localization of stromelysin gene expression in atherosclerotic plaques by in situ hybridization. Proc Natl Acad Sci U S A. 1991;88:8154–8.
9. Galis ZS, Khatri JJ. Matrix metalloproteinases in vascular remodeling and atherogenesis: the good, the bad and the ugly. Circ Res. 2002;90:251–62.
10. Loree HM, Kamm RD, Stringfellow RG, Lee RT. Effects of fibrous cap thickness on peak circumferential stress in model atherosclerotic vessels. Circ Res. 1992;71:850–8.

11. Little WC, Constantinescu M, Applegate RJ, Kutcher MA, Burrows MT, Kahl FR, Santamore WP. Can coronary angiography predict the site of a subsequent myocardial infarction in patients with mild-to-moderate coronary artery disease? Circulation. 1986;78:1157.
12. Nobuyoshi M, Tanaka M, Nosaka H, Kimura T, Yokoi H, Hamasaki N, Kim K, Shindo T, Kimura K. Progression of coronary atherosclerosis: is coronary spasm related to progression? J Am Coll Cardiol. 1991;18:904–10. https://doi.org/10.1016/0735-1097.
13. Falk E, Shah PK, Fuster V. Coronary plaque disruption. Circulation. 1995;92:657–71. https://doi.org/10.1161/01.cir.92.3.657.91)90745-u.
14. Ambrose JA, Tannenbaum MA, Alexopoulos D, Hjemdahl-Morsen CE, Leavy J, Weiss M, Borrico S, Gorlin R, Fuster V. Angiographic progression of coronary artery disease and the development of myocardial infarction. J Am Coll Cardiol. 1988;12:56–62.
15. Giroud D, Li JM, Meier B, Rutishauer W. Relation of the site of acute myocardial infarction to the most severe coronary arterial stenosis at prior angiography. Am J Cardiol. 1992;69:729–32. https://doi.org/10.1016/0002-9149(92)90495-k.
16. Stone GW, Maehara A, Lansky AJ, de Bruyne B, Cristea E, Mintz G, Mehran R, McPherson J, Farhat N, Marso SP, Parise H, Templin B, for the PROSPECT Investigators. A prospective natural-history study of coronary atherosclerosis. N Engl J Med. 2011;364:226–35.
17. Constantinides P. Plaque fissures in human coronary thrombosis. J Atheroscler Res. 1996;6:1–17.
18. Davies MJ, Thomas AC. Plaque fissuring: the cause of acute myocardial infarction causing sudden ischaemic death, and crecendo angina. Br Heart J. 1985;53:363–73.
19. Steffel J, Luscher TF, Tanner FC. Tissue factor in cardiovascular diseases: molecular mechanism and clinical implications. Circulation. 2006;113:722–31. https://doi.org/10.1161/CIRCULATIONAHA.105.567297.
20. DeWood MA, Spores J, Notske R, Mouser LT, Burroughs R, Golden MS, Lang HT. Prevalence of total coronary occlusion during the early hours of transmural myocardial infarction. N Engl J Med. 1980;303:897–902. https://doi.org/10.1056/NEJM198010163031601.
21. Sherman CT, Litvack F, Grundfest W, et al. Coronary angioscopy in patients with unstable angina pectoris. N Engl J Med. 1986;315:913–9.
22. Muller JE, Abela GS, Nesto RW, Tofler GH. Triggers, acute risk factors and vulnerable plaques: the lexicon of a new frontier. J Am Coll Cardiol. 1994;23:809–13. https://doi.org/10.1016/0735-1097(94)90772-2.
23. Schaar JA, Muller JE, Falk E, et al. Terminology for high-risk and vulnerable coronary artery plaques. Eur Heart J. 2004;25:1077–82.
24. Janoudi A, Shamoun FE, Kalavakunta JK, Abela GS. Cholesterol crystal induced arterial inflammation and destabilization of atherosclerotic plaque. Eur Heart J. 2016;37:1959–67. https://doi.org/10.1093/eurheartj/ehv653.
25. Kolodgie FD, Burke AP, Nakazawa G, Cheng Q, Xu X, Virmani R. Free cholesterol in atherosclerotic plaques: where does it come from? Curr Opin Lipidol. 2007;18:500–7.
26. Small DM. George Lyman Duff memorial lecture. Progression and regression of atherosclerotic lesions. Insights from lipid physical biochemistry. Arterioscler Thromb Vasc Biol. 1988;8:103–29.
27. Guyton JR, Klemp KF. Transitional features in human atherosclerosis: intimal thickening, cholesterol clefts, and cell loss in human aortic fatty streaks. Am J Pathol. 1993;143:1444–57.
28. Virmani R, Kolodgie FD, Burke AP, Farb A, Schwartz SM. Lessons from sudden coronary death: a comprehensive morphological classification scheme for atherosclerotic lesions. Arterioscler Thromb Vasc Biol. 2000;20:1262–75. https://doi.org/10.1161/01.atv.20.5.1262.
29. Nasiri M, Janoudi A, Vanderberg AFM, Flegler C, Flegler S, Abela GS. Role of cholesterol crystals in atherosclerosis is unmasked by altering tissue preparation methods. Microsc Res Tech. 2015;78:969–74. https://doi.org/10.1002/jemt.22560.
30. Abela GS. Cholesterol crystals piercing the arterial plaque and intima trigger local and systemic inflammation. J Clin Lipidol. 2010;4:156–64. https://doi.org/10.1016/j.jacl.2010.03.003.

31. Muller JE, Tofler GH, Stone PH. Circadian variation and triggers of onset of acute cardiovascular disease. Circulation. 1989;79:733–43.
32. Libby P. Inflammation in atherosclerosis. Arterioscler Thromb Vasc Biol. 2012;32:2045–51. https://doi.org/10.1161/ATVBAHA.108.179705.
33. Virchow R. Cellular pathology as based upon physiological and pathological histology (translated by frank chance from 2nd German edition). London: John Churchill; 1860. p. 360.
34. Ross R. Atherosclerosis: an inflammatory disease. N Engl J Med. 1999;340:115–26.
35. Libby P. The changing landscape of atherosclerosis. Nature. 2021;592:524. https://doi.org/10.1038/s41586-021-03392-8.
36. Galis ZS, Sukhova GK, Lark MW, Libby P. Increased expression of matrix metalloproteinases and matrix degrading activity in vulnerable regions of human atherosclerotic plaques. J Clin Invest. 1994;94:2494–503. https://doi.org/10.1172/JCI117619.
37. Lendon CL, Davies MJ, Born GV, Richardson PD. Atherosclerotic plaque caps are locally weakened when macrophages density is increased. Atherosclerosis. 1991;87(1):87–90.
38. Naghavi M, Libby P, Falk E, et al. From the vulnerable plaque to the vulnerable patient. Circulation. 2003;108:1664–72.
39. Goldstein JA, Demetriou D, Grines CL, Pica M, Shoukfeh M, O'Neill WW. Multiple complex coronary plaques in patients with acute myocardial infarction. N Engl J Med. 2000;343:915–22.
40. Rossi A, Franceschini L, Fusaro M, et al. Carotid atherosclerotic plaque instability in patients with acute myocardial infarction. Int J Cardiol. 2006;111:263–6.
41. Barger AC, Beeuwkes R 3rd, Lainey LL, Silverman KJ. Hypothesis: vasa vasorum and neovascularization of human coronary arteries. A possible role in the pathophysiology of atherosclerosis. N Engl J Med. 1984;310:175–7.
42. MacIsaac AI, Thomas JD, Topol EJ. Towards the quiescent coronary plaque. JACC. 1993;22:1228–41.
43. Casscells W, Hathorn B, David M, Krabach T, Vaughn WK, McAllister HA, Bearman G, Willerson JT. Thermal detection of cellular infiltrates in living atherosclerotic plaques: possible implication of thermal detection of cellular infiltrates in living atherosclerotic plaques: possible implications for plaque rupture and thrombosis. Lancet. 1996;347(9013):1422–3.
44. Kellner-Weibel G, Jerome WG, et al. Effect of intracellular free cholesterol accumulation on macrophage viability: a model for foam cell death. Arterioscler Thromb Vasc Biol. 1998;18:423–31.
45. Geng Y-J, Phillips JE, Mason RP, Casscells SW. Cholesterol crystallization and macrophage apoptosis: implication for atherosclerotic plaque instability and rupture. Biochem Pharmacol. 2003;66:1485–92.
46. Shi C, Kim T, Steiger S, Mulay SR, Klinkhammer BM, Bäuerle T, Melica ME, Romagnani P, Möckel D, Baues M, Yang L, Brouns SLN, Heemskerk JWM, Braun A, Lammers T, Boor P, Anders H-J. Crystal clots as therapeutic target in cholesterol crystal embolism. Circ Res. 2020;126:e37–52.
47. Aschoff A. Zur Morphologie der lipoiden Substanzen. Über Entwicklungs-Wachstums-und Altersvorgänge an den Gefäßen. Path Anat. 1909;47:1.
48. Kramsch DM, Franzblau C, Hollander W. The protein and lipid composition of arterial elastin and its relationship to lipid accumulation in the atherosclerotic plaque. J Clin Invest. 1971;50:1660–77.
49. Fantini J, Barrantes FJ. How cholesterol interacts with membrane proteins: an exploration of cholesterol-binding sites including CRAC, CARC, and tilted domains. Front Physiol. 2013;4:31. https://doi.org/10.3389/fphys.2013.00031.
50. Fahed AC, Sfa RM, Haddad FF, Bitar FF, Andary RR, Arabi MT, Azar ST, Nemer G. Homozygous familial hypercholesterolemia in Lebanon: a genotype/phenotype correlation. Mol Genet Metab. 2011;102:181–8.

51. Baumer Y, McCurdy S, Weatherby TM, Mehta NN, Halvherr S, Halbherr P, Yamazaki N, Boisvert WA. Hyperlipideia-induced cholesterol crystal production by endothelial cells promotes atherogenesis. Nat Commun. 2017;8:1129.

52. Mason RP, Jacob RF. Membrane microdomains and vascular biology emerging role in atherogenesis. Circulation. 2003;107:2270–3.

53. Samstad EO, Niyonzima N, Nymo S, Aune MH, Ryan L, Bakke SS, Lappegård KT, Brekke OL, Lambris JD, Damås JK, Latz E, Mollnes TE, Espevik T. Cholesterol crystals induce complement-dependent inflammasome activation and cytokine release. J Immunol. 2014;192:2837–45. https://doi.org/10.4049/jimmunol.1302484.

54. Varsano N, Fargion I, Wolf SG, Leiserowitz L, Addadi L. Formation of 3D cholesterol crystals from 2D nucleation sites in lipid bilayer membranes: implications for atherosclerosis. J Am Chem Soc. 2015;137:1601–7.

55. Vedre A, Pathak DR, Crimp M, Lum C, Koochesfahani M, Abela GS. Physical factors that trigger cholesterol crystallization leading to plaque rupture. Atherosclerosis. 2008;203:89–96.

56. Abela GS, Aziz K, Vedre A, Pathak D, Talbott JD, DeJong J. Effect of cholesterol crystals on plaques and intima in arteries of patients with acute coronary and cerebrovascular syndromes. Am J Cardiol. 2009;103:959–68.

57. Abela GS, Kalavakunta JK, Janoudi A, Leffler D, Dhar G, Salehi N, Cohn J, Shah I, Karve M, Kotaru VPK, Gupta V, David S, Narisetty KK, Rich M, Vanderberg A, Pathak DR, Shamoun FE. Frequency of cholesterol crystals in culprit coronary artery aspirate during acute myocardial infarction and their relation to inflammation and myocardial injury. Am J Cardiol. 2017;120:1699–707. https://doi.org/10.1016/j.amjcard.2017.07.075.

58. Patel R, Janoudi A, Vedre A, Aziz K, Tamhane U, Rubinstein J, Abela OG, Berger K, Abela GS. Plaque rupture and thrombosis is reduced by lowering cholesterol levels and crystallization with ezetimibe and is correlated with FDG-PET. Arterioscler Thromb Vasc Biol. 2011;31:2007–14.

59. Xu J, Lu X, Shi G-P. Vasa Vasorum in atherosclerosis and clinical significance. Int J Mol Sci. 2015;16:11574–608. https://doi.org/10.3390/ijms160511574.

60. Dunmore BJ, McCarthy MJ, Naylor AR, Brindle NP. Carotid plaque instability and ischemic symptoms are linked to immaturity of microvessels within plaques. J Vasc Surg. 2007;45:155–9.

61. Kaartinen M, Penttila A, Kovanen PT. Mast cells accompany microvessels in human coronary atheromas: implications for intimal neovascularization and hemorrhage. Atherosclerosis. 1996;123:123–31.

62. Zemplenyi T, Crawford DW, Cole MA. Adaptation to arterial wall hypoxia demonstrated in vivo with oxygen microcathodes. Atherosclerosis. 1989;76:173–9.

63. Al-Handawi MB, Commins P, Prasad Karothu D, Raj G, Li L, Naumov P. Mechanical and crystallographic analysis of cholesterol crystals puncturing biological membranes. Chem A Eur J. 2018;24:11493–7.

64. Lundber B. Chemical composition and physical state of lipid deposits in atherosclerosis. Atherosclerosis. 1985;56:93–110.

65. Jandacek RJ, Webb MR, Mattson FH. Effect of an aqueous phase on the solubility of cholesterol in an oil phase. J Lipid Res. 1977;18:203–10.

66. Luo Y, et al. Modeling of mechanical stress exerted by cholesterol crystallization on atherosclerotic plaques. PloS One. 2016;11(5):e0155117. https://doi.org/10.1371/journal.pone.0155117.

67. Davies MJ, Richardson PD, Woolf N, Katz DR, Mann J. Risk of thrombosis in human atherosclerotic plaques—role of extracellular lipid, macrophage, and smooth-muscle cell content. Br Heart J. 1993;69(5):377–81. PMID: 8518056.

68. Richardson PD, Davies MJ, Born GVR. Influence of plaque configuration and stress-distribution on fissuring of Coronary atherosclerotic plaques. Lancet. 1989;2(8669):941–4. PMID: 2571862.

69. Frink RJ. Parallel cholesterol crystals: a sign of impending plaque rupture? J Invasive Cardiol. 2010;22(9):406–11. PMID: 20814046.
70. Qin Z, Cao M, Xi X, Zhang Y, Wang Z, Zhao S, Tian Y, Xu Q, Yu H, Tian J, Yu B. Cholesterol crystals in non-culptrin plaques of STEMI patients: a 3-vessel OCT study. Int J Cardiol. 2022;364:162. https://doi.org/10.1016/j.ijcard.2022.06.016.
71. Tofler GH, Brezinski D, Schafer AI, Czeisler CA, Rutherford JD, Wilich SN, Gleason SN, Williams GH, Muller JE. Current morning increase in platelet aggregability and the risk of myocardial infarction and sudden death. N Engl J Med. 1987;316:1514–8.
72. Gerber Y, Jacobsen SJ, Killian JM, Weston SA, Roger VL. Seasonability and daily weather conditions in relation to myocardial infarction and sudden cardiac death in Olmsted County, Minnesota 1979 to 2002. J Am Coll Cardiol. 2006;48:287–92.
73. Franklin BA, George P, Henry R, Gordon S, Timmis GC, O'Neill WW. Acute myocardial infarction after manual or automated snow removal. Am J Cardiol. 2001;87:1282–3.
74. Li J, Ley K. Lymphocyte migration into atherosclerotic plaque. Arterioscler Thromb Vasc Biol. 2015;35(1):40–9. https://doi.org/10.1161/ATVBAHA.114.303227.
75. Leistner DM, Kränkel N, Meteva D, Abdelwahed YS, Seppelt C, Stähli BE, Rai H, Skurk C, Lauten A, Mochmann H-C, Fröhlich G, Rauch-Kröhnert U, Flores E, Riedel M, Sieronski L, Kia S, Strässler E, Haghikia A, Dirks F, Steiner JK, Mueller DN, Volk H-D, Klotsche J, Joner M, Libby P, Landmesser U. Differential immunological signature at the culprit site distinguishes acute coronary syndrome with intact from acute coronary syndrome with ruptured fibrous cap: results from the prospective translational OPTICO-ACS study. Eur Heart J. 2020;41:3549–60. https://doi.org/10.1093/eurheartj/ehaa703.
76. Cardiosource American College of Cardiology: Annual Scientific Session 2006 March 11–14. Atlanta GA. Plaque Rupture by Cholesterol Crystallization—A Novel Concept for Acute Coronary Syndrome: Interviewee: George S. Abela, MD, FACC; Interviewer: C Richard Conti, MD, MACC.
77. Abela GS, Aziz K. Plaques are ruptured by cholesterol crystals during myocardial infarction. Scanning. 2006;28:59.
78. Düewell P, Kono H, Rayner KJ, Sirois CM, Vladimer G, Bauernfeind FG, Abela GS, Franchi L, Nuñez G, Schnurr M, Espevik T, Lien E, Fitzgerald KA, Rock KL, Moore KJ, Wright SD, Hornung V, Latz E. NLRP3 inflammasomes are required for atherogenesis and activated by cholesterol crystals. Nature. 2010;464:1357–61. https://doi.org/10.1038/nature08938.
79. Rajamaki K, Lappalainen J, Oorni K, Valimaki E, Matikainen S, Kovanen PT, Eklund KK. Cholesterol crystals activate the NLRP3 inflammasome in human macrophages: a novel link between cholesterol metabolism and inflammation. PloS One. 2010;5(7):e11765. https://doi.org/10.1371/journal.pone.0011765.
80. Martinon F, Pétrilli V, Mayor A, Tardivel A, Tschopp J. Gout-associated uric acid crystals activate the NALP3 inflammasome. Nature. 2006;440(7081):237–41. https://doi.org/10.1038/nature04516.
81. Grebe A, Latz E. Cholesterol crystals and inflammation. Curr Rheumatol Rep. 2013;15(3):313. https://doi.org/10.1007/s11926-012-0313-z.
82. Nidorf SM, Fiolet A, Abela GS. Viewing atherosclerosis through a crystal lens: how the evolving sturture of cholesterol crystals in atheroscleritc plaque alters its stability. J Clin Lipidol. 2020;14:619–30.
83. Cipolletta E, Tata LJ, Nakafero G, Avery AJ, Mamas MA, Abhishek A. Association between gout flare and subsequent cardiovascular events. JAMA. 2022;328:440–50. https://doi.org/10.1001/jama.2022.11390.
84. Gadeela N, Rubinstein J, Tamhane U, Huang R, Pathak DR, Hosein HA, Rich M, Dhar G, Abela GS. The impact of circulating cholesterol crystals on vasomotor function: implications for no-reflow phenomenon. JACC Cardiovasc Interv. 2011;4:521–9. https://doi.org/10.1016/j.jcin.2011.02.010.
85. Fuster V, Stein B, Ambrose JA, Badimon L, Badimon JJ, Chesebro JH. Atherosclerotic plaque rupture and thrombosis. Evolving concepts. Circulation 1990;82(3 Suppl):II47-59. Coronary

artery spasm. Multiple causes and multiple roles in heart disease. Biochem Pharmacol. 1995;30(49):859–71.

86. Kalsner S, Coronary artery spasm. Multiple causes and multiple roles in heart disease. Biochem Pharmacol. 1995;49:859–71. https://doi.org/10.1016/0006-2952(94)00447-t.

87. Katayama Y, Taruya A, Kashiwagi M, Ozaki Y, Shiono Y, Tanimoto T, Yoshikawa T, Kondo T, Tanaka A. No-reflow phenomenon and in vivo cholesterol crystals combined with lipid core in acute myocardial infarction. Int J Cardiol Heart Vasculature. 2022;38:100953. https://doi.org/10.1016/j.ijcha.2022.100953.

88. Pervaiz MH, Durga S, Ianoudi A, Berger K, Abela GS. PET/CTA detection of muscle inflammation related to cholesterol crystal emboli without arterial obstruction. J Nucl Cardiol. 2018;25:433–40. https://doi.org/10.1007/s12350-017-0826-y.67.

89. Yutani C, Nagano T, Komatsu S, Kodama. Visible-free cholesterol crystal emboli adjacent to microinfarcts in myocardial capillaries and arterioles on H&E—stained frozen sections of an autopsied patient. BMJ Case Rep. 2018;2018:bcr2018225558. https://doi.org/10.1136/bcr-2018-225558.

90. Dey S, Flather MD, Devlin G, et al. Global registry of acute coronary events investigators: sex-related differences in the presentation, treatment and outcomes among patients with acute coronary syndromes: the global registry of acute coronary events. Heart. 2009;95(1):20–6.

91. Mughal MM, Khan MK, DeMarco JK, Majid A, Shamoun F, Abela GS. Symptomatic and asymptomatic carotid artery plaque. Expert Rev Cardiovasc Ther. 2011;9:1315–30.

92. Ota H, Reeves MJ, Zhu DC, et al. Sex differences in patients with asymptomatic carotid atherosclerotic plaque: in vivo 3.0-T magnetic resonance study. Stroke. 2010;41:1630–5.

93. Bots SH, Peteres SAE, Woodward M. Sex differences in coronary heart disease and stroke mortality: a global assessment of the effect of ageing between 1980 and 2010. BMJ Glob Health. 2017;2:e000298. https://doi.org/10.1136/bmjgh-2017-000298.

94. Arbustini E, Dal Bello B, Morbini P, et al. Plaque erosion is a major substrate for coronary thrombosis in acute myocardial infarction. Heart. 1999;82:269–72.

95. Wang E, Al-Abcha A, Osman H, Oladeji A, Boumegouas M, Abela GS. The effect of estrogen and testosterone on cholesterol crystallization. J Clin Lipidol. 2022;16(3):e75–6. https://doi.org/10.1016/j.jacl.2022.05.063.

96. Evans NR, Tarkin JM, Chowdhury MM, Warburton EA, Rudd JHF. PET imaging of atherosclerotic disease: advancing plaque assessment from anatomy to pathophysiology. Curr Atheroscler Rep. 2016;18(6):30. https://doi.org/10.1007/s11883-016-0584-3.

97. Couto RD, Dallan LAO, Lisboa LAF, Mesquita CH, Vinagre CGC, Maranhão RC. Deposition of free cholesterol in the blood vessels of patients with coronary artery disease. A possible novel mechanism for atherogenesis. Lipids. 2007;42:411–8.

98. Luo Y, Guo Y, Wang H, Yu M, Hong K, Li D, Li R, Wen B, Hu D, Chang L, Zhang J, Yang B, Sun D, Schwendeman AS, Chen YE. Phospholipid nanoparticles: therapeutic potentials against atherosclerosis via reducing cholesterol crystals and inhibiting inflammation. EBioMed. 2021;74:103725. https://doi.org/10.1016/j.ebiom.2021.103725.

99. Flores AM, Hosseini-Nassab N, Jarr KU, Ye J, Zhu X, Wirka R, Koh AL, Tsantilas P, Wang Y, Nanda V, Kojima Y, Zeng Y, Lotfi M, Sinclair R, Weissman IL, Ingelsson E, Smith BR, Leeper NJ. Pro-efferocytic nanoparticles are specifically taken up by lesional macrophages and prevent atherosclerosis. Nat Nanotechnol. 2020;15:154–61. Epub 2020 Jan 27. https://doi.org/10.1038/s41565-019-0619-3.

100. Abela GS, Eisenberg JD, Mittleman M, Nesto RW, Leeman D, Zarich S, Waxman S, Prieto A, Manzo KS. Detecting and differentiating white from red coronary thrombus by angiography in angina pectoris and in acute myocardial infarction. Am J Cardiol. 1999;83:94–7.

101. Seeger JM, Abela GS. Angioscopy as an adjunct to arterial reconstructive surgery. J Vasc Surg. 1986;4:315–20.

Infarction Without Plaque Rupture

Rocco Vergallo and Filippo Crea

1 Introduction

For decades, we have known from autopsy studies that the proximate cause of most acute myocardial infarctions (AMIs) is an occlusive thrombosis caused by the frank rupture of a lipid-rich plaque, responsible for approximately two third of cases [1–4]. Subsequent studies revealed other plaque morphologies at the basis of AMI, including plaque erosion and eruptive calcified nodule. Mounting evidence supports the concept that these morphologic substrates are separate entities, with distinct pathogenesis, clinical presentation, and prognosis [5–10]. Yet, when patients with AMI present to the emergency department, we still triage them exclusively based on the presence or absence of ST-segment elevation on electrocardiogram and/or on troponin levels, assess them using coronary angiography, and manage them almost invariably with percutaneous coronary intervention (PCI) [11, 12]. The advent of intravascular imaging, including intravascular ultrasound (IVUS) and optical coherence tomography (OCT), has allowed us to fill these gaps in knowledge, providing new insights into the pathogenesis of AMI in vivo, and yielding a contemporary snapshot of the relative prevalence of these different substrates (Fig. 1) [5, 10]. Recent studies suggest that plaque erosion is responsible for more than one third of

R. Vergallo
Department of Cardiovascular Medicine, Fondazione Policlinico Universitario A. Gemelli IRCCS, Rome, Italy
e-mail: rocco.vergallo@unicatt.it

F. Crea (✉)
Department of Cardiovascular and Pneumological Sciences, Catholic University of the Sacred Heart, Rome, Italy
e-mail: filippo.crea@unicatt.it

G. S. Abela, S. M. Nidorf (eds.), *Cholesterol Crystals in Atherosclerosis and Other Related Diseases*, Contemporary Cardiology,
https://doi.org/10.1007/978-3-031-41192-2_11

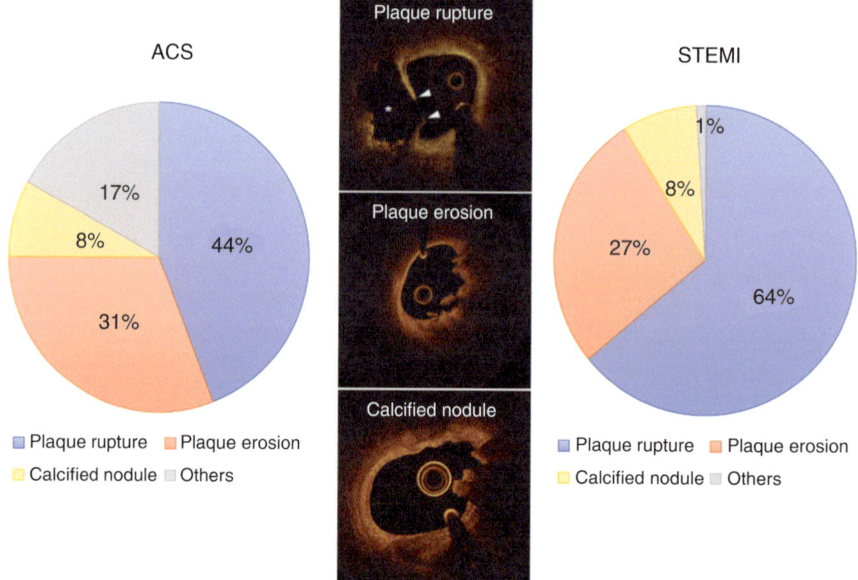

Fig. 1 Prevalence of different culprit plaque phenotypes by intracoronary OCT. Plaque rupture represents the most frequent culprit plaque morphology in patients with ACS, with a prevalence ranging between approximately 45% to 65% based on the clinical presentation (all ACS versus STEMI only). Other culprit plaque morphologies, responsible for about 35% to 55% of cases, include plaque erosion (~30%), calcified nodule (~8%), and others (e.g., spontaneous coronary artery dissection, intraplaque hemorrhage, etc.). (Adapted from Jia et al. J Am Coll Cardiol, 2013;62:1748–1758; and Higuma et al. JACC Cardiovasc Interv 2015;8:1166–1176)

ACS cases, and its prevalence seems to be on the rise probably related to the ongoing modifications of the cardiovascular risk profile of patients, as well as to the efficacy of the contemporary preventive measures (e.g., aggressive lipid-lowering therapies, anti-hypertensive treatments, etc.), which are actively altering the atherosclerotic disease phenotype in humans [13, 14]. Furthermore, initial clinical data suggest that a strategy of potent antithrombotic therapy may stabilize patients with plaque erosion without the need for coronary stenting [15, 16]. While the prognosis of patients with plaque erosion seems to be favorable, patients with AMI caused by a eruptive calcified nodule appears to have a worse clinical outcome, and to respond less favorably to PCI. Cholesterol crystals, by both exacerbating local and systemic inflammation associated with atherosclerosis and directly damaging or perforating the intimal surface of a plaque, may be a key factor not only in the pathogenesis of plaque rupture, but also in that of other culprit plaque morphologies [17, 18]. In this chapter, we will examine the pathobiology, in vivo diagnosis and clinical outcome of patients with AMI without plaque rupture, with particular regard to plaque erosion and eruptive calcified nodule, as well as to other less frequent morphological substrates.

2 Plaque Erosion

2.1 Pathobiology of Plaque Erosion

Coronary thrombosis generated by plaque rupture derives from the contact of the flowing blood with the highly-thrombogenic lipidic core and with tissue factor expressed by macrophages, a cell type that is predominant in plaques typically complicated by fibrous cap disruption [19, 20]. In sharp contrast, altered endothelial shear stress, up-regulation of Toll-like receptor 2, platelet activation, and endothelial denudation followed by luminal thrombosis seem to be the main underlying mechanisms in plaque erosion [19–21] (Fig. 2). Recently, mounting evidence suggests the presence of an alteration of hyaluronan metabolism in patients with AMI

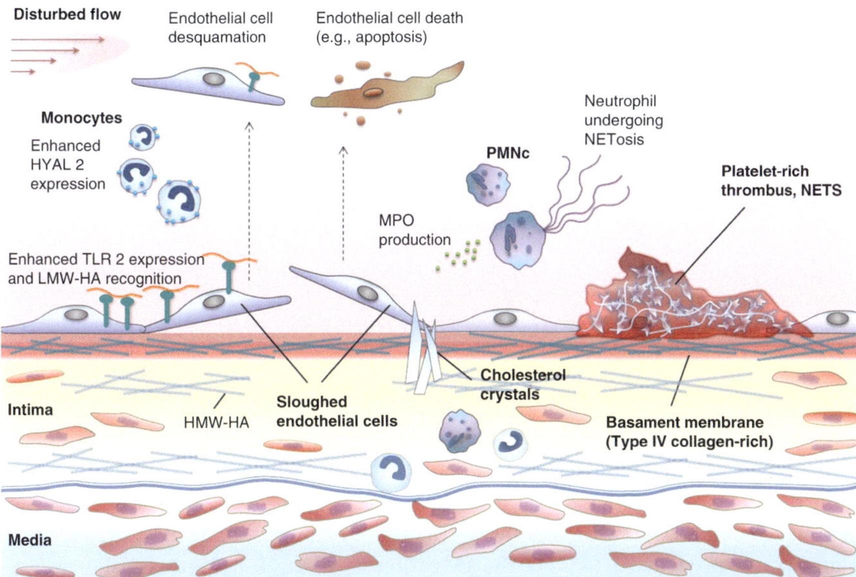

Fig. 2 Pathophysiology of plaque erosion. An overexpression of hyaluronidase 2 (HYAL 2) in peripheral blood mononuclear cell is observed under conditions of altered shear stress. By degrading high-molecular-weight hyaluronan into its proinflammatory 20-kDa isoform, HYAL 2 triggers endothelial cell activation/desquamation and neutrophil recruitment. Neutrophils, in turn, produce web-like structures known as neutrophil extracellular traps (NETs), which entrap platelets and fibrin strands, amplifying thrombus formation. In addition, polymorphonucleates (PMN) also produce myeloperoxidase (MPO), which generates hypochlorous acid exacerbating endothelial cell desquamation and determining apoptosis. Cholesterol crystals can produce plaque volume expansion tearing the fibrous cap and perforating the intima and the endothelium, providing an additional stimulus to thrombus formation. HYAL 2, hyaluronidase 2; TLR 2, toll-like receptor 2; HMW-HA, high-molecular-weight hyaluronan; LMW-HA, low-molecular-weight hyaluronan; MPO, myeloperoxidase; PMN, polymorphonucleates; NETs, neutrophil extracellular traps. (Modified from Vergallo et al. Atherosclerosis 2021;318:45–51)

caused by plaque erosion. Specifically, recent studies demonstrated that genes of hyaluronidase 2 (HYAL2), an enzyme degrading high-molecular-weight hyaluronan into its proinflammatory 20-kDa isoform, and of a specific splicing variant of hyaluronan receptor (i.e., CD44v6) are significantly more expressed in patients with plaque erosion than in those with plaque rupture [9]. The activation of platelets by collagen determines their degranulation with subsequent release of preformed mediators, including proinflammatory cytokines (e.g., CD40L) and chemoattractant (e.g., RANTES) [22, 23]. Neutrophils recruited at the site of plaque erosion produce web-like structures known as neutrophil extracellular traps (NETs), which sustain and amplify thrombosis by entrapping platelets and fibrin strands. Neutrophils also produce myeloperoxidase (MPO), which in turn generates hypochlorous acid exacerbating endothelial cell desquamation and inducing apoptosis [23–26]. Plaque underlying endothelial erosion often contains a necrotic core, which is typically smaller than in plaque rupture. Several local factors can modify the physical status of cholesterol within the necrotic core, including a high saturation, a reduction in temperature, a shift to an alkaline pH and hydration of the cholesterol molecule, favoring its crystallization to a solid state (i.e., cholesterol crystals) [17, 18, 27]. This in turn produce plaque volume expansion that, in the case of plaque fissure, can tear the fibrous cap, determining a frank rupture in the presence of a large lipid pool [28, 29]. In the setting of plaque erosion the role of cholesterol crystallization is less well known although it might contribute to cause endothelial damage (Fig. 2) [17, 18].

2.2 *In Vivo Diagnosis of Plaque Erosion by Intracoronary Imaging*

The advent of intravascular OCT imaging with its unprecedented resolution (10–20 µm), allowed the detection of plaque microstructures including fibrous cap, lipid pool, cholesterol crystals, microchannels, macrophage accumulation, and healing tissue [5, 6, 30–33], and most importantly enabled the in vivo diagnosis of plaque erosion (Fig. 3) [4]. As the detection of a single endothelial layer (i.e., 1–5 µm) is below the OCT resolution, the in vivo diagnosis of plaque erosion is a diagnosis of exclusion [5]. The detection of a fibrous cap without any sign of interruption (i.e., intact fibrous cap) at the culprit lesion differentiates plaque erosion from plaque rupture. When a plaque rupture is present, OCT typically shows a frank discontinuity of the fibrous cap with a communication between plaque cavity and lumen [5, 6]. In contrast, the absence of fibrous cap disruption at the culprit lesion suggests the presence of plaque erosion, in particular if white thrombus and/or irregular intimal surface are detected [5]. When erythrocyte-rich, red thrombus is

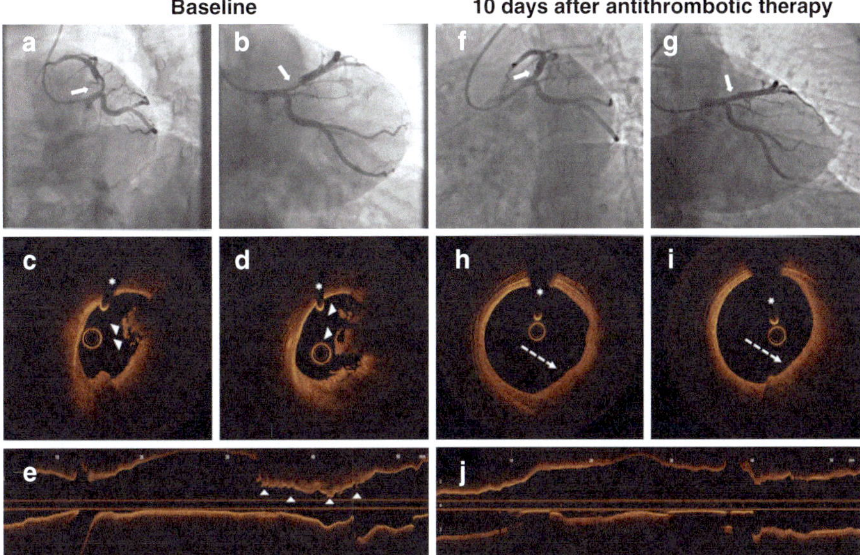

Fig. 3 Representative case of plaque erosion treated conservatively with medical therapy. A 44-year-old man, active smoker, was admitted to the emergency department with a diagnosis of antero-lateral STEMI. Emergency coronary angiography showed a thrombotic lesion of the proximal LAD (**a**, **b**, arrows). OCT imaging disclosed the presence of plaque erosion with large thrombus burden (**c–e**, arrowheads). Thrombus aspiration was performed without stent implantation, and potent antithrombotic therapy with aspirin, ticagrelor, and unfractionated heparin was started. After 10 days of medical therapy, control coronary angiography showed a complete resolution of coronary thrombosis (**f**, **g**, arrows), which was confirmed by OCT imaging, which disclosed the presence of a fibrous plaque without any evidence of fibrous cap disruption or residual thrombus (**h–j**, arrows). Asterisks correspond to wire artifacts

present, which attenuates the OCT light generating a backward shadow, the diagnosis of plaque erosion becomes less definite, but still remains probable if a fibrous cap discontinuity is not evident [5]. OCT imaging studies showed that plaque erosion has an underlying fibrous plaque phenotype in about 60% of cases, while an underlying lipid plaque is present in about 40% of cases [5]. However, lipid burden is significantly smaller in plaque erosion than in plaque rupture, and the prevalence of underlying thin-cap fibroatheroma (TCFA) significantly is lower. While red thrombus is more frequently detected over plaque rupture, white thrombus is the prevalent type of thrombus observed in plaque erosion [5]. A recent OCT study showed the presence of cholesterol crystals in about 35% of culprit plaque erosions (significantly more frequent than in non-culprit plaques), supporting their potential role in the pathogenesis of this plaque complication [34].

2.3 Predictors of Plaque Erosion

Plaque erosion has traditionally been considered a disease of young women with smoking habits. This notion was ascertained from pathological studies in victims of sudden cardiac death (SCD) during the past decades, and thus did not reflect the active change in the cardiovascular risk profile and demographics of ACS patients of the recent years [1–3]. In a contemporary registry of 442 subjects with SCD, plaque erosion was more frequently observed in young victims, independent of sex [35], and a number of OCT investigations confirmed the preferential occurrence of plaque erosion in younger patients, as compared with plaque rupture [5, 36]. In a recent study evaluating the predictors of plaque erosion, an age < 68 years was an independent predictor [odds ratio (OR): 1.56; 95% confidence interval (95% CI): 1.16–2.09] [37]. In this study, most conventional cardiovascular risk factors, such as diabetes mellitus, dyslipidemia, chronic kidney disease, hypertension were less frequent in patients with plaque erosion than in those with plaque rupture [38]. At multivariate analysis, absence of diabetes [OR 1.47 (95% CI: 1.06–1.86), $p = 0.02$] and normal renal function [OR 1.97 (95% CI: 1.32–2.95) $p < 0.001$] were independent predictors of plaque erosion [37]. With regard to the clinical presentations, OCT studies consistently showed a stronger association of plaque erosion with non-ST-segment elevation ACS (NSTE-ACS) than with ST-segment elevation myocardial infarction (STEMI), in sharp contrast with plaque rupture [5, 6, 10].

Angiographic data suggest a less complex and less diffuse atherosclerotic pattern in patients with plaque erosion than in those with plaque rupture [5, 37–39]. Interestingly, plaque erosion has a preferential localization in the left anterior descending artery (LAD), mainly in the proximal and mid segments, often involving a bifurcation [37–41]. This preferential distribution may reflect a distinct local hemodynamic pattern, including altered endothelial shear stress, which may be more characteristic of a vessel with numerous side branches like LAD [42–44]. Recent reports suggest a potential role for high endothelial shear stress in the development of plaque erosion by favoring endothelial damage and thrombogenicity [24, 43, 44]. As compared with patients with plaque rupture, those with plaque erosion also have lower overall atherosclerotic disease burden and lower pancoronary vulnerability [6, 7], which may drive the favorable outcome observed in these patients [10]. Lesions with plaque erosion are typically associated with a "simple" A/B1 lesion phenotype, whereas plaque rupture typically shows a "complex" B2/C lesion phenotype [39]. Furthermore, plaque erosion is less frequently characterized by an angiographic evidence of calcification and thrombus compared with plaque rupture [39, 41]. Of note, thrombus burden measured by dual quantitative coronary angiography analysis has been demonstrated smaller in plaque erosion than in plaque rupture [38]. When focusing on the bio-humoral profile, patients with plaque erosion showed a better lipid profile and lower levels of inflammatory markers than those with plaque rupture [5, 37, 40, 45]. Interestingly, high hemoglobin levels (i.e., >15 g/dL) have been found to be strongly associated with plaque erosion, being an independent predictor (OR 1.48; 95% CI 1.09–2.01, $p = 0.01$), probably related to the increase in blood viscosity associated with hemoconcentration [37, 46]. Ferrante et al. showed high circulating levels of neutrophil-derived myeloperoxidase in patients with plaque erosion, but not in those with plaque rupture [47]. HYAL2 may represent another potential biomarker of plaque erosion [9], as well as surrogate markers of NET formation, such as citrullinated histones or double-stranded DNA [24]. Further studies are needed to identify and validate novel biomarkers aiding a non-invasive point-of-care diagnosis of plaque erosion.

2.4 Treatment and Prognosis of Patients with ACS Caused by Plaque Erosion

Current international guidelines recommend an urgent PCI with stent implantation in patients with STEMI, and often an early invasive strategy with stenting also for a substantial proportion of NSTE-ACS cases [11, 12], and this is reflected into clinical practice. Yet, as described above, the pathobiology of plaque erosion and plaque rupture, along with their clinical presentation, are different [5, 6, 9]. Of importance, these two ACS populations are also different in terms of vascular response to PCI [48, 49], which in turn influences long-term outcome [10]. Our group demonstrated, for the first time, that patients with plaque and erosion have a better clinical outcome than those with plaque rupture, as shown by a lower incidence of the composite endpoint of cardiac death, non-fatal myocardial infarction, unstable angina, and target lesion revascularization [10]. A paradigm shift in the management of ACS focusing on antithrombotic therapies rather than PCI in patients with erosion has been proposed and deserves consideration, as it may avoid the risk of stent failure in these patients, and potentially reduce health care expenses (Fig. 3). The first systematic proof-of-concept study assessing the efficacy and safety of a "conservative" approach in patients with plaque erosion was the EROSION (Effective Anti-Thrombotic Therapy Without Stenting: Intravascular Optical Coherence Tomography-Based Management in Plaque Erosion) study [15]. This OCT study prospectively enrolled 60 patients with ACS due to plaque erosion with a residual vessel stenosis <70% and a TIMI flow grade 3 on angiography, and tested a conservative strategy of potent antithrombotic therapy (i.e., aspirin, ticagrelor, and heparin +/− glycoprotein IIb/IIIa inhibitors) without stenting. Approximately 80% of patients met the primary endpoint of a > 50% reduction of thrombus volume at 1 month, and more than one third had no detectable thrombus [15]. Of note, most patients with plaque erosion managed "conservatively" did not experience major adverse cardiac events up to 1 year, although the study was not powered for this specific aim [16]. In addition to potent antithrombotic therapies, patients with plaque erosion and biomarkers indicating substantive NETosis or alteration of hyaluronan metabolism, may benefit, in the future, from treatments with deoxyribonuclease, inhibitors of peptidyl arginine deiminase-4 (PAD-4), inhibitors of MPO, or drugs interfering with HYAL2 [9, 13, 50, 51], although these hypotheses should be validated in large clinical studies.

3 Eruptive Calcified Nodule

3.1 Pathobiology of Calcified Nodule

Calcified nodules are the least frequent atherosclerotic substrate of coronary thrombosis in patients with AMI, accounting for approximately 5–8% of cases [3–5]. Calcified nodules typically occur in older patients (>60 years), often with chronic kidney disease, without particular between-sex differences [5]. Calcified nodules are predominantly observed in the proximal-mid segments of right coronary artery (RCA), often in the context of severely calcified and tortuous tracts [52]. Recent data from pathology specimens show that segments located proximal or distal to the culprit lesion have a greater arc and area of calcium as compared to the culprit sites of calcified nodules, while the area of the calcified necrotic core is larger in the culprit sites of calcified nodules (Fig. 4) [53]. These observations lend support to the hypothesis that calcified nodules represent previous regions of eccentric plaque,

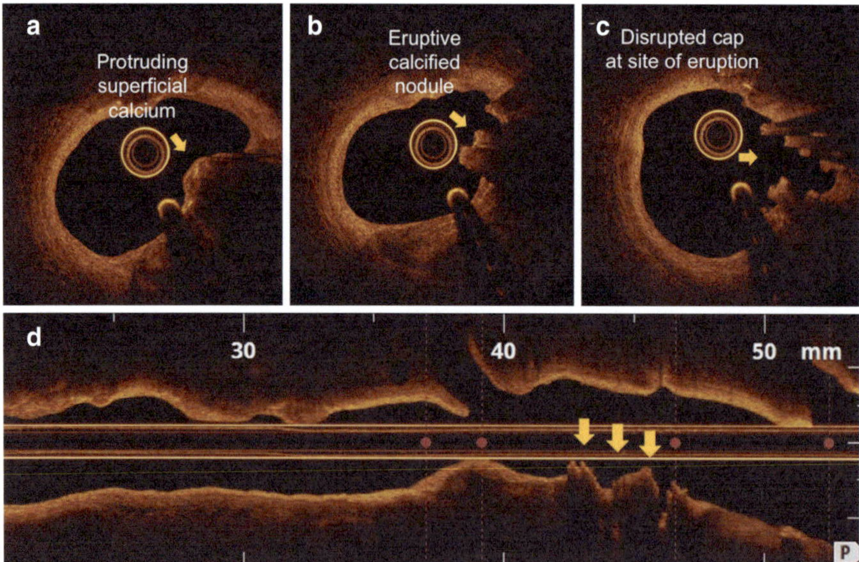

Fig. 4 Representative OCT images of eruptive calcified nodule. Calcified nodules are characterized by superficially located large calcifications, known as "calcium sheets," that locally protrudes into the lumen (**a**, arrow). These protruding nodules are typically located in vessels with tortuous segments exposed to hinge motions, where they can fracture and became eruptive calcified nodules with thrombus formation (**b–d**, arrows)

where the necrotic core calcifies over an area without collagen, and then protrudes due to a lack of tensile strength [52, 53]. In contrast, adjacent areas of sheet calcium are composed of collagen matrix, providing greater strength. During the cardiac cycle, proximal to middle RCA segments have a hinge motion or excessive torsion, and heavily calcified coronary segments adjacent to more flexible and less calcified areas lead to the protrusion of calcified nodules [53, 54].

Although the etiology of plaque calcification remains debated, most data support the notion that progression of calcification in advanced atherosclerotic lesions develops as extension from the external border of the necrotic core involving adjacent smooth muscle cells and collagen-rich extracellular matrix (chapter "Calcium Crystals in Arterial Disease") [55]. Of note, plaque progression occurs when necrotic core merges with calcification sheets extending in the longitudinal direction, eventually determining the development of a fibrocalcific plaque [55, 56]. Calcium fragmentation resulting in nodule formation likely elicits intraplaque hemorrhage caused by damage of the surrounding capillaries and arterioles, as well as the formation of clots involving accumulated fibrin and red blood cells [52]. Hemosiderin deposition with macrophage infiltration may also be observed, depending on the duration of the calcified nodule. Intraplaque hemorrhage is observed in 40% of culprit calcified nodule lesions, highly suggestive of capillary breaks occurring during calcium fragmentation [55]. Although the current study cannot confirm a predisposition toward disruption of a thin fibrous cap, mechanical force exerted by the calcified fragments is likely the underlying mechanism causing the discontinuity of the overlying cap, along with the loss of surface endothelium and overlying platelet/fibrin thrombus [52, 56].

3.2 *In Vivo Diagnosis of Calcified Nodule*

Intracoronary imaging studies using IVUS or OCT provided substantial evidence regarding the morphologic features of calcified nodules and their prevalence in vivo. Three distinct types have been identified: eruptive calcified nodules, superficial calcific sheet, and calcified protrusion (prevalence of 26%, 67%, and 7%, respectively). Eruptive calcified nodules are frequently located in the right coronary arteries, whereas superficial calcific sheet is most frequently found in the left anterior descending coronary arteries. Calcification index is greatest in eruptive calcified nodules, followed by superficial calcific sheet, and smallest in calcified protrusion. The superficial calcific sheet group seem to have the highest peak post-intervention creatine kinase values among the groups [4, 5, 53]. Several studies consistently showed that the in vivo prevalence of calcified nodules in patients with ACS is comparable to that observed in subjects dying from SCD, ranging between 3% and 8.0% [4, 5]. The majority of calcified nodules is characterized by superficially located large calcifications, known as "calcium sheets," that locally protrudes into the lumen, and are typically characterized by negative remodeling [53]. The eruption of calcified nodules may cause endothelial disruption and thrombus formation. Intravascular imaging studies provide additional data in support of this notion by showing that calcified nodules are associated with greater hinge motion on angiogram and are most frequently detected in the mid right coronary artery [4, 53]. Repeated cyclic mechanical forces acting on the coronary region exposed to hinge movements over a prolonged time might determine weakening of the calcified plate and its subsequent fracture [52]. Calcified nodules are frequently covered by fibrin, which is likely to derive from surrounding damaged capillaries. Local hemodynamic factors, including high endothelial shear stress in proximity of a calcified nodule, may also cause local flow turbulence which in turn activates procoagulant factors favoring thrombosis [57]. Typically, eruptive calcified nodules have been associated with a higher prevalence of red rather than white thrombus both in pathology and in vivo studies [52]. The presence of calcified nodules has been consistently associated with older age and renal dysfunction [4, 5]. Previous analyses from the 3-vessel Providing Regional Observations to Study Predictors of Events in the Coronary Tree (PROSPECT) study using virtual histology-IVUS showed a prevalence of calcified nodule at the non-culprit lesions of about 17% per artery [58]. Although the prevalence of cholesterol crystals has been shown to be higher in plaque rupture than in non-ruptured plaques, they can be observed in almost 30% of calcified nodules [4, 29].

3.3 Treatment and Prognosis of Patients with ACS Caused by Calcified Nodule

Patients with AMI caused by eruptive calcified nodules have an unfavorable clinical outcome with a risk to have a major adverse cardiovascular event about eight times higher than those without this culprit plaque morphology [53, 59]. Eruptive calcified nodules are detected more frequently in older patients and in those with three-vessel disease and with greater plaque vulnerability, suggesting that they may represent a marker of more advanced and high-risk atherosclerotic disease [58]. The adoption of an intense secondary prevention with aggressive medical therapy (e.g., potent antithrombotic drugs, aggressive lipid-lowering therapies) to stabilize atherosclerosis may be a reasonable solution in this setting [59]. In contrast, PCI of these lesions is often challenging as it is associated with higher risk of stent underexpansion. Aggressive lesion preparation should be considered when treating calcified nodules, particularly when they are in the context of large calcified plaques with a maximum calcium angle >180°, a maximum thickness >0.5 mm, and length >5 mm [60].

4 Other Causes of Myocardial Infarction Without Plaque Rupture

4.1 Spontaneous Coronary Artery Dissection

Spontaneous coronary artery dissection (SCAD) is a less frequent cause of ACS, predominantly affecting young to middle-aged women, including a minority during or following pregnancy [61, 62]. It is characterized by the formation of a false lumen in the tunica media of the coronary artery wall, which can lead to an external compression of the true lumen [62]. The pathophysiology of SCAD remains largely unknown, although an association of this morphological substrate with arteriopathies, especially fibromuscular dysplasia, has been observed in previous studies. A couple of pathogenic hypotheses have been proposed: (1) the "inside-out" mechanism proposes that a "tear" in the intimal tunica and in the endothelium favors the accumulation of blood into the media; (2) the "outside-in" mechanism proposes that a microvessel rupture occurring within the vessel wall is the *primum movens.*" [62] Although fenestrated and nonfenestrated dissections may represents different entities, they are likely to be two expressions of the same pathological process. This concept is supported by the frequent observation of coronary arteries simultaneously affected by nonfenestrated and fenestrated dissections, separated by areas of structurally normal vessel (Fig. 5) [63, 64]. When a coronary dissection is nonfenestrated, the false lumen appears pressurized, determining an expansion of the external elastic lamina (EEL), an increase of the false lumen volume, and a more severe stenosis. When the differential pressure exceeds the intimal yield stress, a disruption of the vessel wall separating true and false lumen occurs, with a depressurization of the dissection. While SCAD preferentially occurs in normal vessels, some cases develop in vessels with mild atherosclerosis, where cholesterol crystals may tear the intima and the endothelium and cause the accumulation of blood in the false lumen [64].

4.2 Intraplaque Hemorrhage

Intraplaque hemorrhage (IPH) is an infrequent and elusive cause of AMI, which is considered one of the pathological mechanisms responsible for accelerated plaque progression [65]. IPH typically lacks thrombus and is characterized by a layered pattern suggestive of previous healing episodes. At IVUS imaging, IPH can be observed as a deep "black" area, with sharp borders confined within the plaque. The surrounding plaque generally shows a bright speckling pattern with echolucent regions suggestive of plaque inflammation [65]. At OCT imaging, IPH is characterized by a distinct area of low backscattering and relatively low signal with clusters

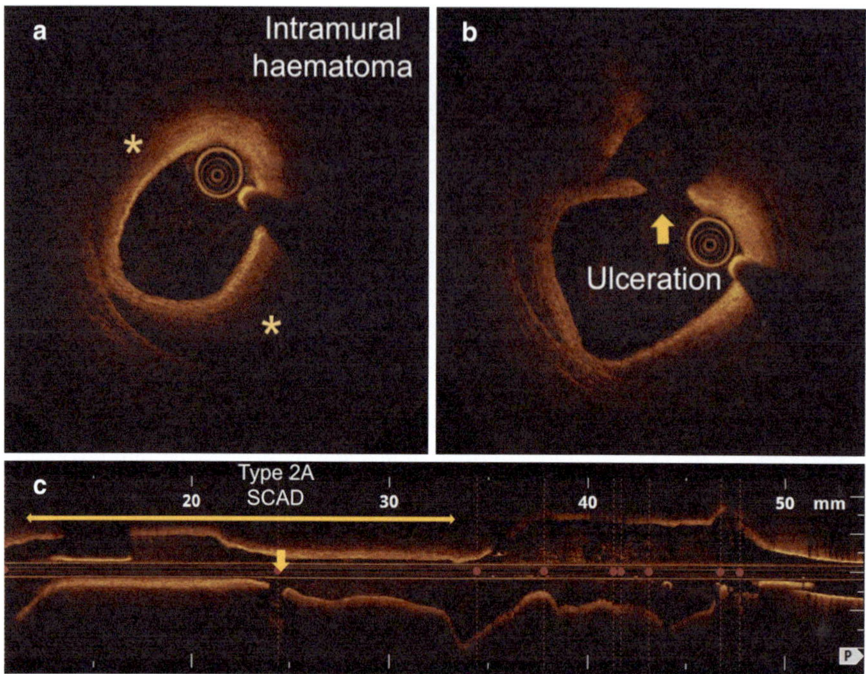

Fig. 5 Representative OCT images of spontaneous coronary artery dissection (SCAD). Representative OCT images of SCAD in a 43-year-old woman without conventional cardiovascular risk factors presenting with a diagnosis of NSTEMI. OCT imaging showed a fenestrated type 2A dissection, with evidence of intramural hematoma in the false lumen (**a**, asterisks) compressing the true lumen. When the differential pressure exceeded the intimal yield stress, a disruption of the vessel wall separating true and false lumen occurred with evidence of a large ulceration of the vessel wall (**b, c**, arrows) allowing the hematoma to depressurize

of macrophages and cholesterol crystals appearing as bright spots [65, 66]. A layered pattern suggestive of previous plaque healing, as well as disrupted and leaking microchannels can be observed in the context of an IPH. It is important to notice that even IPH might be caused by a similar process of cholesterol crystal expansion that can pierce through the vasa vasorum [18, 66, 67].

5   Conclusions

Plaque rupture is still considered the leading cause of AMI. Yet, growing evidence indicates that other etiologies are involved in a substantial proportion of AMI (up to 40%), including plaque erosion, calcified nodules, SCAD and IPH. While the presence of cholesterol crystals is more frequent in plaque rupture, they might play a pathological role also in other causes of AMI without disruption, by directly piercing or tearing the arterial intima and/or exacerbating inflammation. Plaques with cholesterol crystals invading fibrous caps detected by advanced intracoronary imaging techniques should be considered as a novel marker of high-risk plaques, and might became an important therapeutic target in patients with AMI.

Disclosures None.

References

1. Farb A, Burke AP, Tang AL, et al. Coronary plaque erosion without rupture into a lipid core. A frequent cause of coronary thrombosis in sudden coronary death. Circulation. 1996;93:1354–63. https://doi.org/10.1161/01.cir.93.7.1354.
2. Arbustini E, Dal Bello B, Morbini P, et al. Plaque erosion is a major substrate for coronary thrombosis in acute myocardial infarction. Heart. 1999;82:269–72. https://doi.org/10.1136/hrt.82.3.269.
3. Virmani R, Kolodgie FD, Burke AP, Farb A, Schwartz SM. Lessons from sudden coronary death: a comprehensive morphological classification scheme for atherosclerotic lesions. Arterioscler Thromb Vasc Biol. 2000;20:1262–75. https://doi.org/10.1161/01.atv.20.5.1262.
4. Higuma T, Soeda T, Abe N, et al. A combined optical coherence tomography and intravascular ultrasound study on plaque rupture, plaque erosion, and calcified nodule in patients with ST-segment elevation myocardial infarction: incidence, morphologic characteristics, and outcomes after percutaneous coronary intervention. JACC Cardiovasc Interv. 2015;8:1166–76. https://doi.org/10.1016/j.jcin.2015.02.026.
5. Jia H, Abtahian F, Aguirre AD, et al. In vivo diagnosis of plaque erosion and calcified nodule in patients with acute coronary syndrome by intravascular optical coherence tomography. J Am Coll Cardiol. 2013;62:1748–58. https://doi.org/10.1016/j.jacc.2013.05.071.
6. Vergallo R, Ren X, Yonetsu T, et al. Pancoronary plaque vulnerability in patients with acute coronary syndrome and ruptured culprit plaque: a 3-vessel optical coherence tomography study. Am Heart J. 2014;167:59–67. https://doi.org/10.1016/j.ahj.2013.10.011.
7. Sugiyama T, Yamamoto E, Bryniarski K, et al. Nonculprit plaque characteristics in patients with acute coronary syndrome caused by plaque erosion vs plaque rupture: a 3-vessel optical coherence tomography study. JAMA Cardiol. 2018;3:207–14. https://doi.org/10.1001/jamacardio.2017.5234.
8. Hu S, Yonetsu T, Jia H, et al. Residual thrombus pattern in patients with ST-segment elevation myocardial infarction caused by plaque erosion versus plaque rupture after successful fibrinolysis: an optical coherence tomography study. J Am Coll Cardiol. 2014;63:1336–8. https://doi.org/10.1016/j.jacc.2013.11.025.
9. Pedicino D, Vinci R, Giglio AF, et al. Alterations of Hyaluronan metabolism in acute coronary syndrome: implications for plaque erosion. J Am Coll Cardiol. 2018;72:1490–503. https://doi.org/10.1016/j.jacc.2018.06.072.
10. Niccoli G, Montone RA, Di Vito L, et al. Plaque rupture and intact fibrous cap assessed by optical coherence tomography portend different outcomes in patients with acute coronary syndrome. Eur Heart J. 2015;36:1377–84. https://doi.org/10.1093/eurheartj/ehv029.
11. Ibanez B, James S, Agewall S, et al. 2017 ESC guidelines for the management of acute myocardial infarction in patients presenting with ST-segment elevation. Rev Esp Cardiol (Engl Ed). 2017;70:1082. https://doi.org/10.1016/j.rec.2017.11.010.
12. Roffi M, Patrono C, Collet JP, et al. 2015 ESC guidelines for the management of acute coronary syndromes in patients presenting without persistent ST-segment elevation: task force for the Management of Acute Coronary Syndromes in patients presenting without persistent ST-segment elevation of the European Society of Cardiology (ESC). Eur Heart J. 2016;37:267–315. https://doi.org/10.1093/eurheartj/ehv320.

13. Libby P, Pasterkamp G, Crea F, Jang IK. Reassessing the mechanisms of acute coronary syndromes. Circ Res. 2019;124:150–60. https://doi.org/10.1161/CIRCRESAHA.118.311098.
14. Partida RA, Libby P, Crea F, Jang IK. Plaque erosion: a new in vivo diagnosis and a potential major shift in the management of patients with acute coronary syndromes. Eur Heart J. 2018;39:2070–6. https://doi.org/10.1093/eurheartj/ehx786.
15. Jia H, Dai J, Hou J, et al. Effective anti-thrombotic therapy without stenting: intravascular optical coherence tomography-based management in plaque erosion (the EROSION study). Eur Heart J. 2017;38:792–800. https://doi.org/10.1093/eurheartj/ehw381.
16. Xing L, Yamamoto E, Sugiyama T, et al. EROSION study (effective anti-thrombotic therapy without stenting: intravascular optical coherence tomography-based Management in Plaque Erosion): a 1-year follow-up report. Circ Cardiovasc Interv. 2017;10:e005860. https://doi.org/10.1161/CIRCINTERVENTIONS.117.005860.
17. Abela GS, Aziz K, Vedre A, et al. Effect of cholesterol crystals on plaques and intima in arteries of patients with acute coronary and cerebrovascular syndromes. Am J Cardiol. 2009;103:959–68. https://doi.org/10.1016/j.amjcard.2008.12.019.
18. Abela GS. Cholesterol crystals piercing the arterial plaque and intima trigger local and systemic inflammation. J Clin Lipidol. 2010;4:156–64. https://doi.org/10.1016/j.jacl.2010.03.003.
19. Crea F, Liuzzo G. Pathogenesis of acute coronary syndromes. J Am Coll Cardiol. 2013;61:1–11. https://doi.org/10.1016/j.jacc.2012.07.064.
20. Libby P. Mechanisms of acute coronary syndromes and their implications for therapy. N Engl J Med. 2013;368:2004–13. https://doi.org/10.1056/NEJMra1216063.
21. Vergallo R, Jang IK, Crea F. New prediction tools and treatment for ACS patients with plaque erosion. Atherosclerosis. 2021;318:45–51. https://doi.org/10.1016/j.atherosclerosis.2020.10.016.
22. Martinod K, Wagner DD. Thrombosis: tangled up in NETs. Blood. 2014;123:2768–76. https://doi.org/10.1182/blood-2013-10-463646.
23. Badimon L, Vilahur G. Neutrophil extracellular traps: a new source of tissue factor in athero-thrombosis. Eur Heart J. 2015;36:1364–6. https://doi.org/10.1093/eurheartj/ehv105.
24. Quillard T, Araujo HA, Franck G, et al. TLR2 and neutrophils potentiate endothelial stress, apoptosis and detachment: implications for superficial erosion. Eur Heart J. 2015;36:1394–404. https://doi.org/10.1093/eurheartj/ehv044.
25. Franck G, Mawson T, Sausen G, et al. Flow perturbation mediates neutrophil recruitment and potentiates endothelial injury via TLR2 in mice: implications for superficial erosion. Circ Res. 2017;121:31–42. https://doi.org/10.1161/CIRCRESAHA.117.310694.
26. Doring Y, Soehnlein O, Weber C. Neutrophil extracellular traps in atherosclerosis and Atherothrombosis. Circ Res. 2017;120:736–43. https://doi.org/10.1161/CIRCRESAHA.116.309692.
27. Vedre A, Pathak DR, Crimp M, Lum C, Koochesfahani M, Abela GS. Physical factors that trigger cholesterol crystallization leading to plaque rupture. Atherosclerosis. 2008;203:89–96. https://doi.org/10.1016/j.atherosclerosis.2008.06.027.
28. Katayama Y, Tanaka A, Taruya A, et al. Feasibility and clinical significance of in vivo cholesterol crystal detection using optical coherence tomography. Arterioscler Thromb Vasc Biol. 2020;40:220–9. https://doi.org/10.1161/ATVBAHA.119.312934.
29. Nishimura S, Ehara S, Hasegawa T, et al. Cholesterol crystal as a new feature of coronary vulnerable plaques: an optical coherence tomography study. J Cardiol. 2017;69:253–9. https://doi.org/10.1016/j.jjcc.2016.04.003.
30. Vergallo R, Uemura S, Soeda T, et al. Prevalence and predictors of multiple coronary plaque ruptures: in vivo 3-vessel optical coherence tomography imaging study. Arterioscler Thromb Vasc Biol. 2016;36:2229–38. https://doi.org/10.1161/ATVBAHA.116.307891.
31. Vergallo R, Porto I, D'Amario D, et al. Coronary atherosclerotic phenotype and plaque healing in patients with recurrent acute coronary syndromes compared with patients with long-term clinical stability: an in vivo optical coherence tomography study. JAMA Cardiol. 2019;4:321–9. https://doi.org/10.1001/jamacardio.2019.0275.
32. Fracassi F, Crea F, Sugiyama T, et al. Healed culprit plaques in patients with acute coronary syndromes. J Am Coll Cardiol. 2019;73:2253–63. https://doi.org/10.1016/j.jacc.2018.10.093.

33. Yonetsu T, Suh W, Abtahian F, et al. Comparison of near-infrared spectroscopy and optical coherence tomography for detection of lipid. Catheter Cardiovasc Interv. 2014;84:710–7. https://doi.org/10.1002/ccd.25084.

34. Cao M, Wu T, Zhao J, et al. Focal geometry and characteristics of erosion-prone coronary plaques in vivo angiography and optical coherence tomography study. Front Cardiovasc Med. 2021;8:709480. https://doi.org/10.3389/fcvm.2021.709480.

35. Yahagi K, Davis HR, Arbustini E, Virmani R. Sex differences in coronary artery disease: pathological observations. Atherosclerosis. 2015;239:260–7. https://doi.org/10.1016/j.atherosclerosis.2015.01.017.

36. Prati F, Uemura S, Souteyrand G, et al. OCT-based diagnosis and management of STEMI associated with intact fibrous cap. JACC Cardiovasc Imaging. 2013;6:283–7. https://doi.org/10.1016/j.jcmg.2012.12.007.

37. Yamamoto E, Yonetsu T, Kakuta T, et al. Clinical and laboratory predictors for plaque erosion in patients with acute coronary syndromes. J Am Heart Assoc. 2019;8:e012322. https://doi.org/10.1161/JAHA.119.012322.

38. Tian J, Vergallo R, Jia H, et al. Morphologic characteristics of eroded coronary plaques: a combined angiographic, optical coherence tomography, and intravascular ultrasound study. Int J Cardiol. 2014;176:e137–9. https://doi.org/10.1016/j.ijcard.2014.07.204.

39. Vergallo R, Porto I, De Maria GL, et al. Dual quantitative coronary angiography accurately quantifies intracoronary thrombotic burden in patients with acute coronary syndrome: comparison with optical coherence tomography imaging. Int J Cardiol. 2019;292:25–31. https://doi.org/10.1016/j.ijcard.2019.04.060.

40. Dai J, Xing L, Jia H, et al. In vivo predictors of plaque erosion in patients with ST-segment elevation myocardial infarction: a clinical, angiographical, and intravascular optical coherence tomography study. Eur Heart J. 2018;39:2077–85. https://doi.org/10.1093/eurheartj/ehy101.

41. Kim HO, Kim CJ, Kurihara O, et al. Angiographic features of patients with coronary plaque erosion. Int J Cardiol. 2019;288:12–6. https://doi.org/10.1016/j.ijcard.2019.03.039.

42. Vergallo R, Papafaklis MI, Yonetsu T, et al. Endothelial shear stress and coronary plaque characteristics in humans: combined frequency-domain optical coherence tomography and computational fluid dynamics study. Circ Cardiovasc Imaging. 2014;7:905–11. https://doi.org/10.1161/CIRCIMAGING.114.001932.

43. Vergallo R, Papafaklis MI, D'Amario D, et al. Coronary plaque erosion developing in an area of high endothelial shear stress: insights from serial optical coherence tomography imaging. Coron Artery Dis. 2019;30:74–5. https://doi.org/10.1097/MCA.0000000000000673.

44. Yamamoto E, Thondapu V, Poon E, et al. Endothelial shear stress and plaque erosion: a computational fluid dynamics and optical coherence tomography study. JACC Cardiovasc Imaging. 2019;12:374–5. https://doi.org/10.1016/j.jcmg.2018.07.024.

45. Niccoli G, Montone RA, Cataneo L, et al. Morphological-biohumoral correlations in acute coronary syndromes: pathogenetic implications. Int J Cardiol. 2014;171:463–6. https://doi.org/10.1016/j.ijcard.2013.12.238.

46. Papaioannou TG, Stefanadis C. Vascular wall shear stress: basic principles and methods. Hellenic J Cardiol. 2005;46:9–15.

47. Ferrante G, Nakano M, Prati F, et al. High levels of systemic myeloperoxidase are associated with coronary plaque erosion in patients with acute coronary syndromes: a clinicopathological study. Circulation. 2010;122:2505–13. https://doi.org/10.1161/CIRCULATIONAHA.110.955302.

48. Soeda T, Higuma T, Abe N, et al. Morphological predictors for no reflow phenomenon after primary percutaneous coronary intervention in patients with ST-segment elevation myocardial infarction caused by plaque rupture. Eur Heart J Cardiovasc Imaging. 2017;18:103–10. https://doi.org/10.1093/ehjci/jev341.

49. Hu S, Wang C, Zhe C, et al. Plaque erosion delays vascular healing after drug eluting stent implantation in patients with acute coronary syndrome: an in vivo optical coherence tomography study. Catheter Cardiovasc Interv. 2017;89:592–600. https://doi.org/10.1002/ccd.26943.

50. Franck G, Mawson TL, Folco EJ, et al. Roles of PAD4 and NETosis in experimental atherosclerosis and arterial injury: implications for superficial erosion. Circ Res. 2018;123:33–42. https://doi.org/10.1161/CIRCRESAHA.117.312494.

51. Soehnlein O, Bazioti V, Westerterp M. A Pad 4 Plaque erosion. Circ Res. 2018;123:6–8. https://doi.org/10.1161/CIRCRESAHA.118.313110.
52. Torii S, Sato Y, Otsuka F, et al. Eruptive calcified nodules as a potential mechanism of acute coronary thrombosis and sudden death. J Am Coll Cardiol. 2021;77:1599–611. https://doi.org/10.1016/j.jacc.2021.02.016.
53. Sugiyama T, Yamamoto E, Fracassi F, et al. Calcified plaques in patients with acute coronary syndromes. JACC Cardiovasc Interv. 2019;12(6):531–40. https://doi.org/10.1016/j.jcin.2018.12.013.
54. Puentes J, Garreau M, Lebreton H, Roux C. Understanding coronary artery movement: a knowledge-based approach. Artif Intell Med. 1998;13:207–37. https://doi.org/10.1016/s0933-3657(98)00031-1.
55. Mori H, Torii S, Kutyna M, et al. Coronary artery calcification and its progression: what does it really mean? JACC Cardiovasc Imaging. 2018;11:127–42. https://doi.org/10.1016/j.jcmg.2017.10.012.
56. Otsuka F, Sakakura K, Yahagi K, Joner M, Virmani R. Has our understanding of calcification in human coronary atherosclerosis progressed? Arterioscler Thromb Vasc Biol. 2014;34:724–36. https://doi.org/10.1161/ATVBAHA.113.302642.
57. Hoshino T, Chow LA, Hsu JJ, et al. Mechanical stress analysis of a rigid inclusion in distensible material: a model of atherosclerotic calcification and plaque vulnerability. Am J Physiol Heart Circ Physiol. 2009;297:H802–10. https://doi.org/10.1152/ajpheart.00318.2009.
58. Xu Y, Mintz GS, Tam A, et al. Prevalence, distribution, predictors, and outcomes of patients with calcified nodules in native coronary arteries: a 3-vessel intravascular ultrasound analysis from providing regional observations to study predictors of events in the coronary tree (PROSPECT). Circulation. 2012;126:537–45. https://doi.org/10.1161/CIRCULATIONAHA.111.055004.
59. Prati F, Gatto L, Fabbiocchi F, et al. Clinical outcomes of calcified nodules detected by optical coherence tomography: a sub-analysis of the CLIMA study. EuroIntervention. 2020;16:380–6. https://doi.org/10.4244/EIJ-D-19-01120.
60. Fujino A, Mintz GS, Matsumura M, et al. A new optical coherence tomography-based calcium scoring system to predict stent underexpansion. EuroIntervention. 2018;13:e2182–9. https://doi.org/10.4244/EIJ-D-17-00962.
61. Chan N, Premawardhana D, Al-Hussaini A, et al. Pregnancy and spontaneous coronary artery dissection: lessons from survivors and nonsurvivors. Circulation. 2022;146:69–72. https://doi.org/10.1161/CIRCULATIONAHA.122.059635.
62. Kim ESH. Spontaneous coronary-artery dissection. N Engl J Med. 2020;383:2358–70. https://doi.org/10.1056/NEJMra2001524.
63. Alfonso F, Paulo M, Gonzalo N, et al. Diagnosis of spontaneous coronary artery dissection by optical coherence tomography. J Am Coll Cardiol. 2012;59:1073–9. https://doi.org/10.1016/j.jacc.2011.08.082.
64. Jackson R, Al-Hussaini A, Joseph S, et al. Spontaneous coronary artery dissection: pathophysiological insights from optical coherence tomography. JACC Cardiovasc Imaging. 2019;12:2475–88. https://doi.org/10.1016/j.jcmg.2019.01.015.
65. Hernando Salazar C, Escaned J, Gonzalo N. Acute coronary syndrome caused by intraplaque hemorrhage. Rev Esp Cardiol (Engl Ed). 2019;72:776. https://doi.org/10.1016/j.rec.2018.06.028.
66. Antuna P, Cuesta J, Bastante T, et al. Diagnosis of Intraplaque hemorrhage by high-definition intravascular ultrasound and optical coherence tomography. JACC Cardiovasc Interv. 2020;13:1960–2. https://doi.org/10.1016/j.jcin.2020.05.027.
67. Mughal MM, Khan MK, DeMarco JK, Majid A, Shamoun F, Abela GS. Symptomatic and asymptomatic carotid artery plaque. Expert Rev Cardiovasc Ther. 2011;9:1315–30. https://doi.org/10.1586/erc.11.120.

Athero-Embolism: A Manifestation of Atherosclerosis

Rohan M. Prasad, Adolfo Martinez Salazar, Majid Yavari, George S. Abela, and Christopher Hanson

1 Introduction

Although athero-embolism associated with the release of cholesterol crystals into the systemic circulation was first described at autopsy over 150 years ago, the first autopsy series to examine this issue was not reported for another 100 years [1, 2].

In 1945 Flory systematically examined the aorta and arteries of several visceral organs looking specifically for the evidence of cholesterol crystal (CC) embolization in 267 patients with a mean age of 65 years who had died from myocardial infarction without clinical evidence of athero-embolism, and from these studies he made a number of important observations [3]. First, Flory confirmed that atherosclerotic plaque was invariably present in the aorta of patients dying of myocardial infarction. Second, he noted that in 57 patients, (~20%) the atherosclerotic plaques in the aorta appeared eroded, and some were partially covered by mural thrombus. Third, he found aggregates of CCs occluding medium and small arteries (measuring 20–200 µm) in 9 patients; 2 had mild erosions in the aorta and 7 had advanced

R. M. Prasad · A. M. Salazar · M. Yavari
Department of Internal Medicine, Sparrow Hospital, Michigan State University,
Lansing, MI, USA
e-mail: prasadr1@msu.edu; mart2580@msu.edu; yavarim1@msu.edu

G. S. Abela (✉)
Department of Medicine, Division of Cardiovascular Medicine, Michigan State University,
East Lansing, MI, USA
e-mail: abela@msu.edu

C. Hanson
College of Human Medicine, Sparrow Thoracic Cardiovascular Institute, Sparrow Hospital,
Michigan State University, Lansing, MI, USA
e-mail: christopher.hanson@sparrow.org

G. S. Abela, S. M. Nidorf (eds.), *Cholesterol Crystals in Atherosclerosis and Other Related Diseases*, Contemporary Cardiology,
https://doi.org/10.1007/978-3-031-41192-2_12

atherosclerotic erosions. Thus, although the incidence of athero-emboli in this cohort was low (3.1%), in those with advanced aortic atherosclerosis it was much higher (~13%) albeit not clinically evident. Fourth, he noted the presence of foreign body giant cells in the intima of vessels occluded by CCs. Finally, he noted that the only visceral organ with anatomical changes associated with arterial occlusion were the kidneys, where the renal parenchyma was atrophic with depressed wedge-shaped cortical areas consistent with ischemic injury [3].

Flory then extended his research and injected atherosclerotic plaque content that included CCs, fat, and blood cells directly into the ear veins of two rabbits. In one rabbit sacrificed at 24 h, masses of CCs, leukocytes, and red blood cells were found to have occluded the small arteries in the lungs. In the second rabbit sacrificed at 7 days, many small pulmonary arteries still contained CCs, however, the leukocytes and other debris were no longer present, and the intima of these vessels appeared hyperplastic and contained foreign giant cells. Flory concluded that the CCs within the peripheral vessels found in patients at autopsy had not developed de novo, but rather had embolized from more proximal eroded atherosclerotic lesions and summarized his thoughts by stating that … *the mass of CCs mixed with lipid and thrombus material is torn loose (from eroded plaques) by the flow of blood and is carried into the medium-sized or small arteries where it lodges. Surrounding this embolism, thrombus forms and organizes and eventually recanalization of the thrombus takes place between the CCs* [3].

Subsequent bench and in vivo reports in more recent years have confirmed each of his observations and have provided greater insight into the mechanism by which CCs contribute to ischemic and inflammatory injury following embolization [2, 4–6].

The aorto-iliac arteries are the most common source of CCs emboli into the lower limbs triggering the cholesterol crystal embolic syndrome [7]. Moreover, the carotid arteries are also an important origin site of CC emboli that can lead to impairment of the cerebral and retinal blood flow. These changes promote an ischemic and inflammatory processes that can lead to severe complications, including transient ischemic attacks, strokes, and blindness [8]. CC emboli can vary in size (50–200 μm) and shape allowing them to lodge into capillaries, and small arteries (Fig. 1).

In vivo human imaging studies in the last 5 years by Komatsu et al. using non-obstructive general angioscopy to "survey the atherosclerotic landscape" of the aorta in patients with coronary disease and have confirmed that this technique provides the most sensitive means of detecting and characterizing aortic atherosclerotic plaque in vivo [9]. Initially they identified and described a range of appearances of atherosclerotic plaque typically seen at autopsy, including the invariable finding of atherosclerotic lesions with features consistent with spontaneous plaque rupture (SRAPs). (Chapter "Detecting Cholesterol Crystals Clinically in Spontaneous Aortic Plaque Rupture"). Some SRAPs were clearly seen to affect the plaque cap, as evidenced by erosion, fissuring, rupture, and ulceration, while others that involved non-cap regions of the plaque were evident by discoloration of the atherosclerotic surface consistent with intra-mural hemorrhage. Subsequently they safely harvested

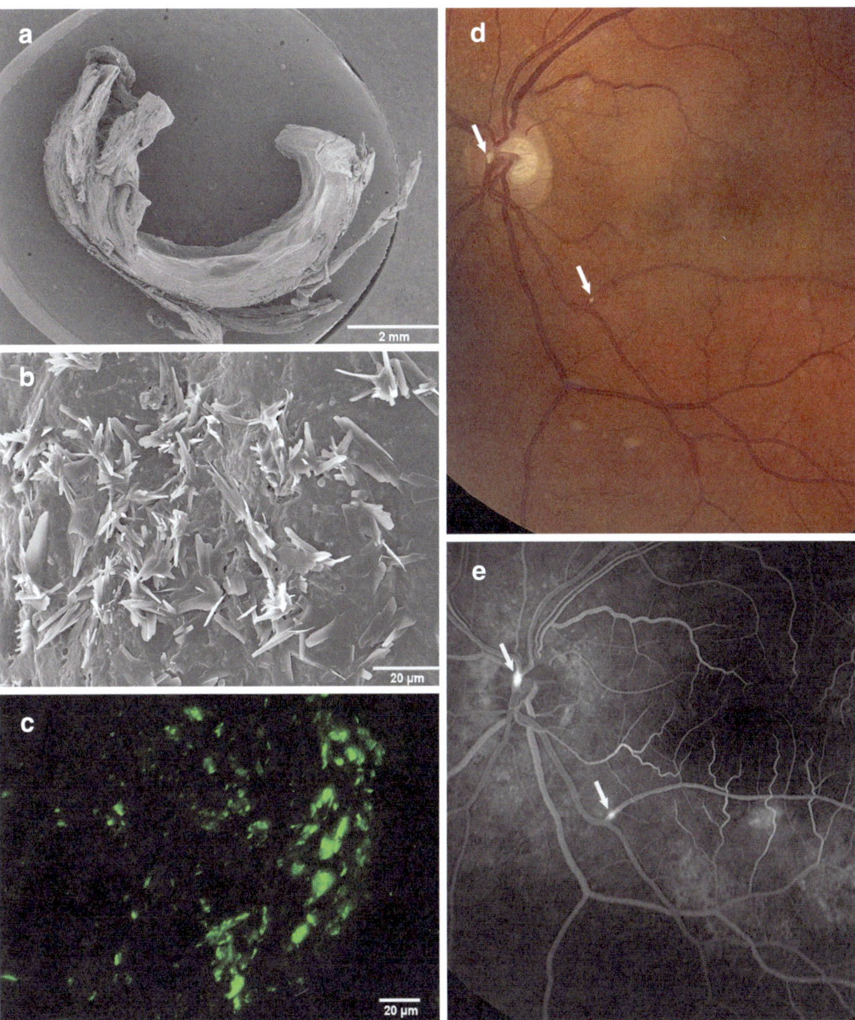

Fig. 1 Images of cholesterol crystal emboli. (**a**) Low power scanning electron micrograph of carotid artery plaque. (**b**) Surface scanning of the plaque demonstrates extensive cholesterol crystals. (**c**) Fluorescence image of cholesterol crystals on the intimal surface of the artery using Bodipy stain for cholesterol crystals (Courtesy of Dr. G. Abela). (**d, e**) Fundoscopy of Hollenhorst plaques of embolized cholesterol crystals in retinal arteries (arrows, Modified from Elizabeth Gauger, MD and Toni Venckus, CRA, University of Iowa; http://webeye.ophth.uiowa.edu/ eyeforum/atlas/pages/Hollenhorst-plaque.htm). (Reproduced with permission [4])

debris from SRAPs that extruded plaque contents and confirmed that it contained large CCs, necrotic gruel with calcium deposits, and cellular infiltrate that mirrored the contents of atherosclerotic plaque as observed by others who used confocal microscopy to examine fresh unprocessed debris obtained from carotid plaques [10, 11].

More recently, Komatsu et al. went one step further and characterized the nature of the cellular infiltrate of the debris associated with the so-called puff-chandelier lesions (plaques with crystals on their surface that glitter with the light shining on them) [12]. This confirmed that aside the presence of large CCs which give the debris its glistening chandelier appearance, its cellular infiltrate stained positive for CD68, NLRP3, IL-1β, and IL-6 typically expressed by activated macrophages. In addition, neutrophils were identified in a significant proportion of specimens. Thus, these data provide strong circumstantial evidence that an innate inflammatory process had been triggered by CCs in these ruptured plaques [13–15].

Together their observations of the atherosclerotic landscape in vivo provide several important insights. Specifically, the finding of large CCs within the debris extruding from some SRAPs speaks to their central role in plaque rupture [12]. Second, the observation that the debris extruding from SRAPs is rich in activated macrophages, and in many instances neutrophils speak to the events that must have occurred in the atherosclerotic bed prior to plaque rupture. Third, the observation that SRAPs associated with extrusion of atherosclerotic debris are common throughout the atherosclerotic landscape of the aorta in patients with coronary disease provides a plausible mechanism whereby the release of atherosclerotic debris into the peripheries can contribute to acute and chronic cerebral, retinal, and renal injury that may in some circumstances be clinically consequential over time [16–18].

2 Athero-Embolism Causes Ischemic Injury

Following plaque rupture, atherosclerotic debris including CCs, leukocytes, and necrotic gruel is released into the systemic circulation. While larger fragments of debris can lodge in small and medium size arteries to cause acute ischemia, smaller fragments of CC can become embedded in the intimal surface of distal vessels and acutely alter vasomotor tone favoring vasospasm [19–21], further promoting ischemic injury.

Abela and his colleagues examined these latter effects of CCs ex vivo using a closed dual perfusion chamber model in which rabbit arteries were placed and perfused using physiologic buffered saline (PBS) [19]. Studies were performed in normal arteries; arteries exposed to polystyrene microspheres and arteries exposed to CCs. By scanning electron microscopy, the intimal surface of arteries exposed to CCs were scrapped and damaged but not those exposed to PBS or microspheres. Using atomic force microscopy to evaluate intimal injury they demonstrated that the arteries exposed to CC had increased roughness due to studding of their surface with CCs. In addition, those arteries exposed to CCs had reduced vasoreactivity that favored vasospasm compared to controls and those exposed to microspheres (Fig. 2).

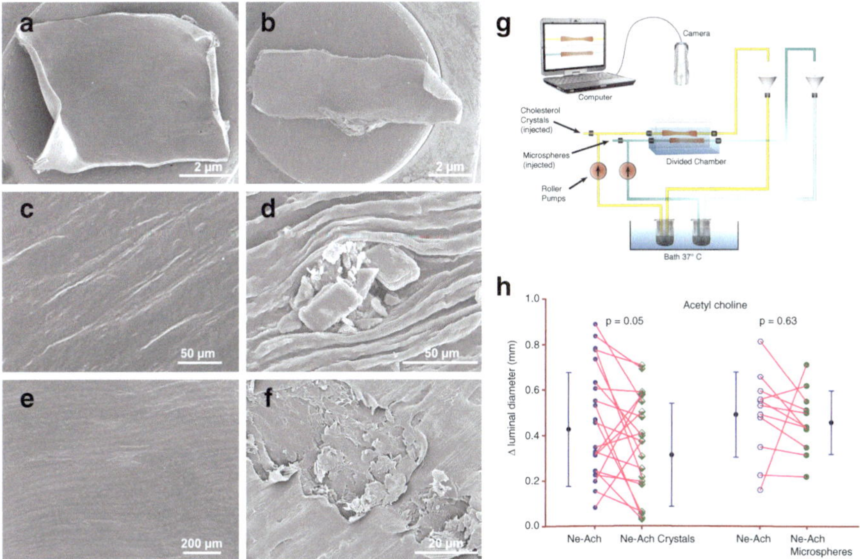

Fig. 2 Scanning electron micrographs of arterial surface with and without crystal injury. (**a, c, e**) Scanning electron micrographs of normal arterial surface with circulating saline. (**b, d, f**) Micrographs of arterial intima with circulating cholesterol crystals demonstrating crystals embedded and disrupting the intimal surface. (**g**) Diagram of dual perfusion chambers demonstrating the flow of normal saline and saline with cholesterol crystals and camera to evaluate arterial diameter and vasomotor activity. (**h**) Graphic demonstrating markedly reduced vasomotor dilatation with acetyl choline with cholesterol crystal exposed arteries compared to normal saline exposed arteries. (Modified and reproduced with permission [19])

3 Cholesterol Crystals in Atherosclerotic Debris Incites Inflammatory Injury

Within 24 h of embolization of atherosclerotic debris into the distal circulation, most of the cellular and necrotic debris is usually cleared, however, larger fragments and aggregates of CCs are difficult to dissolve and remain imbedded in the arterioles and can make their way to the tissues [22, 23]. Here they trigger and immune response after being recognized by hMincle receptors on macrophages and by complement factors C5a and C5b-9 that enhances the expression of endothelial selectins that in turn enhance the ingress of neutrophils and other leukocytes to the vascular and tissue space (Chapter "Atherosclerotic Plaque Morphology and the Conundrum of the Vulnerable Plaque") [24]. Over successive days a foreign body response develops within the vasculature as evidenced by giant cells. In addition, CCs can incite an immune response in the tissues. Together these responses lead to intimal and tissue fibrosis [5].

Abela and his colleagues also confirmed the ability of CCs to incite tissue inflammation independent of ischemic injury in animal models [5]. In their studies, PET/CTA was used to evaluate the effect of CC emboli on muscle injury. Specifically, they examined the thigh muscles in rabbits after intraarterial injection with either CCs, polystyrene microspheres, or normal saline. After 48 h, muscle inflammation and injury were measured by fluorodeoxyglucose uptake using PET/CTA and creatinine phosphokinase (CPK). These studies confirmed that in the absence of thrombotic occlusion, myo-necrosis with the evidence of extensive macrophage infiltrates surrounding muscle, was only evident in those rabbits injected with CCs. The macrophages that were examined at those sites were found to have CC particles within their cytoplasm (Fig. 3).

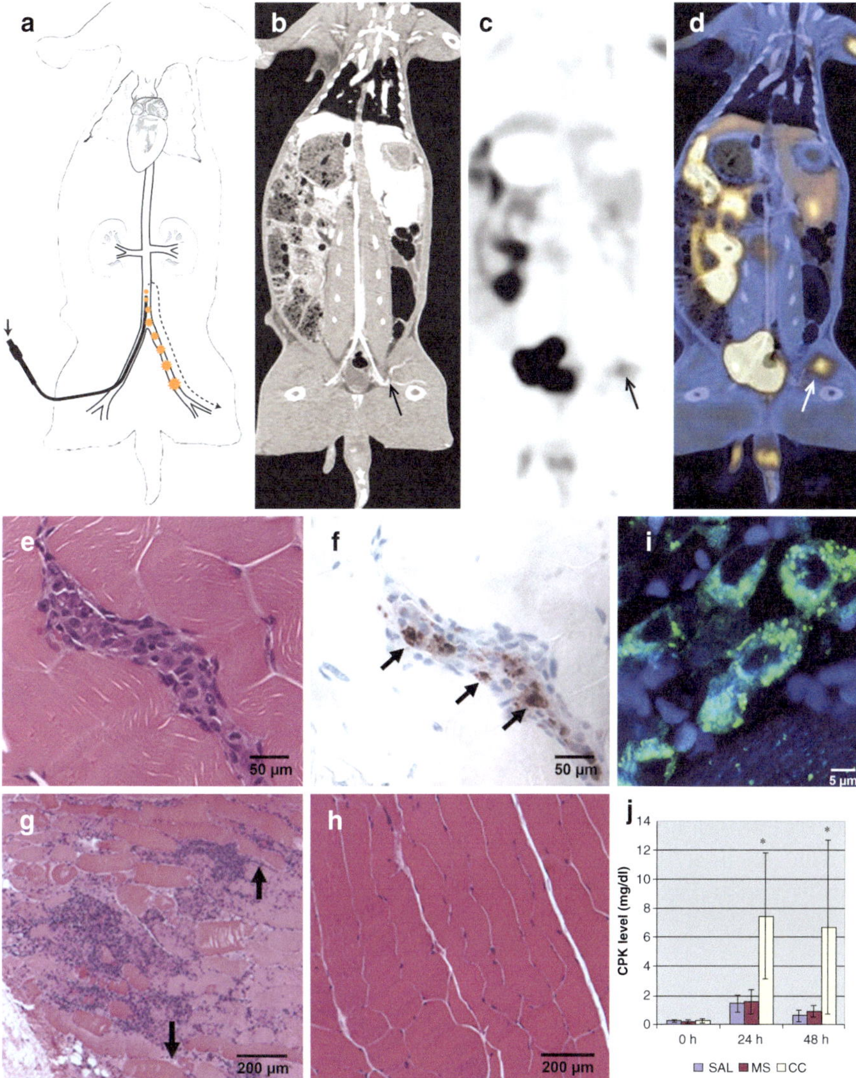

Fig. 3 PET scanning, histology and biomarker demonstrating cholesterol crystal emboli induced myocyte inflammation. (**a**) Diagram of catheter via right femoral artery delivering cholesterol crystals, microspheres, and saline into the left femoral artery in a rabbit model (dotted arrow). (**b**) Computer tomography angiographic image of aorta and iliofemoral arteries. (**c**) PET scan of rabbit with 'hot spot' (black arrow). (**d**) fused PET/CTA image demonstrating the site of inflamed left thigh muscle (white arrow). (**e**) Light micrographs of thigh muscle demonstrating macrophage cell infiltrates. (**f**) brown staining with RAM 11, arrows), (**g**) contraction band necrosis and loss of nuclei (arrows, hematoxylin and eosin). (**h**) Control from normal paraspinous muscle. (**i**) Fluorescence microscopic images of thigh muscle demonstrate macrophages (blue nuclei) with free cholesterol aggregates (green fluorescence) in their cytoplasm. (**j**) Graphic of mean creatinine phosphokinase (CPK) elevation with injection of normal saline (SAL), microspheres (MS), and cholesterol crystals (CC) demonstrating significant increase in CPK only with CCs (ANOVA, *P<0.037). (Modified and reproduced with permission [5])

4 Clinical Presentation

Spontaneous rupture of atherosclerotic plaque may occur in any vascular bed. While plaque rupture in small and medium size arteries typically lead to acute thrombotic occlusion, in some instances the thrombotic response is not occlusive, but embolization of atherosclerotic debris may still occlude the distal microvasculature and lead to ischemic injury due to a no-reflow phenomenon [19, 25–27]. This has been well documented at angiography soon after the onset of myocardial infarction [23]. In fact, a recent report has associated no-reflow with the presence of CCs in the rupture site of the culprit artery [28]. Furthermore, in another report by Yutani et al. using polarizing light demonstrated the presence of CCs emboli in the micro-circulation at sites of small infarcts following a percutaneous coronary intervention in a patient who had died several days following intervention [29] (Fig. 4).

In contrast, plaque rupture in larger arteries including the aorta, carotid, iliac, and femoral arteries may not cause thrombotic occlusion due to the size of their lumen but may still declare themselves as evidenced by distal tissue injury. Small ruptures in the aorta that release a small volume of atherosclerotic debris may cause inconsequential ischemic or inflammatory injury and thus be clinically silent. In contrast, the release of large volumes of atherosclerotic debris from SRAPs in the ascending aorta and cerebral circulation may lead to cerebral and retinal ischemia, while large volumes of debris emanating from SRAPs in the abdominal aorta typically affect the kidneys and leg muscles and skin [2, 4, 17]. In these instances, the skin in the lower limbs typically appear mottled, with a net-like and purple discoloration referred to as livedo reticularis which is believed to be a manifestation of arteriolar vasospasm and venous dilatation. In some instances, ischemic necrosis can occur in the feet [30–32]. Renal injury declares as flank pain, hematuria, and a deterioration in renal function. Although these changes may be acute, renal dysfunction can progress over several weeks due to interstitial nephritis [33, 34] (Fig. 5).

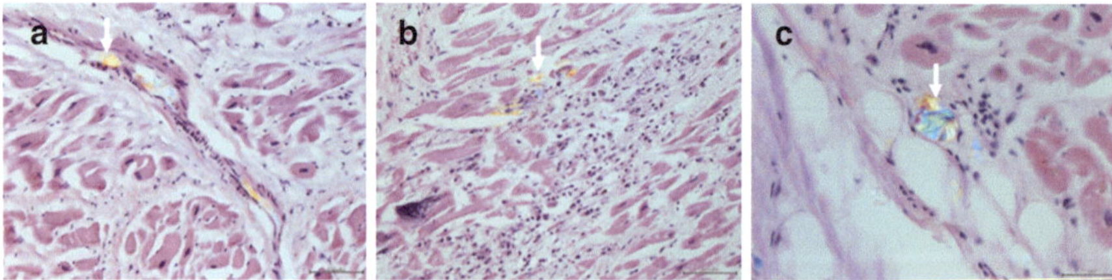

Fig. 4 H&E-stained frozen sections of the myocardial capillaries and arterioles. (**a**) Free cholesterol crystal emboli in the myocardial capillaries and arterioles shown in the frozen sections by using direct polarized light. (**b**) Free cholesterol crystal emboli in the myocardial capillary on H&E-stained frozen sections along the direction of polarized light adjacent to microinfarcts. (**c**) Complete occlusive free cholesterol crystal emboli are occasionally seen in the capillaries on H&E-stained frozen sections along the direction of polarized light adjacent to microinfarcts (arrow). (Modified and reproduced with permission [29])

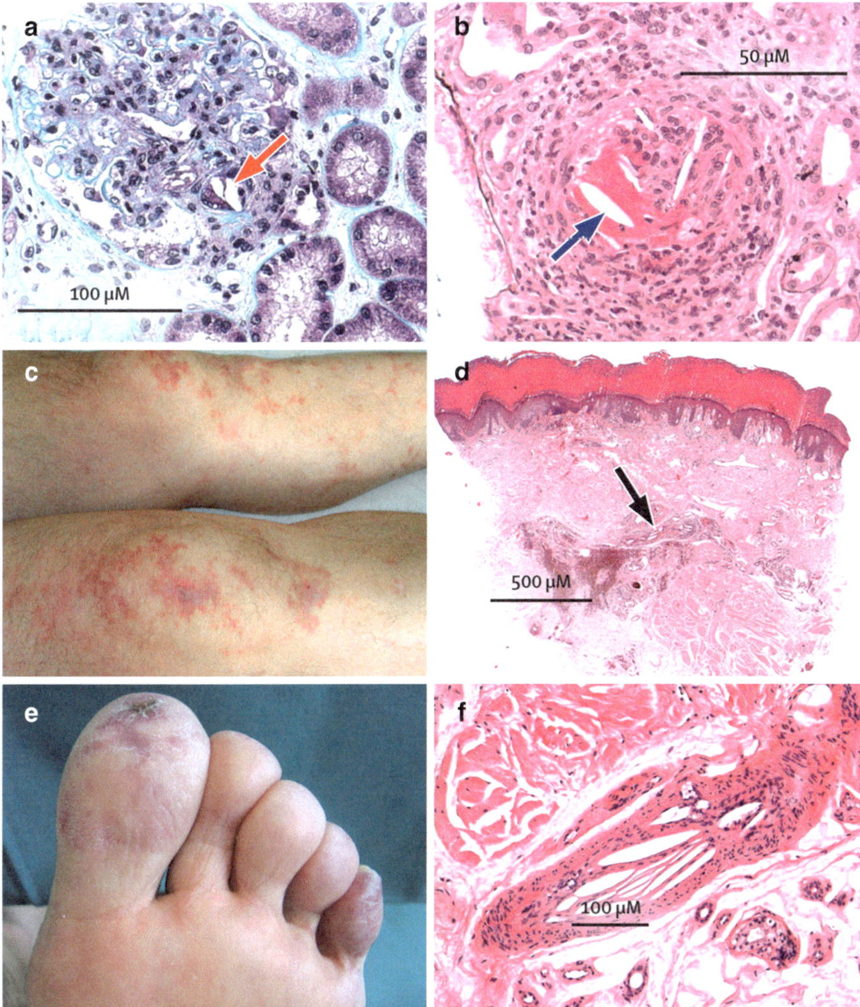

Fig. 5 Histology of cholesterol crystals consistent with a pseudovasculitis with giant cell reaction. (**a**) Intraglomerular renal cholesterol crystals; (**b**) cholesterol crystals in an arcuate artery with encasement of a crystal by a giant cell and pseudovasculitis inflammatory reaction (arrow); (**c**) purpuric lesion over knees; (**d**) skin biopsy with cholesterol crystals; blue toe (**e**) embolic crystals (**f**) in skin arterioles. (Modified and reproduced with permission [35])

The clinical course of the response to athero-embolism therefore depends on the ability of SRAPs to heal. If the SRAPs are extensive, emboli continue to shed debris and the clinical course may appear chronic, resulting in non-specific symptoms that can mimic auto-immune disease or sepsis, including fever, weight loss, myalgia related to myositis or rhabdomyolysis, and elevated inflammatory markers. Although each of these features is non-specific, the presence of livedo reticulitis, an elevation in inflammatory markers and eosinophilia together with the development of renal impairment in a patient with known atherosclerosis helps to secure the diagnosis without the need for tissue biopsy [4, 36] (Fig. 5).

Thus, the clinical consequences of athero-embolism depend on the vascular bed in which the plaque rupture occurred, the extent of atherosclerosis in the affected vessel, the volume and amount of CCs released into the circulation, and the extent of athero-thrombotic response. Since plaque ruptures are known to be common in patients with coronary disease, estimates of the true incidence of *spontaneous* athero-embolism are necessarily limited. Fortunately, despite continuous athero-embolism from SRAPs in the aorta, the incidence of fulminant clinical syndromes is rare, even in patients with extensive aortic atherosclerosis [37].

In contrast, iatrogenic plaque rupture and athero-embolism following intra-vascular diagnostic and interventional procedures including angiography, vascular stenting, percutaneous insertion of aortic valves, and bypass surgery are each well documented to be much more frequent [38]. During vascular intervention the risk of disturbing stable atherosclerotic plaque relates to the degree of existing disease and the duration of the procedure, and the consequences relate to the vascular bed at risk. The use of ultrasound to guide the insertion of tubing into the aorta at the time of heart bypass may reduce the risk of significant plaque injury and stroke, and the distal carriage of athero-embolic debris can be prevented with the use of protection devices during intra-vascular procedures [39, 40].

5 Diagnosis of Cholesterol Crystal Embolic Syndrome

Based on the presenting history and physical exam, CCE should be considered in patients with known atherosclerosis, who undergo a vascular intervention, and then develop acute skin changes, renal failure, Hollenhorst plaques, or abdominal pain [41, 42]. As discussed in the previous sections, depending on the source of the emboli and the presence of end-organ damage, the clinical presentations of each patient can vary, but they are typically generalized and non-specific. While CCE can occur spontaneously, the initial step should be determining if any recent procedures are the inciting event, such as renal artery percutaneous transluminal angioplasty [43].

Laboratory values can be helpful in indicating an inflammatory response, such as leukocytosis with eosinophilia. Fukomoto et al. reported that eosinophil counts (>500/uL) were higher in patients with a CCE after a procedure compared to no CCE. Furthermore, elevated eosinophilia occurred more frequently when accompanied by acute kidney injury (AKI) as a result of CCE [39]. Other labs representing inflammation are elevated C-reactive protein (CRP) and erythrocyte sedimentation rate. Additionally, end-organ damage can be seen in the laboratory values, such as anemia and thrombocytopenia [4, 25, 37]. Skin changes should be carefully noted and evaluated as they can be used as possible source of biopsy [44]. Patients with renal infarcts can present with flank pain and AKI. This can be illustrated via elevated serum lactate dehydrogenase (greater than 600 IU/L) and urine analysis with Hansel's stain showing proteinuria, hematuria, and eosinophiluria [45]. Limb ischemia can eventually lead to muscular damage, elevated levels of creatine phosphokinase, and AKI [5].

Imaging modalities allow us to identify possible sources of CCE, rule out other differentials, and provide possible treatment modalities. As organ damage becomes evident imaging modalities [i.e., ultrasound, computed tomography (CT), and magnetic resonance imaging (MRI)] can be used to help confirm the diagnosis. With acute kidney injury and suspicion of renal infarction, initial ultrasound imaging of the bilateral kidneys and followed by CT angiogram of the renal arteries is the preferred way to diagnose distal renal artery embolism [45]. In the setting of suspected stroke, CT and MRI imaging of the brain is the gold standard. Additionally, imaging studies can be used when bowel and limb ischemia is considered [4, 37].

An important step in CCE diagnosis is evaluating the thoracic aorta for plaque buildup as it is a common source of CCs, especially plaques that are larger than 4 mm, mobile, non-calcified, or lipid-laden. CT and MRI allow for comprehensive imaging of the aorta. Gadolinium-enhanced 3-dimensional magnetic resonance angiogram is useful for imaging the ascending aorta. Transesophageal echocardiography (TEE) can evaluate the thoracic aorta and valvular lesions but it is invasive and cannot completely image the thoracic aorta and distal portion of the ascending aorta. Pervaiz et al. compared injecting CC versus controls of microspheres and normal saline in 22 New Zealand white rabbits. They evaluated CC-induced inflammation by F-18 fluorodeoxyglucose (FDG) positron emission tomography and computed tomography angiography (PET/CTA). The study suggested that PET/CTA can detect inflammation via macrophage infiltration and necrosis without the obstruction of arterial flow [5] (Fig. 2).

The gold standard for diagnosis of CCE is a biopsy, where different stages of CCE and its associated damages can be observed. Tissues that can be considered are skin, kidney, muscle, bowel, and bone marrow. Skin biopsy is the safest option as it is minimally invasive and has a high sensitivity value of 92%. Histologically, the feature of CCE in skin biopsies is biconvex and needle-shaped spaces where the CC resides within arterioles. When prepared under liquid nitrogen, CC in the skin can be seen as double refraction under polarized light. In regard to kidney biopsies, ischemic injury, infarction, and focal and crescentic glomerulonephritis can be seen. The kidney damage from CCE has a patchy distribution; therefore, biopsy has a low sensitivity of 75% [46–48].

When CCE is considered a diagnosis, it is important to rule out the other possible etiologies by a thorough history and physical exam along with laboratory and imaging studies. The typical workup to evaluate for thromboembolism in patients with stroke and infective endocarditis was described above [45]. Left atrial myxoma should also be ruled out by echocardiography [37]. When evaluating a patient with creatinine following a procedure, contrast-induced AKI should always be considered, but it can be distinguished as above. Drug-induced interstitial nephritis is also a possibility depending on the management the patient received prior to and after the procedure [37]. Furthermore, vasculitis can mimic CCE including polyarteritis nodosa, systemic lupus erythematosus, rheumatoid arthritis, Takayasu's arteritis, and Henoch-Schonlein purpura. Therefore, a comprehensive auto-immune workup and biopsies would help in distinguishing these from CCE [37].

6   Prevention and Treatment of Unstable Atherosclerotic Plaques

Since the consequences of plaque rupture can be severe and life threatening, patients with atherosclerosis should be aggressively treated with therapies with the proven ability to reduce the risk of plaque rupture and atherothrombosis, including anti-platelet therapy, lipid lowering therapies, and low dose colchicine [17]. In addition, for patients undergoing vascular intervention, emboli protection devices should be considered during the procedure whenever possible, and surface ultrasound should be used to assist with preparation of the ascending aorta at the time of bypass surgery [37, 49].

Following plaque rupture, stenting specific lesions in medium size arteries has proven beneficial in patients with unstable, symptomatic coronary, and carotid disease. In contrast, in settings in which plaque rupture within the aorta has led to widespread athero-embolism, stenting of extensive aortic atherosclerotic plaque carries considerable risk and is not usually recommended unless the culprit plaque is believed to be infra-renal [50, 51].

No medical therapy has proven useful in reversing ischemic or inflammatory injury related to athero-embolism, including high dose steroids alone or with cyclophosphamide. If the syndrome is short lived, supportive measures including hemodialysis may be of value, however, if the syndrome is chronic or extensive, the prognosis is grave especially if there is mesenteric involvement leading to fulminant bowel ischemia or pancreatitis [52, 53].

Anticoagulation and thrombolytics have been relatively contra-indicated in patients with CCE [54]. The concern is related to possible worsening of the condition by greater release of CCs that were trapped in a thrombus sealing off a ruptured plaque or possibly bleeding into the plaque with extrusion into the circulation [55–58]. However, it is rare to develop CCE by just anticoagulation but rather an underlying event such as a vascular intervention could be the trigger leading to CCs release [37, 59, 60]. Overall, the presence of CCE after a thrombolytic event seems to carry a high morbidity and mortality [61, 62].

7   Conclusion

Athero-embolism consequent to plaque rupture or direct plaque injury at the time of vascular intervention is a systemic manifestation of atherosclerosis which may present in a number of ways. Spontaneous rupture of atherosclerotic plaques consistently occurs once the disease is advanced. In small and medium size arteries ruptures typically lead to athero-thrombotic occlusion, but in some instances, athero-embolism in of itself contributes to ischemic injury. Following spontaneous rupture of plaque in larger vessels including the carotid, iliac, and femoral arteries and aorta, atherosclerotic debris lodges in the distal circulation and leads to immediate ischemic injury. CCs within the debris that cannot be dissolved subsequently incites inflammation in the local vasculature and tissues. Most often spontaneous plaque ruptures in the aorta are clinically silent, however, small recurrent plaque ruptures lead to a chronic syndrome that may mimic a vasculitis and lead to chronic end-organ injury. In some instances, the extent of spontaneous plaque rupture is significant and leads to a fulminant syndrome affecting multiple tissues and organs including the skin, muscles, kidneys, and the mesenteric circulation which are more common in patients undergoing intra-vascular intervention. Although secondary prevention therapies and care at the time of vascular intervention may reduce the risk of plaque trauma, there is no known effective therapy for the sequelae related to athero-embolism.

References

1. Panum PL. Experimentelle Beitrage zur Lehre von der Embolie. Virchows Arch Pathol Anat Physiol. 1862;25:308–10.
2. Kronzon I, Saric M. Cholesterol embolization syndrome. Circulation. 2010;122:631–41. https://doi.org/10.1161/CIRCULATIONAHA.109.886465.
3. Flory CM. Arterial occlusions produced by emboli from eroded aortic atheromatous plaques. Am J Pathol. 1945;21:549–65.
4. Ghanem F, Vodnala D, Kalavakunta JK, et al. Cholesterol crystal embolization following plaque rupture: a systemic disease with unusual features. J Biomed Res. 2017;31:82–94. https://doi.org/10.7555/JBR.31.20160100.
5. Pervaiz MH, Durga S, Janoudi A, Berger K, Abela GS. PET/CTA detection of muscle inflammation related to cholesterol crystal emboli without arterial obstruction. J Nucl Cardiol. 2018;25:433–40. https://doi.org/10.1007/s12350-017-0826-y.
6. Rapp J, Mang X, Neumann M, Hong M, Hollenbeck K, Liu J. Microemboli composed of cholesterol crysals disrupt the blood-brain barrier and reduce cognition. Stroke. 2008;39:2354–61. https://doi.org/10.1161/STROKEAHA.107.496737.
7. Baumann DS, McGraw D, Rubin BG, et al. An institutional experience with arterial atheroembolism. Ann Vasc Surg. 1994;8:258–65. https://doi.org/10.1007/BF02018173.
8. Laloux P, Brucher JM. Lacunar infarctions due to cholesterol emboli. Stroke. 1991;22:1440–4. https://doi.org/10.1007/BF02018173.
9. Komatsu S, Yutani C, Ohara T, et al. Angioscopic evaluation of spontaneously ruptured aortic plaques. J Am Coll Cardiol. 2018;71:2893–902. https://doi.org/10.1016/j.jacc.2018.03.539.
10. Abela GS, Aziz K, Vedre A, Pathak DR, Talbott JD, Dejong J. Effect of cholesterol crystals on plaques and intima in arteries of patients with acute coronary and cerebrovascular syndromes. Am J Cardiol. 2009;103:959–68.
11. Nasiri M, Huang R, Janoudi A, Vanderberg A, Flegler C, Flegler S, Abela GS. Unraveling the role of cholesterol crystals in plaque rupture by altering the method of tissue preparation. Microsc Res Tech. 2015;78:969–74.
12. Komatsu S, Yutani C, Takahashi S, Mitsuhiko T, Ohara T, Hirayama A, Kodama K. Debris collected in-situ from spontaneously ruptured atherosclerotic plaque invariably contains large cholesterol crystals and evidence of activation of innate inflammation: insights from non-obstructive general angioscopy. Atherosclerosis. 2022;352:96–102. https://doi.org/10.1016/j.atherosclerosis.2022.03.010.

13. Düewell P, Kono H, Rayner KJ, et al. NLRP3 inflammasomes are required for atherogenesis and activated by cholesterol crystals. Nature. 2010;464:1357–61. https://doi.org/10.1038/nature08938.
14. Rajamäki K, Lappalainen J, Öörni K, Välimäki E, Matikainen S, Kovanen PT, Eklund KK. Cholesterol crystals activate the NLRP3 Inflammasome in human macrophages: a novel link between cholesterol metabolism and inflammation. PloS One. 2010;5:e11765. https://doi.org/10.1371/journal.pone.0011765.
15. Freigang S, Ampenberger F, Spohn G, Heer S, Shamshiev AT, Kisielow J, Hersberger M, Yamamoto M, Bachmann MF, Kopf M. Nrf2 is essential for cholesterol crystal-induced inflammasome activation and exacerbation of atherosclerosis. Eur J Immunol. 2011;41:2040–51.
16. Bunt TJ. The clinical significance of the asymptomatic Hollenhorst plaque. J Vasc Surg. 1986;4:559–62.
17. Scolari F, Ravani P, Pola A, et al. Predictors of renal and patient outcomes in atheroembolic renal disease: a prospective study. J Am Soc Nephrol. 2003;14:1584–90.
18. Gravastrand GS, Steinkjer B, Halvorsen B, et al. Cholesterol crystals induce coagulation activation through complement-dependent expression of monocytic tissue factor. J Immunol. 2019;203:853–63. https://doi.org/10.4049/jimmunol.1900503.
19. Gadeela N, Rubinstein J, Tamhane U, et al. The impact of circulating cholesterol crystals on vasomotor function: implications for no-reflow phenomenon. J Am Coll Cardiol Intv. 2011;4:521–9. https://doi.org/10.1016/j.jcin.2011.02.010.
20. Niccoli G, Burzotta F, Galiuto L, Crea F. Nyocaridal no-reflow in humans. J Am Coll Cardiol. 2009;54:281–92.
21. Swartz RS, Burke A, Farb A, Kaye D, Lesser JR, Henry TD, Virmani R. Microemboli and microvascular obstruction in acute coronary thrombosis and sudden coronary death: relation to epicardial plaque histology. J Am Coll Cardiol. 2009;54:2167–73.
22. Kealy WF. Atheroembolism. J Clin Pathol. 1978;31:984–9.
23. Komatsu S, Yutani C, Takahashi S, Kodama K. Acute myocardial infarction caused by distal embolization from a proximal ruptured plaque. J Am Coll Cardiol Case Rep. 2020;2:33–4. https://doi.org/10.1016/j.jaccas.2019.11.042.
24. Nidorf SM, Fiolet A, Abela GS. Viewing atherosclerosis through a crystal lens: how the evolving structure of cholesterol crystals in atherosclerotic plaque alters its stability. J Clin Lipidol. 2020;14:619–30. https://doi.org/10.1016/j.jacl.2020.07.003.
25. Rezkalla SH, Kloner RA. No-reflow phenomenon. Circulation. 2002;105:656–62.
26. Fischell TA, Subraya RG, Ashraf K, Perry B, Haller S. "Pharmacologic" distal protection using prophylactic, intragraft nicardipine to prevent no-reflow and non–Q-wave MI during elective saphenous vein graft intervention. J Invasive Cardiol. 2007;19:58–62.
27. Abela GS, Kalavakunta JK, Janoudi A, et al. Frequency of cholesterol crystals in culprit coronary artery aspirate during acute myocardial infarction and their relation to inflammation and myocardial injury. Am J Cardiol. 2017;120:1699–707. https://doi.org/10.1016/j.amjcard.2017.07.075.
28. Katayama Y, Taruya A, Kashiwagi M, et al. No-reflow phenomenon and in vivo cholesterol crystals combined with lipid core in acute myocardial infarction. IJC Heart Vasc. 2022;38:100953. https://doi.org/10.1016/j.ijcha.2022.100953.
29. Yutani C, Nagano T, Komatsu S, Kodama K. Visible-free cholesterol crystal emboli adjacent to microinfarcts in myocardial capillaries and arterioles on H&E stained frozen sections of an autopsied patient. BMJ Case Rep. 2018;2018:bcr2018225558. https://doi.org/10.1136/bcr-2018-225558.
30. Falanga V, Fine MJ, Kapoor WN. The cutaneous manifestations of cholesterol crystal embolization. Arch Dermatol. 1986;122:1194–8.
31. Donohue KG, Saap L, Falanga V. Cholesterol crystal embolization: an atherosclerotic disease with frequent and varied cutaneous manifestations. J Eur Acad Dermatol Venereol. 2003;17:504–11. https://doi.org/10.1046/j.1468-3083.2003.00710.x.

32. Tartari F, Altobrando AD, Merli Y, et al. Blue toe syndrome: a challenging diagnosis. Indian J Dermatol. 2019;64:506–7.

33. Singh NP, Gupta AK, Kaur G. Atheroembolic renal disease. Indian J Nephrol. 2020;30:1–2.

34. Greenberg A, Bastacky SI, Iqbal A, Borochovitz D, Johnson JP. Focal segmental glomerulosclerosis associated with nephrotic syndrome in cholesterol atheroembolism: clinicopathological correlations. Am J Kidney Dis. 1997;29:334–44.

35. Scolari F, Ravani P. Atheroembolic renal disease. Lancet. 2010;375(9726):1650–60. https://doi.org/10.1016/SO140-6736(09)62073-0.

36. Haygood TA, Fessel WJ, Strange DA. Atheromatous microembolism simulating polymyositis. JAMA. 1968;203:423–5.

37. Ozkok A. Cholesterol-embolization syndrome: current perspectives. Vasc Health Risk Manag. 2019;15:209–20.

38. Scolari F, Ravani P, Gaggi R, et al. The challenge of diagnosing atheroembolic renal disease: clinical features and prognostic factors. Circulation. 2007;116:298. https://doi.org/10.1161/CIRCULATIONAHA.106.680991.

39. Fukumoto Y, Tsutsui H, Tsuchihashi M, et al. The incidence and risk factors of cholesterol embolization syndrome, a complication of cardiac catheterization: a prospective study. J Am Coll Cardiol. 2003;42:211–6.

40. Doty JR, Wilentz RE, Salazar JD, Hruban RH, Cameron DE. Atheroembolism in cardiac surgery. Ann Thorac Surg. 2003;75:1221–6. https://doi.org/10.1016/S0003-4975(02)04712-4.

41. Jucgla A, Moresco F, Muniesa C, Moreno A, Vidaller A. Cholesterol embolism: still an unrecognized entity with a high mortality rate. J Am Acad Dermatol. 2006;55:786–93. https://doi.org/10.1016/j.jaad.2006.05.012.

42. Saric M, Kronzon I. Cholesterol embolization syndrome. Curr Opin Cardiol. 2011;26:472–9. https://doi.org/10.1097/HCO.0b013e32834b7fdd.

43. Tanaka H, Yamana H, Matsui H, Fushimi K, Yasunaga H. Proportion and risk factors of cholesterol crystal embolization after cardiovascular procedures: a retrospective national database study. Heart Vessels. 2020;35:1250–5. https://doi.org/10.1007/s00380-020-01593-1.

44. Imai N, Zamami R, Kimura K. Cutaneous cholesterol embolization syndrome. Indian J Dermatol Venereol Leprol. 2015;81:38.

45. Lyaker MR, Tulman DB, Dimitrova GT, Pin RH, Papadimos TJ. Arterial embolism. Int J Crit Illn Inj Sci. 2013;3:77–87.

46. Frock J, Bierman M, Hammeke M, Reyes A. Atheroembolic renal disease: experience with 22 patients. Nebr Med J. 1994;79:317–21.

47. Meyrier A, Buchet P, Simon P, Fernet M, Rainfray M, Callard P. Atheromatous renal disease. Am J Med. 1988;85:139–46. https://doi.org/10.1016/S0002-9343(88)80332-2.

48. Eliot RS, Kanjuh VI, Edwards JE. Atheromatous embolism. Circulation. 1964;30:611–8.

49. Bangalore S, Bhatt D. Embolic protection devices. Circulation. 2014;129:e470–6. https://doi.org/10.1161/CIRCULATIONAHA.114.010240.

50. Matchett W, McFarland D, Eidt J, Moursi M. Blue toe syndrome: treatment with intra-arterial stents and review of therapies. J Vasc Interv Radiol. 2000;11:585–92. https://doi.org/10.1016/S1051-0443(07)61610-8.

51. Müller MD, Lyrer PA, Brown MM, Bonati LH. Carotid artery stenting versus endarterectomy for treatment of carotid artery stenosis. Stoke. 2020;52:e3–5. https://doi.org/10.1161/STROKEAHA.120.030521Stroke.

52. Yucel A, Kart-Koseoglu H, Demirhan B, Ozdemir F. Cholesterol crystal embolization mimicking vasculitis: success with corticosteroid and cyclophosphamide therapy in two cases. Rheumatol Int. 2006;26:454–60. https://doi.org/10.1007/s00296-005-0012-4.

53. Belenfant X, Meyrier A, Jacquot C. Supportive treatment improves survival in multivisceral cholesterol crystal embolism. Am J Kidney Dis. 1999;33:840–50.

54. Cortez AF, Sakuma TH, Lima RB, et al. Cholesterol crystal embolization caused by anticoagulant therapy. Int J Dermatol. 2009;48:989–90.
55. Kassirer JP. Atheroembolic renal disease. N Engl J Med. 1969;280:812–8.
56. Lye WC, Cheah JS, Sinniah R. Renal cholesterol embolic disease. Case report and review of the literature. Am J Nephrol. 1993;13:489–93.
57. Mayo RR, Swartz RD. Redefining the incidence of clinically detectable atheroembolism. Am J Med. 1996;100:524–9.
58. Thadhani RI, Camargo CA Jr, Xavier RJ, Fang LS, Bazari H. Atheroembolic renal failure after invasive procedures. Natural history based on 52 histologically proven cases. Medicine. 1995;74:350–8.
59. Scolari F, Tardanico R, Zani R, et al. Cholesterol crystal embolism: a recognizable cause of renal disease. Am J Kidney Dis. 2000;36:1089–109.
60. Fine MJ, Kapoor W, Falanga V. Cholesterol crystal embolization: a review of 221 cases in the English literature. Angiology. 1987;38:769–84.
61. Hitti WA, Wali RK, Weinman EJ, Drachenberg C, Briglia A. Cholesterol embolization syndrome induced by thrombolytic therapy. Am J Cardiovasc Drugs. 2008;8:27–34.
62. Varis J, Kuusniemi K, Jarvelainen H. Cholesterol microembolization syndrome: a complication of anticoagulant therapy. Can Med Assoc J. 2010;182:931–3. https://doi.org/10.1503/cmaj.090919.

The Role of Cholesterol Crystals in the Development and Progression of Degenerative Valve Disease

Khalid Saeed Al-Asad, Nadine El-Ayache, Abdullah Al-Abcha, and George S. Abela

1 Structure of the Cardiac Skeleton and Heart Valves

The cardiac skeleton consists of four rings of dense connective tissue that surround the mitral and tricuspid valves and extend to the origins of the aorta and the pulmonary trunk thus providing support for the heart valves and electrically isolating the atria and the ventricles. The surface of valve leaflets is endothelialized and normal endothelial function reduces the risk of valvulitis and thrombosis. The body of the leaflets are composed of three layers of highly organized extracellular matrix including, a layer of fibrillar collagen that provides strength to the valvular structure; a middle layer that is primarily composed of proteoglycans that provides leaflet compressibility; and an elastic layer that facilitates valve motion by allowing extension and recoil [1–3] (Fig. 1).

A variety of conditions may affect valve leaflets, however, in the western world, "age-related" degenerative disease is the most common form of valvular disease which is increasing in prevalence due to increased longevity of the general population. This chapter examines the role of CCs in degenerative valve disease [4–6].

K. S. Al-Asad · N. El-Ayache · A. Al-Abcha
Division of Internal Medicine, Department of Medicine, College of Human Medicine, Michigan State University, East Lansing, MI, USA

Sparrow Hospital, Lansing, MI, USA
e-mail: saeedala@msu.edu; al-abcha.abdullah@mayo.edu

G. S. Abela (✉)
Department of Medicine, Division of Cardiovascular Medicine, Michigan State University, East Lansing, MI, USA
e-mail: abela@msu.edu

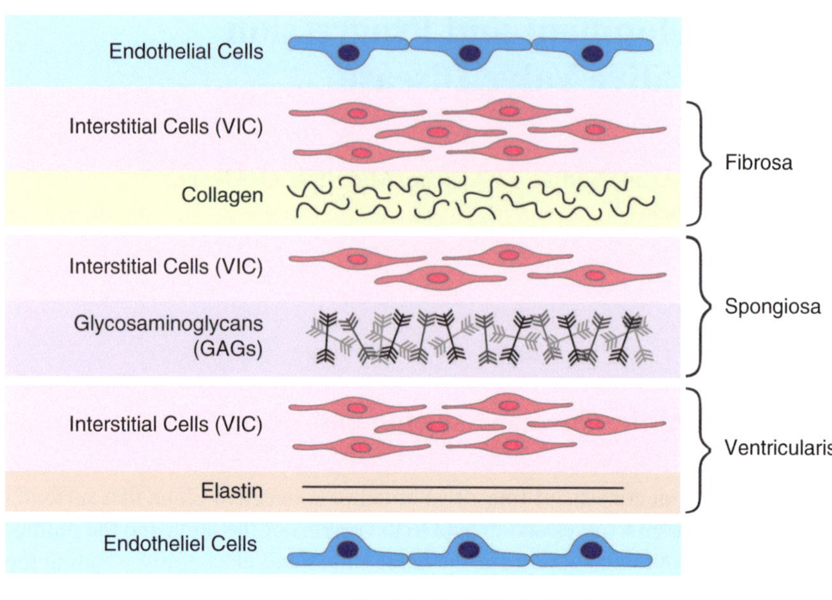

Fig. 1 Cellular architecture of a normal aortic valve. (Reproduced with permission [3])

2 Pathophysiology of Degenerative Valve Disease

The process of valvular degeneration associated with fibrosis and calcification of the cardiac skeleton shares similarities with the atherosclerotic process. Accordingly, it is generally believed that shear stress and systemic pressure contribute to the initial endothelial injury to the leaflets that predisposes to the deposition of lipoproteins into the subendothelial space. It has become increasingly clear that the ongoing injury to the leaflets likely results from incessant injury induced by cholesterol crystals (CCs) in the leaflets that cannot be cleared but can continue to grow and aggregate [7–9] (Fig. 2). Because the architecture and fibrous nature of the leaflets stands in contrast to that of the arterial wall, it initially restricts the capacity for large lipid pools to accumulate, which may explain why degenerative valve disease develops more slowly than atherosclerosis.

Animal and human studies confirm that a lipid rich diet and hypercholesterolemia predispose to the formation of CCs in both native and prosthetic tissue heart valves (Fig. 3) [6, 7, 10]. Physical factors, including a few degrees centigrade change in temperature within physiologic limits, as well as higher pH can facilitate the formation of CCs [11]. In addition, CCs in the valve matrix may act as a nidus for the formation and deposition of calcium phosphate crystals [7, 12–14] (Fig. 4).

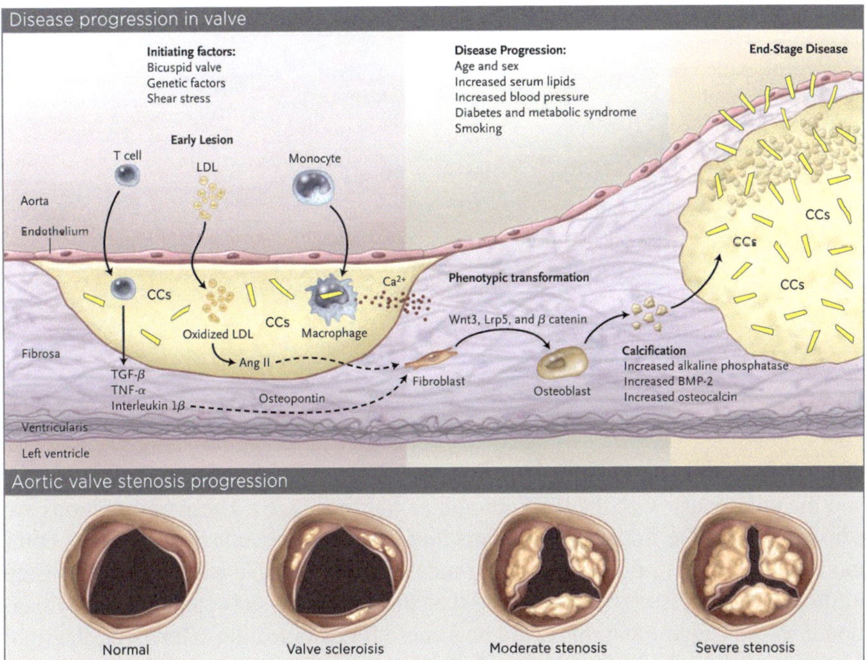

Fig. 2 Inflammatory process in degenerative aortic valve disease. (top) Histology of the early lesion is characterized by a subendothelial accumulation of oxidized low-density lipoprotein (LDL), production of angiotensin (Ang) II, and inflammation with T lymphocytes and macrophages. Cholesterol crystals (CCs) are seen early in the lipid accumulation followed by more dense formations of CCs in the advanced lipid deposits with perforation of the valve surface that triggers an inflammatory response. Disease progression then occurs by local production of proteins, such as osteopontin, osteocalcin, and bone morphogenic protein 2 (BMP-2), which mediate tissue calcification; activation of inflammatory signaling pathways, including tumor necrosis factor α (TNF-α), tumor growth factor β (TGF-β), the complement system, C-reactive protein, NLRP3 inflammasome, and interleukin-1β. Changes in tissue matrix include the accumulation of tenascin C, and upregulation of matrix metalloproteinase 2 and alkaline phosphatase activity. In addition, leaflet fibroblasts undergo phenotypic transformation into osteoblasts, regulated by the Wnt3–Lrp5–β catenin signaling pathway. Microscopic accumulations of extracellular calcification (Ca²⁺) are present early in the disease process, with progressive calcification and areas of frank bone formation in end-stage disease. (bottom) The corresponding changes in aortic-valve anatomy are viewed from the aortic side with the valve open in systole. (Reproduced with permission [9])

In an atherosclerotic rabbit model that evaluated the effect of a lipid rich diet on both atherosclerosis and aortic valve diseases, the accumulation of cholesterol in the aortic leaflets was associated with the formation of CCs, the evidence of CC induced leaflet trauma, macrophage infiltration of valvular tissues and a systematic inflammatory response as evidenced by an increase in C-reactive protein [7] (Fig. 5). In the atherosclerotic rabbit model (Group I, only fed high cholesterol diet), the amount of cholesterol content in the aortic valve far exceeded the amount of cholesterol in the other cardiac valves with the mitral following as a far second, tricuspid as third

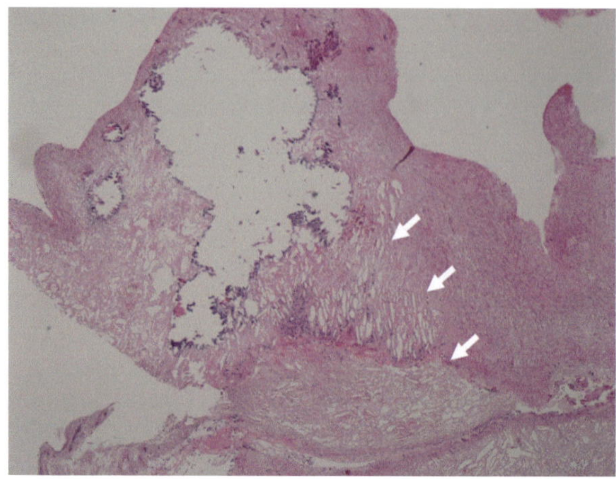

Fig. 3 Hematoxylin and eosin stain of bioprosthetic leaflet demonstrating cholesterol crystal deposition as empty finger-like projections with calcification and chronic inflammation (original magnification ×40) (arrows). (Reproduced with permission [10])

and the pulmonary with the least amount as fourth (Fig. 6). These observations are consistent with the findings in humans that degenerative valve disease most commonly affects the aortic valve. In the model, the aortic valve was the most densely infiltrated by cholesterol and knowing that cholesterol crystals can trigger calcification it would suggest that this could be a cause for calcification. Moreover, the right heart valves had the least amount of cholesterol and are known to have the least amount of calcification.

Thus, CCs that form within the endothelial and deeper layers of the leaflets can trigger traumatic and inflammatory injury that leads to progressive fibrosis and calcification of the leaflets that in turn restricts their excursion and leads to progressive valvular dysfunction. As in other tissues, rapid formation, growth, and aggregation of CCs can cause traumatic injury that in the leaflets results in endothelial injury and damage to its fibrous layers [14–16]. Once released into the matrix of the leaflets, CCs that cannot be cleared predispose to chronic inflammation due to the activation of various cytokines and inflammation molecules including the NLRP3 inflammasome; the expression of interleukins including IL-1β, IL-6, IL-18; the recruitment and activation of leukocytes including macrophages and T-cells; frustrated phagocytosis; the release of lytic enzymes including super-oxide, MMP, and the expression of TNF and RANKL which promote myo-fibroblastic and osteoblastic activity which promotes mineralization and calcification of the leaflets [17–21] (Fig. 2).

A number of risk factors that accelerate atherosclerosis also appear to accelerate valvular degeneration including increasing age; hypertension; elevated LDLc and Lp(a); diabetes; gout; chronic kidney disease, and an elevated absolute neutrophil count. In addition, ACE and Chymase are known to be expressed in calcific valves resulting in increased production of angiotensin II and collagen within the leaflets [22–24].

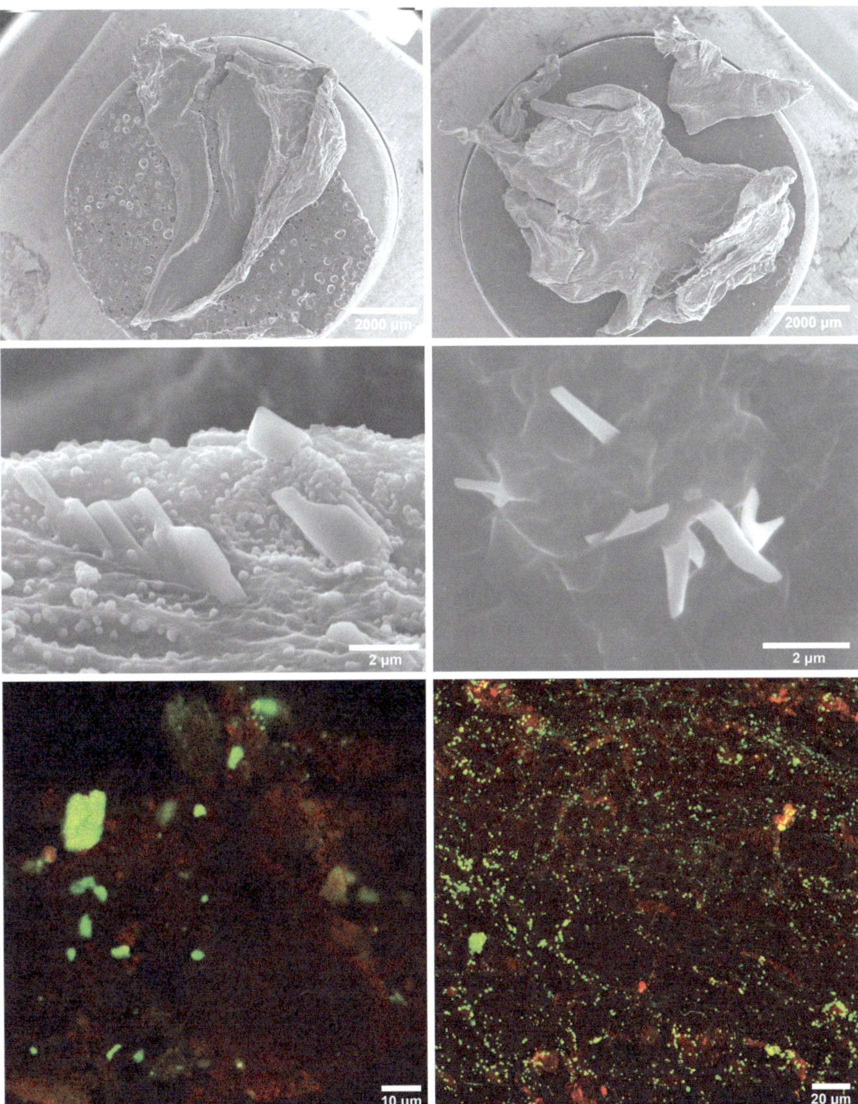

Fig. 4 (Top) Scanning electron micrographs of human aortic (left) and mitral (right) valves with cholesterol crystals that appear to be emerging from the surface of the valves. Fluorescence microscopy demonstrates cholesterol crystals at the valve surface in fresh unprocessed tissue (bodipy staining cholesterol crystals green and Ac-LDL counter-stained endothelium red). (Bottom) Crystallography demonstrates the presence of three calcium peaks on the aortic valve. (Reproduced with permission [7])

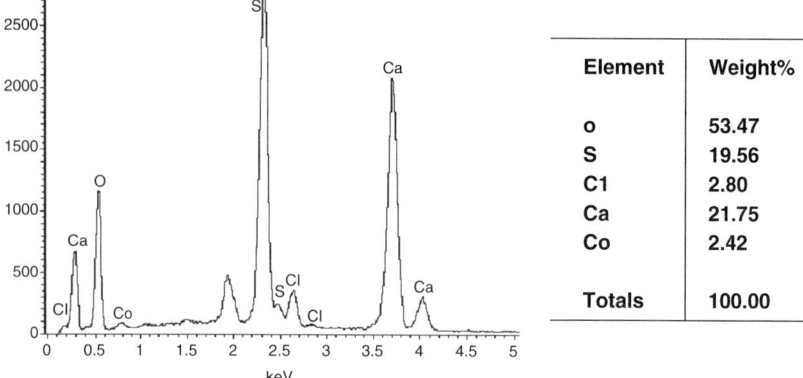

Fig. 4 (continued)

Several genetic mutations have also been associated with valvular degeneration including variants of NOTCH1 and GATA-5 which have been associated with bicuspid aortic valves; variants of NOTCH1, RUNX2 (osteogenic transcription factor) and CACNA1C (voltage-dependent calcium channel subunit) that promote valvular mineralization, and a single-nucleotide polymorphism (SNP) in the LP(a) gene (Lipoprotein a) that has been associated with aortic stenosis likely enhances the uptake of cholesterol into the leaflets [21, 22].

Other distinct forms of valvular heart disease are also driven by inflammatory processes which typically present at a young age but may be accelerated later in life by the CC induced changes described above in susceptible patients [25]. In rheumatic fever, valvulitis that leads to sclerosis is initiated by an abnormal immune response after the exposure to Group A β-hemolytic streptococci (GAS). Antigen mimicry is the cornerstone of the pathophysiology of the disease where antibodies formed by the humoral and cellular immune response against GAS cross-react with tissue antigens in the heart, joints, and the skin resulting in inflammation, and injury to these tissues [26].

In *autoimmune connective tissue diseases* including rheumatoid arthritis, systemic lupus erythematosus, and ankylosing spondylitis, valvulitis is mediated by the adaptive immune system but does not involve autoantibodies directly targeting cardiac antigens [27, 28]. Rather it is caused by the deposition of autoimmune complexes that interact with different adhesion molecules and receptors on the valvular endothelium that then initiates and propagates inflammatory injury [29, 30].

Several *medications* have also been associated with degenerative valve disease, including ergotamine, methysergide, cabergoline, pergolide, fenfluramine, dexfenfluramine, phentermine as well as certain recreational drugs such as MDMA (3,4-methylenedioxymethamphetamine or ecstasy) which act, partially or fully, to agonize the serotonergic 5-hydroxytryptamine 2B receptors on the valvular endothelium resulting in cellular proliferation and tissue fibrosis [31, 32].

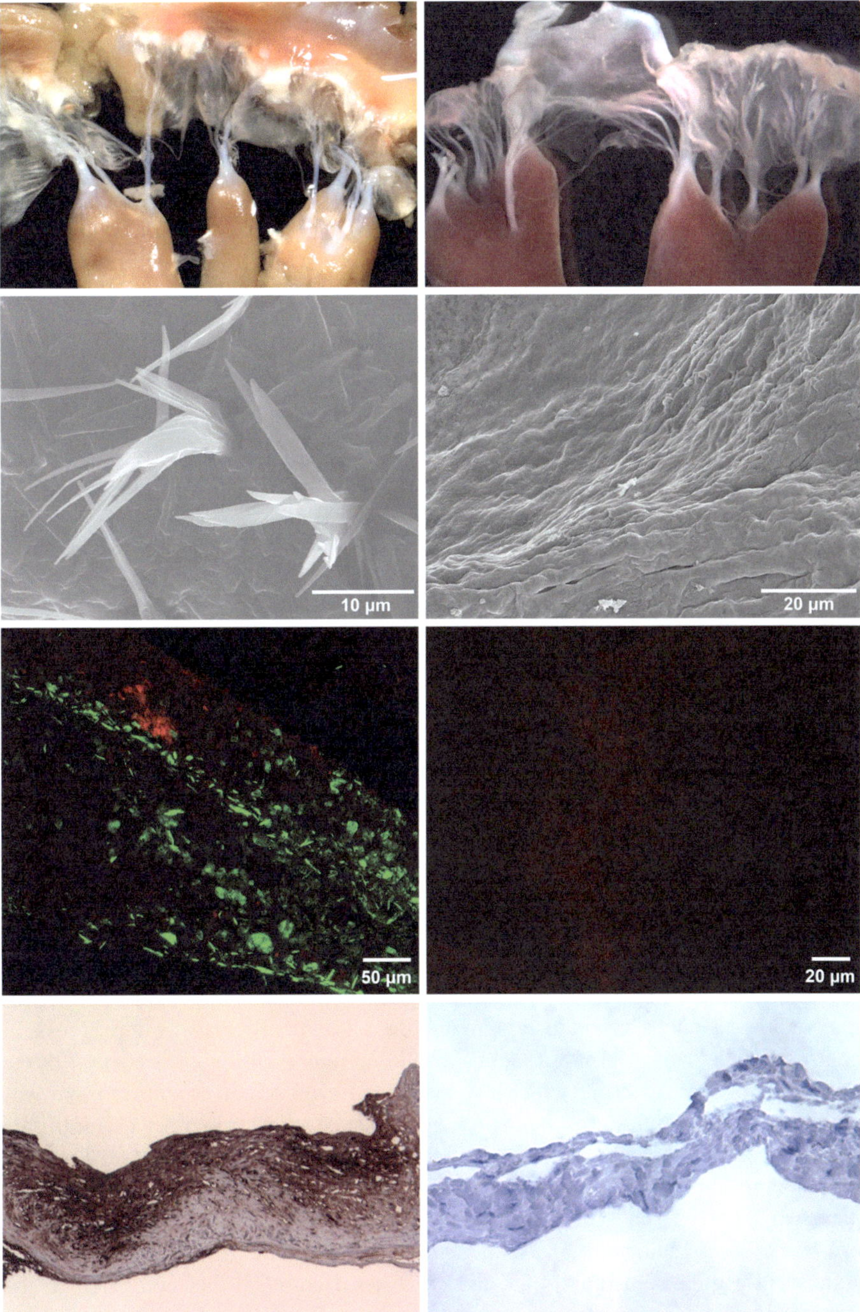

Fig. 5 (Left) Gross valve images, scanning electron micrographs, fluorescence microscopy, and RAM 11 staining of atherosclerotic rabbit mitral valve demonstrating discolored and thickened mitral valve with cholesterol crystals perforating the valve surfaces and macrophage infiltration (brown color). (Right) Gross valve images, scanning electron micrographs and fluorescence microscopy of normal valve from non-atherosclerotic rabbit without evidence of cholesterol crystals or macrophages. (Reproduced with permission [7])

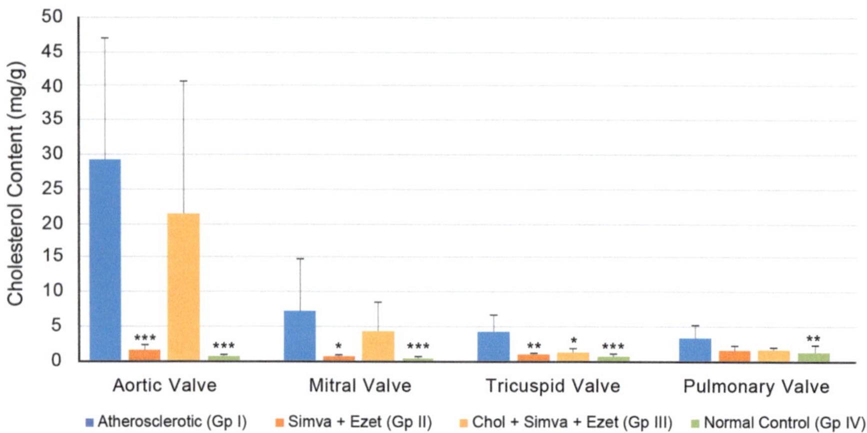

Fig. 6 Cholesterol content of rabbit aortic, mitral, tricuspid, and pulmonary valves. Group I—High cholesterol diet only; Group II—Treatment with simvastatin and ezetimibe *concurrent with* high cholesterol diet; Group III—Treatment with simvastatin and ezetimibe initiated 6 months *after* the initiation of high cholesterol diet; Group IV—Controls.—Normal diet, and no treatment. (***$p < 0.001$; **$p < 0.01$; *$p < 0.05$). (Reproduced with permission [7])

3 The Effect of Lipid Lowering Therapy for Degenerative Valve Disease

Since atherosclerosis and degenerative valve disease share the same risk factors and have a similar pathogenesis, it might be expected that lipid lowering therapy could slow the progression of valvular heart disease. Disappointingly, prospective randomized clinical trials using statins and a combination of statins with ezetimibe demonstrated that aggressive lipid lowering over several years (mean 3.5 years) had no effect on the progression of mild to moderate aortic stenosis [33, 34].

In keeping with these clinical observations, studies in an atherosclerotic rabbit model also demonstrated that lipid lowering therapy was unable to slow the degenerative process once CCs were evident and the sclerotic process was in progress. In contrast, in the same animal model *in which the native valves were normal at the outset* when lipid lowering with simvastatin and ezetimibe was started there was significantly less cholesterol deposition and absence of inflammatory cell infiltrate [7] (Fig. 6). The percent valve area of staining with RAM 11 as a marker for macrophage infiltrate, the untreated atherosclerotic group had 29–36% infiltration compared to 0.0–0.1% in both the normal control group and the simvastatin and ezetimibe combination group. Also, C-reactive protein (CRP) serum levels were significantly greater in rabbits fed the cholesterol enriched diet compared to the group that was fed the cholesterol enriched diet but also given simvastatin and ezetimibe combination (10,519 ± 10,947 vs. 2720 ± 2193 ng/mL, $p = 0.03$).

The lack of effect by lipid lowering therapy on aortic valve disease in humans stands in contrast to its observed benefits in atherosclerosis. This discordance may reflect the fact that cardiovascular (CV) trials have measured the effect of lipid lowering therapy by assessing the incidence of MACE events that relate to acute plaque rupture rather than an effect on the sclerotic progress. In this regard it is notable that statins accelerate rather than reduce the rate of coronary calcification which may negate their potential to slow degenerative valve disease [35]. Another reason could be that once cholesterol is crystalized it is difficult to mobilize by HDLc, the only known endogenous agent with ability to dissolve CCs [36]. Thus, if HDLc cannot contact the crystals because they are deeply embedded within the valve matrix, then it is not likely for it to be effective and similarly, statins which have also been found to dissolve cholesterol crystals, physical contact is critical for them to be effective [37].

No matter the reason for the lack of effect of lipid therapy on the progression of aortic stenosis, the observations from clinical and animal studies suggest that in order to slow the progression of degenerative valve disease, it may be more important to inhibit inflammation induced by CCs. Although aggressive lipid lowering does not affect the degenerative process in heart valves once it is in progress, its ability to reduce the uptake of cholesterol and the development of CCs in normal heart valves raises the possibility that early initiation of lipid lowering therapy in patients with familial lipid disorders may delay the premature development of both atherosclerosis and degenerative valve disease. Thus, early and long-term use of statins and lipid lowering may have an impact on prevention of valve calcification and stenosis if started much earlier in life and prior to the development of advanced valve disease including mild to moderate valve stenosis.

4   CCs May Enhance the Risk of Bacterial Endocarditis

Bacterial attachment to the valves is the first step in the pathogenesis of endocarditis and it has been demonstrated that bacteria have a predilection for adherence to sclerotic heart valves (Chapter "Activation of Systemic- and Intracellular Complement by Cholesterol Crystals"). Microscopic studies of sclerotic valves have shown not only the presence of cholesterol crystals in abundance but have also shown these crystals to perforate the surrounding fibrous tissue making them exposed to the surface [7]. Furthermore, it was demonstrated that bacteria interact with these crystals via certain (yet undefined) adhesions molecules and can dissolve those crystals to utilize cholesterol for metabolism. All these findings lead to the hypothesis that CCs not only increase the risk of endocarditis due to endothelial injury, but that also act as a nidus for bacterial adherence that can attach to and metabolize them [38].

Although lipid lowering does not appear to have a clinically meaningful effect on the rate of progression of aortic valve disease, there is evidence that patients taking statins at the time of developing endocarditis have a reduced risk of systemic embolism and an improved long-term prognosis [38].

5 Summary

Cholesterol crystals that form in native and prosthetic heart valves may trigger traumatic and inflammatory injury that predisposes to chronic degenerative change that over time leads to valvular dysfunction. Furthermore, CC induced injury to the valve surface may predispose to endocarditis, as when exposed to the circulation they may act as "landing sites" for bacteria that can attach to and grow on them while using them as a source of cholesterol to support their own metabolism.

While lipid lowering therapy may reduce CCs formation in normal cardiac valves that may in turn reduce the likelihood of developing degenerative valve disease, it does not slow progression of the degenerative process once it is in progress. This suggests that over time, the inflammatory process induced by CCs becomes the main driver of valvular degeneration and raises the possibility that therapies that inhibit CC induced inflammation may slow the progression of degenerative valve disease.

References

1. Saremi F, Sánchez-Quintana D, Mori S, Muresian H, Spicer DE, Hassani C, Anderson RH. Fibrous skeleton of the heart: anatomic overview and evaluation of pathologic conditions with CT and MR imaging. Radiographics. 2017;37:1330–51.
2. Misfeld M, Sievers H-H. Heart valve macro- and microstructure. Philos Trans R Soc Lond B Biol Sci. 2007;362:1421–36.
3. Rajamannan NM, Evans FJ, Aikawa E, Grande-Allen J, Demer LL, Heistad DD, Simmons CA, Masters KS, Mathieu P, Obrien KD, Schoen FJ, Towler DA, Yoganathan AP, Otto CM. Calcific aortic valve disease: not simply a degenerative process. Circulation. 2011;124:1783. https://doi.org/10.1161/CIRCULATIONAHA.110.006767.
4. Riddle JM, Magilligan DJ, Stein PD, Ford H. Surface topography of stenotic aortic valves by scanning electron microscopy. Circulation. 1980;61:496. http://ahajournals.org.
5. Leask RL, Jain N, Butany J. Endothelium and valvular diseases of the heart. Microsc Res Tech. 2003;60:129–37.
6. Abramowitz Y, Jilaihawi H, Chakravarty T, Mack MJ, Makkar RR. Mitral annulus calcification. J Am Coll Cardiol. 2015;66:1934.
7. El-Khatib LA, de Feijter-Rupp H, Janoudi A, Fry L, Kehdi M, Abela GS. Cholesterol induced heart valve inflammation and injury: efficacy of cholesterol lowering treatment. Open Heart. 2020;7:e001274.
8. Cho KI, Sakuma I, Sohn IS, Jo SH, Koh KK. Inflammatory and metabolic mechanisms underlying the calcific aortic valve disease. Atherosclerosis. 2018;277:60–5.
9. Otto C. Calcific aortic stenosis. N Engl J Med. 2008;359:1395–7.
10. Price L, Sniderman A, Omerglu A, Lachapelle K. Bioprosthetic valve degeneration due to cholesterol deposition in a patient with normal lipid profile. Can J Cardiol. 2007;23:233–4.
11. Vedre A, Pathak DR, Crimp M, Lum C, Koochesfahani M, Abela GS. Physical factors that trigger cholesterol crystallization leading to plaque rupture. Atherosclerosis. 2008;203:89–96.
12. Dorozhkina E, Dorozhkin S. In vitro crystallization of carbonateapatite on cholesterol from a modified simulated body fluid. Colloids Surf A Physicochem Eng Asp. 2003;223:231–7. https://doi.org/10.1016/S0927-7757(03)00221-8.

13. Laird DF, Mucalo MR, Yokogawa Y. Growth of calcium hydroxyapatite (ca-HAp) on cholesterol and cholestanol crystals from a simulated body fluid: a possible insight into the pathological calcifications associated with atherosclerosis. J Colloid Interface Sci. 2006;295:348–63. https://doi.org/10.1016/j.jcis.2005.09.013.
14. Goody PR, Hosen MR, Christmann D, Niepmann ST, Zietzer A, Adam M, Bönner F, Zimmer S, Nickenig G, Jansen F. Aortic valve stenosis: from basic mechanisms to novel therapeutic targets. Arterioscler Thromb Vasc Biol. 2020;40:885–900.
15. Abela GS, Aziz K. Cholesterol crystals rupture biological membranes and human plaques during acute cardiovascular events: a novel insight into plaque rupture by scanning electron microscopy. Scanning. 2006;28:1–10.
16. Al-Handawi MB, Commins P, Karothu DP, Raj G, Li L, Naumov P. Mechanical and crystallographic analysis of cholesterol crystals puncturing biological membranes. Chem A Eur J. 2018;24:11493–7.
17. Nadra I, Mason JC, Philippidis P, Florey O, Smythe CDW, McCarthy GM, Landis RC, Haskard DO. Proinflammatory activation of macrophages by basic calcium phosphate crystals via protein kinase C and MAP kinase pathways. Circ Res. 2005;96:1248–56.
18. Düewell P, Kono H, Rayner KJ, Sirois CM, Vladimer G, Bauernfeind FG, Abela GS, Franchi L, Nuñez G, Schnurr M, Espevik T, Lien E, Fitzgerald KA, Rock KL, Moore KJ, Wright SD, Hornung V, Latz E. NLRP3 inflammasomes are required for atherogenesis and activated by cholesterol crystals. Nature. 2010;464:1357–61. https://doi.org/10.1038/nature08938.
19. Rajamaki K, Lappalainen J, O'orni K, Valimaki E, Matikainen S, Kovanen PT, Eklund KK. Cholesterol crystals activate the NLRP3 inflammasome in human macrophages: a novel link between cholesterol metabolism and inflammation. PloS One. 2010;5(7):e11765. https://doi.org/10.1371/journal.pone.0011765.8.
20. Kelley N, Jeltema D, Duan Y, He Y. The NLRP3 inflammasome: an overview of mechanisms of activation and regulation. Int J Mol Sci. 2019;20:3328.
21. Broeders W, Bekkering S, Messaoudi S, Joosten LAB, van Royen N, Riksen NP. Innate immune cells in the pathophysiology of calcific aortic valve disease: lessons to be learned from atherosclerotic cardiovascular disease? Basic Res Cardiol. 2022;117:28. https://doi.org/10.1007/s00395-022-00935-6.
22. Chen HY, Engert JC, Thanassoulis G. Risk factors for valvular calcification. Curr Opin Endocrinol Diabetes Obes. 2019;26:96–102.
23. O'Donnell A, Yutzey KE. Mechanisms of heart valve development and disease. Development. 2020;147:147.
24. Lindman BR, Clavel MA, Mathieu P, Iung B, Lancellotti P, Otto CM, Pibarot P. Calcific aortic stenosis. Nat Rev Dis Primers. 2016;2:16006.
25. Buleu F, Sirbu E, Caraba A, Dragan S. Heart involvement in inflammatory rheumatic diseases: a systematic literature review. Medicina (Kaunas). 2019;55:249.
26. Marijon E, Mirabel M, Jouven X, Georges Pompidou Hospital E, Marijon E, Mirabel M, Celermajer DS, Jouven X. Rheumatic heart disease. Lancet. 2012;379:953. www.thelancet.com.
27. Liu J, Frishman WH. Nonbacterial thrombotic endocarditis: pathogenesis, diagnosis, and management. Cardiol Rev. 2016;24:244–7.
28. Hurrell H, Roberts-Thomson R, Prendergast BD. Non-infective endocarditis. Heart. 2020;106:1023–9.
29. Breed ER, Binstadt BA. Autoimmune valvular carditis. Curr Allergy Asthma Rep. 2015;15:491.
30. Perlroth MG. Connective tissue diseases and the heart. JAMA. 1975;231:410–2. https://doi.org/10.1001/jama.1975.03240160072038.
31. Cosyns B, Droogmans S, Rosenhek R, Lancellotti P. Drug-induced valvular heart disease. Heart. 2013;99:7–12.
32. Bhattacharyya S, Schapira AH, Mikhailidis DP, Davar J. Drug-induced fibrotic valvular heart disease. Lancet. 2009;374:577–85.

33. Rossebø AB, Pedersen TR, Boman K, Brudi P, Chambers JB, Egstrup K, Gerdts E, Gohlke-Bärwolf C, Holme I, Kesäniemi A, Malbecq W, Nienaber CA, et al. Intensive lipid lowering with simvastatin and ezetimibe in aortic stenosis. N Engl J Med. 2008;359:1343–56. https://doi.org/10.1056/NEJMoa0804602.

34. Chan KL, Teo K, Dumesnil JG, Ni A, Tam J, For the ASTRONOMER Investigators. Effect of lipid lowering with Rosuvastatin on progression of aortic stenosis. Circulation. 2010;121:306–14.

35. Zhang X, Xiao J, Wang L, Xiaoping J. Statins accelerate coronary calcification and reduce the risk of cardiovascular events. Cardiol Rev. 2022. https://doi.org/10.1097/CRD.0000000000000438.

36. Abdulla YH, Adams CW. The action of human high density lipoprotein on cholesterol crystals. Part 2. Biochemical observations. Atherosclerosis. 1978;31:473–80.

37. Abela GS, Vedre A, Janoudi A, Huang R, Durga S, Tamhane U. Effect of statins on cholesterol crystallization and atherosclerotic plaque stabilization. Am J Cardiol. 2011;107:1710–7.

38. Boumegouas M, Raju M, Gardiner J, Hammer N, Saleh Y, Al-Abcha A, Kalra A, Abela GS. Interaction between bacteria and cholesterol crystals: implications for endocarditis and atherosclerosis. PloS One. 2022;17:e0263847.

Part VI
Cholesterol Crystals and Inflammation

Activation of Systemic- and Intracellular Complement by Cholesterol Crystals

Nathalie Niyonzima, Claudia Kemper, Bente Halvorsen, Tom Eirik Mollnes, and Terje Espevik

N. Niyonzima
Department of Cancer Research and Molecular Medicine, Center of Molecular Inflammation Research (CEMIR), Norwegian University of Science and Technology (NTNU), Trondheim, Norway

C. Kemper
Complement and Inflammation Research Section (CIRS), National Heart, Lung, and Blood Institute (NHLBI), National Institutes of Health (NIH), Bethesda, MD, USA

B. Halvorsen
Institute of Clinical Medicine, University of Oslo, Oslo, Norway

Research Institute of Internal Medicine, Oslo University Hospital, Rikshospitalet, Oslo, Norway

T. E. Mollnes
Department of Cancer Research and Molecular Medicine, Center of Molecular Inflammation Research (CEMIR), Norwegian University of Science and Technology (NTNU), Trondheim, Norway

Department of Immunology, Oslo University Hospital, Rikshospitalet, University of Oslo, Oslo, Norway

Research Laboratory, Nordland Hospital, Bodø, Norway

T. Espevik (✉)
Department of Cancer Research and Molecular Medicine, Center of Molecular Inflammation Research (CEMIR), Norwegian University of Science and Technology (NTNU), Trondheim, Norway

Central Norway Regional Health Authority, St. Olavs Hospital HF, Trondheim, Norway
e-mail: terje.espevik@ntnu.no

© The Author(s), under exclusive license to Springer Nature Switzerland AG 2023
G. S. Abela, S. M. Nidorf (eds.), *Cholesterol Crystals in Atherosclerosis and Other Related Diseases*, Contemporary Cardiology,
https://doi.org/10.1007/978-3-031-41192-2_14

233

1 Introduction

Atherosclerosis is a chronic inflammatory disease where immune cells respond locally to accumulating lipids in the vessel wall. The resulting lesions are characterized by the presence of cholesterol crystals (CC) which is a hallmark of the disease. Deposition of CC occurs when cholesterol accumulation in the vessel wall exceeds the amount that macrophages can eliminate [1]. CC generation is initiated when oxidized low-density lipoprotein (LDL) is endocytosed by CD36 expressed on macrophages and then nucleates intracellularly the crystallization of this lipid to CC [2]. In the Apo-E mice (which are atherosclerosis prone when exposed to a high fat, Western diet), small CC appear as early as 2 weeks after the start of an atherogenic diet [3]. CC constitute an essential danger signal that incites inflammatory responses by cells residing in the atherosclerotic plaque, contributing to the development and progression of atherosclerosis and its complications like myocardial infarction and ischemic stroke [4, 5].

The innate immune system uses a range of immune sensors called pattern recognition receptors (PRRs), also termed pattern recognition molecules (PRMs), to initiate and control inflammatory responses. PRRs detect microbial conserved substances, the so-called pathogen associated molecular patterns (PAMPs) and endogenous molecules released from cell- and tissue damage, named alarmins or damage-associated molecular patterns (DAMPs) [6]. Several families of PRRs have been identified and their subcellular localization varies and reflects their various biological roles. The Toll-like receptors (TLRs) and C-type lectin receptors (CLRs) are located on the plasma membrane and on internal membranes (e.g., endosome, lysosome, or endoplasmic reticulum). The cytosol contains receptors such as the Retinoic acid-inducible gene (RIG)-I-like receptors (RLRs) and nucleotide binding oligomerization domain receptors NOD-like receptors (NLRs) [7, 8]. The complement system is another pattern recognition system that operates both extracellularly [9] and intracellularly [10]. The sensing of PAMPs or DAMPs by PRRs leads to the transcription, expression, and/or cleavage-activation of pro-inflammatory cytokines, chemokines, type I interferons (IFNs), or antimicrobial peptides and proteins that modulate inflammatory signaling [11]. Phagocytosis of CC causes lysosomal damage, and this is sensed by the NACHT, LRR, and PYD domains-containing protein 3 (NLRP3) inflammasome, leading to the release of interleukin (IL)-1β [3]. Also, the AIM2 inflammasome has been shown to exacerbates atherosclerosis [12]. IL-1β is upregulated across atherosclerotic disorders and is associated with disease severity and outcome [13, 14]. More recently, a large clinical trial on IL-1β inhibition by canakinumab, a monoclonal antibody against IL-1β, revealed a significant reduced risk of recurrent cardiovascular events, clearly underpinning the important role of IL-1β in atherosclerotic disorders [15]. Importantly, the detailed mechanisms of enhanced release of IL-1β as well as the role of CC-induced NLRP3 inflammasome activation in clinical atherosclerosis are still not fully understood. It is clear, however, that the complement system plays an important role in controlling the NLRP3 pathways and CC-induced inflammatory responses, including a selective complement C5a (C5a)-dependent release of IL-1β [16–18].

2   The Complement System

2.1   *Canonical Functions of Plasma-Derived Complement*

The complement system represents one of the oldest arms of our immune system. Discovered more than 100 years ago by Jules Bordet, the complement system was defined as a liver-derived and serum-circulating system of proteins that are specialized in detecting and removing microorganisms that have breached the protective host barriers [19]. The blood, lymph, and intestinal fluid-circulating complement proteins are with few exception mainly synthesized in the liver in inactive pro-enzyme state and the receptors and regulators are expressed on all immune cells. The recognition of microorganisms that have successfully passed host barriers by the PRR components of the complement system leads to the activation of circulating complement proteins in serine-protease cascade reactions leading to the removal of intruders [20–22] (Fig. 1a). There are three different complement activation pathways: the classical (CP), alternative (AP), and lectin (LP) pathways; all converging at the generation of C3- and C5-convertase complexes that cleave C3 into the anaphylatoxin C3a and opsonin C3b, or cleave C5 into anaphylatoxins C5a and into C5b [21].

The PRM C1q in the CP activates complement by recognizing molecules such as immunoglobulins (IgM or IgG) bound to their antigen, or pentraxins (e.g., C-reactive protein; CRP) as well as distinct structures on microbes or on stressed or apoptotic cells. C1q forms a complex with the serine proteases C1r and C1s ($C1qr_2s_2$) which then cleaves C4 into C4a and the opsonin C4b. The cleavage leads to covalent binding of C4b on cell surface thus mediating opsonization. Subsequently C2 binds to C4b deposited on cell surfaces and this leads to cleavage of C2 into the C2a and C2b fragments, which cumulate in the formation of the classical pathway C3 convertase: C4bC2b which can cleave C3 and initiate downstream complement activation [23, 24].

The LP shares some similarities with the CP but is initiated through mannose-binding lectin (MBL), ficolins (Ficolin-1 to 3), and collectins (CL-10 and CL-11) which recognize various carbohydrate structures [25–27]. Furthermore, the LP uses MBL-associated serine proteases (MASP-1 and MASP-2) while the CP uses C1r and C1s to exert downstream complement activation [28]. MASP-1 and -2 cleave C4 into C4a and C4b and C2 into C2a and C2b fragments. The C2b fragment remains attached to C4b fragment generating the C3 convertase C4bC2b [29].

In contrast to the CP and LP, the initial step of AP activation is mediated by the thioester activation within C3 by polysaccharide hydroxyl groups or water [30], nucleating the formation of a protease complex. C3 is inactive in its native form. C3 molecules are spontaneously and at low levels hydrolyzed into C3 (H_2O), exposing new binding sites. This initial AP convertase is assembled via interaction between C3(H_2O) and Factor B to form the enzymatic complex C3 (H_2O)Bb, that cleaves C3 into C3a and C3b and generates the final AP convertase C3bBb. More C3b will bind to FB generating more AP convertase complex, $C3b_nBb$, thereby amplifying complement response [31]. The alternative pathway C3 convertase is stabilized by the only positive complement regulator, properdin (C3b$_n$BbP) [32].

The deposition of C5b on a pathogen or target surface initiates the formation of the membrane attack complex (MAC) which may lead to cytolysis, but alternatively and probably more important to inflammation, by a sublytic attack on nucleated cell leading to cell activation [33]. Opsonization by C3b promotes phagocytosis of pathogens by immune cells [21, 22]. Cleavage products of C3 (e.g., C3a, C3b, iC3b, and C3dg) can relay signals that alarm cells from the innate and adaptive immunity through interaction with specific receptors (e.g., C3aR, CR1, CR2, CR3, CR4, and CRIg). The anaphylatoxins C3a and C5a stimulate their G-protein coupled receptors (GPCRs) C3aR and C5aR1 and 2 expressed on innate immune cells, and this triggers their migration towards the site of site of infection [9].

Fig. 1 (a) Plasma- or liver derived complement. Liver-derived, serum circulating complement is the first line of defence against pathogens. It can be activated through three pathways: the classical (CP), the lectin (LP) and the alternative (AP) pathway. The formation of C3 convertases (C4bC2a for the CP and LP, and C3bBb for AP) leads to the generation of the opsonin C3b and the anaphylatoxin C3a. The C5 convertase formation (C4bC2aC3b for CP and LP, and C3bBbC3b for the AP) leads to C5b and anaphylatoxin C5a generation, with C5b initiating the formation of the membrane attack complex (MAC) which is inserted into cells infected by bacteria or virus for lysis. The system is equiped with fluid-phase and cell-bound regulators; C1 inhibitor (C1-INH) which inhibits the functions of C1r, C1s and mannan-binding lectin-associated serine protease 2 (MASP2). C3b (and C4b) are inactivated by the serine protease complement Factor I and one of several cofactor proteins (CD46 and complement receptor type 1 (CR1) or fluid-phase Factor H and C4b-binding protein (C4BP)). Convertases are regulated through disassembly by regulators that have decay-accelerating activity—surface-bound CD55 and CR1 or fluid-phase Factor H and C4BP — and the formation of the MAC is controlled at the level of C8 and C9 by CD59 on the cell surface, and the soluble sC5b-9 incorporates vitronectin and clusterin to cover the lipophilc sites to keep the complex soluble. (Figure created with BioRender.com) (b) Non canonical complement in T cells. Autocrine complement activation is triggered when activating signals (T cell receptor on antigen-presenting cells (not shown) initiate secretion of complement proteins C3, C5, factor B, and factor D located in cellular storages, leading to C3 and C5 convertase formation in the extracellular space as well as on the cell surface—and the generation of C3a, C3b, C5b, and C5a (1). T cell and other immune competent cells express intracellular complement which occurs continuously through C3 cleavage by the protease cathepsin L. The resulting C3a fragment engages the intracellular receptor C3aR, localized on the lysosomes, which sustains tonic mammalian target of rapamycin (mTOR) activation and T cell survival (2). Upon T cell activation, complement proteins are shuttled on the surface where they bind to their respective receptors on the T cell surface and signaling through C3aR and CD46 then drives granzyme B production in CTLs and Th1 induction in CD4+ T cells through reprogramming of cell metabolism with increased glycolysis, OXPHOS and subsequently Th1 induction with interferon (IFN)-γ secretion. C5 is also processed intracellularly by a C5 convertase into C5a and C5b, and this process is increased through CD46 signaling. Intracellular C5a binds to the intracellular C5aR1, which triggers ROS activation and subsequent NLRP3 inflammasome assembly and intrinsic IL-1β secretion that sustains Th1 induction by producing IFNγ (3). (Figure created with BioRender.com)

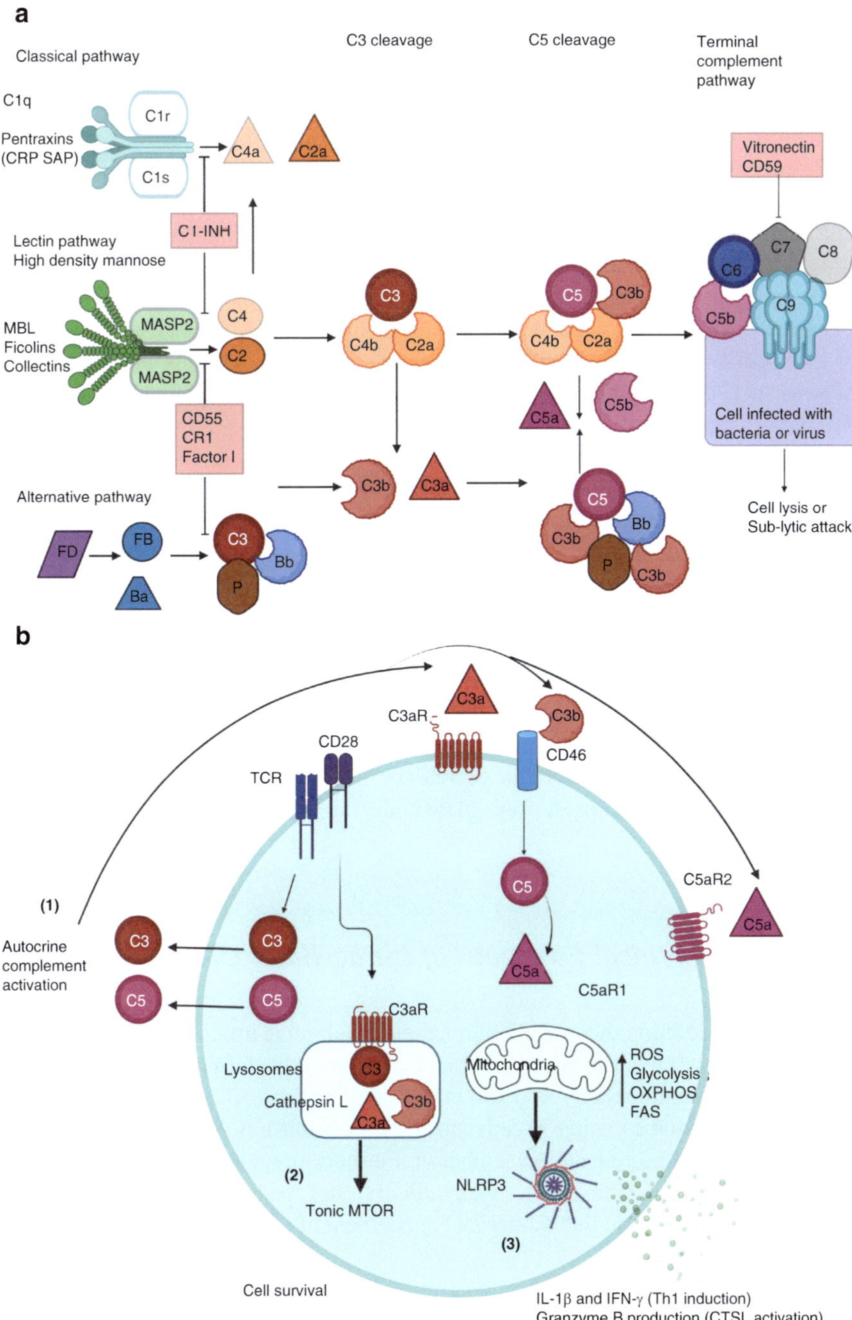
a
Classical pathway
C3 cleavage
C5 cleavage
Terminal complement pathway
C1q
Pentraxins (CRP SAP)
C1r
C1s
C4a
C2a
Vitronectin CD59
C1-INH
Lectin pathway
High density mannose
C6
C7
C8
C9
C5b
MBL
Ficolins
Collectins
MASP2
MASP2
C4
C2
C3
C4b C2a
C5 C3b
C4b C2a
C5a
C5b
Cell infected with bacteria or virus
CD55
CR1
Factor I
C3b C3a
C5
C3b P C3b
Bb
Alternative pathway
FD
FB
Ba
C3 Bb
P
Cell lysis or Sub-lytic attack

b
C3a
C3b
C3aR
CD28
CD46
TCR
C5
C5aR2
(1)
Autocrine complement activation
C3
C5
C3
C5
C5a
C5a
C5aR1
C3aR
Lysosomes
Cathepsin L
C3
C3a C3b
Mitochondria
ROS
Glycolysis
OXPHOS
FAS
(2)
Tonic MTOR
NLRP3
(3)
Cell survival
IL-1β and IFN-γ (Th1 induction)
Granzyme B production (CTSL activation)

C5aR1 binding to C5a leads to the activation of multiple intracellular signaling pathways including extracellular signal-regulated kinase (ERK) 1/2, protein kinase B (PKB), mitogen-activated protein kinase (MAPK), and phosphoinositide 3-kinase (PI3K) [34, 35]. C5aR2 has both pro- and anti-inflammatory activities through the regulation of C5a-induced C5aR1 signaling via recruitment of β-arrestin 2 [36, 37].

Besides its key functions in combatting infections, the role of complement in inflammation goes beyond mere killing of invading pathogen and initiating the general inflammatory reaction. The complement system is also central to the recognition of damage-associated molecular patterns (DAMPs) or self-altered which cause sterile inflammation or ultimately restoration of tissues. For example, the DAMPs that are released after tissue damage and consist of debris and molecules released by necrotic cells recruit phagocytes that can remove these noxious entities safely. Among such dangerous self-derived antigens sensed by complement system are also protein aggregates or crystalline cholesterol or monosodium uric acid [16, 38–41]. The discovery that the complement system recognizes self-altered molecules with subsequent instruction of the innate immune system shows that complement not only works to contain tissue injury during pathogens clearing, but also actively contributes to tissue homeostasis during sterile inflammation.

Complement as a recognition system of both PAMPs and DAMPs has been shown to cross-talk intensively with the TLR system [42]. We have shown in several studies that a combined inhibition of complement, e.g., C3 or C5, and the TLRs, e.g., CD14 as a co-receptor for several of these receptors, including TLR4, TLR2, and others [43] was substantially more effective than the single inhibition of each of the systems [44]. This is in contrast to what we observed with CC, where complement was solely responsible for the secondary cytokine response [16, 18, 45]. This highlights complement as a key player in the innate immune response in atherosclerosis.

2.2 Non-Canonical Functions of Intracellular Complement

Early work on defining the role of complement in adaptive immunity challenged the notion that complement is solely liver and plasma derived. While plasma-derived complement is undoubtably crucial in the recognition of pathogens and their removal, initial studies using T cells and APCs demonstrated that these cells can secrete C3 and C5 proteins upon activation. Furthermore, autocrine generated anaphylatoxins C3a and C5a engage their GPCRs on T cells and APCs, C3aR, and C5aR1, respectively; and that autocrine engagement of the receptors modulates cellular responses [46–48].

It is well acknowledged that almost all cells in the human body can produce complement proteins and express receptors of complement fragments [49, 50] and that complement synthesis occurs in almost all tissues including the kidney [51–53], heart [54], intestine [55–57], and brain [58]. Cleavage products of C3 (e.g., C3a, C3b, iC3b, and C3dg) can relay signals that alarm cells from the innate and adaptive immune system through interaction with specific receptors (e.g., C3aR, CR1, CR2, CR3, CR4, and CRIg). In the same way, the cleavage product of C5, i.e., C5a, can transmit and translate signals into inflammatory responses through activation of C5aR1 [9]. Cellular complement production can be induced by both pro-inflammatory cytokines, chemokines, growth factors, and integrins [18, 59–62], and in turn, the increased complement production can modulate the inflammatory responses of immune cells [16, 63, 64]. Complement is therefore not only an important danger sensor able to recognize harmful structures, but also a danger transmitter able to translate danger signals into suitable responses by immune and other cells.

Recently, the concept that the functional outcomes of complement activation are dictated by its location has been extended to the cell's interior: human CD4$^+$ and CD8$^+$ T cells express intrinsically C3 and C5 and the intracellularly generated fragments C3a and C5a are needed for T cell survival and normal IFN-γ production, respectively [10, 65, 66] (Fig. 1b). Importantly, signaling of intracellularly generated complement proteins to their intracellular receptors have distinct outcome compared to the cellular responses induced by the same receptors expressed on the cell surface [67]. The intracellularly activated and operative complement system has been termed "the complosome." It has also a rather non-canonical activity as it emerged as central orchestrator of key cell physiological pathways such as metabolism and mitochondrial function – and it does so in cross-talk with other immune sensors such as the NLRP3 inflammasome [10, 67–71]. Specifically, resting human T cells contain intracellular stores of C3 and cathepsin L (CTSL), and C3 is continuously cleaved by CTSL into biologically active C3a and C3b. This intracellularly generated C3a signals through the C3aR expressed on lysosomes and drives tonic mTOR activation required for T cell homeostatic cell survival in the periphery. T cell receptor (TCR) activation initiates the rapid translocation of this intracellular "C3 activation system" to the cell surface where C3a engages the surface expressed C3aR, and C3b, its receptor CD46 [10]. Signaling through C3aR and CD46 then drives IFN-γ secretion and granzyme B production in CD8$^+$ cytotoxic T lymphocytes (CTLs) and T helper type 1 (Th1) induction in CD4$^+$ T cells through reprogramming of cell metabolism [10, 65, 66, 69, 71]. Human T cells also contain an intracellular C5 system. In CD4$^+$ T cells, autocrine CD46 activation upon TCR engagement increases intracellular C5 activation into C5a and C5b and engagement of intracellular C5aR1. Intracellular C5aR1 activation induces the generation of ROS and the formation of the canonical NLRP3 complex. Subsequent intracellular C5a-C5aR1-NLRP3-mediated T cell production of IL-1β sustains IFN-γ induction and regulates the magnitude of Th1 responses, specifically at mucosal interfaces [68].

Although the complosome was initially discovered in T cells, it is now clear that all cells so far assessed (monocytes, macrophages, B cells, myeloid cells, pancreatic β-cells, fibroblasts, and epithelial and endothelial cells) express cell-autonomous complement and that it controls important cell activities (autophagy, cell survival and repair, glycolysis, etc.) across these populations [17, 62, 72–75]. Furthermore, perturbations in the complosome are now connected with a range of hypo- or hyper-inflammatory conditions and important human diseases [17, 62, 68, 72, 73]. Thus, the complosome is of broad biological significance, and together with the liver-derived circulating and locally cell-produced complement arms forms a formidable system to mount adequate responses to extrinsic and intrinsic intruders and dangers.

3 Activation of the Complement System by Cholesterol Crystals

3.1 Functions of Extracellular Plasma-Derived Complement

Earlier studies in 1980s demonstrated that CC have the potential to activate complement [76–78]. These were the first indications that CC could directly activate the immune system. Immunization of mice with of cholesterol-containing liposomes and lipid A as an adjuvant led to the production of antibodies against CC [79]. It was also reported that patients with ulcerated atherosclerosis have IgG antibodies against crystalline cholesterol that could activate the CP of complement [76], demonstrating that crystalline cholesterol was an immunogen. The mechanisms of how CC initiate complement activation were recently clarified showing that the CP, LP and AP all cooperate in the recognition of CC [16, 80]. Furthermore, it was also recently shown that complement opsonization of CC not only induces phagocytosis but also rather unexpectedly, aids in priming the CC sensing cells [16]. Subsequent more detailed in vitro analyses then demonstrated that components of the CP bind to CC and trigger formation of complement sC5b-9 in plasma: IgM-mediated C1q binding to CC leads to complement activation [80] and this response is attenuated in C1-depleted serum [16]. Additionally, components of the LP recognition molecules such as Ficolin-2 and MBL can directly bind CC presumably through recognition of the hydroxyl groups on CC. The same study showed that Ficolin-2-mediated binding of MASP-2 to CC, and that this complex leads to the activation-induced deposition of C4b onto CC [80]. The importance of this initial CP and LP-mediated complement "seed activation" is considerable as it enables deposition of C3b on CC, and with this the highly effective amplification loop of the complement cascade. Indeed, the high amount of the C3bBbP convertase complexes are detected in human serum incubated with CC [16]. Overall, CC that are opsonized with complement are more potent complement activation propagators compared to non-opsonized CC, suggesting that complement opsonization by C3b (via the CP or AP) facilitates CC-induced inflammation. This hypothesis was corroborated by the finding that addition of non-cell permeable antagonist to C3 (i.e., compstatin) blocked uptake of CC by human monocytes in blood. These data indicated strongly that monocytes and granulocytes employ the integrin complement receptor 3 (CR3, CD11b/CD18) which binds to the opsonin iC3b for the phagocytic uptake of CC [16].

Upon phagocytosis of CC, monocytes respond by secreting pro-inflammatory cytokines like tumor necrosis factor (TNF) and IL-1β in a complement-dependent manner [16]. C5a and TNF in combination act as a potent primer for CC-induced IL-1 β release by increasing *IL1B* transcripts in these disease-driving immune cells. By using a model consisting of human umbilical vein endothelial cells in lepirudin anticoagulated human whole blood we found that CC cause also the activation of endothelial cells: we noted a marked and complement dose-dependent increase in the expression of the adhesion molecules E-selectin and ICAM-1 on the surface of the endothelial cells [45]. The endothelial activation by CC is mediated by complement-dependent TNF release by whole blood monocytes which demonstrate the interplay between complement activation, TNF release, and endothelial cell activation which may occur during cardiovascular disease.

Atherosclerotic plaques contain dense amounts of CC which may be released to the blood and induce thrombosis during atherosclerotic plaque rupture. There is a close link between CC-induced activation of complement and coagulation. In fact, CC start a coagulation cascade through a complement-dependent expression of tissue factor in monocytes [81]. This reveals an important role for CC and plasma complement also in thromboinflammation that occurs during plaque rupture.

3.2   Activation of Complement by CC in Atherosclerotic Plaques

CC are strong complement inducers, and this may represent a mechanism for recruiting immune cells into the atherosclerotic plaques, which leads to local inflammation and progressively to chronic inflammation. Initial reports have identified complement components and activation products in atherosclerotic lesions [82, 83]. It is now acknowledged that complement is highly induced in advanced atherosclerotic lesions, and studies have shown that cells in plaques express complement both at the mRNA and the protein level [84]. Subsequent complement activation and formation of C5b-9 has also been observed in human atherosclerotic lesions [85, 86], and the level of deposition of C5b-9 correlates with the severity of the lesions [87]. This is emphasized by the high level of sC5b-9 in the plasma of patients with carotid plaques, and the prominent presence of complement components C1q, MBL, Ficolin-2, and C5b-9 in human carotid plaques. MBL and C5b-9 are located around "CC clefts" in the necrotic core of carotid plaques (Fig. 2) [18, 80].

The presence of complement proteins in advanced carotid lesions implies that complement activation occurs locally in the arterial wall and may be an integral part of the progression of atherosclerosis. For example, complement binding to CC in the region populated by cell debris and macrophages may promote the growth of lesions by attracting more immune cells to CC and, simultaneously, sustaining a pro-inflammatory phenotype in these cells. If indeed locally produced complement activation products are responsible for the inflammatory propagation of disease, it is not surprising that high levels of complement C3bc, C4bc, and sC5b-9 were found in the plasma from patients with acute coronary syndrome and with carotid plaques,

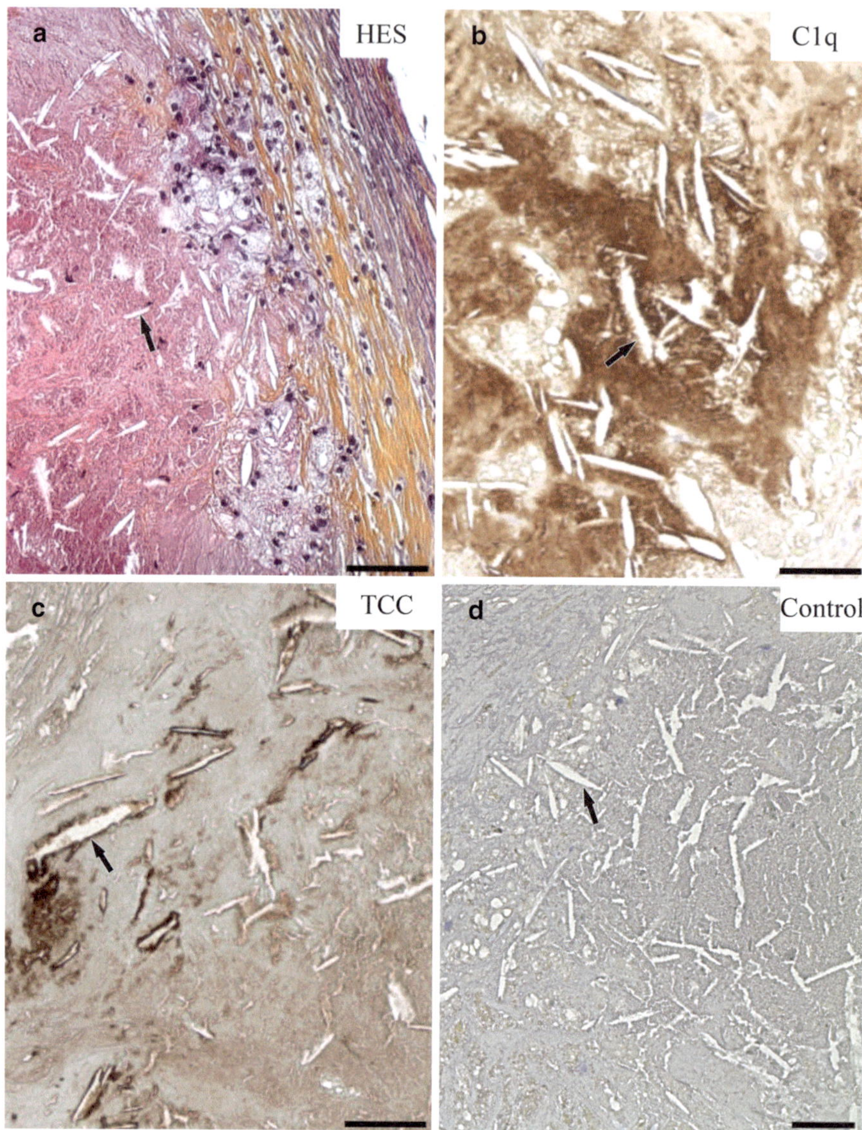

Fig. 2 Accumulation of C1q and TCC around cholesterol crystal clefts in human carotid plaques. Immunohistochemistry was performed on paraffin embedded sectioned plaques which were stained for haematoxylin (HES) (**a**), C1q (**b**), TCC (**c**) and isotype control (**d**) and imaged using EVOS FL auto microscope. One representative image from 3 plaques from 3 patients. Arrows indicate crystal clefts. Scale bar is 50 mm. *C* complement factor, *TCC* terminal C5b-9 complement complex. (From Niyonzima et al. [18])

and that their PBMC express high levels of anaphylatoxins receptors C3aR1, C5aR1, and C5aR2 [18]. These studies solidified the role of CC-induced complement in atherosclerosis and provide solid grounds for the hypothesis that the amplitude of local complement activation is a causal link to disease progression.

It is not only the opsonizing capacity of the complement system that can enhance CC-induced inflammation, but also the anaphylatoxin C5a. C5a induced by CC locally can recruit monocytes via engagement of their surface C5aR1 and also induce the upregulation of the integrin receptor CR3, which then allows phagocytosis of CC; via fostering CC uptake, the surface C5aR1 also supports the production of pro-inflammatory cytokines by blood cells [16]. The importance of CC-C5a axis in the regulation of inflammation is underpinned by the fact that whole blood from rare patients with C5 serum deficiency [88] who suffer from recurrent Neisseria infections fails to produce inflammatory cytokines in response to CC. Ex vivo assessment of whole blood from C5-deficient patients demonstrated that circulating C5 is indeed required to induce optimal IL-1β, TNF, IL-6, and IL-8 by blood monocytes. Reconstitution with purified C5 resulted in a 2.5- to fivefold increase in the CC-induced cytokine secretion by blood monocytes. These findings were corroborated by the findings that addition of a surface antagonist to C5aR1 or an antibody to C5 (i.e., Eculizumab) to whole blood decreased CC-induced IL-1β and TNF by monocytes more than 50%, thus pointing to C5a as an important mediator of these responses. C5a was detected around "CC clefts" in the necrotic core of human carotid arteries where it colocalizes with C5aR1 [89]. Accumulation of C5a and C5aR1 in carotid plaques creates the environment needed for priming of plaque-resident immune cells, and it is thus not surprising that ex vivo exposure of human carotid plaques to CC is sufficient to trigger IL-1β secretion by plaque containing cells [18, 90].

3.3 The Complosome as a Sensor and Inducer of CC-Stimulated Inflammation

Plasma complement derived from the liver is considered as pro-inflammatory and key to the detection and removal of invading pathogens and myeloid cell uptake of CC. However, we have very recently shown that the myeloid cell intracellular complement system also plays an important and specific part in the monocyte and macrophage maladaptive responses underlying atherosclerosis [17]. Specifically, human monocytes in circulation express C5 can generate intracellular C5a and express the C5a receptors C5aR1 and C5aR2. Of note, cell-autonomous complement proteins are not free floating in the cytosol but are confined to subcellular compartment including the Golgi apparatus, the endoplasmic reticulum, endosomes, lysosomes, and mitochondria. While C5 colocalizes with the Golgi, processing of C5 in monocytes into bioactive C5a is a post-Golgi event and is reliant on the formation of an intracellular AP C3/C5 convertase C3bBbC3b. These convertases form preferentially (and not surprisingly) on cellular membranes, such as the inside and outside of the plasma membrane, the endoplasmic reticulum membrane, lysosomal membranes, and the surface of mitochondria [17]. The co-localization of C5a generating convertase and the C5aR1 on mitochondria proved physiologically important to optimal IL-1β production by monocytes upon CC sensing. During sterile inflammation, internalization of CC by human monocytes or macrophages triggers increased transcription of the *CFB* and *IL1B* genes, intracellular cleavage of C5 into C5a and augmented engagement of the mitochondrial C5aR1 (mtC5aR1).

A reduction of C5 activation, for example, by addition of a FB cell permeable inhibitor during monocytes ex vivo stimulation, blocks monocytes release of IL-1β in response to CC. Importantly, the provision of serum purified C5 or C5a to such FB inhibitor treated monocytes does not rescue IL-1β.

CC are DAMPS that are resistant to proteases and CC remain in the tissues over long time. Uptake of CC by myeloid cells such as macrophages results in damaging the lysosomes [3]. The extent of phagocytosis defines the amplitude of damage and consequently inflammation [91]. The inflammatory effect of CC uptake could be influenced by the balance between CC accumulation versus clearance, for example, in early versus late phases of atherosclerosis. While early atherosclerosis may induce moderate NLRP3 activation combined with macrophages ability to remove cholesterol, chronic inflammation shifts the balance towards removal of cholesterol in inflamed tissues and leads to accumulation of crystalline cholesterol and chronic inflammation. Leakage of lysosomal enzymes to the cytosol might damage small organelles such as mitochondria [91]. Targeting the intracellular C5 or C5aR1 (but not cell surface C5aR1) using cell permeable inhibitors or specific siRNA to C5 or C5aR1 blocks IL-1β release from macrophages in response to CC. This is likely an effect of C5a ligation of C5aR1 on mitochondria which leads to ROS production and increased expression of messenger IL1B and consequently release of mature IL-1β [17].

Mice lacking LDLR or ApoE develop atherosclerotic lesions containing CC when fed a high fat diet [3]. By using $LDL^{-/-}C5aR1^{fl/fl}$ *LyzM-cre*$^{-/-}$ (*LDL-Control*) and $LDL^{-/-}C5aR1^{fl/fl}$ *LyzM-cre*$^{+/-}$ (*LDL-mC5aR1*$^{-/-}$), which lack C5aR1 on myeloid cells, we confirmed the in vivo importance of the complosome C5aR1 in atherosclerosis [17]. The inflammatory responses to CC are mainly mediated by myeloid cells, as atherosclerotic mice lacking C5aR1 on myeloid cells have significantly reduced IL-1β. Also, the areas of the atherosclerotic lesions in the aortic tree are significantly decreased in *LDL-Control* (25%) compared to *LDL-mC5aR1*$^{-/-}$ (10%). Quantitative analysis show that the arch and root lesion sizes are significantly decreased in (high fat diet) HFD-fed *LDL-mC5aR1*$^{-/-}$ compared to *LDL-Control* which demonstrate the effect of myeloid C5aR1 on atherogenesis in mice. Dyslipidemia is a risk factor for atherosclerosis development, and analysis revealed that while there was a difference in total cholesterol between the two groups, the levels of triglyceride and lipoprotein profiles (VLDL, LDL, and HDL levels) remain unchanged after HFD treatment. Additionally, analysis of bone marrow derived macrophages (BMDM) from *C5$^{fl/fl}$ LyzM-cre$^{+/-}$* or *C5aR1$^{fl/fl}$ LyzM-cre$^{+/-}$* stimulated with CC show significant reduction in IL-1β secretion. Importantly, provision of serum purified C5 or C5a to BMDM culture does not rescue the secretion of IL-1β [17].

The complosome C5aR1 also exerts effects on human atherosclerotic plaques [17]. A cell permeable inhibitor of C5aR1, but not a cell surface inhibitor, decreases the spontaneous IL-1β release by cells in atherosclerotic plaques. Gene ontology enrichment analysis (GOEA) shows that treatment with the C5aR1 cell permeable inhibitor downregulates almost 453 genes, and further interrogation of the GOEA reveals that targeting the complosome C5aR1 in human plaques affects many key genes in the GO term "inflammatory response," "TNF signaling," and "Complement." Additionally, genes involved in cholesterol metabolism and genes associated to lipid and atherosclerosis are downregulated in plaques when C5aR1 is inhibited. Genes downregulated by the treatment are mainly from CD33+ myeloid cells and CD14+ monocytes confirming our observation in murine macrophages. These data identify the complosome C5a-C5aR1 signaling as a physiological sensor of CC and a master regulator of atherosclerosis.

3.4 The Complosome as a Regulator of Metabolism in Macrophages Exposed to CC

Cellular function requires coordination between different organelles. Mitochondria, ER, and lysosomes are important platforms for metabolism and cell signaling. Mitochondria physically interact with ER through Mitofusin 2, leading to the formation of mitochondria associated membranes (MAM). In inactivated form, NLRP3 resides on Golgi, ER, and cytosol [92, 93]. Upon macrophage activation with NLRP3 inducers such as CC, NLRP3 and ASC colocalize with MAM where they detect increased mitochondrial ROS, a signal for mitochondria activation [92].

NLRP3 recognizes a range of stimuli with different structures, and it is likely that NLRP3 does not recognize each DAMP per se, but ratter recognizes common intracellular changes shared by these DAMPs. Changes in metabolic states might be the signal that is recognized by NLRP3 inflammasome. During infection and inflammation, immune cells undergo a metabolic shift from oxidative phosphorylation (OXPHOS) to glycolysis to meet increased energy demand. Mitochondria constantly respond to changes in energy demand to be able to maintain ATP supplies and at the same time control reactive oxygen species (ROS) production. Macrophage cellular adaptions to tissue environment are driven by specific changes in mitochondrial activity, ATP, and ROS production [94]. Indeed, macrophages in plaques of atherosclerotic patients or in the joint of gout patients have distinct metabolic signatures with high glycolysis and ROS [95].

We have identified C5aR1 in all cell fractions from macrophages including the plasma membrane, cytosol, ER, lysosomes, and other undefined organelles and the outer mitochondrial membrane (mtC5aR1) [17]. The presence of mtC5aR1 was confirmed both by high-resolution microscopy on purified mitochondria and on immune electron microscopy on human monocytes. In purified mitochondria, mtC5aR1 colocalizes with the outer mitochondrial membrane marker TOM20 (Fig. 3), and exogenous stimulation of mtC5aR1 with serum C5a leads to mtROS production suggesting that mtC5aR1 is fully functional. Blocking mtC5aR1 using cell permeable or non-cell permeable receptor antagonists reduced

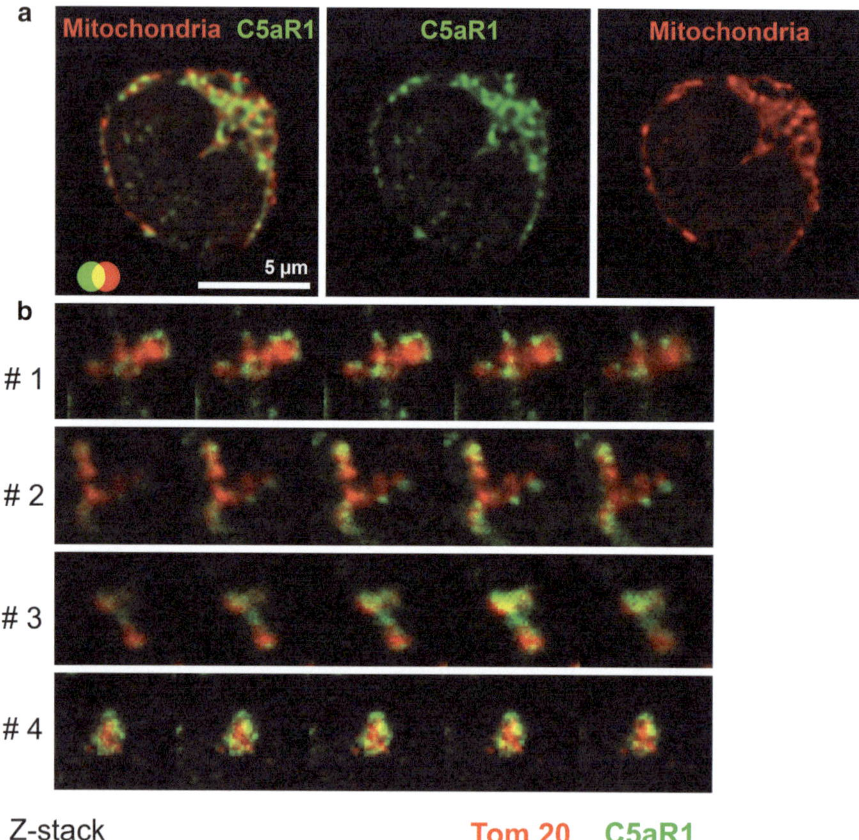

Fig. 3 C5aR1 is located at the mitochondria (**a**) Confocal microscopy of monocytes stained for mitochondria and C5aR1 (**b**) Assessment of C5aR1 and TOM20 expression on mitochondria isolated from human monocytes. (From Niyonzima et al. [17])

mtC5aR1-induced mtROS suggesting that the response is specific to C5aR1. Signaling mediated by mtC5aR1 affects mitochondrial function by reducing ATP and cAMP (which is generated from ATP), both of which have been shown to mediate NLRP3 activation in response to DAMPs including crystals [96]. This indicates an overall inhibitory effect of mtC5aR1 on the mitochondrial electron transport chain (ETC) and OXPHOS.

Assessment of mitochondrial morphology in CC sensing supports a role for the mtC5aR1 in directing mitochondrial dynamics [17]. While mitochondria are randomly spread in resting human monocytes, CC sensing relocates mitochondria to the perinuclear region [17]. Treatment of cells with the C5aR1 cell permeable antagonist results in an increase in the mitochondrial network size, without affecting branch length or size. Assessment of metabolic competence by a Seahorse analyzer revealed that CC sensing by human monocytes leads to significantly augmented glycolysis vs. coupled (ATP-producing) respiration which is downregulated in cells treated with cell permeable C5aR1 inhibitor. Similarly, ex vivo analysis of BMDM deficient in either C5 or C5ar1 also shows reduced mitochondrial ROS generation, glycolysis, and IL-1β secretion upon CC sensing. Consistent with these results, the depletion of intracellular ATP using 2-doxyglucose (2DG) blocks IL-1β production by human monocytes stimulated with CC. Briefly, the complosome C5aR1 positioning on mitochondria is a key in controlling mitochondrial integrity by modulating their dynamic and signaling which shifts ATP production via reverse electron chain flux towards reactive oxygen species (ROS) production and anaerobic glycolysis to favor IL-1β production (Fig. 4). This implies that at steady state, the protein levels of the complosome C5a-C5aR1 are well equilibrated, and that cleavage and ligand-receptor assembly is subject to additional levels of regulations at the transcriptional level, and fully activity requires upregulation of the sensor C5a-C5aR1 axis in response to CC. Thus, the C5-C5aR1 complosome acts as a unique danger sensor of CC suggesting a mechanistic connection between CC, mtC5aR1, mitochondria function, inflammasome activation, and atherosclerosis.

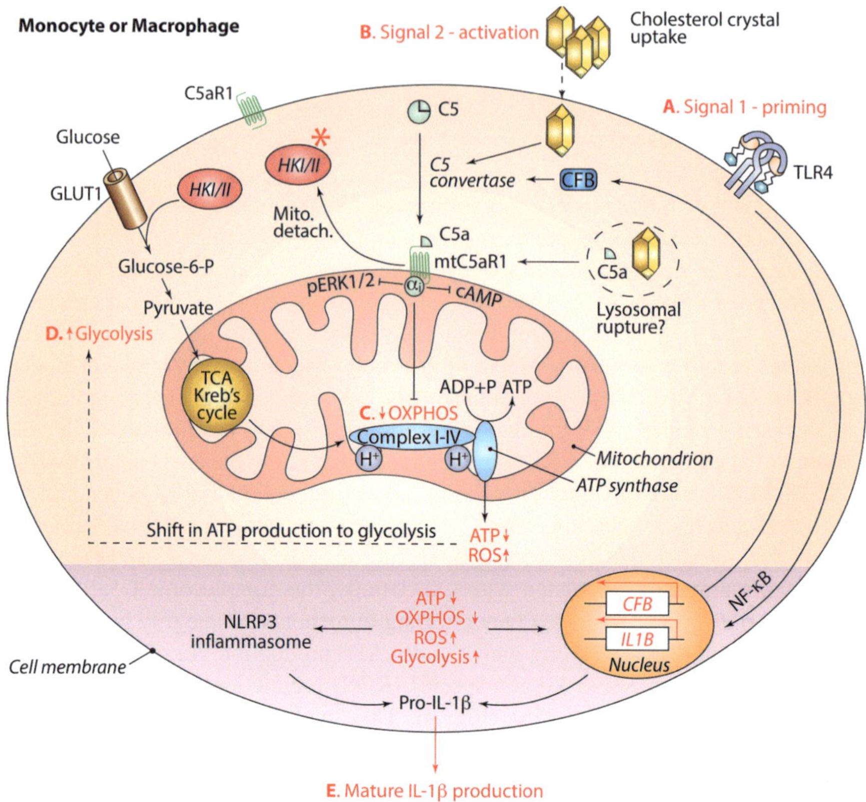

Fig. 4 Mitochondrial C5aR1 contributes to IL-1β production upon CC sensing. Monocytes and macrophages express the C5aR1 constitutively on mitochondria (mtC5aR1), and continuously generate intracellular C5a via an intracellular C5 convertase. TLR4 engagement by endogenous danger signals (for example, modified LDLs) triggers a priming signal 1 (**A**) that induces (increased) transcription of the *IL1B* and *CFB* genes. Uptake of CC amplifies cell-intrinsic C5a production by augmented C5 convertase formation and triggers mtC5aR1 ligation (**B**). mtC5aR1 activation, in a G protein– coupled fashion (αi), reduces mitochondrial ERK1/2 phosphorylation, ATP and cAMP formation, and OXPHOS (**C**) and simultaneously increases ROS production and glycolysis (**D**) via reverse electron transport and also induces detachment of HKI from mitochondria. Together, these events further elevate *IL1B* gene transcription and also provide signal 2 (B) for the assembly of the NLRP3 inflammasome and processing of immature pro–IL-1β into mature IL-1β (**E**). (?) indicates hypothetical provision of C5a to mtC5aR1 via CC-induced lysosomal rupture. (From Niyonzima et al. [17])

4 The C5a-C5aR1 Axis of the Complosome as a Target for Therapy of Cardiovascular Disease

Complement has been identified as an important player in atherosclerosis [97]. The unexpected finding that intracellular C5a and mtC5aR1 drive sensing of CC in myeloid cells may explain why clinical trials aiming at reducing C5a in the plasma of patients with atherosclerosis have failed [98]. The complement receptor C5aR1 is highly expressed in symptomatic carotid plaques, and C5aR1 is more expressed in stable- compared to unstable plaques [17, 18], suggesting that complement stimulates both the severity and the instability of lesions. The intracellular C5a-C5aR1 axis seems to control several levels of CC-induced inflammation including detection of CC, activation of NLRP3 through metabolic reprogramming of macrophages, growth of lesions with increased lipid uptake, and the release of IL-1β, all processes known to work in concert during atherogenesis. The efficacy of inhibiting C5aR1 in reducing inflammatory responses indicates that both intracellular and plasma membrane C5aR1 may be promising targets for treatment of atherosclerosis.

Nevertheless, more data are needed to define the complosome as a therapeutic target. First, it must be clarified whether targeting of the complosome can suppress the growth of advanced atherosclerotic lesions, as this is the stage where most patients are diagnosed with cardiovascular disease. Animal models of atherosclerosis have shown that CC appear quite early in the disease process, and anti-complosome therapy might be a beneficial intervention to prevent inflammatory cell recruitment to the intima and the growth of lesions. Intracellular C5aR1 in myeloid cells plays a role in the development of atherosclerotic lesions, and deletion of C5aR1 led to 50% reduction in atherosclerosis in the entire aorta [17]. Second, more studies are needed to clarify whether inhibition of the complosome may interfere with macrophage functions central to lesion reduction. Lack of myeloid C5aR1 in male mice reduces total cholesterol suggesting that the effect of the knockout on atherosclerosis results in increased cholesterol clearance by macrophages. Thus, macrophage foam cell formation could be reduced by targeting the complosome C5aR1. Results from ex vivo carotid plaques showed that targeting intracellular C5aR1, but not cell surface C5aR1, reduces the expression of the inflammatory cytokine IL-1β. Moreover, gene array analysis showed that targeting the complosome significantly reduced general inflammation in carotid containing plaques, and genes involved in cholesterol metabolism were among the genes that were normalized by the treatment. Altogether, targeting the complosome possesses potent lipid modifying effects and strong anti-inflammatory effects that might attenuate atherosclerosis. These data align very well with recent findings that cyclodextrin promote regression of atherosclerosis in part by reducing intrinsic complement activity in plaque-resident macrophages [99].

Long-term inhibition of the intracellular C5a-C5aR1 axis may not be an attractive strategy because of the risks associated with disabling leukocyte recruitment to homeostatic and inflammatory cues. Will patients treated with inhibitors of intracellular complement for a long period become immunocompromised? Rather than thinking about life-long anti-complement therapy, perhaps we should consider if short term, high intensity blockage of complement activity might offer a significant benefit to patients undergoing acute coronary syndrome. Experimental animal models of arterial injury are needed to investigate if short-term intervention to prevent inflammatory cell recruitment to sites of vascular injury have beneficial effects on the remodeling of the vasculature, without preventing the recruitment of endothelial progenitor cells. Clearly, these are critical issues that need to be addressed before considering the complosome as a therapeutic target in the treatment of atherosclerotic disorders.

References

1. Katz SS, Shipley GG, Small DM. Physical chemistry of the lipids of human atherosclerotic lesions. Demonstration of a lesion intermediate between fatty streaks and advanced plaques. J Clin Invest. 1976;58(1):200–11. https://doi.org/10.1172/jci108450.
2. Sheedy FJ, Grebe A, Rayner KJ, Kalantari P, Ramkhelawon B, Carpenter SB, et al. CD36 coordinates NLRP3 inflammasome activation by facilitating intracellular nucleation of soluble ligands into particulate ligands in sterile inflammation. Nat Immunol. 2013;14(8):812–20. https://doi.org/10.1038/ni.2639.
3. Duewell P, Kono H, Rayner KJ, Sirois CM, Vladimer G, Bauernfeind FG, et al. NLRP3 inflammasomes are required for atherogenesis and activated by cholesterol crystals. Nature. 2010;464(7293):1357–61. https://doi.org/10.1038/nature08938.
4. Kataoka Y, Puri R, Hammadah M, Duggal B, Uno K, Kapadia SR, et al. Cholesterol crystals associate with coronary plaque vulnerability in vivo. J Am Coll Cardiol. 2015;65(6):630–2. https://doi.org/10.1016/j.jacc.2014.11.039.
5. Fujiyoshi K, Minami Y, Ishida K, Kato A, Katsura A, Muramatsu Y, et al. Incidence, factors, and clinical significance of cholesterol crystals in coronary plaque: an optical coherence tomography study. Atherosclerosis. 2019;283:79–84. https://doi.org/10.1016/j.atherosclerosis.2019.02.009.
6. Janeway CA Jr. Approaching the asymptote? Evolution and revolution in immunology. Cold Spring Harb Symp Quant Biol. 1989;54(Pt 1):1–13. https://doi.org/10.1101/sqb.1989.054.01.003.
7. Pandey S, Kawai T, Akira S. Microbial sensing by toll-like receptors and intracellular nucleic acid sensors. Cold Spring Harb Perspect Biol. 2014;7(1):a016246. https://doi.org/10.1101/cshperspect.a016246.
8. Broz P, Dixit VM. Inflammasomes: mechanism of assembly, regulation and signalling. Nat Rev Immunol. 2016;16(7):407–20. https://doi.org/10.1038/nri.2016.58.
9. Kohl J. The role of complement in danger sensing and transmission. Immunol Res. 2006;34(2):157–76. https://doi.org/10.1385/ir:34:2:157.
10. Liszewski MK, Kolev M, Le Friec G, Leung M, Bertram PG, Fara AF, et al. Intracellular complement activation sustains T cell homeostasis and mediates effector differentiation. Immunity. 2013;39(6):1143–57. https://doi.org/10.1016/j.immuni.2013.10.018.
11. Takeuchi O, Akira S. Pattern recognition receptors and inflammation. Cell. 2010;140(6):805–20. https://doi.org/10.1016/j.cell.2010.01.022.
12. Fidler TP, Xue C, Yalcinkaya M, Hardaway B, Abramowicz S, Xiao T, et al. The AIM2 inflammasome exacerbates atherosclerosis in clonal haematopoiesis. Nature. 2021;592(7853):296–301. https://doi.org/10.1038/s41586-021-03341-5.
13. Kirii H, Niwa T, Yamada Y, Wada H, Saito K, Iwakura Y, et al. Lack of interleukin-1beta decreases the severity of atherosclerosis in ApoE-deficient mice. Arterioscler Thromb Vasc Biol. 2003;23(4):656–60. https://doi.org/10.1161/01.atv.0000064374.15232.c3.
14. Jiang X, Wang F, Wang Y, Gistera A, Roy J, Paulsson-Berne G, et al. Inflammasome-driven interleukin-1alpha and interleukin-1beta production in atherosclerotic plaques relates to hyperlipidemia and plaque complexity. JACC Basic Transl Sci. 2019;4(3):304–17. https://doi.org/10.1016/j.jacbts.2019.02.007.

15. Ridker PM, Everett BM, Thuren T, MacFadyen JG, Chang WH, Ballantyne C, et al. Antiinflammatory therapy with Canakinumab for atherosclerotic disease. N Engl J Med. 2017;377(12):1119–31. https://doi.org/10.1056/NEJMoa1707914.

16. Samstad EO, Niyonzima N, Nymo S, Aune MH, Ryan L, Bakke SS, et al. Cholesterol crystals induce complement-dependent inflammasome activation and cytokine release. J Immunol. 2014;192(6):2837–45. https://doi.org/10.4049/jimmunol.1302484.

17. Niyonzima N, Rahman J, Kunz N, West EE, Freiwald T, Desai JV, et al. Mitochondrial C5aR1 activity in macrophages controls IL-1β production underlying sterile inflammation. Sci Immunol. 2021;6(66):eabf2489. https://doi.org/10.1126/sciimmunol.abf2489.

18. Niyonzima N, Bakke SS, Gregersen I, Holm S, Sandanger Ø, Orrem HL, et al. Cholesterol crystals use complement to increase NLRP3 signaling pathways in coronary and carotid atherosclerosis. EBioMedicine. 2020;60:102985. https://doi.org/10.1016/j.ebiom.2020.102985.

19. Jules Bordet OG. Sur l'existence de substances sensibilisatrices dans la plupart des sérums antimicrobiens. Paris: Institut Pasteur; 1901.

20. Merle NS, Noe R, Halbwachs-Mecarelli L, Fremeaux-Bacchi V, Roumenina LT. Complement system part II: role in immunity. Front Immunol. 2015;6:257. https://doi.org/10.3389/fimmu.2015.00257.

21. Merle NS, Church SE, Fremeaux-Bacchi V, Roumenina LT. Complement system part I - molecular mechanisms of activation and regulation. Front Immunol. 2015;6:262. https://doi.org/10.3389/fimmu.2015.00262.

22. Ricklin D, Hajishengallis G, Yang K, Lambris JD. Complement: a key system for immune surveillance and homeostasis. Nat Immunol. 2010;11(9):785–97. https://doi.org/10.1038/ni.1923.

23. Gaboriaud C, Thielens NM, Gregory LA, Rossi V, Fontecilla-Camps JC, Arlaud GJ. Structure and activation of the C1 complex of complement: unraveling the puzzle. Trends Immunol. 2004;25(7):368–73. https://doi.org/10.1016/j.it.2004.04.008.

24. Wallis R, Mitchell DA, Schmid R, Schwaeble WJ, Keeble AH. Paths reunited: initiation of the classical and lectin pathways of complement activation. Immunobiology. 2010;215(1):1–11. https://doi.org/10.1016/j.imbio.2009.08.006.

25. Runza VL, Schwaeble W, Männel DN. Ficolins: novel pattern recognition molecules of the innate immune response. Immunobiology. 2008;213(3–4):297–306. https://doi.org/10.1016/j.imbio.2007.10.009.

26. Kjaer TR, Jensen L, Hansen A, Dani R, Jensenius JC, Dobó J, et al. Oligomerization of Mannan-binding lectin dictates binding properties and complement activation. Scand J Immunol. 2016;84(1):12–9. https://doi.org/10.1111/sji.12441.

27. Garred P, Honoré C, Ma YJ, Rørvig S, Cowland J, Borregaard N, et al. The genetics of ficolins. J Innate Immun. 2010;2(1):3–16. https://doi.org/10.1159/000242419.

28. Yongqing T, Drentin N, Duncan RC, Wijeyewickrema LC, Pike RN. Mannose-binding lectin serine proteases and associated proteins of the lectin pathway of complement: two genes, five proteins and many functions? Biochim Biophys Acta. 2012;1824(1):253–62. https://doi.org/10.1016/j.bbapap.2011.05.021.

29. Garred P, Genster N, Pilely K, Bayarri-Olmos R, Rosbjerg A, Ma YJ, et al. A journey through the lectin pathway of complement-MBL and beyond. Immunol Rev. 2016;274(1):74–97. https://doi.org/10.1111/imr.12468.

30. Sahu A, Kozel TR, Pangburn MK. Specificity of the thioester-containing reactive site of human C3 and its significance to complement activation. Biochem J. 1994;302(Pt 2):429–36. https://doi.org/10.1042/bj3020429.

31. Harboe M, Mollnes TE. The alternative complement pathway revisited. J Cell Mol Med. 2008;12(4):1074–84. https://doi.org/10.1111/j.1582-4934.2008.00350.x.

32. Kemper C, Atkinson JP, Hourcade DE. Properdin: emerging roles of a pattern-recognition molecule. Annu Rev Immunol. 2010;28:131–55. https://doi.org/10.1146/annurev-immunol-030409-101250.

33. Niculescu F, Rus H. Mechanisms of signal transduction activated by sublytic assembly of terminal complement complexes on nucleated cells. Immunol Res. 2001;24(2):191–9. https://doi.org/10.1385/ir:24:2:191.

34. Monk PN, Scola AM, Madala P, Fairlie DP. Function, structure and therapeutic potential of complement C5a receptors. Br J Pharmacol. 2007;152(4):429–48. https://doi.org/10.1038/sj.bjp.0707332.

35. Klos A, Wende E, Wareham KJ, Monk PN. International Union of Basic and Clinical Pharmacology. [corrected]. LXXXVII. Complement peptide C5a, C4a, and C3a receptors. Pharmacol Rev. 2013;65(1):500–43. https://doi.org/10.1124/pr.111.005223.

36. Croker DE, Monk PN, Halai R, Kaeslin G, Schofield Z, Wu MC, et al. Discovery of functionally selective C5aR2 ligands: novel modulators of C5a signalling. Immunol Cell Biol. 2016;94(8):787–95. https://doi.org/10.1038/icb.2016.43.

37. Croker DE, Halai R, Kaeslin G, Wende E, Fehlhaber B, Klos A, et al. C5a2 can modulate ERK1/2 signaling in macrophages via heteromer formation with C5a1 and β-arrestin recruitment. Immunol Cell Biol. 2014;92(7):631–9. https://doi.org/10.1038/icb.2014.32.

38. Khameneh HJ, Ho AW, Laudisi F, Derks H, Kandasamy M, Sivasankar B, et al. C5a regulates IL-1β production and leukocyte recruitment in a murine model of monosodium urate crystal-induced peritonitis. Front Pharmacol. 2017;8:10. https://doi.org/10.3389/fphar.2017.00010.

39. Ratajczak MZ, Adamiak M, Kucia M, Tse W, Ratajczak J, Wiktor-Jedrzejczak W. The emerging link between the complement Cascade and purinergic signaling in stress hematopoiesis. Front Immunol. 2018;9:1295. https://doi.org/10.3389/fimmu.2018.01295.

40. Hong S, Beja-Glasser VF, Nfonoyim BM, Frouin A, Li S, Ramakrishnan S, et al. Complement and microglia mediate early synapse loss in Alzheimer mouse models. Science. 2016;352(6286):712–6. https://doi.org/10.1126/science.aad8373.

41. Gregersen E, Betzer C, Kim WS, Kovacs G, Reimer L, Halliday GM, et al. Alpha-synuclein activates the classical complement pathway and mediates complement-dependent cell toxicity. J Neuroinflammation. 2021;18(1):177. https://doi.org/10.1186/s12974-021-02225-9.

42. Hajishengallis G, Lambris JD. Crosstalk pathways between toll-like receptors and the complement system. Trends Immunol. 2010;31(4):154–63. https://doi.org/10.1016/j.it.2010.01.002.

43. Lee CC, Avalos AM, Ploegh HL. Accessory molecules for toll-like receptors and their function. Nat Rev Immunol. 2012;12(3):168–79. https://doi.org/10.1038/nri3151.

44. Barratt-Due A, Pischke SE, Nilsson PH, Espevik T, Mollnes TE. Dual inhibition of complement and toll-like receptors as a novel approach to treat inflammatory diseases-C3 or C5 emerge together with CD14 as promising targets. J Leukoc Biol. 2017;101(1):193–204. https://doi.org/10.1189/jlb.3VMR0316-132R.

45. Nymo S, Niyonzima N, Espevik T, Mollnes TE. Cholesterol crystal-induced endothelial cell activation is complement-dependent and mediated by TNF. Immunobiology. 2014;219(10):786–92. https://doi.org/10.1016/j.imbio.2014.06.006.

46. Strainic MG, Liu J, Huang D, An F, Lalli PN, Muqim N, et al. Locally produced complement fragments C5a and C3a provide both costimulatory and survival signals to naive CD4+ T cells. Immunity. 2008;28(3):425–35. https://doi.org/10.1016/j.immuni.2008.02.001.

47. Liu J, Miwa T, Hilliard B, Chen Y, Lambris JD, Wells AD, et al. The complement inhibitory protein DAF (CD55) suppresses T cell immunity in vivo. J Exp Med. 2005;201(4):567–77. https://doi.org/10.1084/jem.20040863.

48. Lalli PN, Strainic MG, Yang M, Lin F, Medof ME, Heeger PS. Locally produced C5a binds to T cell-expressed C5aR to enhance effector T-cell expansion by limiting antigen-induced apoptosis. Blood. 2008;112(5):1759–66. https://doi.org/10.1182/blood-2008-04-151068.

49. Passwell J, Schreiner GF, Nonaka M, Beuscher HU, Colten HR. Local extrahepatic expression of complement genes C3, factor B, C2, and C4 is increased in murine lupus nephritis. J Clin Invest. 1988;82(5):1676–84. https://doi.org/10.1172/jci113780.

50. Morgan BP, Gasque P. Extrahepatic complement biosynthesis: where, when and why? Clin Exp Immunol. 1997;107(1):1–7. https://doi.org/10.1046/j.1365-2249.1997.d01-890.x.

51. Welch TR, Beischel LS, Witte DP. Differential expression of complement C3 and C4 in the human kidney. J Clin Invest. 1993;92(3):1451–8. https://doi.org/10.1172/jci116722.
52. Sacks SH, Zhou W, Andrews PA, Hartley B. Endogenous complement C3 synthesis in immune complex nephritis. Lancet. 1993;342(8882):1273–4. https://doi.org/10.1016/0140-6736(93)92362-w.
53. Sacks SH, Zhou W. Locally produced complement and its role in renal allograft rejection. Am J Transplant. 2003;3(8):927–32. https://doi.org/10.1034/j.1600-6143.2003.00175.x.
54. Yasojima K, Schwab C, McGeer EG, McGeer PL. Human heart generates complement proteins that are upregulated and activated after myocardial infarction. Circ Res. 1998;83(8):860–9. https://doi.org/10.1161/01.res.83.8.860.
55. Sugihara T, Kobori A, Imaeda H, Tsujikawa T, Amagase K, Takeuchi K, et al. The increased mucosal mRNA expressions of complement C3 and interleukin-17 in inflammatory bowel disease. Clin Exp Immunol. 2010;160(3):386–93. https://doi.org/10.1111/j.1365-2249.2010.04093.x.
56. Molmenti EP, Ziambaras T, Perlmutter DH. Evidence for an acute phase response in human intestinal epithelial cells. J Biol Chem. 1993;268(19):14116–24.
57. Andoh A, Fujiyama Y, Bamba T, Hosoda S. Differential cytokine regulation of complement C3, C4, and factor B synthesis in human intestinal epithelial cell line, Caco-2. J Immunol. 1993;151(8):4239–47.
58. Veerhuis R, Nielsen HM, Tenner AJ. Complement in the brain. Mol Immunol. 2011;48(14):1592–603. https://doi.org/10.1016/j.molimm.2011.04.003.
59. Shavva VS, Mogilenko DA, Dizhe EB, Oleinikova GN, Perevozchikov AP, Orlov SV. Hepatic nuclear factor 4α positively regulates complement C3 expression and does not interfere with TNFα-mediated stimulation of C3 expression in HepG2 cells. Gene. 2013;524(2):187–92. https://doi.org/10.1016/j.gene.2013.04.036.
60. Gerritsma JS, van Kooten C, Gerritsen AF, van Es LA, Daha MR. Transforming growth factor-beta 1 regulates chemokine and complement production by human proximal tubular epithelial cells. Kidney Int. 1998;53(3):609–16. https://doi.org/10.1046/j.1523-1755.1998.00799.x.
61. Bialas AR, Stevens B. TGF-β signaling regulates neuronal C1q expression and developmental synaptic refinement. Nat Neurosci. 2013;16(12):1773–82. https://doi.org/10.1038/nn.3560.
62. Kolev M, West EE, Kunz N, Chauss D, Moseman EA, Rahman J, et al. Diapedesis-induced integrin signaling via LFA-1 facilitates tissue immunity by inducing intrinsic complement C3 expression in immune cells. Immunity. 2020;52(3):513–27.e8. https://doi.org/10.1016/j.immuni.2020.02.006.
63. Asgari E, Le Friec G, Yamamoto H, Perucha E, Sacks SS, Köhl J, et al. C3a modulates IL-1β secretion in human monocytes by regulating ATP efflux and subsequent NLRP3 inflammasome activation. Blood. 2013;122(20):3473–81. https://doi.org/10.1182/blood-2013-05-502229.
64. Grailer JJ, Bosmann M, Ward PA. Regulatory effects of C5a on IL-17A, IL-17F, and IL-23. Front Immunol. 2012;3:387. https://doi.org/10.3389/fimmu.2012.00387.
65. Arbore G, West EE, Rahman J, Le Friec G, Niyonzima N, Pirooznia M, et al. Complement receptor CD46 co-stimulates optimal human CD8(+) T cell effector function via fatty acid metabolism. Nat Commun. 2018;9(1):4186. https://doi.org/10.1038/s41467-018-06706-z.
66. Kolev M, Le Friec G, Kemper C. Complement—tapping into new sites and effector systems. Nat Rev Immunol. 2014;14(12):811–20. https://doi.org/10.1038/nri3761.
67. West EE, Kunz N, Kemper C. Complement and human T cell metabolism: location, location, location. Immunol Rev. 2020;295:68. https://doi.org/10.1111/imr.12852.
68. Arbore G, West EE, Spolski R, Robertson AA, Klos A, Rheinheimer C, et al. T helper 1 immunity requires complement-driven NLRP3 inflammasome activity in CD4(+) T cells. Science. 2016;352(6292):aad1210. https://doi.org/10.1126/science.aad1210.
69. Kolev M, Dimeloe S, Le Friec G, Navarini A, Arbore G, Povoleri GA, et al. Complement regulates nutrient influx and metabolic reprogramming during Th1 cell responses. Immunity. 2015;42(6):1033–47. https://doi.org/10.1016/j.immuni.2015.05.024.

70. West EE, Kemper C. Complement and T cell metabolism: food for thought. Immunometabolism. 2019;1(T Cell Metabolic Reprogramming):e190006. https://doi.org/10.20900/immunometab20190006.

71. Kolev M, Kemper C. Keeping it all going-complement meets metabolism. Front Immunol. 2017;8:1. https://doi.org/10.3389/fimmu.2017.00001.

72. Yan B, Freiwald T, Chauss D, Wang L, West E, Mirabelli C, et al. SARS-CoV-2 drives JAK1/2-dependent local complement hyperactivation. Sci Immunol. 2021;6(58):eabg0833. https://doi.org/10.1126/sciimmunol.abg0833.

73. King BC, Kulak K, Krus U, Rosberg R, Golec E, Wozniak K, et al. Complement component C3 is highly expressed in human pancreatic islets and prevents β cell death via ATG16L1 interaction and autophagy regulation. Cell Metab. 2019;29(1):202–10.e6. https://doi.org/10.1016/j.cmet.2018.09.009.

74. Kulkarni HS, Elvington ML, Perng YC, Liszewski MK, Byers DE, Farkouh C, et al. Intracellular C3 protects human airway epithelial cells from stress-associated cell death. Am J Respir Cell Mol Biol. 2019;60(2):144–57. https://doi.org/10.1165/rcmb.2017-0405OC.

75. Daugan MV, Revel M, Lacroix L, Sautès-Fridman C, Fridman WH, Roumenina LT. Complement detection in human tumors by immunohistochemistry and immunofluorescence. Methods Mol Biol. 2021;2227:191–203. https://doi.org/10.1007/978-1-0716-1016-9_18.

76. Hammerschmidt DE, Greenberg CS, Yamada O, Craddock PR, Jacob HS. Cholesterol and atheroma lipids activate complement and stimulate granulocytes. A possible mechanism for amplification of ischemic injury in atherosclerotic states. J Lab Clin Med. 1981;98(1):68–77.

77. Seifert PS, Kazatchkine MD. Generation of complement anaphylatoxins and C5b-9 by crystalline cholesterol oxidation derivatives depends on hydroxyl group number and position. Mol Immunol. 1987;24(12):1303–8.

78. Vogt W, von Zabern I, Damerau B, Hesse D, Luhmann B, Nolte R. Mechanisms of complement activation by crystalline cholesterol. Mol Immunol. 1985;22(2):101–6.

79. Swartz GM Jr, Gentry MK, Amende LM, Blanchette-Mackie EJ, Alving CR. Antibodies to cholesterol. Proc Natl Acad Sci U S A. 1988;85(6):1902–6. https://doi.org/10.1073/pnas.85.6.1902.

80. Pilely K, Rosbjerg A, Genster N, Gal P, Pal G, Halvorsen B, et al. Cholesterol crystals activate the lectin complement pathway via Ficolin-2 and mannose-binding lectin: implications for the progression of atherosclerosis. J Immunol. 2016;196(12):5064–74. https://doi.org/10.4049/jimmunol.1502595.

81. Gravastrand CS, Steinkjer B, Halvorsen B, Landsem A, Skjelland M, Jacobsen EA, et al. Cholesterol crystals induce coagulation activation through complement-dependent expression of monocytic tissue factor. J Immunol. 2019;203(4):853–63. https://doi.org/10.4049/jimmunol.1900503.

82. Niculescu F, Rus HG, Vlaicu R. Activation of the human terminal complement pathway in atherosclerosis. Clin Immunol Immunopathol. 1987;45(2):147–55. https://doi.org/10.1016/0090-1229(87)90029-8.

83. Niculescu F, Hugo F, Rus HG, Vlaicu R, Bhakdi S. Quantitative evaluation of the terminal C5b-9 complement complex by ELISA in human atherosclerotic arteries. Clin Exp Immunol. 1987;69(2):477–83.

84. Yasojima K, Schwab C, McGeer EG, McGeer PL. Generation of C-reactive protein and complement components in atherosclerotic plaques. Am J Pathol. 2001;158(3):1039–51. https://doi.org/10.1016/s0002-9440(10)64051-5.

85. Rus HG, Niculescu F, Vlaicu R. Co-localization of terminal C5b-9 complement complexes and macrophages in human atherosclerotic arterial walls. Immunol Lett. 1988;19(1):27–32.

86. Vlaicu R, Rus HG, Niculescu F, Cristea A. Quantitative determinations of immunoglobulins and complement components in human aortic atherosclerotic wall. Med Interne. 1985;23(1):29–35.

87. Niculescu F, Rus HG, Vlaicu R. Immunohistochemical localization of C5b-9, S-protein, C3d and apolipoprotein B in human arterial tissues with atherosclerosis. Atherosclerosis. 1987;65(1–2):1–11. https://doi.org/10.1016/0021-9150(87)90002-5.
88. Lappegard KT, Christiansen D, Pharo A, Thorgersen EB, Hellerud BC, Lindstad J, et al. Human genetic deficiencies reveal the roles of complement in the inflammatory network: lessons from nature. Proc Natl Acad Sci U S A. 2009;106(37):15861–6. https://doi.org/10.1073/pnas.0903613106.
89. Speidl WS, Kastl SP, Hutter R, Katsaros KM, Kaun C, Bauriedel G, et al. The complement component C5a is present in human coronary lesions in vivo and induces the expression of MMP-1 and MMP-9 in human macrophages in vitro. FASEB J. 2011;25(1):35–44. https://doi.org/10.1096/fj.10-156083.
90. Paramel Varghese G, Folkersen L, Strawbridge RJ, Halvorsen B, Yndestad A, Ranheim T, et al. NLRP3 Inflammasome expression and activation in human atherosclerosis. J Am Heart Assoc. 2016;5(5):e003031. https://doi.org/10.1161/jaha.115.003031.
91. Franklin BS, Mangan MS, Latz E. Crystal formation in inflammation. Annu Rev Immunol. 2016;34:173–202. https://doi.org/10.1146/annurev-immunol-041015-055539.
92. Missiroli S, Patergnani S, Caroccia N, Pedriali G, Perrone M, Previati M, et al. Mitochondria-associated membranes (MAMs) and inflammation. Cell Death Dis. 2018;9(3):329. https://doi.org/10.1038/s41419-017-0027-2.
93. Andreeva L, David L, Rawson S, Shen C, Pasricha T, Pelegrin P, et al. NLRP3 cages revealed by full-length mouse NLRP3 structure control pathway activation. Cell. 2021;184(26):6299–312. e22. https://doi.org/10.1016/j.cell.2021.11.011.
94. Weinberg SE, Sena LA, Chandel NS. Mitochondria in the regulation of innate and adaptive immunity. Immunity. 2015;42(3):406–17. https://doi.org/10.1016/j.immuni.2015.02.002.
95. Tumurkhuu G, Shimada K, Dagvadorj J, Crother TR, Zhang W, Luthringer D, et al. Ogg1-dependent DNA repair regulates NLRP3 Inflammasome and prevents atherosclerosis. Circ Res. 2016;119(6):e76–90. https://doi.org/10.1161/circresaha.116.308362.
96. Nomura J, So A, Tamura M, Busso N. Intracellular ATP decrease mediates NLRP3 Inflammasome activation upon Nigericin and crystal stimulation. J Immunol. 2015;195(12):5718–24. https://doi.org/10.4049/jimmunol.1402512.
97. Kiss MG, Binder CJ. The multifaceted impact of complement on atherosclerosis. Atherosclerosis. 2022;351:29. https://doi.org/10.1016/j.atherosclerosis.2022.03.014.
98. Smith PK, Shernan SK, Chen JC, Carrier M, Verrier ED, Adams PX, et al. Effects of C5 complement inhibitor pexelizumab on outcome in high-risk coronary artery bypass grafting: combined results from the PRIMO-CABG I and II trials. J Thorac Cardiovasc Surg. 2011;142(1):89–98. https://doi.org/10.1016/j.jtcvs.2010.08.035.
99. Zimmer S, Grebe A, Bakke SS, Bode N, Halvorsen B, Ulas T, et al. Cyclodextrin promotes atherosclerosis regression via macrophage reprogramming. Sci Transl Med. 2016;8(333):333ra50. https://doi.org/10.1126/scitranslmed.aad6100.

Role of CCs and Their Lipoprotein Precursors in NLRP3 and IL-1β Activation

Kristiina Rajamäki and Katariina Öörni

Abbreviations

Apo	Apolipoprotein
CCs	Cholesterol crystals
DAMPs	Danger-associated molecular patterns
HDL	High density lipoprotein
HFD	High-fat diet
IL	Interleukin
LDL	Low density lipoprotein
LDLR/Ldlr	Low density lipoprotein receptor
NLRP3/Nlrp3	NLR family pyrin domain containing 3
oxLDL	Oxidized low density lipoprotein
PAMPs	Pathogen-associated molecular patterns
TLR	Toll-like receptor

K. Rajamäki (✉)
University of Helsinki, Helsinki, Finland
e-mail: kristiina.rajamaki@helsinki.fi

K. Öörni
Wihuri Research Institute, Helsinki, Finland
e-mail: kati.oorni@wri.fi

257

G. S. Abela, S. M. Nidorf (eds.), *Cholesterol Crystals in Atherosclerosis and Other Related Diseases*, Contemporary Cardiology,
https://doi.org/10.1007/978-3-031-41192-2_15

1   NLRP3 Inflammasome Is Activated in Atherosclerosis

1.1   What Is an Inflammasome?

The term *inflammasome* was coined to describe a pro-inflammatory pathway that controls the proteolytic cleavage of precursor cytokines pro-interleukin(IL)-1β and pro-IL-18 into their biologically active, secreted forms [1]. The cytokine cleavage involves the activation of an inflammatory caspase, caspase-1, within a large cytoplasmic multiprotein scaffold complex that bears resemblance to the apoptosome complex activating apoptotic caspases [2]. Inflammasome activation can also result in a distinct form of pro-inflammatory cell death called *pyroptosis* [3] where the cell releases its cytoplasmic contents—along with the mature cytokines—via plasma membrane pores formed by another caspase-1 cleavage target, gasdermin D. Although inflammasome activity was first described in innate immune cells of the monocyte-macrophage lineage [1], it has been later demonstrated in numerous immune and non-immune cell types in various contexts.

The assembly of an inflammasome can be triggered by several different cytoplasmic pattern recognition receptors that act as sensors for pathogen-associated or danger-associated molecular patterns (PAMPs and DAMPs, respectively) [2]. Accordingly, the composition and regulation of the triggered inflammasome complex varies along with the associated physiological roles that range from host defense, acute inflammation, and sepsis to chronic inflammatory diseases. The most widely studied inflammasome complex is that triggered by the NLR family pyrin domain containing 3 (NLRP3) receptor, in particular owing to the perplexing number of endogenous DAMPs activating this receptor to trigger sterile inflammation [4] (Fig. 1). These include ATP released from necrotic cells [5], extracellular matrix components released upon tissue injury [6, 7], pathological protein aggregates such as amyloid-β in Alzheimer's disease [8] and the islet amyloid polypeptide in type II diabetes [9], obesity-associated danger signals such as palmitate and ceramides [10, 11], and crystallized metabolites such as uric acid crystals in gout [12] and—our main focus here—CCs in atherosclerosis [13, 14]. How such diverse compounds can activate a single receptor is not fully understood, but it is clear that there is no direct interaction between the (often) extracellular stimulus and the cytoplasmic receptor. Instead, NLRP3 is a sensor for certain intracellular perturbations caused by these agents [4].

Before going further into the detailed molecular mechanisms of CC-induced NLRP3 inflammasome activation and contribution of lipoprotein modifications in CC formation (Sects. 2 and 3), we shall first summarize here what is known of the expression and contribution of the NLRP3 inflammasome pathway in progression of atherosclerosis.

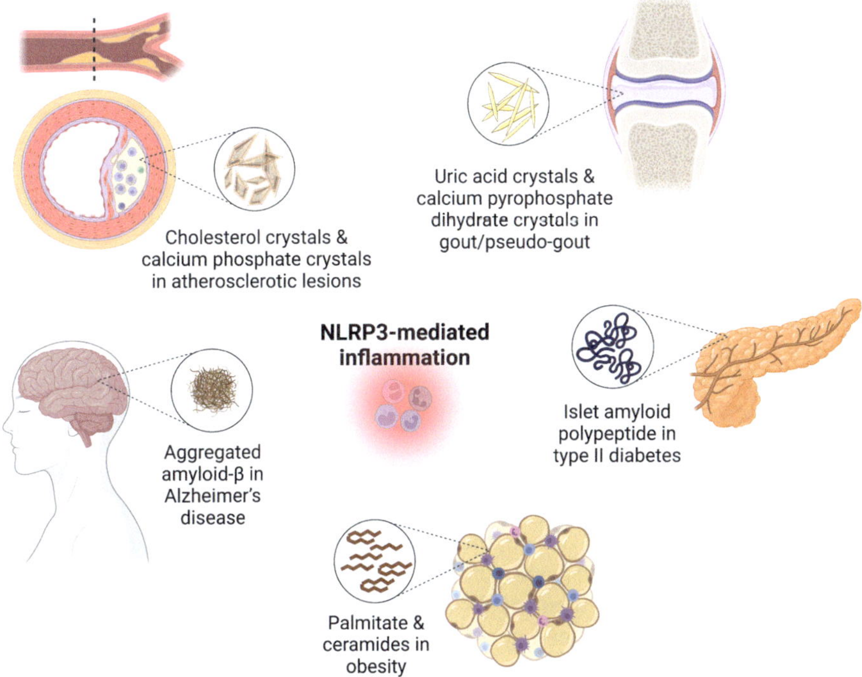

Fig. 1 NLRP3 inflammasome as a mediator of sterile inflammation. Examples of endogenous danger signals triggering inflammation via the NLRP3 inflammasome. See the text for further details. (Created with BioRender.com (2022))

1.2 NLRP3 Inflammasome in Mouse Models of Atherosclerosis

A comprehensive study by Duewell et al. [13] provided compelling evidence towards a proatherogenic role for the Nlrp3 inflammasome. Low density lipoprotein receptor deficient ($Ldlr^{-/-}$) mice were reconstituted with bone marrow deficient in *Nlrp3* receptor, the inflammasome adapter molecule PYD and CARD domain containing (*Pycard*, also known as *Asc*), or *Il1a* and *Il1b*. After 8 weeks on a high-fat diet (HFD), aortic lesion area was strikingly reduced by ~70% in all three models compared to mice receiving wild-type bone marrow. Significant decreases in atherosclerotic lesion area were later demonstrated in apolipoprotein E deficient ($ApoE^{-/-}$) $Casp1^{-/-}$ double knock-out mice [15, 16], after lentiviral silencing of *Nlrp3* in $ApoE^{-/-}$ mice [17], and in $Ldlr^{-/-}$ mice reconstituted with $Casp1/11^{-/-}$ bone marrow [18]. Also decreased necrotic core size, decreased macrophage and lipid content, decreased IL-1β reactivity, and modified immune cell activation were noted in the lesions in these studies. However, a study by Menu et al. crossed $ApoE^{-/-}$ mice with $Nlrp3^{-/-}$, $Pycard^{-/-}$, or $Casp1^{-/-}$ mice and found no difference in atherosclerotic plaque size or composition after 11 weeks of HFD [19]. Differences in the HFD may have played a role, the Menu et al. study using both a high cholesterol content of 1.25% and long diet duration of 11 weeks, combined with the more severe hypercholesterolemia in the $ApoE^{-/-}$ model compared to the $Ldlr^{-/-}$ model [20, 21]. Taken together, the majority of studies in mouse models have supported a proatherogenic role for the Nlrp3 inflammasome.

Further support for the proatherogenic effects of inflammasome activation comes from a plethora of studies exploring the effects of downstream inflammasome effector molecules in atherogenesis. Knock-out of $Il1b$ alone (without simultaneous disruption of IL-1α signaling via the same receptor) attenuated spontaneous atherogenesis in $ApoE^{-/-}$ mice [22], albeit to a lesser degree compared to the $Il1a/b$ double knock-out [13]. Targeting IL-1β with monoclonal antibodies reduced HFD-induced lesions in $ApoE^{-/-}$ mice [23]. Interleukin-1 receptor antagonist deficient mice displayed severe transmural arterial inflammation and lethal aneurysms [24], while IL-1Ra administration in $ApoE^{-/-}$ mice [25] or overexpression in $Ldlr^{-/-}$ mice on HFD [26] reduced the development of early atherosclerotic lesions. Genetic ablation of IL-18 activity in $ApoE^{-/-}$ mice impaired and IL-18 injections aggravated atherosclerotic lesion development [27–29]. Finally, a recent report using $Ldlr$ antisense oligonucleotide-induced hyperlipidemic mice showed cleaved gasdermin D in situ in atherosclerotic lesions and reduced lesion area in $GsdmD^{-/-}$ mice [30].

Beyond local inflammation in atherosclerotic plaques, $Nlrp3$ deficiency in $Ldlr^{-/-}$ mice was reported to block the systemic inflammation and myeloid immune cell hyper-reactivity induced as an early effect of HFD before significant lesion development [31]. Furthermore, Nlrp3 inflammasome plays a role in the development of obesity-induced adipose tissue inflammation and insulin resistance in mouse models [11, 32], thus potentially contributing to risk factors associated with atherosclerosis.

1.3 NLRP3 Inflammasome in Atherosclerotic Human Arterial Wall

Well before the discovery of the NLRP3 inflammasome, IL-1β immunoreactivity was found in macrophages and endothelial cells of coronary arteries of patients with ischemic heart disease and shown to correlate with the severity of coronary atherosclerosis [33]. Similarly, IL-18 and IL-18 receptor subunits were shown to be expressed in situ in human atheromas, and Western blots revealed cleavage of IL-18 and caspase-1 into their active forms in lesions but not in normal tissue [34]. Further reports showed immunoreactivity for the active cleaved form of caspase-1 in macrophages near atherosclerotic plaque lipid cores, colocalizing with IL-1β and with markers of apoptosis and hypoxia [35, 36].

The first study of NLRP3 expression in patients with coronary atherosclerosis showed in aortic samples strong NLRP3 staining that correlated with disease severity and several atherosclerotic risk factors [37]. Further studies showed significantly increased expression of NLRP3, PYCARD/ASC, caspase-1, IL-1β, and IL-18 mRNA and protein directly in carotid artery plaque tissue from carotid endarterectomy in comparison to nonatherosclerotic mesenteric or iliac arteries from a different set of individuals [38, 39]. NLRP3 inflammasome localized primarily in plaque macrophages, and significantly higher NLRP3 levels were found in unstable compared to stable atherosclerotic plaques [38] and in symptomatic compared to asymptomatic patients [39]. We stained NLRP3 inflammasome components in paired early and advanced coronary artery atherosclerotic plaques from the same ten individuals to study changes in expression levels during progression of atherosclerosis [40]. Macrophages in early coronary lesions displayed only occasional PYCARD/ASC and caspase-1 positivity, and very rare positivity for NLRP3. In advanced coronary plaques, lipid-filled foam cell macrophages strongly positive for NLRP3, ASC, and caspase-1 were common near necrotic lipid cores with abundant cholesterol crystal clefts, suggesting increased inflammasome signaling during progression of atherogenesis. A quantitative PCR array further showed significant upregulation of *CASP1*, *IL18*, and *IL1RN* mRNAs in the advanced compared to early lesions [40]. Signs of NLRP3 inflammasome activation are detectable also systemically in patients with cardiovascular disease. Serum levels of IL-1β and IL-18 were shown to be elevated in carotid endarterectomy patients [38] and increased NLRP3 protein levels were found in peripheral blood monocytes from patients with acute coronary syndrome [41].

2 CC-Induced Activation of the NLRP3 Inflammasome

As introduced in Sect. 1, CCs activate the NLRP3 inflammasome resulting in maturation and secretion of the potent pro-inflammatory cytokines IL-1β and IL-18, and this pathway is associated with proatherogenic effects in both mice and men. In this section we will focus on the more detailed mechanisms associated with NLRP3 inflammasome activation by CCs. The emphasis will lie on studies performed in immune cells of the monocyte-macrophage lineage, the major cell type expressing NLRP3 in human atherosclerotic lesions.

2.1 *Priming of the NLRP3 Inflammasome*

While pro-IL-18 is expressed constitutively, pro-IL-1β is absent in resting monocytes and macrophages [42]. Also the NLRP3 receptor is expressed at a limiting level and induction of NLRP3 expression is a prerequisite for subsequent inflammasome assembly [43]. CCs and other canonical inflammasome activators only trigger activation of the NLRP3 receptor, not its expression nor the expression of pro-IL-1β. Thus, a separate priming stimulus is first required to enable sufficient amounts of NLRP3 receptor and pro-IL-1β to accumulate in cells before the pathway can be activated. Priming can be triggered by pro-inflammatory stimuli including Toll-like receptor (TLR) activators and inflammatory cytokines, including IL-1β itself as a positive feedback loop, that activate the NF-κB transcription factor [43]. The priming stimuli are typically ineffective in triggering NLRP3 inflammasome assembly and proteolytic cytokine maturation. Thus, two separate signals are required for full activation of the NLRP3 inflammasome pathway.

In the context of atherosclerosis, many different priming stimuli are likely to contribute. TLRs respond to both PAMPs and DAMPs, and both can be present in the altered tissue microenvironment of atherosclerotic plaques [44]. Potential sterile endogenous priming stimuli include for example many DAMPs released from dying cells, modified low density lipoprotein, oxidized phospholipids, complement factors, and degradation products of extracellular matrix components [44].

2.2 Activation Mechanisms of the NLRP3 Inflammasome by CCs

CCs in atherosclerotic plaques can originate both from extracellular lipid pools and intracellularly within lipid-engorged cells, as discussed in detail in Sect. 3. A seminal study published on CC-induced NLRP3 inflammasome activation examined both routes in detail [13]. Using confocal fluorescence and reflection microscopy, the authors first revealed that microcrystals of cholesterol are detectable within subendothelial macrophages in early diet-induced atherosclerotic lesions in $ApoE^{-/-}$ mice as early as after 2 weeks of HFD. Upon continued atherogenic diet, CCs were detected in necrotic cores but also in subendothelial areas, both inside and outside cells. Abundant cholesterol microcrystals were demonstrated also in human atherosclerotic lesions with this technique. Further experiments in lipopolysaccharide (LPS) -primed cultured mouse macrophages showed robust caspase-1 activation and secretion of mature IL-1β in response to in vitro crystallized CCs, abolished in $Nlrp3^{-/-}$ and $Pycard/Asc^{-/-}$ cells. The authors also demonstrated that oxidized LDL (oxLDL) as a TLR ligand can induce priming of mouse macrophages and also weak IL-1β secretion owing to crystallization of oxLDL-derived cholesterol intracellularly in lysosomes. Our own study published soon after confirmed these findings in LPS-primed primary human monocytes and macrophages stimulated with CCs, where cellular uptake of the crystals triggered IL-1β secretion in an NLRP3 receptor and caspase-1 dependent manner [14]. Of note, both studies showed the complete lack of IL-1β secretion in response to CCs alone, which thus behave as a canonical inflammasome activator.

For extracellularly administered crystals, cellular uptake was a prerequisite for IL-1β secretion, and inhibition or genetic ablation of lysosomal cathepsin B/L resulted in reduced cytokine secretion [13, 14]. Lysosomal destabilization was demonstrated using fluorescent markers in each study. While phagolysosomal damage has emerged as a widely accepted mechanism in NLRP3 inflammasome activation by crystalline and particulate materials, the exact details remain obscure. Lysosome-disrupting agents fail to activate caspase-1 while NLRP3-activating crystals/particles trigger caspase-1 activation in the absence of overt lysosome rupture in a process dependent on multiple lysosomal cathepsins [45, 46]. We showed an additional dependence of the CC-induced IL-1β secretion on potassium efflux [14], another well-established cellular stress signal proposed to convey NLRP3 receptor activation by many activators [47]. Again, the exact mechanisms and possible channel proteins triggering potassium efflux remain obscure for many NLRP3 activators [48]. However, progress has been made in understanding how the NLRP3 receptor might sense the drop in intracellular potassium levels, which may involve a conformational change in the NLRP3 protein and NLRP3-NEK7 interaction acquired as a result of potassium efflux [48]. Interestingly, a *Cd36*-dependent mechanism was later defined for the oxLDL-induced intracellular cholesterol crystallization in mouse macrophages; cholesterol crystallization, caspase-1 activation, and IL-1β immunoreactivity were markedly attenuated in atherosclertic lesions of $ApoE^{-/-}/Cd36^{-/-}$ double knock-out mice, accompanied by reduced lesion size [49].

The intracellular stress signals caused by CC phagocytosis (lysosomal damage and potassium efflux) are sensed by the NLRP3 receptor that upon activation oligomerizes and recruits the adapter molecule PYCARD/ASC to form a large multimolecular complex. ASC, in turn, harbors a caspase activation and recruitment domain (CARD) that interacts with pro-caspase-1, resulting in the autoproteolytic activation of caspase-1 within the complex. This generates an active inflammasome that cleaves its target cytokines IL-1β and IL-18 into their biologically active forms. However, IL-1β and IL-18 lack the signal peptide for classical secretion. Another caspase-1 target, gasdermin D, generates pores into the plasma membrane for cytokine release, and can also trigger pyroptotic cell death [3, 50]. The priming and activation mechanisms of the NLRP3 inflammasome by CCs are summarized in Fig. 2.

2.3 Tissue Microenvironment Modulates CC-Induced NLRP3 Inflammasome Activation

CCs and oxLDL are prominent, lipid-derived danger signals in atherosclerotic plaques, yet they coexist in the lesions with several other factors associated with NLRP3 inflammasome priming or activation. Examples include hypoxia [36], extracellular acidosis [51], extracellular ATP [52], the acute phase protein serum amyloid A [53], activated complement [54], neutrophil-derived proteinase 3 [55], and products of extracellular matrix degradation [6, 7]. These may synergize with or exacerbate CC-induced NLRP3 activation. For example, CCs can be opsonized by complement, which augments their phagocytosis by monocytes and the resulting

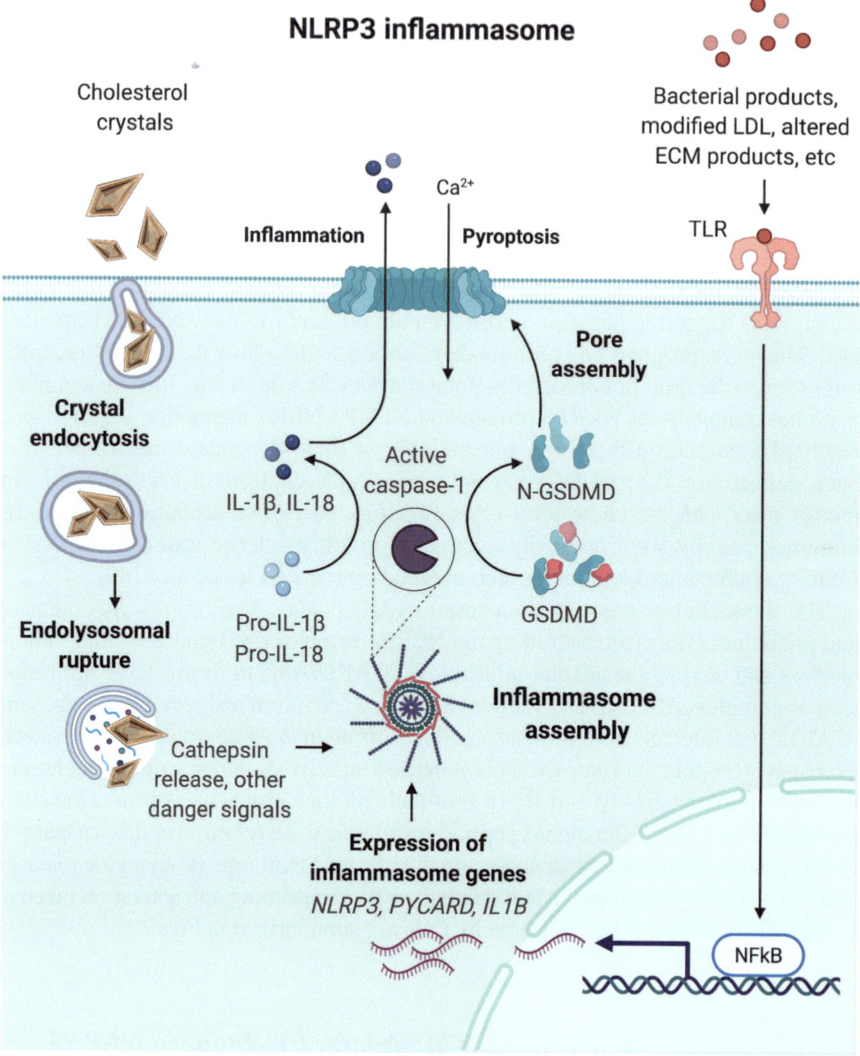

Fig. 2 Activation of the NLRP3 inflammasome by cholesterol crystals. See the text for further details. *ECM* extracellular matrix, *GSDMD* gasdermin D, *IL* interleukin, *LDL* low density lipoprotein, *NF-κB* nuclear factor kappa-light-chain-enhancer of activated B cells, *N-GSDMD* N-terminal fragment of gasdermin D, *NLRP3* NLR family pyrin domain containing 3, *TLR* Toll-like receptor. (Created with BioRender.com; adapted from a template retrieved from BioRender.com (2022))

inflammasome activation [56], as discussed in more detail in the previous chapter. We explored the potential effects of acidification of plaque microenvironment, an independent NLRP3 inflammasome activator, on CC-induced NLRP3 inflammasome activation [51]. A very mildly acidic environment of pH 7.0 that triggered only a modest IL-1β response in macrophages substantially augmented the IL-1β response to CCs. Thus, local acidosis may potentiate NLRP3 inflammasome activation by CCs by creating a sensitizing microenvironment for macrophages. Another interesting example is proteinase 3 released by activated neutrophils, short-lived immune cells found from atherosclerotic lesions. Substantial amounts of pro-IL-1β can be released upon pyroptosis or necrosis of plaque cells into the extracellular space, where proteinase 3 is able to carry out alternative processing of the precursor cytokine into an active form and amplify the local IL-1β response [55]. Chymase released during degranulation of lesional mast cells is another protease reported to extracellularly process pro-IL-1β [57].

3 Lipoprotein Modifications in CC Formation

Circulating low density lipoprotein (LDL) particles are retained in the arterial intima due to their interactions with the dense intimal extracellular matrix and modified by oxidizing agents and enzymes, such as proteases and lipases secreted by the local cells [58]. Such modifications induce lipoprotein aggregation, enhance lipoprotein retention to the extracellular matrix and promote the uptake of the lipoproteins by macrophages, which are converted into foam cells. In the developing lesions, the macrophage foam cells die and form a necrotic lipid core containing the remains of the dead cells and the lipids they contained [59]. The fibrous cap containing collagen and other components of the extracellular matrix becomes progressively thinner due to degradation and reduced synthesis of the matrix components [60]. A thin-cap atherosclerotic lesion usually contains numerous inflammatory cells, a large necrotic core and is vulnerable to rupture [61].

CCs are particularly abundant in the necrotic lipid core of advanced atherosclerotic lesions, but they are seen throughout the lesion development in both experimental and human atherosclerosis [13, 62–65]. The crystals are most often observed as empty clefts in microscopic images [66], but their presence has been verified by spatial lipidomic analysis of human coronary atherosclerotic lesions [67], physicochemical analysis [67–69], and optical coherence tomography [70, 71]. The presence of CCs in atheroclerotic plaques enhances the risk for future cardiovascular events [70]. As discussed in the previous section, CCs are thought to contribute to the inflammatory potential of the lesions. Here, we focus on the upstream events resulting in CC formation within atherosclerotic lesions, summarizing the mechanisms of both extra- and intracellular cholesterol crystallization. We conclude the chapter with a brief introduction into approaches for blocking CC accumulation and CC-induced inflammation in atherosclerotic lesions, topics further discussed in Chapter "Formation of CCs in Endothelial Cells".

3.1 Extracellular Cholesterol Crystallization

In early atherosclerotic lesions, extracellular CCs can be derived from lipoproteins accumulating in the arterial wall, while in advanced atherosclerotic lesions, most of the extracellular CCs are likely derived from dying cells that have released their lipid contents. Generation of CCs from lipoproteins requires lipolysis: cholesterol in the lipoprotein particles is mostly esterified and, for example, each LDL particle contains about 3500 cholesteryl ester molecules in its core [72]. Unless the cholesteryl esters are lipolyzed to free cholesterol and fatty acid molecules, extracellular accumulation of even large amounts of lipoproteins will not induce CC formation. Enzymes capable of cholesteryl ester hydrolysis, such as lysosomal acid lipase, are found extracellularly in atherosclerotic lesions [73]. Hydrolysis of cholesteryl esters has been shown to induce generation of CCs in vitro. Thus, Guarino et al. [74] showed that a combination of sphingomyelinase and cholesterol esterase induces CC nucleation from LDL. We showed that destabilization of LDL surface by oxidation, proteolysis, and hydrolysis by sphingomyelinase or phospholipase A2 promotes lipolysis of the core cholesteryl esters and induces formation of CCs [64, 74]. Such multiply modified lipoproteins are found in human atherosclerotic lesions [75]. Isolation and analysis of extracellular lipoproteins from advanced human atherosclerotic lesions verified that they are derived from apoB-containing lipoproteins via lipolysis and, importantly, are connected to CCs [64]. Uptake of the isolated lipoproteins and CCs, as well as LDL modified in vitro by the combination of phospholipase A2 and lysosomal acid lipase, induced secretion of IL-1β from macrophages.

3.2 Intracellular Cholesterol Crystallization

Macrophages are professional phagocytes that have the potential to take up modified LDL particles via several different mechanisms leading to foam cell formation [76]. A prototype of modified LDL often used in in vitro experiments is oxidized LDL that binds to various scavenger receptors on macrophages. Other uptake mechanisms include Fcγ-receptor -mediated uptake of immune complexes of antibodies bound to oxidized LDL and phagocytosis of aggregated LDL and CCs [14, 77, 78]. Very large LDL aggregates can be taken up via specific surface-connected compartments to which cells can secrete lysosomal enzymes, such as lysosomal acid lipase [79–81]. LDL aggregates are hydrolyzed partially outside the cells after which they are taken up by the cells and hydrolyzed in the lysosomes. Actin polymerization and TLR4 activation drive the intracellular catabolism of the aggregates [79, 82].

Once lipoproteins have reached the lysosomes, their components are hydrolyzed, and cholesteryl ester hydrolysis results in formation of unesterified cholesterol. Accumulation of cholesterol in the lysosomes may lead to its crystallization. Indeed, CD36-mediated uptake of oxidized LDL was shown to result in the formation of

CCs in lysosomes [49]. As described above, this leads to lysosomal destabilization and activation of the NLRP3 inflammasome. Similarly, the uptake of CCs leads to inflammasome activation via lysosomal destabilization [49, 83].

Cholesterol can be transported from lysosomes to the cytoplasm, where it can be re-esterified and packaged into intracellular lipid droplets characteristic of foam cells [84]. Figure 3 summarizes the downstream effects of the uptake of modified

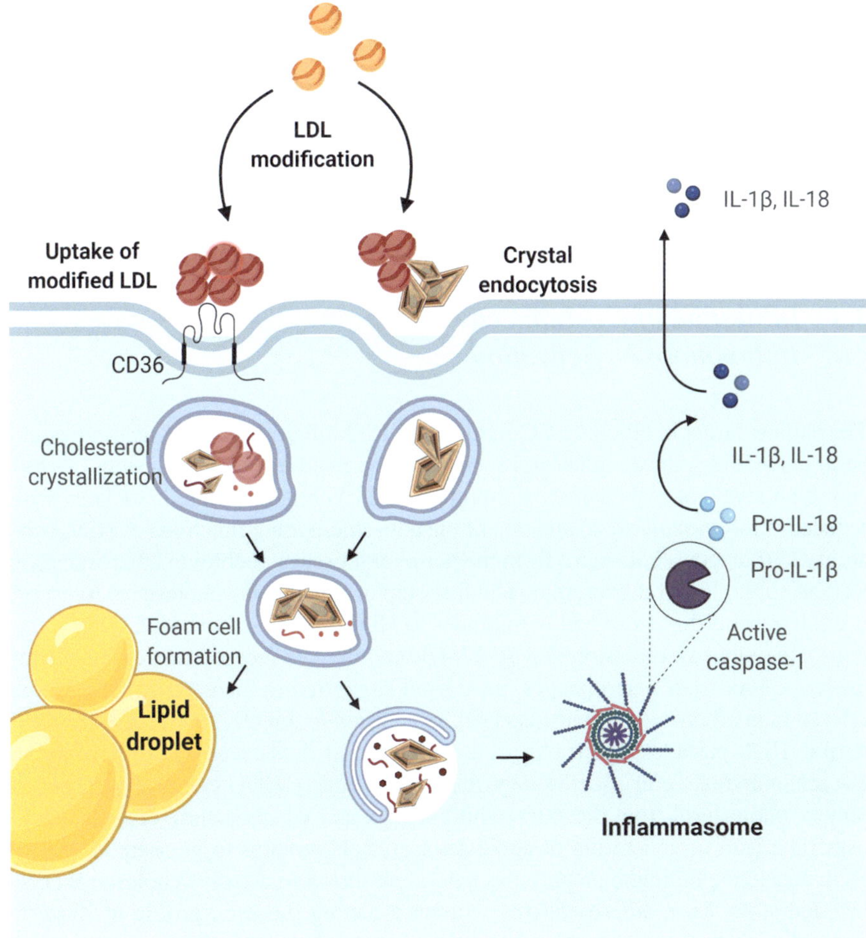

Fig. 3 CCs are formed from modified LDL extra- and intracellularly. Uptake of modified LDL induces CC formation in lysosomes and uptake of both modified LDL and CCs induces foam cell formation. See the text for further details. (Created with BioRender.com; adapted from a template retrieved from BioRender.com (2022))

LDL and CCs. Two major transport proteins responsible for the transport of cholesterol from lysosomes to the cytoplasm are the Niemann-Pick C1 and C2 proteins [85]. Deficiency in these proteins leads to accumulation of cholesterol in the lysosomes and is linked to generation of CCs [86]. Another enzyme controlling cellular homeostasis is Acyl-CoA:Cholesterol Acyltransferase 1 (ACAT1) that esterifies cholesterol, which is then packed into cytoplasmic lipid droplets. If cholesterol re-esterification is not sufficient, unesterified cholesterol will accumulate in the cells. Indeed, inhibition of ACAT1 results in excess production of unesterified cholesterol [87]. Notably, a clinical trial with the ACAT inhibitor pactimibe showed unfavorable effects in patients with coronary disease, where the drug treatment attenuated the regression of atherosclerosis [88].

Most of the studies on CC formation have focused on macrophages and macrophage foam cells. However, recently also endothelial cells and smooth muscle cells have been shown to produce CCs under hyperlipidemic conditions [62, 89]. Interestingly, in *Ldlr*$^{-/-}$ mice, endothelial cells were shown to secrete the generated CCs into the subendothelial space and increase the expression of E-selectin. This promoted monocyte adherence and transmigration, processes important in atherogenesis [89].

3.3   Inhibition of CC-Induced NLRP3 Inflammasome Activation

The earliest target in blocking CC-induced NLRP3 inflammasome activation would be to prevent or reduce cholesterol crystallization in atherosclerotic lesions. To this end, high levels of high density lipoprotein (HDL) cholesterol are associated with reduced cardiovascular risk, and one of the anti-atherogenic functions of HDL is its ability to transport cholesterol from the peripheral tissues, including atherosclerotic lesions, to the liver for excretion. The first step of this reverse cholesterol transport is cholesterol efflux from cell membranes to HDL particles. Low HDL concentrations and reduced expression of *ABCA1/ABCG1*, the two receptors involved in cholesterol efflux from macrophages, have been suggested to increase inflammasome activation in atherosclerotic lesions [90]. In addition to directly transporting cholesterol to HDL particles, macrophages are also able to shed excess cholesterol to the extracellular matrix in specific deposits [91]. Whether HDL particles are able to remove cholesterol from the extracellular matrix and whether these deposits could over time lead to generation of cholesterol crystals remains to be seen. However, HDL-like phospholipid nanoparticles have been shown to dissolve cholesterol crystals and slow down atherosclerosis without affecting the lipid profile of *ApoE*$^{-/-}$ mice [92, 93]. Similarly, the treatment of *ApoE*$^{-/-}$ mice with cyclodextrin, a compound that increases cholesterol solubility, reduced plaque size and CC burden, dissolving both extra- and intracellular CCs and increasing cholesterol efflux from macrophages [94].

Various factors in plaque microenvironment may modulate the NLRP3 inflammasome activation resulting from cholesterol crystallization. The ketone metabolite β-hydroxybutyrate produced during starvation or low carbohydrate diets [95] and dietary omega-3 fatty acids [96] suppress NLRP3 inflammasome activation in response to various activators (CCs not tested) in cultured monocytes and macrophages, and in vivo in mouse models of inflammatory diseases. In atherosclerotic *ApoE*$^{-/-}$ mice, β-hydroxybutyrate treatment reduced aortic plaque formation without affecting blood lipid profiles [97, 98], the latter study reporting reduced levels of serum IL-1β.

Colchicine, a microtubule inhibitor downregulating multiple inflammatory pathways, was one of the first compounds shown to inhibit crystal-induced NLRP3 inflammasome activation in the context of gout-associated pathogenic crystals [12]. Low-dose colchicine was later found effective in the prevention of cardiovascular events in two clinical trials [99, 100], as discussed in more detail in Chapter "Formation of CCs in Endothelial Cells". Direct inhibition of the NLRP3 receptor has been achieved with two small-molecule inhibitors, MCC950 [101] and CY-09 [102]. These compounds bind to the ATP binding site of the NLRP3 NACHT domain, thus locking the receptor in an inactive conformation and inhibiting inflammasome assembly [102–104]. MCC950 has been shown to reduce atherosclerotic lesion development in *ApoE*$^{-/-}$ mice [105, 106]. Several novel small-molecule compounds predicted to inhibit NLRP3 are currently under study [107]. In addition to CC-induced NLRP3 activation in atherosclerosis, NLRP3 is activated by multiple different DAMPs released during myocardial ischemia reperfusion injury and preclinical studies have shown beneficial effects by NLRP3 inhibitors, yet more studies are warranted owing to some contradicting results [108].

Finally, perhaps the most compelling evidence for the significance of the NLRP3/IL-1β axis in human atherosclerosis comes from a large clinical trial named CANTOS (Canakinumab Anti-Inflammatory Thrombosis Outcomes Study) involving 10,061 patients with previous myocardial infarction [109]. Treatment with the monoclonal IL-1β neutralizing antibody canakinumab significantly lowered the rate of recurrent cardiovascular events compared to placebo, providing strong evidence in support of the central role of inflammation in atherosclerosis and paving the way for further anti-inflammatory treatments.

References

1. Martinon F, Burns K, Tschopp J. The inflammasome: a molecular platform triggering activation of inflammatory caspases and processing of proIL-beta. Mol Cell. 2002;10:417–26.
2. Van Opdenbosch N, Lamkanfi M. Caspases in cell death, inflammation, and disease. Immunity. 2019;50:1352–64.
3. Shi J, et al. Cleavage of GSDMD by inflammatory caspases determines pyroptotic cell death. Nature. 2015;526:660–5.
4. Gong T, Liu L, Jiang W, Zhou R. DAMP-sensing receptors in sterile inflammation and inflammatory diseases. Nat Rev Immunol. 2020;20:95–112.

5. McDonald B, et al. Intravascular danger signals guide neutrophils to sites of sterile inflammation. Science. 2010;330:362–6.
6. Babelova A, et al. Biglycan, a danger signal that activates the NLRP3 inflammasome via toll-like and P2X receptors. J Biol Chem. 2009;284:24035–48.
7. Yamasaki K, et al. NLRP3/cryopyrin is necessary for interleukin-1beta (IL-1beta) release in response to hyaluronan, an endogenous trigger of inflammation in response to injury. J Biol Chem. 2009;284:12762–71.
8. Halle A, et al. The NALP3 inflammasome is involved in the innate immune response to amyloid-beta. Nat Immunol. 2008;9:857–65.
9. Masters SL, et al. Activation of the NLRP3 inflammasome by islet amyloid polypeptide provides a mechanism for enhanced IL-1β in type 2 diabetes. Nat Immunol. 2010;11:897–904.
10. Wen H, et al. Fatty acid-induced NLRP3-ASC inflammasome activation interferes with insulin signaling. Nat Immunol. 2011;12:408–15.
11. Vandanmagsar B, et al. The NLRP3 inflammasome instigates obesity-induced inflammation and insulin resistance. Nat Med. 2011;17:179–88.
12. Martinon F, Pétrilli V, Mayor A, Tardivel A, Tschopp J. Gout-associated uric acid crystals activate the NALP3 inflammasome. Nature. 2006;440:237–41.
13. Duewell P, et al. NLRP3 inflammasomes are required for atherogenesis and activated by cholesterol crystals. Nature. 2010;464:1357–61.
14. Rajamäki K, et al. Cholesterol crystals activate the NLRP3 inflammasome in human macrophages: a novel link between cholesterol metabolism and inflammation. PloS One. 2010;5:e11765.
15. Usui F, et al. Critical role of caspase-1 in vascular inflammation and development of atherosclerosis in Western diet-fed apolipoprotein E-deficient mice. Biochem Biophys Res Commun. 2012;425:162–8.
16. Gage J, Hasu M, Thabet M, Whitman SC. Caspase-1 deficiency decreases atherosclerosis in apolipoprotein E-null mice. Can J Cardiol. 2012;28:222–9.
17. Zheng F, Xing S, Gong Z, Mu W, Xing Q. Silence of NLRP3 suppresses atherosclerosis and stabilizes plaques in apolipoprotein E-deficient mice. Mediators Inflamm. 2014;2014:1–8.
18. Hendrikx T, et al. Bone marrow-specific caspase-1/11 deficiency inhibits atherosclerosis development in Ldlr(−/−) mice. FEBS J. 2015;282:2327–38.
19. Menu P, et al. Atherosclerosis in ApoE-deficient mice progresses independently of the NLRP3 inflammasome. Cell Death Dis. 2011;2:e137.
20. Ishibashi S, et al. Hypercholesterolemia in low density lipoprotein receptor knockout mice and its reversal by adenovirus-mediated gene delivery. J Clin Invest. 1993;92:883–93.
21. Zhang SH, Reddick RL, Piedrahita JA, Maeda N. Spontaneous hypercholesterolemia and arterial lesions in mice lacking apolipoprotein E. Science. 1992;258:468–71.
22. Kirii H, et al. Lack of interleukin-1beta decreases the severity of atherosclerosis in ApoE-deficient mice. Arterioscler Thromb Vasc Biol. 2003;23:656–60.
23. Bhaskar V, et al. Monoclonal antibodies targeting IL-1 beta reduce biomarkers of atherosclerosis in vitro and inhibit atherosclerotic plaque formation in apolipoprotein E-deficient mice. Atherosclerosis. 2011;216:313–20.
24. Nicklin MJH, Hughes DE, Barton JL, Ure JM, Duff GW. Arterial inflammation in mice lacking the interleukin 1 receptor antagonist gene. J Exp Med. 2000;191:303–12.
25. Elhage R, et al. Differential effects of interleukin-1 receptor antagonist and tumor necrosis factor binding protein on fatty-streak formation in apolipoprotein E-deficient mice. Circulation. 1998;97:242–4.
26. Devlin CM, Kuriakose G, Hirsch E, Tabas I. Genetic alterations of IL-1 receptor antagonist in mice affect plasma cholesterol level and foam cell lesion size. Proc Natl Acad Sci U S A. 2002;99:6280–5.
27. Mallat Z, et al. Interleukin-18/interleukin-18 binding protein signaling modulates atherosclerotic lesion development and stability. Circ Res. 2001;89:E41–5.

28. Elhage R, et al. Reduced atherosclerosis in interleukin-18 deficient apolipoprotein E-knockout mice. Cardiovasc Res. 2003;59:234–40.
29. Whitman SC, Ravisankar P, Daugherty A. Interleukin-18 enhances atherosclerosis in apolipoprotein E(−/−) mice through release of interferon-gamma. Circ Res. 2002;90:E34–8.
30. Opoku E, et al. Gasdermin D mediates inflammation-induced defects in reverse cholesterol transport and promotes atherosclerosis. Front Cell Dev Biol. 2021;9:715211.
31. Christ A, et al. Western Diet Triggers NLRP3-Dependent innate immune reprogramming. Cell. 2018;172:162–175.e14.
32. Stienstra R, et al. Inflammasome is a central player in the induction of obesity and insulin resistance. Proc Natl Acad Sci U S A. 2011;108:15324–9.
33. Galea J, et al. Interleukin-1 beta in coronary arteries of patients with ischemic heart disease. Arterioscler Thromb Vasc Biol. 1996;16:1000–6.
34. Gerdes N, et al. Expression of interleukin (IL)-18 and functional IL-18 receptor on human vascular endothelial cells, smooth muscle cells, and macrophages. J Exp Med. 2002;195:245–57.
35. Geng YJ, Libby P. Evidence for apoptosis in advanced human atheroma. Colocalization with interleukin-1 beta-converting enzyme. Am J Pathol. 1995;147:251–66.
36. Folco EJ, Sukhova GK, Quillard T, Libby P. Moderate hypoxia potentiates interleukin-1β production in activated human macrophages. Circ Res. 2014;115:875–83.
37. Zheng F, Xing S, Gong Z, Xing Q. NLRP3 inflammasomes show high expression in aorta of patients with atherosclerosis. Heart Lung Circ. 2013;22:746–50.
38. Shi X, Xie W-L, Kong W-W, Chen D, Qu P. Expression of the NLRP3 Inflammasome in carotid atherosclerosis. J Stroke Cerebrovasc Dis. 2015;24:2455–66.
39. Paramel Varghese G, et al. NLRP3 Inflammasome expression and activation in human atherosclerosis. J Am Heart Assoc. 2016;5:e003031.
40. Rajamäki K, et al. p38δ MAPK: a novel regulator of NLRP3 Inflammasome activation with increased expression in coronary atherogenesis. Arterioscler Thromb Vasc Biol. 2016;36:1937–46.
41. Afrasyab A, et al. Correlation of NLRP3 with severity and prognosis of coronary atherosclerosis in acute coronary syndrome patients. Heart Vessels. 2016;31:1218–29.
42. Puren AJ, Fantuzzi G, Dinarello CA. Gene expression, synthesis, and secretion of interleukin 18 and interleukin 1 are differentially regulated in human blood mononuclear cells and mouse spleen cells. Proc Natl Acad Sci. 1999;96:2256–61.
43. Bauernfeind FG, et al. Cutting edge: NF-kappaB activating pattern recognition and cytokine receptors license NLRP3 inflammasome activation by regulating NLRP3 expression. J Immunol. 2009;183:787–91.
44. Zimmer S, Grebe A, Latz E. Danger signaling in atherosclerosis. Circ Res. 2015;116:323–40.
45. Lima H Jr, et al. Role of lysosome rupture in controlling Nlrp3 signaling and necrotic cell death. Cell Cycle. 2013;12:1868–78.
46. Orlowski GM, et al. Frontline science: multiple cathepsins promote inflammasome-independent, particle-induced cell death during NLRP3-dependent IL-1β activation. J Leukoc Biol. 2017;102:7–17.
47. Muñoz-Planillo R, et al. K⁺ efflux is the common trigger of NLRP3 inflammasome activation by bacterial toxins and particulate matter. Immunity. 2013;38:1142–53.
48. Xu Z, et al. Distinct molecular mechanisms underlying potassium efflux for NLRP3 Inflammasome activation. Front Immunol. 2020;11:609441.
49. Sheedy FJ, et al. CD36 coordinates NLRP3 inflammasome activation by facilitating intracellular nucleation of soluble ligands into particulate ligands in sterile inflammation. Nat Immunol. 2013;14:812–20.
50. Heilig R, et al. The Gasdermin-D pore acts as a conduit for IL-1β secretion in mice. Eur J Immunol. 2018;48:584–92.
51. Rajamäki K, et al. Extracellular acidosis is a novel danger signal alerting innate immunity via the NLRP3 inflammasome. J Biol Chem. 2013;288:13410–9.

52. Mariathasan S, et al. Cryopyrin activates the inflammasome in response to toxins and ATP. Nature. 2006;440:228–32.
53. Niemi K, et al. Serum amyloid a activates the NLRP3 inflammasome via P2X7 receptor and a cathepsin B-sensitive pathway. J Immunol. 2011;186:6119–28.
54. Laudisi F, et al. Cutting edge: the NLRP3 inflammasome links complement-mediated inflammation and IL-1β release. J Immunol. 2013;191:1006–10.
55. Coeshott C, et al. Converting enzyme-independent release of tumor necrosis factor alpha and IL-1beta from a stimulated human monocytic cell line in the presence of activated neutrophils or purified proteinase 3. Proc Natl Acad Sci U S A. 1999;96:6261–6.
56. Samstad EO, et al. Cholesterol crystals induce complement-dependent inflammasome activation and cytokine release. J Immunol. 2014;192:2837–45.
57. Mizutani H, Schechter N, Lazarus G, Black RA, Kupper TS. Rapid and specific conversion of precursor interleukin 1 beta (IL-1 beta) to an active IL-1 species by human mast cell chymase. J Exp Med. 1991;174:821–5.
58. Öörni K, Kovanen PT. Aggregation susceptibility of low-density lipoproteins—a novel modifiable biomarker of cardiovascular risk. J Clin Med Res. 2021;10:1769.
59. Borén J, et al. Low-density lipoproteins cause atherosclerotic cardiovascular disease: pathophysiological, genetic, and therapeutic insights: a consensus statement from the European atherosclerosis society consensus panel. Eur Heart J. 2020;41:2313–30.
60. Virmani R, Burke AP, Kolodgie FD, Farb A. Pathology of the thin-cap fibroatheroma: a type of vulnerable plaque. J Interv Cardiol. 2003;16:267–72.
61. Bentzon JF, Otsuka F, Virmani R, Falk E. Mechanisms of plaque formation and rupture. Circ Res. 2014;114:1852–66.
62. Ho-Tin-Noé B, et al. Cholesterol crystallization in human atherosclerosis is triggered in smooth muscle cells during the transition from fatty streak to fibroatheroma. J Pathol. 2017;241:671–82.
63. Baumer Y, et al. Hyperlipidemia-induced cholesterol crystal production by endothelial cells promotes atherogenesis. Nat Commun. 2017;8:1129.
64. Lehti S, et al. Extracellular lipids accumulate in human carotid arteries as distinct three-dimensional structures and have proinflammatory properties. Am J Pathol. 2018;188:525–38.
65. Baumer Y, Mehta NN, Dey AK, Powell-Wiley TM, Boisvert WA. Cholesterol crystals and atherosclerosis. Eur Heart J. 2020;41:2236–9.
66. Stary HC, et al. A definition of advanced types of atherosclerotic lesions and a histological classification of atherosclerosis. A report from the committee on vascular lesions of the council on arteriosclerosis, American Heart Association. Arterioscler Thromb Vasc Biol. 1995;15:1512–31.
67. Lehti S, et al. Spatial distributions of lipids in atherosclerosis of human coronary arteries studied by time-of-flight secondary ion mass spectrometry. Am J Pathol. 2015;185:1216–33.
68. Bogren H, Larsson K. An x-ray-diffraction study of crystalline cholesterol in some pathological deposits in man. Biochim Biophys Acta. 1963;75:65–9.
69. Suhalim JL, et al. Characterization of cholesterol crystals in atherosclerotic plaques using stimulated Raman scattering and second-harmonic generation microscopy. Biophys J. 2012;102:1988–95.
70. Fujiyoshi K, et al. Incidence, factors, and clinical significance of cholesterol crystals in coronary plaque: an optical coherence tomography study. Atherosclerosis. 2019;283:79–84.
71. Shi X, et al. Cholesterol crystals are associated with carotid plaque vulnerability: an optical coherence tomography study. J Stroke Cerebrovasc Dis. 2020;29:104579.
72. Hevonoja T, Pentikäinen MO, Hyvönen MT, Kovanen PT, Ala-Korpela M. Structure of low density lipoprotein (LDL) particles: basis for understanding molecular changes in modified LDL. Biochim Biophys Acta. 2000;1488:189–210.
73. Hakala JK, et al. Lysosomal enzymes are released from cultured human macrophages, hydrolyze LDL in vitro, and are present extracellularly in human atherosclerotic lesions. Arterioscler Thromb Vasc Biol. 2003;23:1430–6.

74. Guarino AJ, Tulenko TN, Wrenn SP. Cholesterol crystal nucleation from enzymatically modified low-density lipoproteins: combined effect of sphingomyelinase and cholesterol esterase. Biochemistry. 2004;43:1685–93.
75. Torzewski M, et al. Enzymatic modification of low-density lipoprotein in the arterial wall: a new role for plasmin and matrix metalloproteinases in atherogenesis. Arterioscler Thromb Vasc Biol. 2004;24:2130–6.
76. Witztum JL. You are right too! J Clin Invest. 2005;115:2072–5.
77. Kruth HS. Sequestration of aggregated low-density lipoproteins by macrophages. Curr Opin Lipidol. 2002;13:483–8.
78. Mineo C. Lipoprotein receptor signalling in atherosclerosis. Cardiovasc Res. 2020;116:1254–74.
79. Grosheva I, Haka AS, Qin C, Pierini LM, Maxfield FR. Aggregated LDL in contact with macrophages induces local increases in free cholesterol levels that regulate local actin polymerization. Arterioscler Thromb Vasc Biol. 2009;29:1615–21.
80. Haka AS, et al. Monocyte-derived dendritic cells upregulate extracellular catabolism of aggregated low-density lipoprotein on maturation, leading to foam cell formation. Arterioscler Thromb Vasc Biol. 2015;35:2092–103.
81. Singh RK, et al. Degradation of aggregated LDL occurs in complex extracellular subcompartments of the lysosomal synapse. J Cell Sci. 2016;129:1072–82.
82. Singh RK, et al. TLR4 (toll-like receptor 4)-dependent signaling drives extracellular catabolism of LDL (low-density lipoprotein) aggregates. Arterioscler Thromb Vasc Biol. 2020;40:86–102.
83. Rajamäki K, et al. Cholesterol crystals activate the NLRP3 inflammasome in human monocytes and macrophages. Chem Phys Lipids. 2010;163:S27–8.
84. Brown MS, Goldstein JL. Lipoprotein metabolism in the macrophage: implications for cholesterol deposition in atherosclerosis. Annu Rev Biochem. 1983;52:223–61.
85. Ory DS. The niemann-pick disease genes; regulators of cellular cholesterol homeostasis. Trends Cardiovasc Med. 2004;14:66–72.
86. Kruth HS. Lipoprotein cholesterol and atherosclerosis. Curr Mol Med. 2001;1:633–53.
87. Amengual J, et al. Short-term Acyl-CoA:Cholesterol Acyltransferase inhibition, combined with apoprotein A1 overexpression, promotes atherosclerosis inflammation resolution in mice. Mol Pharmacol. 2021;99:175–83.
88. Nissen SE, et al. Effect of ACAT inhibition on the progression of coronary atherosclerosis. N Engl J Med. 2006;354:1253–63.
89. Baumer Y, et al. Ultramorphological analysis of plaque advancement and cholesterol crystal formation in Ldlr knockout mouse atherosclerosis. Atherosclerosis. 2019;287:100–11.
90. Tall AR, Westerterp M. Inflammasomes, neutrophil extracellular traps, and cholesterol. J Lipid Res. 2019;60:721–7.
91. Jin X, et al. Macrophages shed excess cholesterol in unique extracellular structures containing cholesterol microdomains. Arterioscler Thromb Vasc Biol. 2018;38:1504–18.
92. Chung B-H, et al. Phosphatidylcholine-rich acceptors, but not native HDL or its apolipoproteins, mobilize cholesterol from cholesterol-rich insoluble components of human atherosclerotic plaques. Biochim Biophys Acta. 2005;1733:76–89.
93. Luo Y, et al. Phospholipid nanoparticles: therapeutic potentials against atherosclerosis via reducing cholesterol crystals and inhibiting inflammation. EBioMedicine. 2021;74:103725.
94. Zimmer S, et al. Cyclodextrin promotes atherosclerosis regression via macrophage reprogramming. Sci Transl Med. 2016;8:333ra50.
95. Youm Y-H, et al. The ketone metabolite β-hydroxybutyrate blocks NLRP3 inflammasome–mediated inflammatory disease. Nat Med. 2015;21:263–9.
96. Yan Y, et al. Omega-3 fatty acids prevent inflammation and metabolic disorder through inhibition of NLRP3 inflammasome activation. Immunity. 2013;38:1154–63.
97. Krishnan M, et al. β-Hydroxybutyrate impedes the progression of Alzheimer's disease and atherosclerosis in ApoE-deficient mice. Nutrients. 2020;12:471.

98. Zhang S-J, et al. Ketone body 3-hydroxybutyrate ameliorates atherosclerosis via receptor Gpr109a-mediated calcium influx. Adv Sci. 2021;8:2003410.
99. Nidorf SM, Eikelboom JW, Budgeon CA, Thompson PL. Low-dose colchicine for secondary prevention of cardiovascular disease. J Am Coll Cardiol. 2013;61:404–10.
100. Tardif J-C, et al. Efficacy and safety of low-dose colchicine after myocardial infarction. N Engl J Med. 2019;381:2497–505.
101. Coll RC, et al. A small-molecule inhibitor of the NLRP3 inflammasome for the treatment of inflammatory diseases. Nat Med. 2015;21:248–55.
102. Jiang H, et al. Identification of a selective and direct NLRP3 inhibitor to treat inflammatory disorders. J Exp Med. 2017;214:3219–38.
103. Coll RC, et al. MCC950 directly targets the NLRP3 ATP-hydrolysis motif for inflammasome inhibition. Nat Chem Biol. 2019;15:556–9.
104. Tapia-Abellán A, et al. MCC950 closes the active conformation of NLRP3 to an inactive state. Nat Chem Biol. 2019;15:560–4.
105. van der Heijden T, et al. NLRP3 inflammasome inhibition by MCC950 reduces atherosclerotic lesion development in apolipoprotein E-deficient mice-brief report. Arterioscler Thromb Vasc Biol. 2017;37:1457–61.
106. Zeng W, et al. The selective NLRP3 inhibitor MCC950 hinders atherosclerosis development by attenuating inflammation and pyroptosis in macrophages. Sci Rep. 2021;11:19305.
107. Sebastian-Valverde M, et al. Discovery and characterization of small-molecule inhibitors of NLRP3 and NLRC4 inflammasomes. J Biol Chem. 2021;296:100597.
108. Silvis MJM, et al. Immunomodulation of the NLRP3 inflammasome in atherosclerosis, coronary artery disease, and acute myocardial infarction. J Cardiovasc Transl Res. 2021;14:23–34.
109. Ridker PM, et al. Antiinflammatory therapy with canakinumab for atherosclerotic disease. N Engl J Med. 2017;377:1119–31.

Molecular Pathomechanisms of Crystal-Induced Disorders

Chongxu Shi, Shrikant R. Mulay, Stefanie Steiger, and Hans-Joachim Anders

1 Introduction

Outer and inner surfaces of the human body are exposed to crystalline microparticles from all around the environment. In particular dust, sands, and powders cause lung injury, corneal damage or epithelial irritation in skin wounds and intestinal ulcers. In addition, human metabolism involves ions forming salts and calculi, especially in excretory ducts. Indeed, kidney and biliary stone disease are highly prevalent. Besides, bone minerals can form extraosseous calcifications, e.g., in the vascular wall, and lipid particles and crystals enrich in luminal plaques of the aging arteries. Certain metabolites crystallize in joints and periarticular tissue arthritis and cause episodes of pain or chronic disability. Although, serum proteins effectively inhibit crystallization, crystals can occur in the circulation during malaria and upon rupture of large atherosclerotic plaques. Other microparticles in the human body originate from implants made of metal or synthetic materials can trigger local inflammation and foreign body responses (Fig. 1).

The biology of such "crystallopathies" is poorly explored. The traditional concept was based on a macrophage-driven foreign body reaction, whereby macrophages are unable to clear such microparticles via phagocytosis and lysosomal breakdown; thus, leading to the formation of granulomas as an attempt to encapsulate the particle, conceptually like encapsulating the pathogen in tuberculosis

C. Shi · S. Steiger · H.-J. Anders (✉)
Division of Nephrology, Department of Internal Medicine IV, University Hospital of LMU, Munich, Germany
e-mail: hjanders@med.uni-muenchen.de

S. R. Mulay
Division of Pharmacology, CSIR-Central Drug Research Institute, Lucknow, India

G. S. Abela, S. M. Nidorf (eds.), *Cholesterol Crystals in Atherosclerosis and Other Related Diseases*, Contemporary Cardiology, https://doi.org/10.1007/978-3-031-41192-2_16

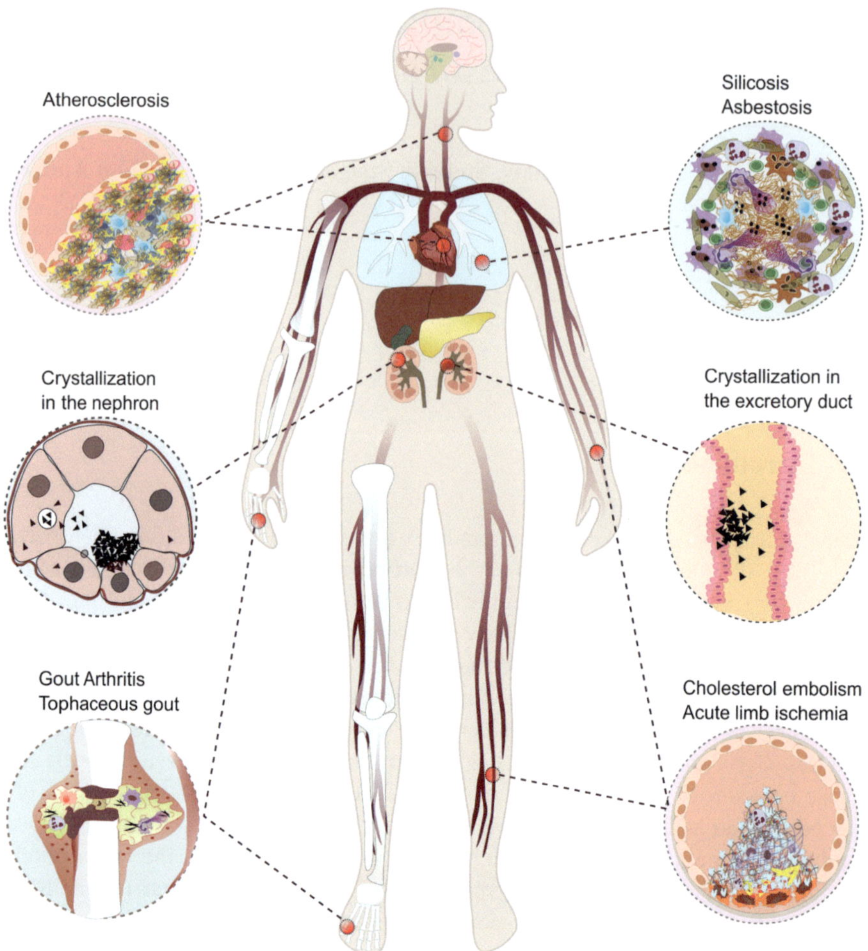

Fig. 1 Physiology and pathology of crystal-induced human diseases. Crystals that form within the human body or enter from the environment trigger many cellular and physiological processes. 1) Free cholesterol in the blood can crystalize and accumulate in arterial walls, forming atherosclerotic plaques in the intima; cholesterol crystals can also directly trigger local inflammatory response forming blood clots. 2) Elevated uric acid levels in the blood form monosodium urate crystals that accumulate in the joints, causing acute gout attacks and chronic tophaceous gout. 3) Crystal nephropathies, crystal deposit in the tubular lumen that lead to tubular cell death, or in the excretory duct. 4) Exposure to environmental pollutants, such as silica, asbestos fiber, results in the accumulation of crystals in the lungs and triggers an inflammatory response, forming granulomas in the lung. (Reproduced with permission [3])

[1]. Chronic lesions as silicosis, tophaceous gout and cholesterol embolism supported this concept. However, the last two decades, an increasing number of discoveries in "crystal biology" have been observed that demonstrate a more complex picture and can explain far more clinical phenomena [2]. For example,

dissecting crystallopathies into those causing (a) acute necroinflammation, (b) chronic inflammation and tissue remodeling, and (c) obstruction by crystalline masses that better cover the broad spectrum of clinical presentations by sharing similar or identical crystal-induced tissue responses [2]. Acute necroinflammation involves crystal-induced inflammation and cell necrosis [3], while chronic lesions involve granuloma formation, low-grade inflammation, and tissue fibrosis. Obstruction by crystalline masses involves mechanisms of crystal aggregation, adhesion, crystal growth to the size of calculi [4], and obstruction of vessels by thrombosis and excretory ducts by muscular spasms. In this chapter we present some examples of paradigmatic diseases, highlighting some of the newer insights into crystal biology in the context of disease symptoms and consequences for human health.

2 Cholesterol Crystal-Related Inflammation in Vessels

2.1 Atherosclerosis

Atherosclerosis, a chronic inflammatory vascular disease, is characterized by fatty-fibrous material retained in the intima of an artery wall. It is the most common underlying cause of cardiovascular disease and associated with high morbidity and mortality worldwide. Atherosclerotic plaque formation is a dynamic process. Low-density lipoprotein cholesterol (LDL-C) accumulating in the arterial intima initiates the development of atherosclerosis [5, 6]. Following that, endothelial cells recruit leukocytes to the site via adhesion molecules, such as vascular cell adhesion protein-1 (VCAM-1), immune cell adhesion protein-1 (ICAM-1) [7, 8]. In addition to infiltration to the intima, leukocytes can also proliferate within the lesion [9]. Other factors (like semaphorins) can also promote leukocyte's constant existence in the atherosclerotic plaque by lessening their efflux [10]. Meanwhile, endothelial cells release cytokines such as granulocyte macrophage- (GM) and macrophage (M)-colony stimulating factor (CSF) that trigger monocyte differentiation into macrophages. Lipoproteins continuously gather to the atherosclerotic plaque promoting foam cell formation [10]. Monocyte-derived macrophages are considered as precursors of lipid-loaded foam cells in atheromata. In the arterial intima, trapped foam cells lose their migratory capacity and die [11]. Dead foam cells form a necrotic core in the advanced plaque consisting of apoptotic and necrotic cells, cholesterol crystals (CC), and other extracellular material. Various Toll-like receptors (TLRs) recognize pathogen- and damage-associated molecular patterns (PAMPs, and DAMPs), such as modified LDL and its products. In atherosclerotic lesions, macrophages get activated by the nuclear factor-$\kappa\beta$ (NF-$\kappa\beta$) signaling pathway. Such activated macrophages express TLR2 and TLR4 and bind LDL [12–14] (Fig. 2).

Fig. 2 Pathogenesis of atherosclerosis. (**a**) Innate immune responses in atherosclerosis. LDL retention in the intima initiates atherosclerosis development, where they can undergo oxidative and other modifications that can render them pro-inflammatory and immunogenic. Accumulation of LDL leads to the upregulation of adhesion molecules on the endothelial surface and recruitment of monocytes to the forming lesion. In the subendothelial space, monocytes differentiate into macrophages in response to M-CSF and GM-CSF produced by endothelial cells. These macrophages express scavenger receptor can uptake lipoproteins leads to the formation of foam cells. Cholesterol crystals form in foam cells and activate the NLRP3 inflammasome, resulting in release of IL-1β, which stimulates smooth muscle cells to produce IL-6. Both IL-1β and IL-6 exert proinflammatory effects. T lymphocytes also enter the intima and regulate functions of the innate immune cells as well as the endothelial and SMCs. As the lesion advances, SMCs and macrophages can undergo cell death including apoptosis. The debris from dead and dying cells accumulates, forming the necrotic lipid-rich core of the atheroma. (**b**) Modified lipoproteins and cholesterol crystals induce NLRP3 inflammasome activation. The expression of NLRP3 components and pro-IL-1β can be triggered by cellular uptake of oxLDL. OxLDL uptake can lead to the formation of cholesterol crystals in the lysosomes, with ensuing lysosomal destabilization and release of cathepsin B from disrupted lysosomes. The release of unesterified cholesterol from the disrupted lysosomes causes an increase in the content of unesterified cholesterol in intracellular membranes and can thereby cause NLRP3 activation. Regardless of the activation mechanism, formation of the NLRP3 complex induces autocleavage and activation of caspase 1. Active caspase 1 can then cleave pro-IL-1β and the constitutively expressed pro-IL-1β to mature IL-1β. LDL: lowdensity lipoprotein, M-CSF: macrophage-colony stimulating factor, GM-CSF: granulocyte-macrophage colony-stimulating factor, TLR: Toll-like receptor, oxLDL: oxidized LDL, IL: interleukin. (Reproduced with permission [15])

In addition to monocyte-derived macrophages, activated T cells are largely present in the plaque lesions, indicating that they might be involved in the atherosclerotic plaque growth and evolution [16–18]. CD4+ helper T (TH) cells are the main adaptive effector cells in atherosclerotic plaques [19]. TH1 cells typically secrete interferon γ (IFNγ) that can promote atherosclerosis via modulating monocytes infiltration and foam cell formation, while TH2 and regulatory T (Treg) cells counterbalance the inflammatory response via secretion of anti-inflammatory cytokines, such as IL-5, IL-10, IL-13 [20–22]. Other studies suggested that Treg cells secrete transforming growth factor β (TGF-β) having a plaque-stabilizing effect via promoting interstitial collagen synthesis [18, 23]. Emerging evidence indicates that LDL particles can activate both innate and adaptive immune responses in atherosclerosis. CCs formed in the early stage can activate NOD-like receptor family pyrin domain-containing 3 (NLRP3) to secret mature interleukin (IL)-1β triggering the innate immune system [24] (Fig. 2). An atherosclerotic rabbit model has confirmed that reducing serum cholesterol levels can significantly reduce CC content in the intima, plaque rupture, and thrombosis [25].

To prevent atherogenesis, a healthy lifestyle to reduce LDL-C and lipid levels is the ideal primary therapy (primordial prevention), which can target multiple risk factors and has beneficial effects at any stage of atherosclerotic disease [26, 27]. The lipid-lowering therapy particularly targets, primarily LDL- C, remains a vital role in

a) Innate immune responses in atherosclerosis

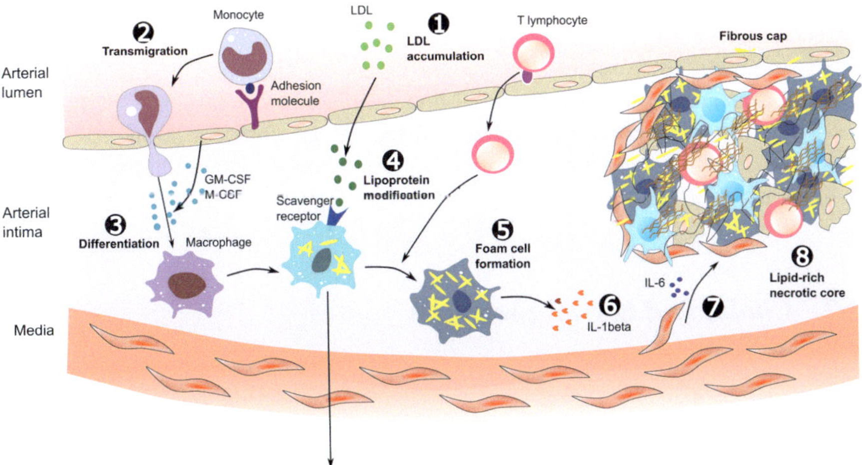

b) Modified lipoproteins and cholesterol crystals induce inflammasome activation

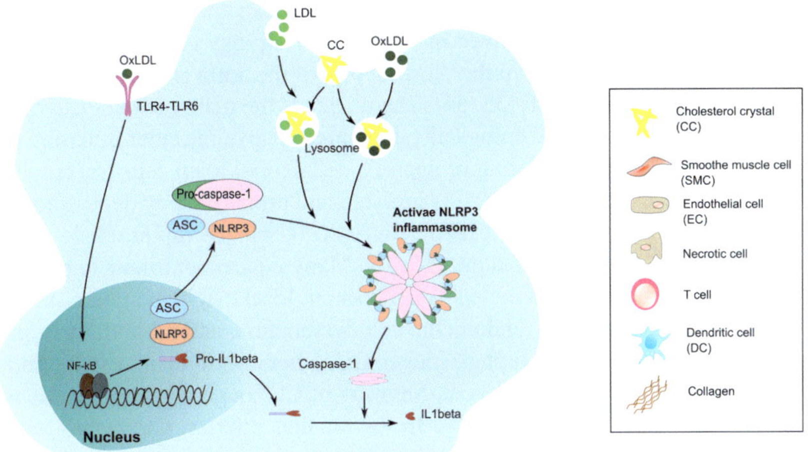

managing atherosclerotic disease [28, 29]. In experimental models of atherosclerosis, vaccination against modified LDL particles significantly prevent disease progression [30, 31].

In summary, atherosclerosis is caused by an accumulation of LDL-C in the intima of the arterial wall and the lipid-driven inflammatory response (particularly monocyte-driven macrophage) is essential for the development of atherosclerotic lesions. With time, the atherosclerotic plaque can become more fibrous and accumulate calcium mineral.

2.2 *Cholesterol Crystal Embolism*

Cholesterol crystal embolism (CCE) is a unique version of arterio-arterial embolization. Autopsy studies revealed an incidence of spontaneous CCE ranging from 1% to 3.4% [32]. Blunt trauma, catheterization, and cardiovascular surgery also cause traumatic plaque rupture [33, 34]. CCE is characterized by multiple microemboli composed of CCs and plaque debris mobilized to a variety of tissues and organs. Several key elements are involved in the pathophysiology of CCE. Advanced atherosclerotic plaques present in the thoracic part of the aorta and other large arteries represent the source of CCE [35, 36]. The plaque is the main pathological manifestation of atherosclerosis. Histologically, the fibrous cap of the atherosclerotic plaque covers a necrotic core consisting of necrotic cell debris, foam cells (macrophages), and various lipids (like CCs). CCE is initiated and propagated by deprivation of the fibrous cap. Spontaneous or mechanically induced plaque rupture dislocates CCs from the deposits inside the plaque [32, 37]. Many factors contribute to plaque vulnerability, such as adhesion molecule expression, local cytokine release, monocyte and macrophage activation, endothelial cell dysfunction, and the activity of proteolytic enzymes [38]. Plaque rupture lodges CC material into distal small arteries as the third step for CCE development. Showers of CC lodge in small arteries with a diameter between 100 and 200 μm. In the smaller arteries, CC emboli not only mechanically restrict blood flow but also provoke the coagulation process by activating platelets. CC emboli can injure the vascular endothelial lining releasing tissue factor and extracellular DNA, followed by platelet activation and aggregation. Meanwhile, activated platelets also trigger local inflammation, all together progressing to intravascular thrombus formation. Ultimately, the result is a partial or complete occlusion of the arterial lumen and signs of tissue ischemia [39] (Fig. 3). Platelets and extracellular DNA play a critical role in obstruction formation. Histopathological studies suggest that the NLRP3 inflammasome and neutrophils are additional central elements of CCE-induced acute tissue ischemic inflammation [39]. CCs are visible only in cryofixed biopsy specimens under polarized light. Within the lumen of obstructed vessels, classic ovoid, or needle-shaped clefts are observed in routinely processed biopsy specimens as CCs have washed away [40]. CCE may affect multiple organs or tissues, including the kidneys, the

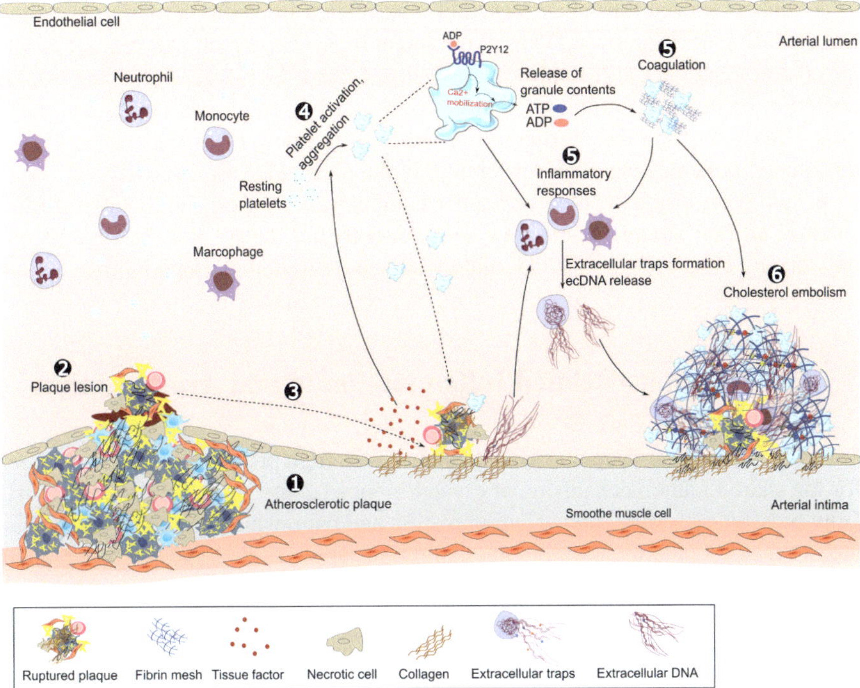

Fig. 3 Pathophysiology of cholesterol crystal embolism (CCE). Atherosclerotic plaque in the proximal artery is the premise for CCE development. CCE is initiated by plaque rupture followed by dislocating CC into distal small arteries. In the smaller arteries, CC emboli alone do not yet restrict blood flow but trigger local clot formation by activating platelets. CC emboli can damage vascular walls releasing tissue factor and extracellular DNA, followed by platelet activation and aggregation. Meanwhile, activated platelets can also trigger an immune response, all together progress to intravascular thrombus formation. Ultimately, the result is a partial or complete occlusion of the arterial lumen causing ischemic necrosis. (Reproduced with permission [15])

gastrointestinal tract, the skin, and the lower limbs. The brain is considered the most vulnerable site upon CCE.

Although CCE has been recognized as a separate clinical disorder for many years, there is still no specific therapy for this syndrome [41]. As CCE is a complication of atherosclerosis, modifications of risk factors such as tobacco use, diabetes mellitus, hypertension, and serum LDL levels should be undertaken. Treatment goals are aimed at alleviating end-organ damage and preventing further occurrence of CCE. Some evidence showed that statin therapy decreases the risk for CCE [42]. Until today, no randomized trial with statin therapy in patients with severe aortic plaques has been undertaken [43]. There is no direct clinical evidence for routine use of antiplatelet agents to prevent the recurrence of CCE, and the relationship between CCE and thrombolytic and anticoagulation therapy remains controversial. While an animal model of CCE showed that the antiplatelet agent clopidogrel as well as heparin or the thrombolytic agent urokinase significantly decrease

CCE-related arterial thrombus formation and related ischemic tissue injury in the acute phase [39]. Moreover, DNase I treatment improved crystal clot-related vascular obstructions via the thrombolytic effect of DNase I [39]. However, neutrophil depletion or necrosis inhibitor therapies only prevent end-organ damage without vital effects on thrombus formation. Therefore, the new therapeutic strategy for thrombotic patients may consider rebuilding the plasma DNase I activity.

In summary, inside the blood stream, CC induce clotting, especially upon getting stuck in arterial vessels where they cause endothelial injury. Not the crystals but only crystal clots obstruct the vasculature and cause ischemic tissue injury.

3 MSU Crystals-Related Inflammation In and Around Joints

Several crystalline arthropathies exist but due to its high prevalence, gout is a model for the shared pathomechanisms of crystal-induced acute necroinflammation [44]. Gout presents as a crescendo of inflammation and pain, which has been long attributed to the pro-inflammatory effects that monosodium urate (MSU) crystals elicit on mononuclear phagocytes in cell culture. In 2005, a landmark study by Martinon and colleagues unraveled that the NLRP3 inflammasome, a macromolecular complex in the cellular cytosol, is the main caspase-1-activating enzyme that induces the enzymatic activation and secretion of IL-1β, a central element of crystal-induced tissue inflammation [45]. Indeed, specific antagonists of IL-1β entirely abrogate acute inflammation in patients with gouty arthritis, clearly demonstrating the central role of this pathomechanism [46] (Fig. 4). The same mechanism applies to acute and chronic inflammation induced by many other microparticles composed of crystals, proteins, or synthetic materials and is, therefore, a paradigmatic example for a shared pathomechanism across clinically completely diverse disorders [3]. Discovering the NLRP3 inflammasome was only the first step in deciphering the pathophysiology of gout and indeed may mainly occur in macrophages and dendritic cells resident to the synovial joint lining and periarticular tissues [47]. However, the main effector cell in gout is the neutrophil that readily migrates to tissues, where activated resident mononuclear phagocytes sense danger by secreting cytokines and chemokines. When infiltrating neutrophils encounter MSU crystals, they undergo necroptosis, a regulated form of necrosis involving a series of specific kinases subsequently ending in the formation of lytic pores in the outer and inner membranes [48] (Fig. 4). This phenomenon is also not MSU-specific and applies to crystals of all types, sizes, and shapes [49]. Neutrophil necrosis releases nuclear chromatin similar to the release of neutrophil extracellular traps (NETs) and indeed, there may be overlaps between crystal-induced neutrophil necrosis and what has been called NETosis [50]. Such extracellular chromatin releases cytotoxic histones, which join lytic proteases released from neutrophil granules and cytosol altogether producing local tissue injury and inflammation, i.e., necroinflammation [47], during the crescendo of clinical symptoms in the early phase of gouty arthritis (Fig. 4).

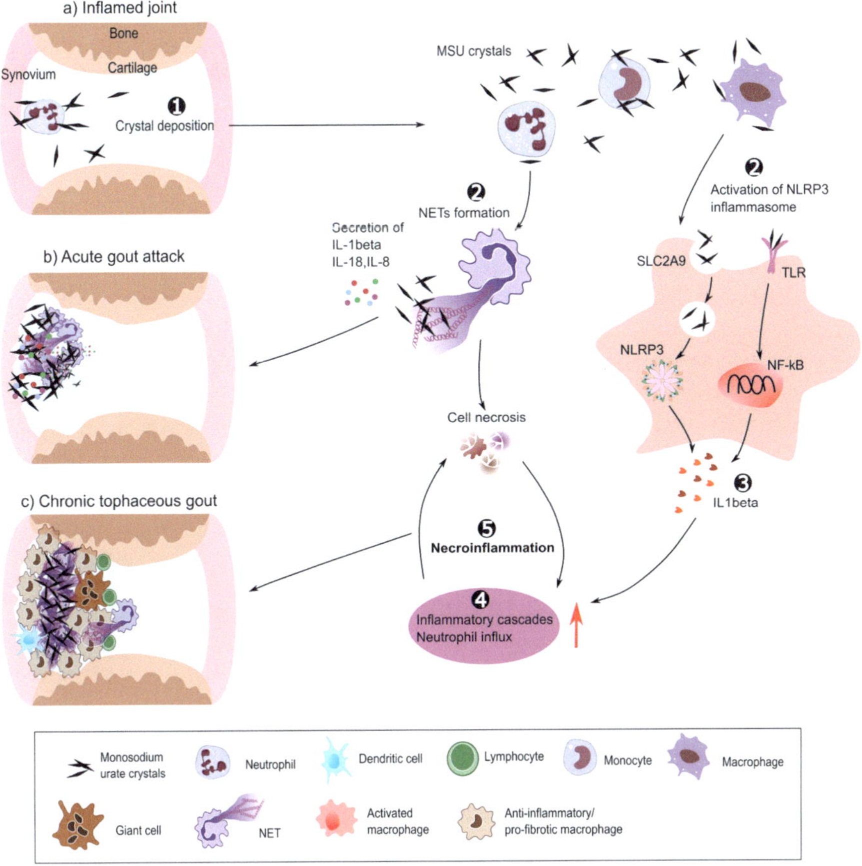

Fig. 4 Crystal tophus formation in the joints. Uric acid supersaturation results in MSU crystal formation. (**a**) MSU crystals have direct cytotoxic effects on resident synoviocytes such as macrophages and epithelial cells. When these cells undergo regulated necrosis, they release DAMPs and alarmins. (**b**) At the onset of an acute gout attack, MSU crystal cause an acute inflammatory response characterized by massive infiltration of immune cells, such as neutrophils, monocytes, and macrophages. Mononuclear phagocytes take up MSU crystals, a process that ultimately activates the NLRP3 inflammasome and IL-1β release. In particular, neutrophils can form NETs and undergo necrosis, release histones, MPO, cytokines, and chemokines. That contributes to the crescendo of the auto-amplification loop of necroinflammation. (**c**) Necrotic neutrophils released proinflammatory factors attracting more neutrophils and more NETs formation. The NETs neutrophils clump together and form aggregates NETs (aggNETs). Macrophages localize around the tophus attempting to clear MSU crystals and aggNETs. This can lead to foreign-body granuloma formation with tophus masses at the center, surrounded by giant cells and epithelioid cell layers. MSU: monosodium urate, DAMP: damage-associated molecular pattern, MPO: myeloperoxidase, NET: neutrophil extracellular trap, IL: interleukin

However, a number of clinical settings indicate a more complex biology of crystal-induced inflammation. For example, MSU crystals are found in joints also outside acute gout attacks in the absence of signs of inflammation. Indeed, the metabolic substrate of MSU crystals, soluble uric acid was found to be a potent inhibitor of crystal-induced inflammation, implying that although hyperuricemia is a risk factor for gout, soluble uric acid also suppresses the activation of the NLRP3 inflammasome by entering the cytosol of immune cells via the urate transporter SLC2A9 [51]. Furthermore, gouty arthritis usually spontaneously resolves within 1 week or so despite MSU crystals still being present in the joint or periarticular tissue. There are several counter-regulatory mechanisms of innate immunity that can explain this phenomenon such as the formation of aggregated NETs that digest released pro-inflammatory mediators as well as phagocytic clearance of NETs by macrophages [52]. In the long run, the crystal may persist in the joint and periarticular tissues as part of aggregated NETs and dead neutrophils, i.e., gouty tophus (Fig. 4). Such a tophus is frequently surrounded by macrophages that compartmentalize the dead neutrophil-crystal mass, conceptually like an abscess membrane [53].

In summary, gout is instrumental to examine several different aspects of crystal biology when dissecting the different phases of the disease involving different immune cell subsets that deal with MSU crystals differently.

4 Silica Crystal-Related Inflammation and Granuloma Formation in the Lung

Acute and prolonged inhalation of occupational microparticles entering interstitial compartments of the lung can lead to pulmonary complications associated with acute and chronic toxic exposure in farmers, flour mill worker, jewelers, or coal, uranium and gold miners, tunnel or quarry workers, and stone dressers [54–56]. Although prevention efforts have been made for many decades, silicosis is a major cause of morbidity and mortality worldwide [57]. Microparticle-related lung disease remains a major health issue in low- and middle-income countries [58–61], but also in developed countries, including USA and Australia [62, 63]. Depending on the dose and duration of exposure, patients can present with various clinical and pathological forms of silicosis, including simple (nodular) or acute (silicoproteinosis) silicosis, and complicated or progressive chronic silicosis [64]. For example, acute silicosis usually results from accidental high-intensity silica exposure and may develop within a few weeks to less than 5 years with dyspnea, cough, fever, and weight loss that may progress to respiratory failure and death. In the lung, silica particles are engulfed by alveolar macrophages via scavenger receptors such as the macrophage receptor with collagenous structure [65], which causes acute inflammation and cytotoxicity (Fig. 5). The inflammatory response is associated with cell death, autophagy, formation of NETs as well as release of reactive oxygen species (ROS) and pro-inflammatory cytokines such as NLRP3 inflammasome-mediated IL-1β and tumor necrosis factor (TNF)-α by epithelial cells and alveolar macrophages [49, 66–68]. This in turn provokes further recruitment of alveolar macrophages, a perpetual cycle known as necroinflammation leading to accelerated alveolitis and fibrosis [69] (Fig. 5). Dendritic cells exhibit cellular activation and

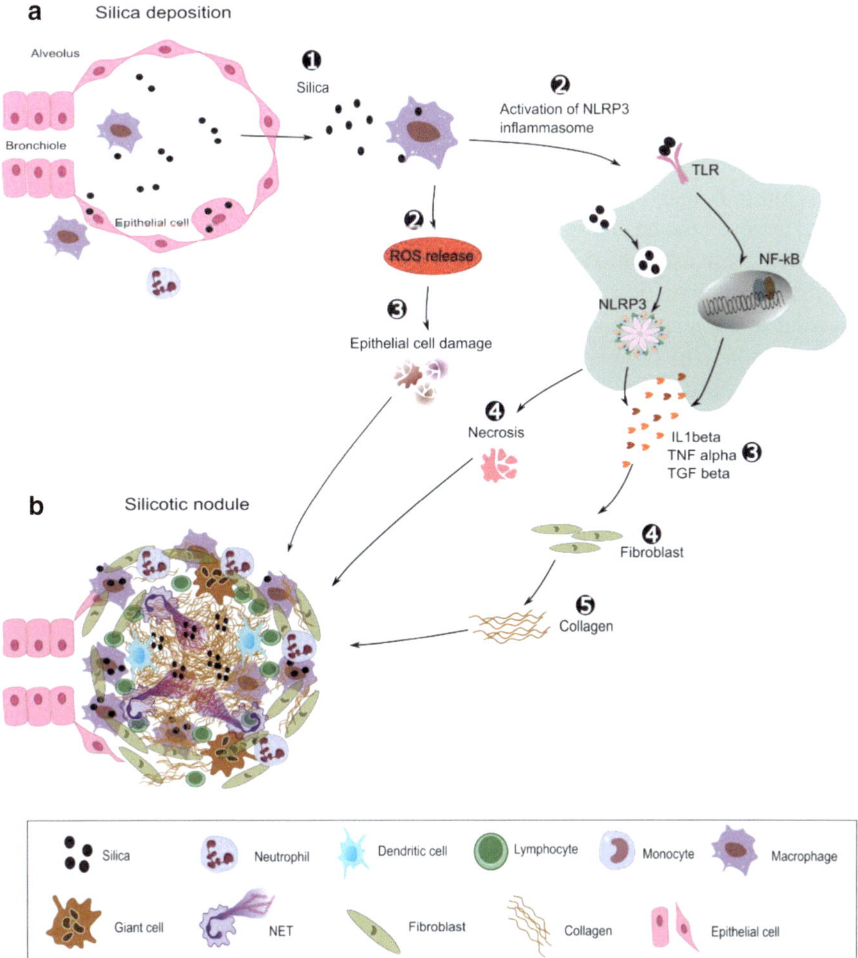

Fig. 5 Microparticle-induced granuloma formation in the lung. Microparticles (like silica) have direct cytotoxic effects on epithelial cells and alveolar macrophages generating ROS that disrupt the cell membrane and release lysosomal enzymes causing tissue damage (**a**). Silica activates transcriptional factors (NF-κβ) in macrophages that trigger inflammatory and fibrotic processes. The release of cytokines and chemokines recruits polymorphonuclear and mononuclear cells to alveolar spaces and around the silica particles, which contribute to the formation of granulomas. During silica-induced inflammation, epithelial cells and alveolar macrophages secrete IL-1β triggering fibroblasts activation and collagen deposition. Once fibroblasts are recruited to the damage site, TGF-β release induces local collagen deposition. Also TNF-α release leads to fibroblast activation and proliferation. Prolonged silica exposure can eventually cause the formation of interstitial silicotic nodules (**b**), which contain macrophages, lymphocytes, and fibroblasts with disorganized collagen patches. These silicotic nodules cause progressive lung fibrosis and reduction of lung volume. ROS: reactive oxygen species, IL: interleukin, TGF: transforming growth factor, TNF: tumor necrosis factor

migrate from the alveoli into the lung parenchyma in mice [70]. In a mouse model, Treg cells can exert modulatory functions both directly by expressing cytotoxic T lymphocyte antigen 4 during the inflammatory phase and indirectly by secreting TGF-β1, osteopontin, and IL-4 during the fibrotic stage [71–74]. Data suggest a potential role of lung epithelial cells in vivo and in vitro dependent and independent of NF-Kβ [75]. Profibrotic mediators can also induce epithelial to mesenchymal transition in human bronchial epithelial cells and such effect is enhanced by IL-1β [76]. However, the exact roles of TGF-β1 and IL-1β in silicosis remain unknown.

Chronic silicosis has a long latency, usually over 20 years, and is associated with persistent inflammation and particle overload, at which alternatively activated M2 alveolar macrophages cannot accommodate further silica particles from the lung; hence, leading to progressive massive fibrosis with excess collagen deposition, fibroblast proliferation, and crystal granuloma formation [77] (Fig. 5). Indeed, granuloma formation in interstitial silicotic nodules is a form of discrete and organized microparticle compartmentalization due to free silica particles distributed in the interstitium [78, 79]. Such granulomas have a core of activated phagocytes, mainly pro-inflammatory M1 macrophages, and an outer aspect of anti-inflammatory and profibrotic immune cells (macrophages, dendritic cells, and lymphocytes), which promote remodeling and interstitial fibrosis of the surrounding healthy tissue. Histopathological images of the lung from T cell-deficient mice that were exposed to microparticles were described as diffuse inflammation throughout the parenchyma but no visible granulomas [80]. Although this finding supports the view that T cells may play a role in initiating granuloma formation [81], T cells and granulomas may have nothing to do with the progression of lung inflammation but rather granulomas (M1 macrophages) simply sequester silica particles [82]. Evidence suggests that granuloma formation in chronic silicosis is associated with the presence of anti-apoptotic factors, including soluble Fas and Fas ligand [83–85], unlike in acute silicosis [86].

Silicosis-related immune dysfunction has been associated with several disorders, including an increased risk for infections [64, 87], lung malignancy [88–90], chronic obstructive pulmonary disease [91], and autoimmune diseases such as rheumatoid arthritis, systemic lupus erythematosus and scleroderma [92]. As yet, no proven curative treatment for silicosis exists [59]. For managing acute silicosis, whole lung lavage might remove silica particles, macrophages and soluble mediators from the lung and relieve symptoms [93], but sustained improvement of long-term outcomes or mortality has not been shown in clinical trials. Several immunosuppressive and anti-fibrotic drugs [94–96], tyrosine kinase inhibitors, e.g., bosutinib [97], dasatinib [98], or cell-based therapies [99, 100] were tested to attenuate pulmonary inflammation and fibrosis in experimental silicosis, but are yet to progress to human clinical trials. For young patients with acute respiratory failure, lung transplantation remains the only option. Further efforts are needed to improve the quality of life and slow deterioration of silicosis.

In summary, acute silicosis is characterized by interstitial inflammation, apoptosis, alveolar epithelial cell hyperplasia and the development of pulmonary lesions, while chronic silicosis is associated with silicotic nodules and massive pulmonary fibrosis. Thus, it is important to dissect the molecular mechanisms for developing effective therapies and for managing the various forms of silicosis differently.

5 Calcium Oxalate and MSU Crystals-Related Inflammation in Kidneys

During the urine formation process, most of the water is reabsorbed from the fluid filtered by the glomerulus. When mineral concentrations are high and the amount of fluid is low, this process results in supersaturation of minerals and promotes their crystallization within the tubular lumen, leading to the development of type II (tubular lumen) and type III (renal pelvis) crystal nephropathies [101]. Crystallization of minerals, proteins, and drugs contributes to kidney injury in many different ways, e.g., via direct or indirect cytotoxicity involving regulated necrosis of kidney cells, or via inducing intrarenal inflammation. An autoamplification loop between inflammation and regulated necrosis further aggravates kidney injury and contributes to kidney dysfunction. The reaction of kidney cells to crystalline particles is usually driven by their size, e.g., tubular cells phagocytose crystals of <10 μm in size and attempt to digest them within lysosomes [102]. During this process, amorphous calcium crystals release calcium that induces tubular necrosis via activation of calpains [103]. If the particles cannot be digested, they destabilize the lysosomal membrane causing the release of lysosomal enzymes into the cytosol, which triggers cellular stress [104]. Such cellular stress culminates in mitochondrial dysfunction and ROS formation, subsequently resulting in either enhanced autophagy [19] or regulated necrosis via receptor-interacting protein kinase (RIPK)-3 and mixed lineage kinase-like (MLKL)-mediated necroptosis [105, 106], glutathione peroxidase (GPX)-4-mediated ferroptosis [107], or cyclophilin (Cyp) D-mediated mitochondrial permeability transition-related necrosis [108]. Furthermore, crystal-induced tubular necrosis may cause the release of extracellular histones, a cytotoxic DAMP [109]. The strong basic charge of extracellular histones triggers necrosis of neighboring cells that may aggravate kidney injury during crystal nephropathies [109, 110] (Fig. 6).

Histones as well as other DAMPs and alarmins released in the extracellular compartment trigger inflammation in the kidneys by activating several pattern recognition receptors present on both kidney immune and parenchymal cells, and thereby, activate the crescendo loop of necroinflammation [110, 111]. Crystals deposited in kidneys can also directly induce inflammation by enhancing NLRP3 inflammasome-mediated IL-1β release from renal mononuclear phagocytes [112, 113]. The crystal-induced NLRP3 activation mainly depends on lowering the potassium concentration within the cytosol either by increasing the efflux or dilution, e.g., cholesterol, silica, and MSU crystals [114, 115]. As explained earlier, cells attempt to digest crystals in the lysosome, which may lead to either calcium release (if crystals are digested) or lysosomal destabilization (if crystals are not digested), both processes result in

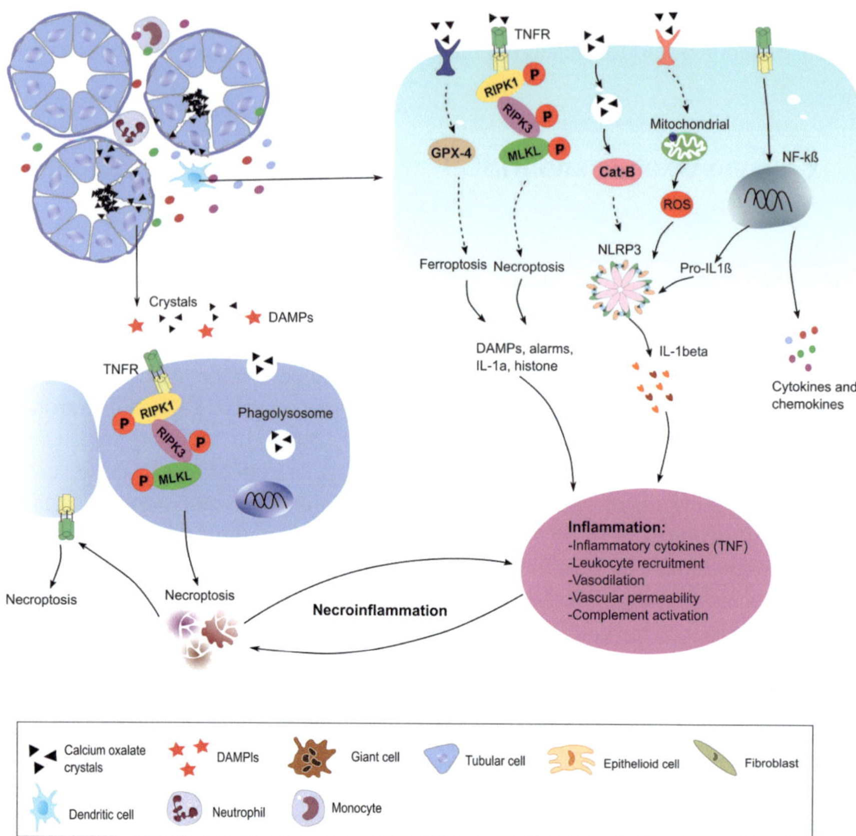

Fig. 6 Molecular mechanisms of crystal-induced necroinflammation. Supersaturation of solutes in the urine leads to the deposition of crystals in the tubular lumen, which activates signaling pathways, resulting in tubular cell death and inflammation. Phagocytosis of crystals causes lysosomal destabilization and release of cathepsin B (cat-B), which cleaves RIPK1, a negative regulator of necroptosis. RIPK1 degradation triggers the formation of the RIPK3–MLKL necrosome complex, resulting in tubular cell necroptosis. Dying tubular cells release numerous DAMPs and alarmins, which initiate inflammation. Dendritic cells and macrophages phagocytose crystals that are present in the interstitial compartment. Also here, lysosomal destabilization releases cat-B and ROS, which activate the NLRP3 inflammasome and induce the secretion of mature IL-1β by dendritic cells, triggering IL-1R-dependent inflammation in the kidney. The TNFR pathway can activate NF-κβ, which contributes to the activation of the inflammasome. RIPK3 and MLKL can also activate the NLRP3 inflammasome. Certain pro-inflammatory cytokines such as TNF can trigger regulated necrosis in kidney cells through the TNFR, leading to further DAMP release. This process leads to an autoamplification loop of crystal-induced necroinflammation. DAMPs such as histones act as a central mediator of the necroinflammation loop as they induce both Toll-like receptor-dependent inflammation and charge-dependent cell necrosis. RIPK: receptor-interacting protein kinase, DAMP: damage-associated molecular pattern, ROS: reactive oxygen species, IL: interleukin, TNFR: tumor necrosis factor receptor, MLKL: mixed lineage kinase domain-like protein

activation of the NLRP3 inflammasome inside professional phagocytes but not in parenchymal cells [116–119]. Lysosomal destabilization releases the lytic protease cathepsin B into the cytosol that induces NLRP3 activation as well as degradation of RIPK1, an endogenous inhibitor of necroptosis, thereby inducing necroptosis and DAMPs release. The calcium released from digested crystals activates the calcium-dependent protease calpain that cleaves pro-IL-1α into mature IL-1α, which may contribute to intrarenal inflammation [3] (Fig. 6).

Interestingly, macrophages surrounding intrarenal crystals undergo a phenotype shift to pro-inflammatory M1 macrophages. These granuloma macrophages contribute to renal inflammation during crystal nephropathies [120]. Furthermore, persistent inflammation also contributes to the development of kidney fibrosis [120–122]. For example, crystal-induced NLRP3 activation augments TGF-β signaling-mediated kidney fibrosis in an inflammasome-independent manner [120, 122]. Also, inflammatory TNFR signaling initiates the adhesion of crystals to the tubular epithelium that subsequently leads to the formation of crystal plug in tubular lumen resulting in obstructive nephropathy [123, 124] (Fig. 6).

In summary, crystals or crystalline particle deposition induce necroinflammation by activating regulated necrosis as well as inflammation within kidneys, and thereby, contributing to kidney injury, inflammation and fibrosis that result in a decline in kidney function.

6 Crystals-Related Inflammation in Excretory Ducts

Excretory ducts are prone to crystallization of minerals, since they excrete concentrated filtrate from body fluids that consist of various mineral ions, and thus, supersaturation-driven crystallization takes place. A classic example of this is the occurrence of stones in the urinary system (nephrolithiasis), ureter (ureterolithiasis), and bladder (cystolithiasis). Apart from supersaturation, several recent reports provide an entirely novel insight, wherein the immune system-mediated response has been implicated to trigger crystallization. For example, a systematic analysis of salivary gland stone, i.e., sialoliths revealed that smaller crystals induce NET formation, subsequently NETs surrounding the smaller crystals leading to the formation of aggregates that provide a niche for further mineralization. This in turn results in the formation of macroscopic sialoliths, which occlude the ducts of salivary glands [125]. A similar mechanism was also proposed for the formation of gall stones [126], and crystallization in pancreatic ducts (pancreatic lithiasis) [127, 128]. The stones formed in the ducts can cause injury mainly by blocking the lumen of the duct and obstructing the flow of the filtrate. This leads to inflammation as characterized by infiltrating leukocytes, increased cytokine production, etc. The crystal-induced NETs also release extracellular DAMPs that may further contribute to inflammation via TLR activation [129]. Furthermore, crystals induce oxidative stress, which contributes to injury and inflammation in the excretory ducts [130, 131].

7 Conclusions

Crystal biology is an expanding field of shared and crystal-specific body responses to crystal exposure. The general conceptual umbrella is that of innate host defense and wound healing. However, especially microparticles corrupt some of the otherwise highly efficient mechanisms of innate host defense, triggering acute and chronic tissue inflammation and tissue destruction [132]. Specific mechanisms relate to the atomic nature of the microparticle and the components released from them, e.g., calcium released from calcium phosphate particles in acidic environments or sodium released from monosodium urate crystals inside phagocytes. Crystal masses of non-aggregating crystals remain soft such as the gout tophus but aggregating crystals that grow to the size of calculi can obstruct excretory ducts and cause painful colic. Vascular obstructions induced by embolic CCs can trigger intravascular thrombosis, ischemia, and tissue necrosis as can large luminal atheroma or severe vascular wall calcifications. The clinical scenarios and presentations may be diverse and followed in different medical disciplines but the similarities in the underlying fundamental biological mechanisms demand a call for interdisciplinary research activities. There is a huge potential to significantly improve the morbidity and mortality of people suffering from "crystallopathies," therefore joining in for a concerted scientific effort to address the many open questions related to crystal nephropathies is not only needed but also promising.

Acknowledgments HJA was supported by the Deutsche Forschungsgemeinschaft (AN372/16-2, 30-1, 27-1) and SS by the Deutsche Forschungsgemeinschaft (STE2437/2-1 and 2-2). SRM is supported by the Council of Scientific and Industrial Research (CSIR)—Central Drug Research Institute (CDRI); Department of Biotechnology (DBT), Government of India (BT/RLF/Reentry/01/2017).

References

1. Molina-Ruiz AM, Requena L. Foreign body granulomas. Dermatol Clin. 2015;33(3):497–523.
2. Mulay SR, Anders H-J. Crystallopathies. N Engl J Med. 2016;374:2465–76.
3. Franklin BS, Mangan MS, Latz E. Crystal formation in inflammation. Annu Rev Immunol. 2016;34:173–202.
4. Worcester EM, Coe FL. Clinical practice. Calcium kidney stones. N Engl J Med. 2010;363:954–63.
5. Skålén K, Gustafsson M, Rydberg EK, Hultén LM, Wiklund O, Innerarity TL, Borén J. Subendothelial retention of atherogenic lipoproteins in early atherosclerosis. Nature. 2002;417:750–4.
6. Williams KJ, Tabas I. The response-to-retention hypothesis of early atherogenesis. Arterioscler Thromb Vasc Biol. 1995;15:551–61.
7. Gimbrone MAJ, García-Cardeña G. Endothelial cell dysfunction and the pathobiology of atherosclerosis. Circ Res. 2016;118:620–36.

8. SenBanerjee S, Lin Z, Atkins GB, et al. KLF2 is a novel transcriptional regulator of endothelial proinflammatory activation. J Exp Med. 2004;199:1305–15.

9. Robbins CS, Hilgendorf I, Weber GF, et al. Local proliferation dominates lesional macrophage accumulation in atherosclerosis. Nat Med. 2013;19:1166–72.

10. Swirski FK, Nahrendorf M, Libby P. The ins and outs of inflammatory cells in atheromata. Cell Metab. 2012;15:135–6.

11. Geng YJ, Libby P. Evidence for apoptosis in advanced human atheroma. Colocalization with interleukin-1 beta-converting enzyme. Am J Pathol. 1995;147:251–66.

12. van Lammeren GW, den Ruijter HM, Vrijenhoek JEP, et al. Time-dependent changes in atherosclerotic plaque composition in patients undergoing carotid surgery. Circulation. 2014;129:2269–76.

13. Quillard T, Franck G, Mawson T, Folco E, Libby P. Mechanisms of erosion of atherosclerotic plaques. Curr Opin Lipidol. 2017;28:434–41.

14. de Winther MPJ, Kanters E, Kraal G, Hofker MH. Nuclear factor kappaB signaling in atherogenesis. Arterioscler Thromb Vasc Biol. 2005;25:904–14.

15. Shi C, Mammadova-Bach E, Li C, Liu D, Anders H-J. Pathophysiology and targeted treatment of cholesterol crystal embolism and the related thrombotic angiopathy. https://doi.org/10.1096/fj.202301316RA.

16. Libby P, Lichtman AH, Hansson GK. Immune effector mechanisms implicated in atherosclerosis: from mice to humans. Immunity. 2013;38:1092–104.

17. Ketelhuth DFJ, Hansson GK. Adaptive response of T and B cells in atherosclerosis. Circ Res. 2016;118:668–78.

18. Nus M, Mallat Z. Immune-mediated mechanisms of atherosclerosis and implications for the clinic. Expert Rev Clin Immunol. 2016;12:1217–37.

19. Jonasson L, Holm J, Skalli O, Bondjers G, Hansson GK. Regional accumulations of T cells, macrophages, and smooth muscle cells in the human atherosclerotic plaque. Arteriosclerosis. 1986;6:131–8.

20. Binder CJ, Hartvigsen K, Chang M-K, Miller M, Broide D, Palinski W, Curtiss LK, Corr M, Witztum JL. IL-5 links adaptive and natural immunity specific for epitopes of oxidized LDL and protects from atherosclerosis. J Clin Invest. 2004;114:427–37.

21. Cardilo-Reis L, Gruber S, Schreier SM, Drechsler M, Papac-Milicevic N, Weber C, Wagner O, Stangl H, Soehnlein O, Binder CJ. Interleukin-13 protects from atherosclerosis and modulates plaque composition by skewing the macrophage phenotype. EMBO Mol Med. 2012;4:1072–86.

22. Mallat Z, Besnard S, Duriez M, et al. Protective role of interleukin-10 in atherosclerosis. Circ Res. 1999;85:e17–24.

23. Libby P, Hansson GK. Inflammation and immunity in diseases of the arterial tree: players and layers. Circ Res. 2015;116:307–11.

24. Duewell P, Kono H, Rayner KJ, et al. NLRP3 inflammasomes are required for atherogenesis and activated by cholesterol crystals. Nature. 2010;464:1357–61.

25. Patel R, Janoudi A, Vedre A, Aziz K, Tamhane U, Rubinstein J, Abela OG, Berger K, Abela GS. Plaque rupture and thrombosis are reduced by lowering cholesterol levels and crystallization with ezetimibe and are correlated with fluorodeoxyglucose positron emission tomography. Arterioscler Thromb Vasc Biol. 2011;31:2007–14.

26. Piepoli MF, Hoes AW, Agewall S, et al. 2016 European guidelines on cardiovascular disease prevention in clinical practice: the sixth joint task force of the European society of cardiology and other societies on cardiovascular disease prevention in clinical practice (constituted by representat). Eur Heart J. 2016;37:2315–81.

27. Chow CK, Jolly S, Rao-Melacini P, Fox KAA, Anand SS, Yusuf S. Association of diet, exercise, and smoking modification with risk of early cardiovascular events after acute coronary syndromes. Circulation. 2010;121:750–8.

28. Ference BA, Ginsberg HN, Graham I, et al. Low-density lipoproteins cause atherosclerotic cardiovascular disease. 1. Evidence from genetic, epidemiologic, and clinical studies. A

consensus statement from the European atherosclerosis society consensus panel. Eur Heart J. 2017;38:2459–72.

29. Baigent C, Blackwell L, Emberson J, et al. Efficacy and safety of more intensive lowering of LDL cholesterol: a meta-analysis of data from 170,000 participants in 26 randomised trials. Lancet. 2010;376:1670–81.

30. Palinski W, Miller E, Witztum JL. Immunization of low density lipoprotein (LDL) receptor-deficient rabbits with homologous malondialdehyde-modified LDL reduces atherogenesis. Proc Natl Acad Sci U S A. 1995;92:821–5.

31. Zhou X, Caligiuri G, Hamsten A, Lefvert AK, Hansson GK. LDL immunization induces T-cell-dependent antibody formation and protection against atherosclerosis. Arterioscler Thromb Vasc Biol. 2001;21:108–14.

32. Flory CM. Arterial occlusions produced by emboli from eroded aortic atheromatous plaques. Am J Pathol. 1945;21:549–65.

33. Keeley EC, Grines CL. Scraping of aortic debris by coronary guiding catheters: a prospective evaluation of 1,000 cases. J Am Coll Cardiol. 1998;32:1861–5.

34. Ascione R, Ghosh A, Reeves BC, Arnold J, Potts M, Shah A, Angelini GD. Retinal and cerebral microembolization during coronary artery bypass surgery: a randomized, controlled trial. Circulation. 2005;112:3833–8.

35. Kassirer JP. Atheroembolic renal disease. N Engl J Med. 1969;280:812–8.

36. Scolari F, Ravani P. Atheroembolic renal disease. Lancet. 2010;375:1650–60.

37. Fine MJ, Kapoor W, Falanga V. Cholesterol crystal embolization: a review of 221 cases in the English literature. Angiology. 1987;38:769–84.

38. Soufi M, Sattler AM, Maisch B, Schaefer JR. Molecular mechanisms involved in atherosclerosis. Herz. 2002;27:637–48.

39. Shi C, Kim T, Steiger S, et al. Crystal clots as therapeutic target in cholesterol crystal embolism. Circ Res. 2020;126:e37. https://doi.org/10.1161/CIRCRESAHA.119.315625.

40. Saric M, Kronzon I. Cholesterol embolization syndrome. Curr Opin Cardiol. 2011;26:472–9.

41. Tunick PA, Nayar AC, Goodkin GM, Mirchandani S, Francescone S, Rosenzweig BP, Freedberg RS, Katz ES, Applebaum RM, Kronzon I. Effect of treatment on the incidence of stroke and other emboli in 519 patients with severe thoracic aortic plaque. Am J Cardiol. 2002;90:1320–5.

42. Tunick PA, Kronzon I. Embolism from the aorta: atheroemboli and thromboemboli. Curr Treat Options Cardiovasc Med. 2001;3:181–6.

43. Smith SCJ, Allen J, Blair SN, et al. AHA/ACC guidelines for secondary prevention for patients with coronary and other atherosclerotic vascular disease: 2006 update: endorsed by the National Heart, Lung, and Blood Institute. Circulation. 2006;113:2363–72.

44. Kuo C-F, Grainge MJ, Zhang W, Doherty M. Global epidemiology of gout: prevalence, incidence and risk factors. Nat Rev Rheumatol. 2015;11:649–62.

45. Martinon F, Petrilli V, Mayor A, Tardivel A, Tschopp J. Gout-associated uric acid crystals activate the NALP3 inflammasome. Nature. 2006;440:237–41.

46. Schlesinger N, Alten RE, Bardin T, Schumacher HR, Bloch M, Gimona A, Krammer G, Murphy V, Richard D, So AK. Canakinumab for acute gouty arthritis in patients with limited treatment options: results from two randomised, multicentre, active-controlled, double-blind trials and their initial extensions. Ann Rheum Dis. 2012;71:1839–48.

47. Desai J, Steiger S, Anders H-J. Molecular pathophysiology of gout. Trends Mol Med. 2017;23:756–68.

48. Desai J, Kumar SV, Mulay SR, et al. PMA and crystal-induced neutrophil extracellular trap formation involves RIPK1-RIPK3-MLKL signaling. Eur J Immunol. 2016;46:223–9.

49. Desai J, Foresto-Neto O, Honarpisheh M, Steiger S, Nakazawa D, Popper B, Buhl EM, Boor P, Mulay SR, Anders H-J. Particles of different sizes and shapes induce neutrophil necroptosis followed by the release of neutrophil extracellular trap-like chromatin. Sci Rep. 2017;7:15003.

50. Desai J, Mulay SR, Nakazawa D, Anders H-J. Matters of life and death. How neutrophils die or survive along NET release and is "NETosis" = necroptosis? Cell Mol Life Sci. 2016;73:2211–9.

51. Ma Q, Honarpisheh M, Li C, Sellmayr M, Lindenmeyer M, Böhland C, Romagnani P, Anders H-J, Steiger S. Soluble uric acid is an intrinsic negative regulator of monocyte activation in monosodium urate crystal-induced tissue inflammation. J Immunol. 2020;205:789–800.

52. Schauer C, Janko C, Munoz LE, et al. Aggregated neutrophil extracellular traps limit inflammation by degrading cytokines and chemokines. Nat Med. 2014;20(5):511–7. https://doi.org/10.1038/nm.3547; Supplementary Figure 1 : In vitro-generated aggregates share characteristics of NETs. Representative immunofluorescence images of cryosections prepared fro.

53. Chhana A, Dalbeth N. The gouty tophus: a review. Curr Rheumatol Rep. 2015;17:19.

54. Mlika M, Adigun R, Bhutta BS. Silicosis. In: StatPearls. Treasure Island (FL): StatPearls Publishing; 2021.

55. Hoy RF, Chambers DC. Silica-related diseases in the modern world. Allergy. 2020;75:2805–17.

56. Richardson DB, Rage E, Demers PA, et al. Mortality among uranium miners in North America and Europe: the pooled uranium miners analysis (PUMA). Int J Epidemiol. 2020;50:633. https://doi.org/10.1093/ije/dyaa195.

57. Greenberg MI, Waksman J, Curtis J. Silicosis: a review. Dis Mon. 2007;53:394–416.

58. Ndlovu N, Nelson G, Vorajee N, Murray J. 38 years of autopsy findings in South African mine workers. Am J Ind Med. 2016;59:307–14.

59. Leung CC, Yu ITS, Chen W. Silicosis. Lancet. 2012;379:2008–18.

60. Akgun M, Araz O, Akkurt I, Eroglu A, Alper F, Saglam L, Mirici A, Gorguner M, Nemery B. An epidemic of silicosis among former denim sandblasters. Eur Respir J. 2008;32:1295–303.

61. Carneiro APS, Barreto SM, Siqueira AL, Cavariani F, Forastiere F. Continued exposure to silica after diagnosis of silicosis in Brazilian gold miners. Am J Ind Med. 2006;49:811–8.

62. Blackley DJ, Halldin CN, Laney AS. Continued increase in prevalence of coal workers' pneumoconiosis in the United States, 1970-2017. Am J Public Health. 2018;108:1220–2.

63. Zosky GR, Hoy RF, Silverstone EJ, Brims FJ, Miles S, Johnson AR, Gibson PG, Yates DH. Coal workers' pneumoconiosis: an Australian perspective. Med J Aust. 2016;204:414–8.

64. Rimal B, Greenberg AK, Rom WN. Basic pathogenetic mechanisms in silicosis: current understanding. Curr Opin Pulm Med. 2005;11:169–73.

65. Biswas R, Hamilton RFJ, Holian A. Role of lysosomes in silica-induced inflammasome activation and inflammation in absence of MARCO. J Immunol Res. 2014;2014:304180, 1.

66. Barnes H, Goh NSL, Leong TL, Hoy R. Silica-associated lung disease: an old-world exposure in modern industries. Respirology. 2019;24:1165–75.

67. Gossart S, Cambon C, Orfila C, Séguélas MH, Lepert JC, Rami J, Carré P, Pipy B. Reactive oxygen intermediates as regulators of TNF-alpha production in rat lung inflammation induced by silica. J Immunol. 1996;156:1540–8.

68. Hamilton RFJ, Thakur SA, Holian A. Silica binding and toxicity in alveolar macrophages. Free Radic Biol Med. 2008;44:1246–58.

69. Huaux F. New developments in the understanding of immunology in silicosis. Curr Opin Allergy Clin Immunol. 2007;7:168–73.

70. Beamer CA, Holian A. Antigen-presenting cell population dynamics during murine silicosis. Am J Respir Cell Mol Biol. 2007;37:729–38.

71. Mossman BT, Churg A. Mechanisms in the pathogenesis of asbestosis and silicosis. Am J Respir Crit Care Med. 1998;157:1666–80.

72. Olbrück H, Seemayer NH, Voss B, Wilhelm M. Supernatants from quartz dust treated human macrophages stimulate cell proliferation of different human lung cells as well as collagen-synthesis of human diploid lung fibroblasts in vitro. Toxicol Lett. 1998;96–97:85–95.

73. Liu F, Liu J, Weng D, Chen Y, Song L, He Q, Chen J. CD4+CD25+Foxp3+ regulatory T cells depletion may attenuate the development of silica-induced lung fibrosis in mice. PLoS One. 2010;5:e15404.

74. Nau GJ, Guilfoile P, Chupp GL, Berman JS, Kim SJ, Kornfeld H, Young RA. A chemoattractant cytokine associated with granulomas in tuberculosis and silicosis. Proc Natl Acad Sci U S A. 1997;94:6414–9.
75. van Berlo D, Knaapen AM, van Schooten F-J, Schins RP, Albrecht C. NF-kappaB dependent and independent mechanisms of quartz-induced proinflammatory activation of lung epithelial cells. Part Fibre Toxicol. 2010;7:13.
76. Doerner AM, Zuraw BL. TGF-beta1 induced epithelial to mesenchymal transition (EMT) in human bronchial epithelial cells is enhanced by IL-1beta but not abrogated by corticosteroids. Respir Res. 2009;10:100.
77. Liu G, Cheresh P, Kamp DW. Molecular basis of asbestos-induced lung disease. Annu Rev Pathol. 2013;8:161–87.
78. Hnizdo E, Vallyathan V. Chronic obstructive pulmonary disease due to occupational exposure to silica dust: a review of epidemiological and pathological evidence. Occup Environ Med. 2003;60:237–43.
79. Langley RJ, Kalra R, Mishra NC, Hahn FF, Razani-Boroujerdi S, Singh SP, Benson JM, Peña-Philippides JC, Barr EB, Sopori ML. A biphasic response to silica: I. Immunostimulation is restricted to the early stage of silicosis in Lewis rats. Am J Respir Cell Mol Biol. 2004;30:823–9.
80. Beamer CA, Migliaccio CT, Jessop F, Trapkus M, Yuan D, Holian A. Innate immune processes are sufficient for driving silicosis in mice. J Leukoc Biol. 2010;88:547–57.
81. Co DO, Hogan LH, Il-Kim S, Sandor M. T cell contributions to the different phases of granuloma formation. Immunol Lett. 2004;92:135–42.
82. Kawasaki H. A mechanistic review of silica-induced inhalation toxicity. Inhal Toxicol. 2015;27:363–77.
83. Tomokuni A, Aikoh T, Matsuki T, Isozaki Y, Otsuki T, Kita S, Ueki H, Kusaka M, Kishimoto T, Ueki A. Elevated soluble Fas/APO-1 (CD95) levels in silicosis patients without clinical symptoms of autoimmune diseases or malignant tumours. Clin Exp Immunol. 1997;110:303–9.
84. Langley RJ, Mishra NC, Peña-Philippides JC, Hutt JA, Sopori ML. Granuloma formation induced by low-dose chronic silica inhalation is associated with an anti-apoptotic response in Lewis rats. J Toxicol Environ Health A. 2010;73:669–83.
85. Otsuki T, Sakaguchi H, Tomokuni A, et al. Detection of alternatively spliced variant messages of Fas gene and mutational screening of Fas and Fas ligand coding regions in peripheral blood mononuclear cells derived from silicosis patients. Immunol Lett. 2000;72:137–43.
86. Borges VM, Falcão H, Leite-Júnior JH, et al. Fas ligand triggers pulmonary silicosis. J Exp Med. 2001;194:155–64.
87. Park HH, Girdler-Brown BV, Churchyard GJ, White NW, Ehrlich RI. Incidence of tuberculosis and HIV and progression of silicosis and lung function impairment among former Basotho gold miners. Am J Ind Med. 2009;52:901–8.
88. Silica, some silicates, coal dust and para-aramid fibrils. IARC Monogr Eval Carcinog Risks Hum. 1997;68:1–475.
89. Lacasse Y, Martin S, Gagné D, Lakhal L. Dose-response meta-analysis of silica and lung cancer. Cancer Causes Control. 2009;20:925–33.
90. Satpathy SR, Jala VR, Bodduluri SR, Krishnan E, Hegde B, Hoyle GW, Fraig M, Luster AD, Haribabu B. Crystalline silica-induced leukotriene B4-dependent inflammation promotes lung tumour growth. Nat Commun. 2015;6:7064.
91. Rushton L. Chronic obstructive pulmonary disease and occupational exposure to silica. Rev Environ Health. 2007;22:255–72.
92. Shtraichman O, Blanc PD, Ollech JE, Fridel L, Fuks L, Fireman E, Kramer MR. Outbreak of autoimmune disease in silicosis linked to artificial stone. Occup Med (Lond). 2015;65:444–50.
93. Stafford M, Cappa A, Weyant M, Lara A, Ellis JJ, Weitzel NS, Puskas F. Treatment of acute silicoproteinosis by whole-lung lavage. Semin Cardiothorac Vasc Anesth. 2013;17:152–9.
94. Zhang H, Sui J-N, Gao L, Guo J. Subcutaneous administration of infliximab-attenuated silica-induced lung fibrosis. Int J Occup Med Environ Health. 2018;31:503–15.

95. Wollin L, Maillet I, Quesniaux V, Holweg A, Ryffel B. Antifibrotic and anti-inflammatory activity of the tyrosine kinase inhibitor nintedanib in experimental models of lung fibrosis. J Pharmacol Exp Ther. 2014;349:209–20.

96. Abdelaziz RR, Elkashef WF, Said E. Tadalafil reduces airway hyperactivity and protects against lung and respiratory airways dysfunction in a rat model of silicosis. Int Immunopharmacol. 2016;40:530–41.

97. Carneiro PJ, Clevelario AL, Padilha GA, Silva JD, Kitoko JZ, Olsen PC, Capelozzi VL, Rocco PRM, Cruz FF. Bosutinib therapy ameliorates lung inflammation and fibrosis in experimental silicosis. Front Physiol. 2017;8·159.

98. Cruz FF, Horta LFB, de Maia LA, Lopes-Pacheco M, da Silva AB, Morales MM, Gonçalves-de-Albuquerque CF, Takiya CM, de Castro-Faria-Neto HC, PRM R. Dasatinib reduces lung inflammation and fibrosis in acute experimental silicosis. PLoS One. 2016;11:e0147005.

99. Bandeira E, Oliveira H, Silva JD, et al. Therapeutic effects of adipose-tissue-derived mesenchymal stromal cells and their extracellular vesicles in experimental silicosis. Respir Res. 2018;19:104.

100. Lopes-Pacheco M, Bandeira E, Morales MM. Cell-based therapy for silicosis. Stem Cells Int. 2016;2016:5091838.

101. Mulay SR, Anders HJ. Crystal nephropathies: mechanisms of crystal-induced kidney injury. Nat Rev Nephrol. 2017;13:226–40.

102. Tan M, Epstein W. Polymer formation during the degradation of human light chain and Bence-Jones proteins by an extrct of the lysosomal fraction of normal human kidney. Immunochemistry. 1972;9:9–16.

103. Liu Z, Xiao Y, Chen W, Wang Y, Wang B, Wang G, Xu X, Tang R. Calcium phosphate nanoparticles primarily induce cell necrosis through lysosomal rupture: the origination of material cytotoxicity. J Mater Chem B. 2014;2:3480–9.

104. Huang D, Zhou H, Gao J. Nanoparticles modulate autophagic effect in a dispersity-dependent manner. Sci Rep. 2015;5:14361.

105. Mulay SR, Desai J, Kumar SV, et al. Cytotoxicity of crystals involves RIPK3-MLKL-mediated necroptosis. Nat Commun. 2016;7:10274.

106. Liu W, Chen B, Wang Y, et al. RGMb protects against acute kidney injury by inhibiting tubular cell necroptosis via an MLKL-dependent mechanism. Proc Natl Acad Sci. 2018;115:E1475–84.

107. Linkermann A, Skouta R, Himmerkus N, et al. Synchronized renal tubular cell death involves ferroptosis. Proc Natl Acad Sci U S A. 2014;111:16836–41.

108. Mulay SR, Honarpisheh MM, Foresto-Neto O, et al. Mitochondria permeability transition versus necroptosis in oxalate-induced AKI. J Am Soc Nephrol. 2019;30:1857. https://doi.org/10.1681/ASN.2018121218.

109. Allam R, Scherbaum CR, Darisipudi MN, et al. Histones from dying renal cells aggravate kidney injury via TLR2 and TLR4. J Am Soc Nephrol. 2012;23:1375–88.

110. Anders HJ. Necroptosis in acute kidney injury. Nephron. 2018;139:342–8.

111. Mulay SR, Linkermann A, Anders H-J. Necroinflammation in kidney disease. J Am Soc Nephrol. 2016;27:27–39.

112. Linkermann A, Stockwell BR, Krautwald S, Anders H-J. Regulated cell death and inflammation: an auto-amplification loop causes organ failure. Nat Rev Immunol. 2014;14:759–67.

113. Mulay SR, Kulkarni OP, Rupanagudi KV, et al. Calcium oxalate crystals induce renal inflammation by NLRP3-mediated IL-1β secretion. J Clin Invest. 2013;123:236–46.

114. Kiyotake R, Oh-Hora M, Ishikawa E, Miyamoto T, Ishibashi T, Yamasaki S. Human mincle binds to cholesterol crystals and triggers innate immune responses. J Biol Chem. 2015;290:25322–32.

115. Hari A, Zhang Y, Tu Z, Detampel P, Stenner M, Ganguly A, Shi Y. Activation of NLRP3 inflammasome by crystalline structures via cell surface contact. Sci Rep. 2014;4:7281.

116. Gross O, Yazdi AS, Thomas CJ, Masin M, Heinz LX, Guarda G, Quadroni M, Drexler SK, Tschopp J. Inflammasome activators induce interleukin-1α secretion via distinct

pathways with differential requirement for the protease function of caspase-1. Immunity. 2012;36:388–400.

117. Hornung V, Bauernfeind F, Halle A, Samstad EO, Kono H, Rock KL, Fitzgerald KA, Latz E. Silica crystals and aluminum salts activate the NALP3 inflammasome through phagosomal destabilization. Nat Immunol. 2008;9:847–56.

118. Halle A, Hornung V, Petzold GC, Stewart CR, Monks BG, Reinheckel T, Fitzgerald KA, Latz E, Moore KJ, Golenbock DT. The NALP3 inflammasome is involved in the innate immune response to amyloid-beta. Nat Immunol. 2008;9:857–65.

119. Heneka MT, Kummer MP, Stutz A, et al. NLRP3 is activated in Alzheimer's disease and contributes to pathology in APP/PS1 mice. Nature. 2013;493:674–8.

120. Anders HJ, Suarez-Alvarez B, Grigorescu M, et al. The macrophage phenotype and inflammasome component NLRP3 contributes to nephrocalcinosis-related chronic kidney disease independent from IL-1–mediated tissue injury. Kidney Int. 2018;93:753–60.

121. Sellmayr M, Hernandez Petzsche MR, Ma Q, et al. Only hyperuricemia with crystalluria, but not asymptomatic hyperuricemia, drives progression of chronic kidney disease. J Am Soc Nephrol. 2020;31:2773–92.

122. Ludwig-Portugall I, Bartok E, Dhana E, et al. An NLRP3-specific inflammasome inhibitor attenuates crystal-induced kidney fibrosis in mice. Kidney Int. 2016;90:525–39.

123. Mulay SR, Eberhard JN, Desai J, et al. Hyperoxaluria requires TNF receptors to initiate crystal adhesion and kidney stone disease. J Am Soc Nephrol. 2017;28:761–8.

124. Klinkhammer BM, Djudjaj S, Kunter U, et al. Cellular and molecular mechanisms of kidney injury in 2,8-dihydroxyadenine nephropathy. J Am Soc Nephrol. 2020;31:799–816.

125. Schapher M, Koch M, Weidner D, et al. Neutrophil extracellular traps promote the development and growth of human salivary stones. Cell. 2020;9:2139. https://doi.org/10.3390/cells9092139.

126. Muñoz LE, Boeltz S, Bilyy R, et al. Neutrophil extracellular traps initiate gallstone formation. Immunity. 2019;51:443–450.e4.

127. Leppkes M, Maueröder C, Hirth S, et al. Externalized decondensed neutrophil chromatin occludes pancreatic ducts and drives pancreatitis. Nat Commun. 2016;7:10973.

128. Kravets OV, Danilenko IA, Smorodska OM, Piddubnyi AM, Zakorko I-MS, Danilchenko SN, Moskalenko RA, Kononenko MG, Romaniuk AM. Morphological and crystal chemical characteristic of pancreatic lithiasis. Wiad Lek. 2018;71:237–41.

129. Li Y, Cao X, Liu Y, Zhao Y, Herrmann M. Neutrophil extracellular traps formation and aggregation orchestrate induction and resolution of sterile crystal-mediated inflammation. Front Immunol. 2018;9:1559.

130. Sharma M, Kaur T, Singla SK. Role of mitochondria and NADPH oxidase derived reactive oxygen species in hyperoxaluria induced nephrolithiasis: therapeutic intervention with combinatorial therapy of N-acetyl cysteine and apocynin. Mitochondrion. 2016;27:15–24.

131. Khan SR, Canales BK, Dominguez-Gutierrez PR. Randall's plaque and calcium oxalate stone formation: role for immunity and inflammation. Nat Rev Nephrol. 2021;17:417. https://doi.org/10.1038/s41581-020-00392-1.

132. Mulay SR, Steiger S, Shi C, Anders H-J. A guide to crystal-related and nano- or microparticle-related tissue responses. FEBS J. 2019;287:818. https://doi.org/10.1111/febs.15174.

Omega-3 Fatty Acids Influence Membrane Cholesterol Distribution and Crystal Formation in Models of Atherosclerosis

Samuel C. R. Sherratt, Peter Libby, Deepak L. Bhatt, and R. Preston Mason

Abbreviations

AA   Arachidonic acid
CVD   Cardiovascular disease
DHA   Docosahexaenoic acid
EPA   Eicosapentaenoic acid
IPE   Icosapent ethyl
n3-FA   Omega-3 fatty acids

S. C. R. Sherratt
Department of Molecular, Cellular, and Biomedical Sciences, University of New Hampshire, Durham, NH, USA

Elucida Research LLC, Beverly, MA, USA
e-mail: ssherratt@elucidaresearch.com

P. Libby
Department of Medicine, Cardiovascular Division, Brigham and Women's Hospital, Harvard Medical School, Boston, MA, USA
e-mail: plibby@bwh.harvard.edu

D. L. Bhatt
Mount Sinai Heart, Icahn School of Medicine at Mount Sinai Health System, New York, NY, USA
e-mail: deepak.bhatt@mountsinai.org

R. P. Mason (✉)
Elucida Research LLC, Beverly, MA, USA

Department of Medicine, Cardiovascular Division, Brigham and Women's Hospital, Harvard Medical School, Boston, MA, USA
e-mail: rpmason@elucidaresearch.com

G. S. Abela, S. M. Nidorf (eds.), *Cholesterol Crystals in Atherosclerosis and Other Related Diseases*, Contemporary Cardiology, https://doi.org/10.1007/978-3-031-41192-2_17

1 Overview

Cholesterol crystals commonly localize in atherosclerotic lesions where they promote inflammation and disease progression. These crystals are distributed throughout the necrotic lipid core as well as areas associated with active macrophage recruitment, suggesting an early role in lesion development. Cholesterol crystal formation typically begins in the cell membrane—the site where cholesterol concentrates while serving essential structural and functional roles. When membrane cholesterol levels rise above a critical point, cholesterol will self-associate into its own nanodomains, which disrupt membrane function and nucleate the formation of extracellular crystals. Membrane lipid oxidation also favors cholesterol domain and crystal formation, especially under conditions of hyperglycemia. In the cytosol, cholesterol crystals activate inflammasomes and associated pathways following lysosomal damage, resulting in cytokine activation and inflammatory responses. These crystals can undergo rapid expansion, extending into the extracellular space of the atherosclerotic lesion, resulting in cell death and ultimately fibrous cap disruption. Omega-3 fatty acids (n3-FAs) mitigate these effects as they readily incorporate into cell membranes, and influence cholesterol distribution, lipid raft formation, and sterol crystallization. Eicosapentaenoic acid (EPA), in particular, inhibits cholesterol domain formation due to its potent antioxidant and membrane stabilizing effects. Clinical trials have shown that EPA can reduce composite CV events in statin-treated, high-risk patients while reducing plaque volume and increasing fibrous cap thickness. Other long-chain fatty acids such as docosahexaenoic acid (DHA) or mixed EPA/DHA formulations did not produce these benefits. Understanding the mechanisms by which EPA disrupts cholesterol crystal formation will provide novel insights into the cardioprotective effects of these agents and their role in treating CV disease.

2 Essential Role of Cholesterol in Membrane Structure and Cellular Function

Cellular cholesterol associates almost exclusively with membranes, where it influences phospholipid bilayer width, lipid dynamics, raft formation, and protein function [1, 2]. In the plasma membrane, cholesterol serves an integral structural role, providing lateral stability to various transmembrane ion channels and signal transduction proteins. Due to its highly planar and rigid sterol backbone, cholesterol reduces acyl chain trans-gauche isomerization in neighboring phospholipids, resulting in a concentration-dependent increase in membrane width and density [2–4]. These changes in acyl chain packing constraints also influence the movement and activity of transmembrane proteins in a reversible manner as observed in models of hypercholesterolemia [5–7]. One study showed that cholesterol can modulate the activity of calcium-activated potassium channels, promoting a transition from open to closed state as a result of increasing the lateral stress exerted on transmembrane helices in the membrane bilayer [8]. Cholesterol also influences other membrane properties, including water permeability, fluidity, intrinsic curvature, viral fusion, and endosome formation [9].

Plasma membrane lipid rafts, which serve as platforms for various signal transduction proteins, contain 3–5 times the amount of cholesterol than other areas of the membrane. These rafts are also enriched in sphingolipids that have favorable interactions with cholesterol due to their highly saturated hydrocarbon chains and complex headgroup structures [10]. These rafts float laterally through the more fluid, phospholipid-enriched lipid bilayer and can cluster to form enlarged domains. Certain key proteins localize preferentially to lipid rafts, such as the insulin receptor, which forms a functional dimer only after it is incorporated into certain lipid rafts [11]. Rafts also concentrate ligands and receptors necessary for a wide variety of cell signaling pathways, including Src-family kinase-induced phosphorylation cascades and glycosylphosphatidylinositol (GPI)-anchored protein-dependent actions [12]. Lipid rafts also sequester growth factor receptors as well as antigen receptors in immune cells such as T cells, B cells, mast cells, and basophils [13, 14]. Loss of raft integrity disrupts cytokine secretion triggered by inflammatory stimuli as well as B cell and T cell activation. The polyunsaturated fatty acid (PUFA) content of membrane phospholipids strongly influences cholesterol-enriched lipid rafts and their signaling protein [15–18].

Lipoproteins carry cholesterol through the circulation and deliver it to cells by receptor-mediated endocytosis [19]. Each low-density lipoprotein (LDL) particle contains approximately 1500 molecules of cholesteryl ester compressed into a hydrophobic core, surrounded by a polar phospholipid monolayer and a single apolipoprotein B (ApoB) molecule. Upon endocytosis, the LDL particles combine with intracellular lysosomes where hydrolysis liberates cholesterol from cholesteryl ester for use in membrane synthesis. As excessive cholesterol is toxic, cells such as macrophages use acetyl-coenzyme A (CoA) cholesterol acyltransferases (ACATs) to convert excess cholesterol back to cholesteryl esters for storage in cytoplasmic inclusions [20, 21].

The enzymes responsible for cholesterol synthesis are regulated in a coordinated fashion based on intracellular cholesterol concentrations. If cholesterol levels in the cell are too high, the expression of LDL receptors as well as HMG CoA reductase, the rate-limiting enzyme in cholesterol biosynthesis, declines; if cholesterol levels are too low, the expression of these proteins are increased (Fig. 1). The transcription factor sterol regulatory element-binding protein-2 (SREBP-2) in the endoplasmic reticulum (ER) regulates membrane cholesterol levels [22]. Low intracellular cholesterol concentrations below 5% of total ER lipids (molar basis) activate SREBP-2 by several proteolytic cleavage steps in the Golgi apparats, ultimately promoting the transcription of genes in the nucleus that modulate cholesterol synthesis and uptake from external sources [23]. The transcription factor nuclear factor erythroid 2 related factor-1 (Nrf1) is an essential regulator of cholesterol homeostasis in the ER [24]. Nrf1 detects changes in ER cholesterol content through a transmembrane binding domain that regulates its location, processing and activation.

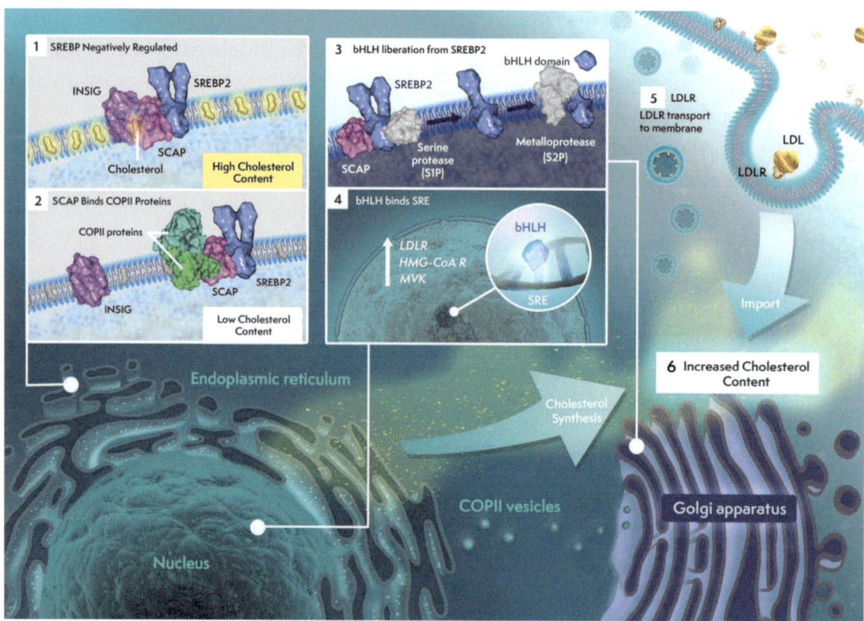

Fig. 1 Intracellular Cholesterol Content Depends on Tight Regulation of Sterol Regulating Element-Binding Protein 2 (SREBP-2). (1) When intracellular cholesterol content is sufficient to facilitate normal cellular function, SREBP2 is sequestered to the endoplasmic reticulum though binding SREBP cleavage-activating protein (SCAP). This complex remains anchored to the ER because SCAP binds to membrane cholesterol, which in turn causes a conformational change to allow SCAP to bind to insulin-induced gene 1 (INSIG). (2) When the intracellular concentration drops (measured by total sterol in the ER), there is insufficient cholesterol in the ER to bind SCAP and thus the SCAP-INSIG complex dissociates. SCAP is then open to binding COP-II proteins in anticipation of transport to the Golgi apparatus via COP-II vesicles. (3) In the Golgi, two sequential proteases cleave SREBP2 to liberate the basic helix-loop-helix (bHLH) domain. (4) The bHLH domain then travels to the nucleus where it binds the sterol regulatory element (SRE) and induces transcription of proteins necessary for de novo cholesterol synthesis and extracellular cholesterol uptake, including HMG-CoA reductase (*HMG-CoA R*), melovonate kinase (*MVK*), and the LDL receptor (*LDLR*). (5) Newly synthesized LDLR is transported to the cell membrane where is binds LDL particles in circulation and facilitates their endocytosis. (6) The net result of this mechanism is increased intracellular cholesterol, which will eventually increase the cholesterol content in the ER to bind SCAP and terminate this process

When cholesterol levels exceed cell requirements, it is packaged as cholesteryl esters in intracellular lipid droplets. Hydrolases can convert these esters back to free cholesterol, as needed, before incorporation into membranes. Importantly, the non-polar, esterified form of cholesterol cannot partition into the membrane lipid bilayer. As cells do not degrade cholesterol, efflux from cellular membranes is essential for maintaining normal sterol levels in a process called reverse cholesterol transport. High-density lipoprotein (HDL), which consists of the apolipoprotein A-I (ApoA-I) protein and a lipid core containing a higher ratio of cholesterol to triglycerides as compared to LDL, can serve as an acceptor for the exported cholesterol. The transport of plasma membrane cholesterol to extracellular HDL particles depends on ATP-binding cassette (ABC) transporters or by passive diffusion across a cholesterol gradient. Lipid rafts and caveolae can coordinate and facilitate cholesterol release to external lipoproteins [25]. To complete reverse cholesterol transport, HDL returns the sterol to the liver for excretion in the bile or to steroidogenic tissues that synthesize steroidal hormones [9]. In addition to hormones, metabolism of cholesterol leads to essential bile acids, vitamin D, and oxysterols [26].

3 Endothelial Dysfunction Leads to LDL Retention and Promotes Inflammatory Changes

Impaired endothelial dysfunction can promote the entry and retention of LDL particles in the arterial intima, triggering macrophage- and T cell-mediated inflammatory changes, and resulting in early plaque development [27]. LDL lipid oxidation results in the deamination of lysine residues on ApoB and formation of reactive aldehydes. Scavenger receptors on macrophages bind modified LDL, mediating LDL uptake and foam cell formation [28]. The foam cells trigger an inflammatory reaction through the release of various pro-inflammatory factors and cytokines [29, 30]. Increased risk for acute coronary syndromes, ischemic events, and metabolic disorders are associated with circulating levels of oxidized forms of LDL [31–34]. Oxidized LDL also shifts endothelial conditions from an anti-inflammatory and anti-thrombotic state to pro-inflammatory environment as evidenced by increased production of potent vasoconstrictors, including endothelin-1, angiotensin II, thromboxane A_2, and prostaglandin H2.

Endothelial dysfunction associated with increased levels of oxidized LDL can also involve reduced nitric oxide (NO) bioavailability [35–37]. As an inhibitor of platelet aggregation and leukocyte adhesion, NO is a key signaling molecule generated by the dimeric enzyme, NO synthase (NOS), which catalyzes the oxidation of L-arginine into L-citrulline. In the presence of oxidized LDL, endothelial NOS (eNOS) dimers become uncoupled due to an inadequate supply of co-factors such as tetrahydrobiopterin. Under these conditions, eNOS donates electrons to molecular oxygen to produce superoxide (O_2^-) rather than NO [38, 39]. Excess levels of O_2^- can directly facilitate an increase in oxidized LDL.

The eNOS molecule is regulated by caveolin proteins, which are palmitoylated transmembrane proteins with a hairpin-like structure that binds tightly to cholesterol [40]. One of the three caveolin isoforms, caveolin-1, binds eNOS and inhibits its activation by competing with calcium calmodulin while also modulating various inflammatory responses. As a calcium regulatory protein, calmodulin is essential for eNOS function but also attenuates its activity following phosphorylation in endothelial cells [41]. Changes in the cholesterol content of caveolae influences caveolin-1 expression and NO production in aortic endothelial cells [42]. Additionally, the inhibition of cholesterol synthesis with a statin has been shown to increase eNOS activity by reducing caveolin-1 expression and other post-transcriptional mechanisms [43]. Statins also modulate eNOS and reduce inflammation through increased expression of Kruppel-like factor 2 (KLF2) [44, 45]. These findings suggest that endothelial dysfunction associated with hypercholesterolemia can be reversed by inhibiting cholesterol biosynthesis and modulating eNOS function. EPA also contributes to caveolae-mediated improvements in NO bioavailability by modifying the lipid content and structural properties of caveolae, leading to caveolin-1 displacement and enhanced eNOS activity [37, 46].

4 Origins and Inflammatory Effects of Cholesterol Crystals

Cholesterol crystals comprise an abundant and pathologic component of atherosclerotic plaques [47–49]. Lesions with increased levels of lipid accumulation and large quantities of crystals are among the most vulnerable to rupture and provoke adverse ischemic events [50, 51]. Nascent lesions can also contain cholesterol crystals, suggesting that these structures accumulate much earlier in plaque development than previously thought [52–54]. Available data suggest that cholesterol crystals form in macrophage-derived foam cells following excessive accumulation of cholesterol [55, 56] as well as potentially starting as extracellular lipid in the matrix of the plaque [57]. Once a critical mass is reached, an intracellular nucleating event occurs, leading to cholesterol crystallization [58]. In mouse macrophages, inhibition of cholesterol esterification by blocking ACAT leads to the rapid accumulation of free, monomeric cholesterol and crystal formation (Fig. 2) [55]. Exclusion of an extracellular acceptor such as HDL accelerates this process [55]. Unlike membrane cholesterol, which can be easily transferred to extracellular acceptors, cholesterol crystals resist removal even by phagocytotic mechanisms [59].

Disruptions in the biosynthesis, transportation and metabolism of cholesterol lead to various diseases such as atherosclerosis and lipid storage disorders. In lipid-laden, macrophage-derived foam cells, cholesterol crystals result from excessive sterol accumulation or disruption in the regulation of cholesterol esterification [20]. Under hypercholesterolemic conditions, excessive cholesterol accumulation in membranes of vascular smooth muscle cells and macrophages leads to the formation of cholesterol domains, a precursor to cholesterol crystals, as shown in animal and membrane-based models of atherosclerosis [3, 60–62]. Tulenko et al. studied the effects of cholesterol enrichment in aortic smooth muscle cells obtained ex vivo from rabbits with diet-induced atherosclerosis [3]. After exposure to a Western (cholesterol-enriched) diet for up to 13 weeks, the cholesterol content measured in aortic smooth muscle cell membranes increased substantially from a typical level of ~30 mol% to over 50 mol% over time of exposure to diet. These membranes were isolated and further examined using X-ray diffraction approaches, which demonstrated immiscible cholesterol monohydrate domains or "bilayers" with a highly reproducible periodicity of 34 Å. The molecular dimensions associated with the cholesterol bilayer phase corresponded to a tail-to-tail arrangement of cholesterol as

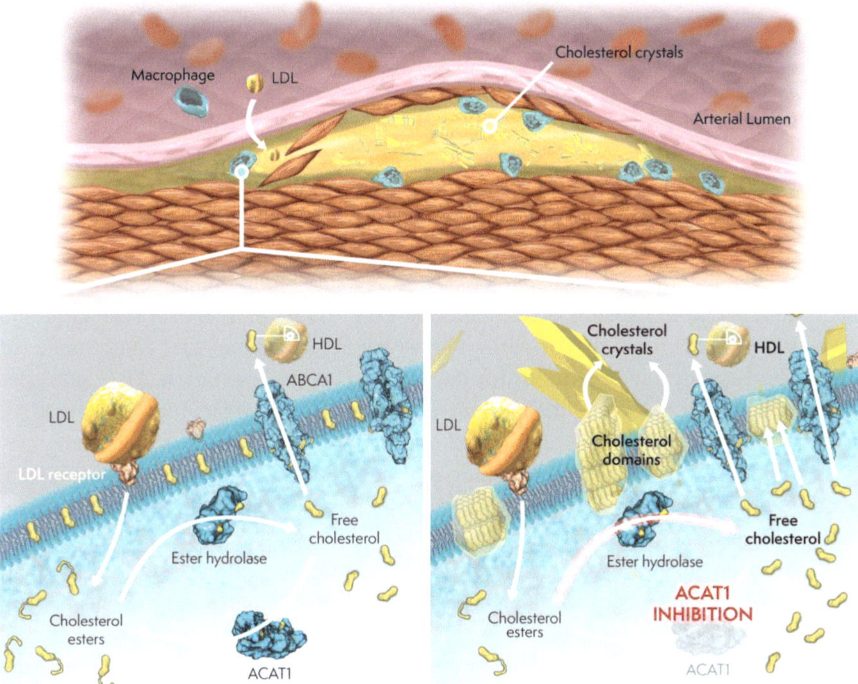

Fig. 2 ACAT inhibition increases free cholesterol content and induces membrane cholesterol domain formation. During atherosclerosis, LDL particles can pass through the endothelium and accumulate in the arterial intima. Macrophages phagocytose these LDL particles, eventually forming macrophage foam cells. Cells maintain cholesterol homeostasis within the cell through ester hydrolase enzymes and acetyl CoA cholesterol acyltransferase (ACAT) enzymes: ester hydrolase enzymes remove the ester moeity from cholesterol esters (from LDL) to form free cholesterol, and ACAT esterifies free cholesterol. Because excess free cholesterol can be toxic, it can be stored intracellularly as cholesterol esters via ACAT activity or it can be effluxed from the cell via ATP binding cassette 1 (ABCA1) to extracellular acceptors. Accumulation of excess free cholesterol in the cell membrane induces the formation of cholesterol domains, which in turn form nucleation sites for larger extracellular cholesterol crystals. In vitro experiments have shown that inhibition of ACAT leads to formation of such domains and cholesterol crystals due to excessive free cholesterol in the cell membrane

the long axis of cholesterol monohydrate was shown to be 17 Å in previous X-ray crystallographic analyses [63]. The formation of cholesterol domains was reproduced in membranes reconstituted as binary mixtures of phospholipid and cholesterol at levels replicating disease conditions. Oxidized sterols such as 7-ketocholesterol also produced similar membrane domains, which exhibited a slightly larger periodicity of 35.4 Å due to the differing chemical structure [64]. Oxidized sterols also form toxic extracellular crystals that trigger apoptosis with dimensions that differ only slightly from that of non-oxidized crystals [65].

Cholesterol crystals also localize in murine macrophage-derived foam cells incubated with an ACAT inhibitor and deprived of any extracellular acceptors of free cholesterol for up to 5 days [66]. X-ray diffraction approaches have shown that cell membranes can develop reproducible cholesterol domains after exposure to treatment for only 31 h. The formation of intracellular crystals follows, as the crystals extend quickly into the extracellular space, increase in size and assume various morphologies, including plates, needles, or helices [66]. Other studies have shown such crystals to be cytotoxic and highly resistant to pharmacologic intervention due to their inert properties and stability under various experimental conditions. In the atheroma, the sharp tips and edges of these crystals can damage cellular components leading to expansion of the necrotic core, damage to the fibrous cap, and eventual plaque rupture [67–69]. These studies indicate the importance of cholesterol-focused interventions for interrupting crystal formation. Therapies specifically targeted at events that trigger membrane cholesterol domain formation, such as oxidative stress and cholesterol enrichment, are essential for reducing cardiovascular (CV) risk. Among the interventions that may reduce cholesterol crystal accumulation, administration of cyclodextrin has demonstrated some beneficial actions experimentally [70].

Duewell et al. used a novel microscopic technique to demonstrate that small cholesterol crystals appear in early, diet-induced atherosclerotic lesions in atherosclerosis-prone (apolipoprotein E-deficient) mice. These crystals were found to cause lysosomal damage in phagocytes in vitro resulting in the activation of the nucleotide-binding oligomerization domain (NOD)-like receptor containing pyrin domain 3 (NLRP3) inflammasome (Fig. 3) [52]. This complex, which often requires multiple danger signals prior to activation, recruits the adapted apoptosis-associated speck-like protein containing a caspase recruitment domain (CARD) (ASC), which converts procaspase-1 into caspase-1 which converts the inactive pro- forms of interleukins (IL)-1β and IL-18 to their mature biologically functional forms [71, 72]. There appear to be several mechanisms of activation for the NLRP3 inflammasome depending on the inflammatory stimulus. Phagocytosis of cholesterol crystals results in the rupture of phagolysosomes and release of their proteolytic contents—most notably the proteases cathepsin B and L, which in turn activate the NLRP3 inflammasome [52, 73]. In mice the lack of NLRP3- or cathepsin protease subjected to the same high-cholesterol diet, highly attenuates the inflammatory and atherosclerotic effects of these crystals [52].

Cholesterol crystals can also induce the release of neutrophil extracellular traps (NETs) from neutrophils in a manner dependent on reactive oxygen species (ROS). These structures can promote the amplification and propagation of thrombosis [74]. NETs in turn signal the release of IL-1β through the NLRP3 inflammasome [75]. NETs also bear IL-1 alpha which can activate endothelial cells [76]. NETs localize in atherosclerotic lesions isolated from high-fat diet-exposed, ApoE-deficient mice; and genetic knockout of key NET production enzymes in some studies reduces arterial lesions to an extent similar to that observed in NLRP3-specific knockout strains [75]. This observation strengthens the connection between cholesterol crystals and NLRP3-dependent inflammatory signaling within the atheroma.

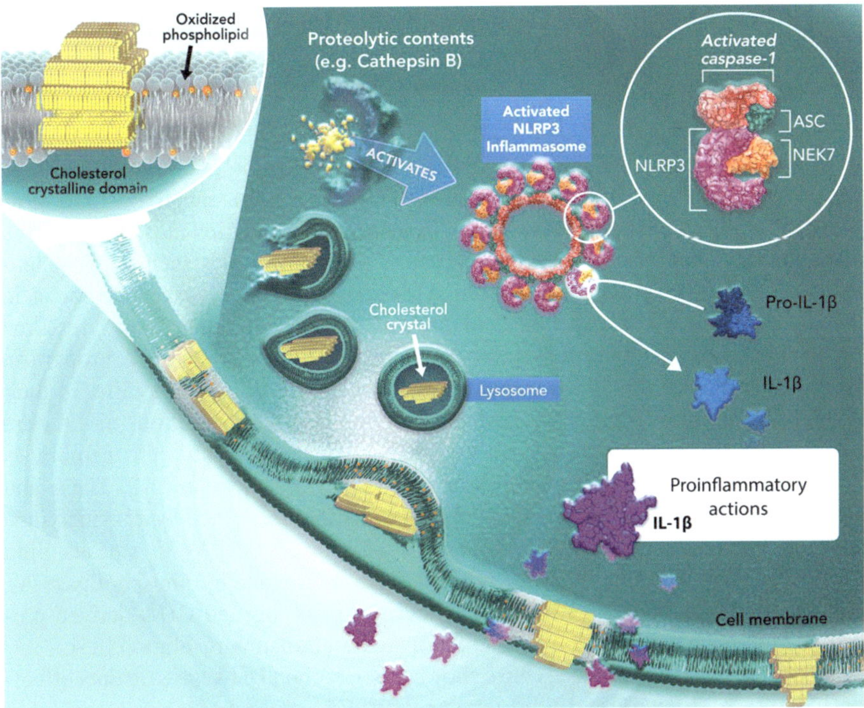

Fig. 3 Assembly of the NLRP3 Inflammasome can be Initiated by Cholesterol Crystals, Resulting in Cytokine Release. The NOD-LLR and pyrin domain-containing protein 3 (NLRP3) inflammasome assembles following stimulation from multiple external signals. Among these are cholesterol crystals, which can degrade and rupture lysosomes as they are destined for degradation. As a result, proteolytic contents such as cathepsin B are released from the lysosome into the cytosol, leading to the NLRP3 assembly. NLRP3 recruits NIMA-related kinase 7 (NEK7), the adapted apoptosis-associated speck-like protein containing a caspase (ASC), and procaspase-1 which is then converted into activated caspase-1. It is the activated caspase which converts pro-interleukins (IL)-1β and pro-IL-18 to their active functional forms for release

ROS generated from pathogen- and damage-associated molecular patterns (PAMPs and DAMPs, respectively) can also initiate inflammasome activation [72]. Microtubules play a key role in NLRP3 inflammasome activation by facilitating the aggregation of the various components in response to inflammatory stimuli; thus inhibitors of tubulin polymerization such as colchicine may offer additional anti-inflammatory effects [77]. Indeed, the Low-Dose Colchicine (LoDoCo 1 and 2) trials showed significant reductions in composite cardiovascular events in patients with coronary disease while the Colchicine Cardiovascular Outcomes Trial (COLCOT) trial showed similar effects in patients with recent myocardial infarction receiving low-dose colchicine on top of statin use [78–80].

5 Effects of Omega-3 Fatty Acids on Membrane Structure and Cholesterol Distribution

Omega-3 fatty acids (n3-FAs) accumulate in circulating red blood cells in proportion to dietary intake [81, 82]. Following absorption in the gut, n3-FAs travel to tissues throughout the body in triglyceride (TG)-rich lipoproteins like VLDL or as free fatty acids bound to plasma albumin [82–84]. n3-FAs carried in lipoproteins are also typically converted into cholesteryl esters or phospholipids such as phosphatidylcholine and phosphatidylethanolamine [84]. Two n3-FAs, eicosapentaenoic acid (EPA; 20:5) and docosahexaenoic acid (DHA; 22:6) have dominated much research because of their putative anti-atherothrombotic and cardioprotective properties. Obtained from oily fish like sardines and anchovies, EPA and DHA differ in their chemical structure by only two carbons and one double bond. Both n3-FAs are incorporated into phospholipids in the ER and transported into cell membranes where they influence lipid dynamics and structural organization [18]. These and other n3-FAs also participate in intracellular signaling, facilitated by enzymes such as cyclooxygenases and lipoxygenases, which convert n3-FAs to various lipid metabolites following their release from the cell membrane by phospholipase A_2. Several lipid metabolites, including EPA-derived resolvins and DHA-derived protectins, influence gene expression and facilitate inflammation resolution [85].

X-ray diffraction approaches have shown that EPA and DHA have distinct effects on membrane structure and lipid organization. EPA, in both free fatty acid and phospholipid-associated forms, normalizes membrane lipid structural order and preserves normal cholesterol distribution [18, 86]; DHA, however, reconstituted in similar forms, promotes membrane lipid disorder and the segregation of cholesterol into discrete domains [87]. Treatment with both n3-FAs resulted in little change in membrane structure as compared to their separate effects. These distinct biophysical effects may contribute directly to the differences observed for EPA and DHA in various clinical studies [88].

The disparate effects of EPA and DHA on cholesterol-dependent, membrane physical properties were confirmed using micropipette aspiration techniques [89]. This approach permits the controlled application of force to the membrane surface and the measurement of the apparent expansion modulus (K_{app}), a surrogate for membrane elasticity. In membranes prepared with normal levels of cholesterol, DHA reduced the K_{app} and promoted cholesterol domain formation. By sequestering cholesterol from bulk lipid, DHA reduces van der Wall interactions between cholesterol and phospholipid acyl chain segments, effectively reducing the energy required to stretch the membrane. In contrast, EPA promoted a normal, homogenous distribution of cholesterol in the membrane bilayer and a higher K_{app} [89].

Fluorescence polarization techniques have substantiated the separate effects of EPA and DHA on membrane dynamics [87]. Changes in membrane fluidity were measured in the absence or presence of EPA and DHA by monitoring the apparent rotational correlation time (ARCT) of the fluorescent probe, 1,6-diphenyl-1,3,5-hexatriene (DPH). DHA significantly increased ARCT in a dose-dependent manner, while EPA had no significant effect on ARCT values over a broad range of concentrations (1–10 mol%). These data indicate that DHA, unlike EPA, promotes membrane cholesterol aggregation and domain formation, leading to cholesterol crystal formation.

6 Effects of Omega-3 Fatty Acids on Membrane Lipid Oxidation and Cholesterol Crystal Formation During Hyperglycemia

Oxidative damage to unsaturated phospholipid acyl segments leads to deleterious changes in membrane structure, including lipid redistribution, cholesterol domain formation, and changes in bilayer width [60, 90–92]. n3-FAs can mitigate the effects of oxidative stress by trapping and stabilizing free radicals via their acyl chain-associated, conjugated double bonds, which are optimally positioned to block free radical propagation in the membrane hydrocarbon core. EPA has very potent antioxidant properties and significantly reduces lipid oxidation in cholesterol-enriched model membranes as well as in ApoB-containing lipoprotein particles [62, 87, 93, 94]. TG lowering agents and other long-chain fatty acids were tested in the same studies and shown to be relatively ineffective. In patients with elevated TG levels, EPA significantly reduced circulating levels of oxidized LDL as compared to placebo alone [95]. DHA can exert some antioxidant effects, but these actions attenuate with time due to rapid isomerization that lead to disruption in adjacent phospholipid acyl chains and inefficient reduction of free radical propagation through the membrane lipid bilayer [18, 93, 96–98]. The sub-nanosecond rates of isomerization have correlation times ranging from 80 picoseconds (ps) near the carbonyl group to a mere 8 ps near the terminal methyl group as determined by nuclear magnetic resonance (NMR) relaxation measurements [99]. The antioxidant effects of EPA increase when combined with the atorvastatin active metabolite, which occupies the same membrane location as EPA and facilitates further resonance stabilization of ROS through the statin's aromatic ring structures [60, 94, 100, 101].

The lipid membrane antioxidant effects of EPA also apply under conditions of hyperglycemia. High glucose levels increase ROS production and the formation of carbonyl species and other products of lipid degradation [62, 91]. Such effects associate with discrete changes in lipid order and structural organization, leading to increased cell permeability and loss of membrane function [102, 103]. Prolonged exposure to glucose also promotes membrane cholesterol aggregation, domain formation, and the extracellular deposition of cholesterol crystals as observed in the atheroma [62, 91]. The ability of glucose to promote lipid oxidation and cholesterol crystalline domain formation appear to be unique as it was not reproduced by other monosaccharides (e.g., mannose) at comparable concentrations [60, 91]. In fact, glucose has certain properties that make it more reactive with singlet oxygen and other ROS to form glucose radicals [104, 105]. By virtue of its potent free radical scavenging effects, EPA can abrogate the effects of glucose-induced oxidation, blocking lipid peroxidation and cholesterol crystal formation in a dose-dependent manner [62]. The atorvastatin active metabolite also blocks lipid oxidation and cholesterol crystal formation under hyperglycemic conditions [60].

7 Clinical Implications of EPA Effects on Cholesterol Organization

The ability of EPA to interfere with cholesterol crystal formation and its associated effects on inflammation and endothelial cell function may contribute to its clinical benefits in CV trials [106]. The Reduction of Cardiovascular Events with Icosapent Ethyl–Intervention Trial (REDUCE-IT) showed that administration of a highly purified EPA ethyl ester formulation, icosapent ethyl (IPE), at 4 g/day, significantly reduced risk of composite CV events by 25% in at-risk patients with elevated TG levels (>150 mg/dL) [107]. The risk reductions observed in the REDUCE-IT did not relate to TG lowering (19.7% decrease) but more likely due a combination of pleiotropic actions [108–110]. Serum EPA levels correlated more strongly with CV outcomes than did other traditional biomarkers such as LDL cholesterol, HDL cholesterol, and high-sensitivity C-reactive protein [111]. The reductions in events were also independent of statin choice that included high intensity agents such as rosuvastatin and atorvastatin [112]. Other large CV trials and clinical imaging studies using IPE formulations have yielded results consistent with REDUCE-IT while also providing mechanistic insights [113–116].

By contrast, clinical studies using EPA/DHA combination therapy, in the form of prescription or dietary supplement products, have not demonstrated favorable CV outcomes [117–121]. In the Long-Term Outcomes Study to Assess Statin Residual Risk with Epanova in High Cardiovascular Risk Patients with Hypertriglyceridemia (STRENGTH) trial, free carboxylic acid formulations of EPA and DHA (4 g/day combined) had no significant effect on primary CV outcomes despite reducing TG levels by 19% as compared to placebo [122]. This was consistent with the neutral effects observed with other TG lowering agents, such as niacin and fenofibrate, when combined with statin therapy [123–126]. The Pemafibrate to Reduce Cardiovascular Outcomes by Reducing Triglycerides in Patients with Diabetes (PROMINENT) trial was conducted to test pemafibrate, a selective peroxisome proliferator-activated receptor alpha modulator (SPPARM-α), on CV events in statin-treated patients with type 2 diabetes and mild to moderate hypertriglyceridemia (200–499 mg/dL) [127]. Pemafibrate reduces median TG levels between 40–50% compared with placebo in regulatory studies. Despite more potent TG lowering activity compared to fenofibric acid derivatives, PROMINENT recently halted due to futility at the recommendation of the independent data monitoring committee [128]. These findings indicate that TG lowering does not add incremental benefit over reductions in ApoB using intensive statin therapy. Mendelian randomization analyses of variants that associated TG-rich lipoprotein and LDL levels with CV risk confirm that absolute changes in ApoB levels were the best indicator of risk reduction [129]. Thus, the clinical benefits with EPA may arise from its particular physicochemical properties, including the ability to inhibit cholesterol domain and crystal formation, as opposed to TG lowering actions alone [130].

Studies of plaque progression in high-risk patients with well-established coronary atherosclerosis reinforce the improved CV outcomes with EPA and provide mechanistic insights [113–116, 131, 132]. In the Combination Therapy of Eicosapentaenoic Acid and Pitavastatin for Coronary Plaque Regression Evaluated by Integrated Backscatter Intravascular Ultrasonography (CHERRY) trial, patients received pitavastatin alone or pitavastatin plus IPE and followed prospectively for 6–8 months to determine effects on coronary plaque regression and features ascribed to stabilization [114]. Coronary plaque volume and composition were measured using integrated backscatter intravascular ultrasound (IB-IVUS). Treatment with both IPE and pitavastatin reduced total atheroma volume, increased fibrous cap thickness, and reduced plaque macrophage levels as compared to pitavastatin alone. These changes correlated with an increase in the ratio of EPA to arachidonic acid (AA), a largely pro-inflammatory omega-6 fatty acid. These two fatty acids compete for binding at the *sn*-2 position of phospholipids in the cell membrane and are both hydrolyzed by phospholipase A_2 (PLA_2), which releases them back into the cytosol for use in numerous signaling and metabolic pathways.

As noted above, subsequent enzymatic processing of EPA produces a series of active metabolites known as eicosanoids, which have disparate downstream effects depending on their fatty acid source. For example, during inflammatory challenge, AA is converted by cyclooxygenase (COX) and lipoxygenase (LOX) into prostaglandin E2 and leukotriene B4, respectively, both of which are potent, pro-inflammatory signaling molecules. By contrast, EPA is acted on by COX to produce the anti-inflammatory signaling molecule prostacyclin and various bioactive mediators, including resolvin E1, which have potent pro-revolving and immunoregulatory effects [133, 134]. These and other studies indicate that the EPA/AA ratio plays an important role in maintaining inflammatory homeostasis. Clinically, the EPA/AA ratio is a well-established predictor of CV risk [135]. Various clinical trials, including JELIS, MARINE, and ANCHOR, have also shown that IPE treatment increase the EPA/AA ratio [81, 113, 136]. Together with laboratory findings, these observations suggest that EPA facilitates coronary plaque stabilization, in part, through anti-inflammatory mechanisms that offset the effects of enhanced AA metabolism due to plaque incorporation and direct effects on dendritic cells and T-lymphocytes [137, 138].

A computed tomographic angiographic study assessed the effects of IPE intervention on plaque evolution in statin-treated patients with coronary disease and dyslipidemia in the randomized, double-blind, placebo-controlled Effect of Vascepa on Improving Coronary Atherosclerosis in People With High Triglycerides Taking Statin Therapy (EVAPORATE) trial [116]. In the placebo arm, low attenuation plaque (LAP) volume increased 109% compared to baseline over the 18-month study period. In the IPE treatment arm (4 g/day), LAP volume decreased 17%

compared to baseline ($P = 0.006$) over the same time period, an effect consistent with overall plaque *regression*. LAP has particular clinical significance as LAP burden strongly predicts fatal versus nonfatal myocardial infarction [139]. The effects observed with IPE in EVAPORATE agreed with other measurements of plaque volume, including total plaque, which fell compared to placebo (−9% vs. 11%, respectively; $p = 0.002$) [106]. These changes in indices of plaque vulnerability did not associate with TG levels or other lipid changes and persisted after multivariable adjustment of risk factors [116]. Importantly, the HEARTS trial investigated the effects of an EPA/DHA mixed formulation on non-calcified plaque volume in statin-treated patients with established coronary artery disease [117]. The results showed no significant reduction in plaque volume, consistent with the lack of clinical benefit observed in outcome trials. Together with CHERRY and other imaging trials, these data provide strong evidence that IPE treatment provides incremental benefit on top of statin to reduce CV events, facilitated, in part, by a reduction in plaque burden and vulnerability in high-risk and dyslipidemic patients.

8 Conclusion

Cholesterol crystals are early contributors to inflammation, atherogenesis, and eventual plaque erosion, including the rupture of the fibrous cap. These crystals develop through various pathways that interrupt normal cholesterol metabolism, including excessive accumulation of cholesterol in cell membranes as well as lipid oxidation associated with hyperglycemia and other risk factors. Intracellular cholesterol crystals activate the NLRP3 inflammasome leading to the release of the active forms of the pro-inflammatory cytokines IL-1β and IL-18 and consequent inflammatory changes. Given their role in the formative stages of atherosclerosis, blocking the biogenesis of intravascular cholesterol crystals represents a promising area of therapeutic intervention. EPA holds particular promise as it stabilizes membrane cholesterol distribution and prevents cholesterol crystalline domain formation under disease-like conditions in vitro—an effect not replicated by other fatty acids or TG lowering agents. These basic, physicochemical properties may explain, in part, the significant reduction in CV events and plaque volume observed with EPA in high-risk CV patients.

Acknowledgments The authors wish to thank Robert F. Jacob, Ph.D., Elucida Research LLC, for providing editorial assistance and Luke Groothoff, Elucida Research LLC, for preparing figure artwork.

Disclosures RPM has received grant/research support from Amarin Pharma Inc., HLS Therapeutics, Lexicon and the Cleveland Clinic. DLB discloses the following relationships— Advisory Board: AngioWave, Bayer, Boehringer Ingelheim, Cardax, CellProthera, Cereno Scientific, Elsevier Practice Update Cardiology, High Enroll, Janssen, Level Ex, Medscape Cardiology, Merck, MyoKardia, NirvaMed, Novo Nordisk, PhaseBio, PLx Pharma, Regado Biosciences, Stasys; Board of Directors: AngioWave (stock options), Boston VA Research

drugs, currently focusing on cancer therapeutics. Dr. Libby's interests were reviewed and are managed by Brigham and Women's Hospital and Mass General Brigham in accordance with their conflict-of-interest policies. FUNDING Dr. Libby receives funding support from the National Heart, Lung, and Blood Institute (1R01HL134892 and 1R01HL163099-01), the RRM Charitable Fund and the Simard Fund SCRS has no disclosures to report.

Funding Sources None.

References

1. Paukner K, Králová Lesná I, Poledne R. Cholesterol in the cell membrane—an emerging player in atherogenesis. Int J Mol Sci. 2022;23:533.
2. Subczynski WK, Pasenkiewicz-Gierula M, Widomska J, Mainali L, Raguz M. High cholesterol/low cholesterol: effects in biological membranes: a review. Cell Biochem Biophys. 2017;75:369–85.
3. Tulenko TN, Chen M, Mason PE, Mason RP. Physical effects of cholesterol on arterial smooth muscle membranes: evidence of immiscible cholesterol domains and alterations in bilayer width during atherogenesis. J Lipid Res. 1998;39:947–56.
4. Chakraborty S, Doktorova M, Molugu TR, Heberle FA, Scott HL, Dzikovski B, et al. How cholesterol stiffens unsaturated lipid membranes. Proc Natl Acad Sci. 2020;117:21896–905.
5. Paragh G, Kovács É, Seres I, Keresztes T, Balogh Z, Szabó J, et al. Altered signal pathway in granulocytes from patients with hypercholesterolemia. J Lipid Res. 1999;40:1728–33.
6. Fang Y, Mohler ER, Hsieh E, Osman H, Hashemi SM, Davies PF, et al. Hypercholesterolemia suppresses inwardly rectifying K+ channels in aortic endothelium in vitro and in vivo. Circ Res. 2006;98:1064–71.
7. Lee AG. How lipids affect the activities of integral membrane proteins. Biochim Biophys Acta. 2004;1666:62–87.
8. Chang HM, Reitstetter R, Mason RP, Gruener R. Attenuation of channel kinetics and conductance by cholesterol: an interpretation using structural stress as a unifying concept. J Membr Biol. 1995;143:51–63.
9. Yang S-T, Kreutzberger AJB, Lee J, Kiessling V, Tamm LK. The role of cholesterol in membrane fusion. Chem Phys Lipids. 2016;199:136–43.
10. Lingwood D, Simons K. Lipid rafts as a membrane-organizing principle. Science. 2010;327:46–50.
11. Bickel PE. Lipid rafts and insulin signaling. Am J Physiol Endocrinol Metab. 2002;282:E1–10.
12. Simons K, Toomre D. Lipid rafts and signal transduction. Nat Rev Mol Cell Biol. 2000;1:31–9.
13. Pike LJ. Growth factor receptors, lipid rafts and caveolae: an evolving story. Biochim Biophys Acta. 2005;1746:260–73.
14. Varshney P, Yadav V, Saini N. Lipid rafts in immune signalling: current progress and future perspective. Immunology. 2016;149:13–24.
15. Brzustowicz MR, Cherezov V, Caffrey M, Stillwell W, Wassall SR. Molecular organization of cholesterol in polyunsaturated membranes: microdomain formation. Biophys J. 2002;82:285–98.
16. Kucerka N, Marquardt D, Harroun TA, Nieh MP, Wassall SR, de Jong DH, et al. Cholesterol in bilayers with PUFA chains: doping with DMPC or POPC results in sterol reorientation and membrane-domain formation. Biochemistry. 2010;49:7485–93.
17. Kucerka N, Marquardt D, Harroun TA, Nieh MP, Wassall SR, Katsaras J. The functional significance of lipid diversity: orientation of cholesterol in bilayers is determined by lipid species. J Am Chem Soc. 2009;131:16358–9.
18. Sherratt SCR, Juliano RA, Copland C, Bhatt DL, Libby P, Mason RP. Eicosapentaenoic acid and docosahexaenoic acid containing phospholipids have contrasting effects on membrane structure. J Lipid Res. 2021;100106:100106.

19. Goldstein Joseph L, Brown MS. A century of cholesterol and coronaries: from plaques to genes to statins. Cell. 2015;161:161–72.
20. Brown MS, Ho YK, Goldstein JL. The cholesteryl ester cycle in macrophage foam cells. Continual hydrolysis and re-esterification of cytoplasmic cholesteryl esters. J Biol Chem. 1980;255:9344–52.
21. Basu SK, Goldstein JL, Anderson GW, Brown MS. Degradation of cationized low density lipoprotein and regulation of cholesterol metabolism in homozygous familial hypercholesterolemia fibroblasts. Proc Natl Acad Sci. 1976;73:3178–82.
22. Goldstein JL, DeBose-Boyd RA, Brown MS. Protein sensors for membrane sterols. Cell. 2006;124:35–46.
23. Radhakrishnan A, Goldstein JL, McDonald JG, Brown MS. Switch-like control of SREBP-2 transport triggered by small changes in ER cholesterol: a delicate balance. Cell Metab. 2008;8:512–21.
24. Widenmaier SB, Snyder NA, Nguyen TB, Arduini A, Lee GY, Arruda AP, et al. NRF1 is an ER membrane sensor that is central to cholesterol homeostasis. Cell. 2017;171:1094–109.e15.
25. Gallegos AM, McIntosh AL, Atshaves BP, Schroeder F. Structure and cholesterol domain dynamics of an enriched caveolae/raft isolate. Biochem J. 2004;382:451–61.
26. Hu J, Zhang Z, Shen W-J, Azhar S. Cellular cholesterol delivery, intracellular processing and utilization for biosynthesis of steroid hormones. Nutr Metab. 2010;7:47.
27. Gimbrone MA, García-Cardeña G. Endothelial cell dysfunction and the pathobiology of atherosclerosis. Circ Res. 2016;118:620–36.
28. Steinberg D, Witztum JL. Oxidized low-density lipoprotein and atherosclerosis. Arterioscler Thromb Vasc Biol. 2010;30:2311–6.
29. Libby P, Ridker PM, Hansson GK. Progress and challenges in translating the biology of atherosclerosis. Nature. 2011;473:317–25.
30. Libby P. The changing landscape of atherosclerosis. Nature. 2021;592:524–33.
31. Ehara S, Ueda M, Naruko T, Haze K, Itoh A, Otsuka M, et al. Elevated levels of oxidized low density lipoprotein show a positive relationship with the severity of acute coronary syndromes. Circulation. 2001;103:1955–60.
32. Walter MF, Jacob RF, Bjork RE, Jeffers B, Buch J, Mizuno Y, et al. Circulating lipid hydroperoxides predict cardiovascular events in patients with stable coronary artery disease: the PREVENT study. J Am Coll Cardiol. 2008;51:1196–202.
33. Walter MF, Jacob RF, Jeffers B, Ghadanfar MM, Preston GM, Buch J, et al. Serum levels of TBARS predict cardiovascular events in patients with stable coronary artery disease: a longitudinal analysis of the PREVENT study. J Am Coll Cardiol. 2004;44:1996–2002.
34. Holvoet P, Kritchevsky SB, Tracy RP, Mertens A, Rubin SM, Butler J, et al. The metabolic syndrome, circulating oxidized LDL, and risk of myocardial infarction in well-functioning elderly people in the health, aging, and body composition cohort. Diabetes. 2004;53:1068–73.
35. Forstermann U, Munzel T. Endothelial nitric oxide synthase in vascular disease: from marvel to menace. Circulation. 2006;113:1708–14.
36. Panza JA, Quyyumi AA, Brush JE, Epstein SE. Abnormal endothelium-dependent vascular relaxation in patients with essential hypertension. N Engl J Med. 1990;323:22–7.
37. Mason RP, Dawoud H, Jacob RF, Sherratt SCR, Malinski T. Eicosapentaenoic acid improves endothelial function and nitric oxide bioavailability in a manner that is enhanced in combination with a statin. Biomed Pharmacother. 2018;103:1231–7.
38. Landmesser U, Dikalov S, Price SR, McCann L, Fukai T, Holland SM, et al. Oxidation of tetrahydrobiopterin leads to uncoupling of endothelial cell nitric oxide synthase in hypertension. J Clin Invest. 2003;111:1201–9.
39. Huk I, Nanobashvili J, Neumayer C, Punz A, Mueller M, Afkhampour K, et al. L-arginine treatment alters the kinetics of nitric oxide and superoxide release and reduces ischemia/reperfusion injury in skeletal muscle. Circulation. 1997;96:667–75.
40. Parton RG, Simons K. The multiple faces of caveolae. Nat Rev Mol Cell Biol. 2007;8:185–94.
41. Greif DM, Sacks DB, Michel T. Calmodulin phosphorylation and modulation of endothelial nitric oxide synthase catalysis. Proc Natl Acad Sci. 2004;101:1165–70.

42. Peterson TE, Poppa V, Ueba H, Wu A, Yan C, Berk BC. Opposing effects of reactive oxygen species and cholesterol on endothelial nitric oxide synthase and endothelial cell Caveolae. Circ Res. 1999;85:29–37.
43. Laufs U, Fata VL, Plutzky J, Liao JK. Upregulation of endothelial nitric oxide synthase by HMG CoA reductase inhibitors. Circulation. 1998;97:1129–35.
44. Parmar KM, Nambudiri V, Dai G, Larman HB, Gimbrone MA Jr, García-Cardeña G. Statins exert endothelial atheroprotective effects via the KLF2 transcription factor. J Biol Chem. 2005;280:26714–9.
45. Bu D-x, Tarrio M, Grabie N, Zhang Y, Yamazaki H, Stavrakis G, et al. Statin-induced Kruppel-like factor 2 expression in human and mouse T cells reduces inflammatory and pathogenic responses. J Clin Invest. 2010;120:1961–70.
46. Li Q, Zhang Q, Wang M, Zhao S, Ma J, Luo N, et al. Eicosapentaenoic acid modifies lipid composition in caveolae and induces translocation of endothelial nitric oxide synthase. Biochimie. 2007;89:169–77.
47. Stary HC, Chandler AB, Dinsmore RE, Fuster V, Glagov S, Insull W, et al. A definition of advanced types of atherosclerotic lesions and a histological classification of atherosclerosis. Circulation. 1995;92:1355–74.
48. Falk E. Pathogenesis of atherosclerosis. J Am Coll Cardiol. 2006;47:C7–12.
49. Virmani R, Kolodgie FD, Burke AP, Farb A, Schwartz SM. Lessons from sudden coronary death. Arterioscler Thromb Vasc Biol. 2000;20:1262–75.
50. Schroeder AP, Falk E. Vulnerable and dangerous coronary plaques. Atherosclerosis. 1995;118:S141–9.
51. Abela GS. Cholesterol crystals piercing the arterial plaque and intima trigger local and systemic inflammation. J Clin Lipidol. 2010;4:156–64.
52. Duewell P, Kono H, Rayner KJ, Sirois CM, Vladimer G, Bauernfeind FG, et al. NLRP3 inflammasomes are required for atherogenesis and activated by cholesterol crystals. Nature. 2010;464:1357–61.
53. Lim RS, Suhalim JL, Miyazaki-Anzai S, Miyazaki M, Levi M, Potma EO, et al. Identification of cholesterol crystals in plaques of atherosclerotic mice using hyperspectral CARS imaging. J Lipid Res. 2011;52:2177–86.
54. Baumer Y, McCurdy S, Weatherby TM, Mehta NN, Halbherr S, Halbherr P, et al. Hyperlipidemia-induced cholesterol crystal production by endothelial cells promotes atherogenesis. Nat Commun. 2017;8:1129.
55. Kellner-Weibel G, Jerome WG, Small DM, Warner GJ, Stoltenborg JK, Kearney MA, et al. Effects of intracellular free cholesterol accumulation on macrophage viability. Arterioscler Thromb Vasc Biol. 1998;18:423–31.
56. Tangirala RK, Jerome WG, Jones NL, Small DM, Johnson WJ, Glick JM, et al. Formation of cholesterol monohydrate crystals in macrophage-derived foam cells. J Lipid Res. 1994;35:93–104.
57. Guyton JR, Klemp KF. The lipid-rich core region of human atherosclerotic fibrous plaques. Prevalence of small lipid droplets and vesicles by electron microscopy. Am J Pathol. 1989;134:705–17.
58. Libby P, Buring JE, Badimon L, Hansson GK, Deanfield J, Bittencourt MS, et al. Atherosclerosis. Nat Rev Dis Primers. 2019;5:56.
59. Small DM. George Lyman duff memorial lecture. Progression and regression of atherosclerotic lesions. Insights from lipid physical biochemistry. Arteriosclerosis. 1988;8:103–29.
60. Mason RP, Walter MF, Day CA, Jacob RF. Active metabolite of atorvastatin inhibits membrane cholesterol domain formation by an antioxidant mechanism. J Biol Chem. 2006;281:9337–45.
61. Ruocco MJ, Shipley GG. Interaction of cholesterol with galactocerebroside and galactocerebroside-phosphatidylcholine bilayer membranes. Biophys J. 1984;46:695–707.
62. Mason RP, Jacob RF. Eicosapentaenoic acid inhibits glucose-induced membrane cholesterol crystalline domain formation through a potent antioxidant mechanism. Biochim Biophys Acta. 2015;1848:502–9.
63. Craven BM. Crystal structure of cholesterol monohydrate. Nature. 1976;260:727–9.

64. Phillips JE, Geng YJ, Mason RP. 7-Ketocholesterol forms crystalline domains in model membranes and murine aortic smooth muscle cells. Atherosclerosis. 2001;159:125–35.
65. Geng YJ, Phillips JE, Mason RP, Casscells SW. Cholesterol crystallization and macrophage apoptosis: implication for atherosclerotic plaque instability and rupture. Biochem Pharmacol. 2003;66:1485–92.
66. Kellner-Weibel G, Yancey PG, Jerome WG, Walser T, Mason RP, Phillips MC, et al. Crystallization of free cholesterol in model macrophage foam cells. Arterioscler Thromb Vasc Biol. 1999;19:1891–8.
67. Abela GS, Aziz K. Cholesterol crystals rupture biological membranes and human plaques during acute cardiovascular events--a novel insight into plaque rupture by scanning electron microscopy. Scanning. 2006;28:1–10.
68. Abela GS, Aziz K. Cholesterol crystals cause mechanical damage to biological membranes: a proposed mechanism of plaque rupture and erosion leading to arterial thrombosis. Clin Cardiol. 2005;28:413–20.
69. Nidorf SM, Fiolet A, Abela GS. Viewing atherosclerosis through a crystal lens: how the evolving structure of cholesterol crystals in atherosclerotic plaque alters its stability. J Clin Lipidol. 2020;14:619–30.
70. Zimmer S, Grebe A, Bakke SS, Bode N, Halvorsen B, Ulas T, et al. Cyclodextrin promotes atherosclerosis regression via macrophage reprogramming. Sci Transl Med. 2016;8:333ra50.
71. Zhao N, Li CC, Di B, Xu LL. Recent advances in the NEK7-licensed NLRP3 inflammasome activation: mechanisms, role in diseases and related inhibitors. J Autoimmun. 2020;113:102515.
72. Martínez GJ, Celermajer DS, Patel S. The NLRP3 inflammasome and the emerging role of colchicine to inhibit atherosclerosis-associated inflammation. Atherosclerosis. 2018;269:262–71.
73. Rajamäki K, Lappalainen J, Oörni K, Välimäki E, Matikainen S, Kovanen PT, et al. Cholesterol crystals activate the NLRP3 inflammasome in human macrophages: a novel link between cholesterol metabolism and inflammation. PLoS One. 2010;5:e11765.
74. Döring Y, Libby P, Soehnlein O. Neutrophil extracellular traps participate in cardiovascular diseases. Circ Res. 2020;126:1228–41.
75. Warnatsch A, Ioannou M, Wang Q, Papayannopoulos V. Neutrophil extracellular traps license macrophages for cytokine production in atherosclerosis. Science. 2015;349:316–20.
76. Folco EJ, Mawson TL, Vromman A, Bernardes-Souza B, Franck G, Persson O, et al. Neutrophil extracellular traps induce endothelial cell activation and tissue factor production through interleukin-1α and cathepsin G. Arterioscler Thromb Vasc Biol. 2018;38:1901–12.
77. Misawa T, Takahama M, Kozaki T, Lee H, Zou J, Saitoh T, et al. Microtubule-driven spatial arrangement of mitochondria promotes activation of the NLRP3 inflammasome. Nat Immunol. 2013;14:454–60.
78. Nidorf SM, Fiolet ATL, Mosterd A, Eikelboom JW, Schut A, Opstal TSJ, et al. Colchicine in patients with chronic coronary disease. N Engl J Med. 2020;383:1838–47.
79. Nidorf SM, Eikelboom JW, Budgeon CA, Thompson PL. Low-dose colchicine for secondary prevention of cardiovascular disease. J Am Coll Cardiol. 2013;61:404–10.
80. Tardif J-C, Kouz S, Waters DD, Bertrand OF, Diaz R, Maggioni AP, et al. Efficacy and safety of low-dose colchicine after myocardial infarction. N Engl J Med. 2019;381:2497–505.
81. Braeckman RA, Manku MS, Bays HE, Stirtan WG, Soni PN. Icosapent ethyl, a pure EPA omega-3 fatty acid: effects on plasma and red blood cell fatty acids in patients with very high triglyceride levels (results from the MARINE study). Prostaglandins Leukot Essent Fatty Acids. 2013;89:195–201.
82. Braeckman RA, Stirtan WG, Soni PN. Pharmacokinetics of eicosapentaenoic acid in plasma and red blood cells after multiple oral dosing with icosapent ethyl in healthy subjects. Clin Pharmacol Drug Dev. 2014;3:101–8.
83. Sawazaki S, Hamazaki T, Yamazaki K, Taki H, Kaneda M, Yano S, et al. Comparison of the increment in plasma eicosapentaenoate concentrations by fish oil intake between young and middle-aged volunteers. J Nutr Sci Vitaminol (Tokyo). 1989;35:349–59.

84. Subbaiah PV, Kaufman D, Bagdade JD. Incorporation of dietary n-3 fatty acids into molecular species of phosphatidyl choline and cholesteryl ester in normal human plasma. Am J Clin Nutr. 1993;58:360–8.

85. Serhan CN. Novel pro-resolving lipid mediators in inflammation are leads for resolution physiology. Nature. 2014;510:92–101.

86. Sherratt SCR, Mason RP. Eicosapentaenoic acid and docosahexaenoic acid have distinct membrane locations and lipid interactions as determined by X-ray diffraction. Chem Phys Lipids. 2018;212:73–9.

87. Mason RP, Jacob RF, Shrivastava S, Sherratt SCR, Chattopadhyay A. Eicosapentaenoic acid reduces membrane fluidity, inhibits cholesterol domain formation, and normalizes bilayer width in atherosclerotic-like model membranes. Biochim Biophys Acta. 2016;1858:3131–40.

88. Mason RP, Libby P, Bhatt DL. Emerging mechanisms of cardiovascular protection for the omega-3 fatty acid eicosapentaenoic acid. Arterioscler Thromb Vasc Biol. 2020;40:1135–47.

89. Jacobs ML, Faizi HA, Peruzzi JA, Vlahovska PM, Kamat NP. EPA and DHA differentially modulate membrane elasticity in the presence of cholesterol. Biophys J. 2021;120:2317–29.

90. Mason RP, Walter MF, Mason PE. Effect of oxidative stress on membrane structure: Small angle x-ray diffraction analysis. Free Radic Biol Med. 1997;23:419–25.

91. Self-Medlin Y, Byun J, Jacob RF, Mizuno Y, Mason RP. Glucose promotes membrane cholesterol crystalline domain formation by lipid peroxidation. Biochim Biophys Acta. 2009;1788:1398–403.

92. Wratten ML, van-Ginkel G, van't Veld AA, Bekker A, van Faassen EE, Sevanian A. Structural and dynamic effects of oxidatively modified phospholipids in unsaturated lipid membranes. Biochemistry. 1992;31:10901–7.

93. Sherratt SCR, Juliano RA, Mason RP. Eicosapentaenoic acid (EPA) has optimal chain length and degree of unsaturation to inhibit oxidation of small dense LDL and membrane cholesterol domains as compared to related fatty acids in vitro. Biochim Biophys Acta Biomembr. 2020;1862:183254.

94. Mason RP, Sherratt SCR, Jacob RF. Eicosapentaenoic acid inhibits oxidation of ApoB-containing lipoprotein particles of different size *in vitro* when administered alone or in combination with atorvastatin active metabolite compared with other triglyceride-lowering agents. J Cardiovasc Pharmacol. 2016;68:33–40.

95. Bays HE, Ballantyne CM, Braeckman RA, Stirtan WG, Soni PN. Icosapent ethyl, a pure ethyl ester of eicosapentaenoic acid: effects on circulating markers of inflammation from the MARINE and ANCHOR studies. Am J Cardiovasc Drugs. 2013;13:37–46.

96. Shaikh SR. Biophysical and biochemical mechanisms by which dietary N-3 polyunsaturated fatty acids from fish oil disrupt membrane lipid rafts. J Nutr Biochem. 2012;23:101–5.

97. Williams JA, Batten SE, Harris M, Rockett BD, Shaikh SR, Stillwell W, et al. Docosahexaenoic and eicosapentaenoic acids segregate differently between raft and nonraft domains. Biophys J. 2012;103:228–37.

98. Shaikh SR, Kinnun JJ, Leng X, Williams JA, Wassall SR. How polyunsaturated fatty acids modify molecular organization in membranes: insight from NMR studies of model systems. Biochim Biophys Acta. 2015;1848:211–9.

99. Soubias O, Gawrisch K. Docosahexaenoyl chains isomerize on the sub-nanosecond time scale. J Am Chem Soc. 2007;129:6678–9.

100. Jacob RF, Walter MF, Self-Medlin Y, Mason RP. Atorvastatin active metabolite inhibits oxidative modification of small dense low-density lipoprotein. J Cardiovasc Pharmacol. 2013;62:160–6.

101. Aviram M, Rosenblat M, Bisgaier CL, Newton RS. Atorvastatin and gemfibrozil metabolites, but not the parent drugs, are potent antioxidants against lipoprotein oxidation. Atherosclerosis. 1998;138:271–80.

102. Borow KM, Nelson JR, Mason RP. Biologic plausibility, cellular effects, and molecular mechanisms of eicosapentaenoic acid (EPA) in atherosclerosis. Atherosclerosis. 2015;242:357–66.

103. Mason RP, Jacob RF. Membrane microdomains and vascular biology: emerging role in atherogenesis. Circulation. 2003;107:2270–3.

104. Jakus V, Rietbrock N. Advanced glycation end-products and the progress of diabetic vascular complications. Physiol Res. 2004;53:131–42.
105. Pennathur S, Heinecke JW. Mechanisms for oxidative stress in diabetic cardiovascular disease. Antioxid Redox Signal. 2007;9:955–69.
106. Mason RP, Sherratt SCR, Eckel RH. Rationale for different formulations of omega-3 fatty acids leading to differences in residual cardiovascular risk reduction. Metab Clin Exp. 2022;130:130.
107. Bhatt DL, Steg PG, Miller M, Brinton EA, Jacobson TA, Ketchum SB, et al. Cardiovascular risk reduction with icosapent ethyl for hypertriglyceridemia. N Engl J Med. 2019;380:11–22.
108. Bhatt DL, Steg PG, Miller M. Cardiovascular risk reduction with icosapent ethyl. N Engl J Med. 2019;380:1678.
109. Mason RP. New insights into mechanisms of action for omega-3 fatty acids in atherothrombotic cardiovascular disease. Curr Atheroscler Rep. 2019;21:2.
110. Bhatt DL, Steg PG, Miller M, Brinton EA, Jacobson TA, Jiao L, et al. Reduction in first and total ischemic events with icosapent ethyl across baseline triglyceride tertiles. J Am Coll Cardiol. 2019;74:1159–61.
111. Pisaniello AD, Nicholls SJ, Ballantyne CM, Bhatt DL, Wong ND. Eicosapentaenoic acid: atheroprotective properties and the reduction of atherosclerotic cardiovascular disease events. Eur Med J. 2020;5:29–36.
112. Singh N, Bhatt DL, Miller M, Steg PG, Brinton EA, Jacobson TA, et al. Consistency of benefit of Icosapent ethyl by background statin type in REDUCE-IT. J Am Coll Cardiol. 2022;79:220–2.
113. Yokoyama M, Origasa H, Matsuzaki M, Matsuzawa Y, Saito Y, Ishikawa Y, et al. Effects of eicosapentaenoic acid on major coronary events in hypercholesterolaemic patients (JELIS): a randomised open-label, blinded endpoint analysis. Lancet. 2007;369:1090–8.
114. Watanabe T, Ando K, Daidoji H, Otaki Y, Sugawara S, Matsui M, et al. A randomized controlled trial of eicosapentaenoic acid in patients with coronary heart disease on statins. J Cardiol. 2017;70:537–44.
115. Nishio R, Shinke T, Otake H, Nakagawa M, Nagoshi R, Inoue T, et al. Stabilizing effect of combined eicosapentaenoic acid and statin therapy on coronary thin-cap fibroatheroma. Atherosclerosis. 2014;234:114–9.
116. Budoff MJ, Bhatt DL, Kinninger A, Lakshmanan S, Muhlestein JB, Le VT, et al. Effect of icosapent ethyl on progression of coronary atherosclerosis in patients with elevated triglycerides on statin therapy: final results of the EVAPORATE trial. Eur Heart J. 2020;41:3925–32.
117. Alfaddagh A, Elajami TK, Ashfaque H, Saleh M, Bistrian BR, Welty FK. Effect of eicosapentaenoic and docosahexaenoic acids added to statin therapy on coronary artery plaque in patients with coronary artery disease: a randomized clinical trial. J Am Heart Assoc. 2017;6:6.
118. Aung T, Halsey J, Kromhout D, Gerstein HC, Marchioli R, Tavazzi L, et al. Associations of omega-3 fatty acid supplement use with cardiovascular disease risks: meta-analysis of 10 trials involving 77 917 individuals. JAMA Cardiol. 2018;3:225–33.
119. Group ASC, Bowman L, Mafham M, Wallendszus K, Stevens W, Buck G, et al. Effects of n-3 fatty acid supplements in diabetes mellitus. N Engl J Med. 2018;379:1540–50.
120. Manson JE, Cook NR, Lee IM, Christen W, Bassuk SS, Mora S, et al. Marine n-3 fatty acids and prevention of cardiovascular disease and cancer. N Engl J Med. 2018;380:23–32.
121. Kalstad AA, Myhre PL, Laake K, Tveit SH, Schmidt EB, Smith P, et al. Effects of n-3 fatty acid supplements in elderly patients after myocardial infarction: a randomized, controlled trial. Circulation. 2021;143:528–39.
122. Nicholls SJ, Lincoff AM, Garcia M, Bash D, Ballantyne CM, Barter PJ, et al. Effect of high-dose Omega-3 fatty acids vs corn oil on major adverse cardiovascular events in patients at high cardiovascular risk: the STRENGTH randomized clinical trial. JAMA. 2020;324:2268–80.
123. Elam MB, Ginsberg HN, Lovato LC, Corson M, Largay J, Leiter LA, et al. Association of fenofibrate therapy with long-term cardiovascular risk in statin-treated patients with type 2 diabetes. JAMA Cardiol. 2017;2:370–80.

124. Effects of combination lipid therapy in type 2 diabetes mellitus. N Engl J Med. 2010;362:1563–74.
125. Effects of extended-release niacin with laropiprant in high-risk patients. N Engl J Med. 2014;371:203–12.
126. Niacin in patients with low HDL cholesterol levels receiving intensive statin therapy. N Engl J Med. 2011;365:2255–67.
127. Pradhan AD, Paynter NP, Everett BM, Glynn RJ, Amarenco P, Elam M, et al. Rationale and design of the pemafibrate to reduce cardiovascular outcomes by reducing triglycerides in patients with diabetes (PROMINENT) study. Am Heart J. 2018;206:80–93.
128. Das Pradhan A, Glynn RJ, Fruchart JC, MacFadyen JG, Zaharris ES, Everett BM, et al. Triglyceride lowering with pemafibrate to reduce cardiovascular risk. N Engl J Med. 2022;387:1923–34.
129. Ference BA, Kastelein JJP, Ray KK, Ginsberg HN, Chapman MJ, Packard CJ, et al. Association of triglyceride-lowering LPL variants and LDL-C–lowering LDLR variants with risk of coronary heart disease. JAMA. 2019;321:364–73.
130. Bhatt DL, Budoff MJ, Mason RP. A revolution in Omega-3 fatty acid research*. J Am Coll Cardiol. 2020;76:2098–101.
131. Kita Y, Watanabe M, Kamon D, Ueda T, Soeda T, Okayama S, et al. Effects of fatty acid therapy in addition to strong statin on coronary plaques in acute coronary syndrome: an optical coherence tomography study. J Am Heart Assoc. 2020;9:e015593.
132. Motoyama S, Nagahara Y, Sarai M, Kawai H, Miyajima K, Sato Y, et al. Effect of Omega-3 fatty acids on coronary plaque morphology - a serial computed tomography angiography study. Circ J. 2021;86:831.
133. Hansen TV, Vik A, Serhan CN. The protectin family of specialized pro-resolving mediators: potent immunoresolvents enabling innovative approaches to target obesity and diabetes. Front Pharmacol. 2019;9:1582.
134. Arita M, Yoshida M, Hong S, Tjonahen E, Glickman JN, Petasis NA, et al. Resolvin E1, an endogenous lipid mediator derived from omega-3 eicosapentaenoic acid, protects against 2,4,6-trinitrobenzene sulfonic acid-induced colitis. Proc Natl Acad Sci. 2005;102:7671–6.
135. Nishizaki Y, Shimada K, Tani S, Ogawa T, Ando J, Takahashi M, et al. Significance of imbalance in the ratio of serum n-3 to n-6 polyunsaturated fatty acids in patients with acute coronary syndrome. Am J Cardiol. 2014;113:441–5.
136. Ballantyne CM, Manku MS, Bays HE, Philip S, Granowitz C, Doyle RT, et al. Icosapent ethyl effects on fatty acid profiles in statin-treated patients with high triglycerides: the randomized, placebo-controlled ANCHOR study. Cardiol Ther. 2019;8:79–90.
137. Nakajima K, Yamashita T, Kita T, Takeda M, Sasaki N, Kasahara K, et al. Orally administered eicosapentaenoic acid induces rapid regression of atherosclerosis via modulating the phenotype of dendritic cells in LDL receptor-deficient mice. Arterioscler Thromb Vasc Biol. 2011;31:1963–72.
138. Sato T, Horikawa M, Takei S, Yamazaki F, Ito TK, Kondo T, et al. Preferential incorporation of administered eicosapentaenoic acid into thin-cap atherosclerotic plaques. Arterioscler Thromb Vasc Biol. 2019;39:1802–16.
139. Williams MC, Kwiecinski J, Doris M, McElhinney P, D'Souza MS, Cadet S, et al. Low-attenuation noncalcified plaque on coronary computed tomography angiography predicts myocardial infarction. Circulation. 2020;141:1452–62.

Part VII

Interaction of CCs with Other Crystalloids and Disease Conditions

Uric Acid in Inflammation and the Pathogenesis of Atherosclerosis: Lessons for Cholesterol from the Land of Gout

Binita Shah, Gary Ho, Sonal Pruthi, Michael Toprover, and Michael H. Pillinger

1 Introduction

Gout is a chronic, inflammatory, crystal-driven condition and patients who suffer from it have increased cardiovascular risk and related comorbidities [1–3]. The biology and management of gout may therefore provide insights relevant to understanding the role that inflammation and other mechanisms play in cardiovascular disease (CVD) both among patients with gout and in the general population. The fact that both gout and CVD are driven in part by crystals [monosodium urate (MSU) for gout, cholesterol for CVD] underline potential similarities and lessons to be learned. Here, we provide an overview of gout, its mechanisms of action and inflammation, and possible lessons for how crystals and chronic inflammation contribute to CVD.

B. Shah · S. Pruthi
Division of Cardiology, NYU Grossman School of Medicine, New York, NY, USA

Section of Cardiology, Margaret Cochran Corbin Campus of the New York Harbor Health Care System, United States Department of Veterans Affairs, Washington, DC, USA

G. Ho · M. Toprover · M. H. Pillinger (✉)
Division of Rheumatology, NYU Grossman School of Medicine, New York, NY, USA

Section of Rheumatology, Margaret Cochran Corbin Campus of the New York Harbor Health Care System, United States Department of Veterans Affairs, Washington, DC, USA
e-mail: Michael.Pillinger@nyulangone.org

G. S. Abela, S. M. Nidorf (eds.), *Cholesterol Crystals in Atherosclerosis and Other Related Diseases*, Contemporary Cardiology,
https://doi.org/10.1007/978-3-031-41192-2_18

2 Gout and Inflammation

2.1 *Overview*

Gout is the most common inflammatory arthritis, affecting approximately 4% of the adult US population [4]. The sine qua non of gout is systemic hyperuricemia, which on a biochemical basis is defined as serum urate (SU) $\geq$6.8 mg/dL, the solubility point at which urate precipitates into MSU crystals at pH 7.4 [5]. Alternative, population-based definitions of hyperuricemia set the threshold as SU two standard deviations or greater above the mean, or typically as >7.0 mg dL in men and >6.0 mg/dL in women. Epidemiologic studies establish the prevalence of hyperuricemia in the USA at approximately 20% of the adult population [4]; estimates around the world vary [6]. When individuals experience hyperuricemia for an extended time, they gradually accrue MSU crystals in tissues, most typically on the surface of cartilage. Eventually, these crystals can trigger the acute, excruciatingly painful inflammatory attacks known as gout flares. The biology of the gout flare is increasingly well understood and reviewed below; the onset of a first gout flare signals the transition from the so-called asymptomatic hyperuricemia to a diagnosis of gout. Early gout flares tend to occur in the first metatarsal phalangeal joint and other joints of the lower extremities; later attacks may occur in almost any joint and may be polyarticular. During flares, inflammatory markers such as C-reactive protein and the erythrocyte sedimentation rate rise precipitously. Even without treatment, early gout flares typically self-resolve in a matter of weeks. It was previously thought that the periods between flares (intercritical periods) represented gouty quiescence; it is now appreciated that between flares most gout patients are subject to low, subclinical levels of chronic ongoing systemic inflammation, presumed to be driven by low-level responses to persistent MSU crystal deposition. If not properly managed, flares become more frequent, and may eventually coalesce into chronic joint swelling and pain. In addition to flares, poorly managed gout patients may experience the formation of nodule-like accretions of MSU crystals, or tophi, in and around joints and soft tissue structures. Tophi are complex structures that include a surrounding inflammatory rind composed of mixed populations of lymphocytes, macrophages and histiocytes, and neutrophils. Tophi also serve as reservoirs of monosodium urate (total body urate burden) that may resist dissolution, and/or support persistent SU levels even as urate lowering drugs are instituted (Fig. 1).

2.2 *Mechanisms of Hyperuricemia*

Hyperuricemic individuals can be broadly categorized into overproducers of urate, underexcreters of urate, or a combination of both. To understand hyperuricemia and its associated pathogenic mechanisms, it is crucial to first examine purine metabolism (Fig. 2). The catabolic end-product of purine nucleic acids (e.g., adenine and

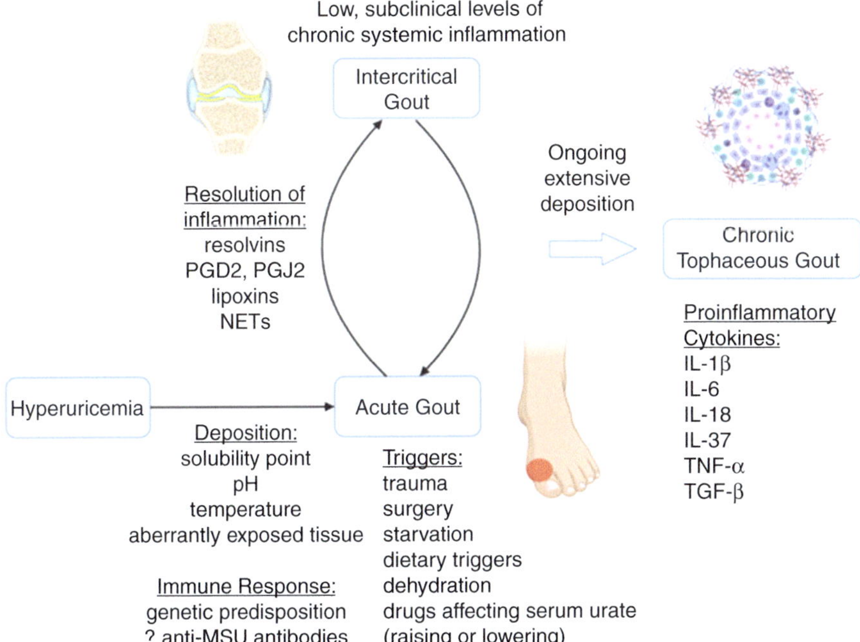

Fig. 1 Hyperuricemia to Gout. The progression from hyperuricemia to the various phases of gout is depicted from left to right. High serum urate levels under the appropriate conditions will deposit within tissues and joints as monosodium urate (MSU), most commonly of the surface of cartilage. Progression to acute gout is characterized by an acute immune response against the MSU, with numerous factors potentially contributing to the hyperuricemia-gout transition. Intercritical gout is defined as the period between gout flares, and characterized by persistence of and potential for accumulating of MSU deposition (depicted in yellow on the surface of the knee cartilage) with associated subclinical inflammation. Chronic tophaceous gout develops in the setting uncontrolled hyperuricemia and extensive MSU deposition. The tophus, which is the hallmark of this stage, houses a microenvironment that promotes the cellular secretion of pro-inflammatory cytokines and induces both local and systemic inflammation, as well as bone and cartilage erosion. (Created with BioRender)

guanine) is uric acid. Thus, the production of urate mainly stems from the degradation of exogenously consumed dietary, and/or endogenously synthesized, purine compounds, which occurs in all cells but is most prevalent in hepatocytes. Dietary sources rich in purine precursors include organ meats and other animal and seafood sources, and beer (owing to its high content of hops) [7]. Accelerated hepatic ATP (adenosine triphosphate) turnover triggered by metabolism of alcohol and/or fructose, along with increased nucleotide turnover in myeloproliferative and lymphoproliferative disorders, are examples of endogenous sources of urate production; a small minority of patients possess genetic mutations that lead to accelerated urate production and are considered primary overproducers. Degradation of purine mononucleotides generates hypoxanthine. Xanthine oxidase catalyzes the conversion of hypoxanthine to xanthine, and xanthine to uric acid [8]. Evolutionarily, humans

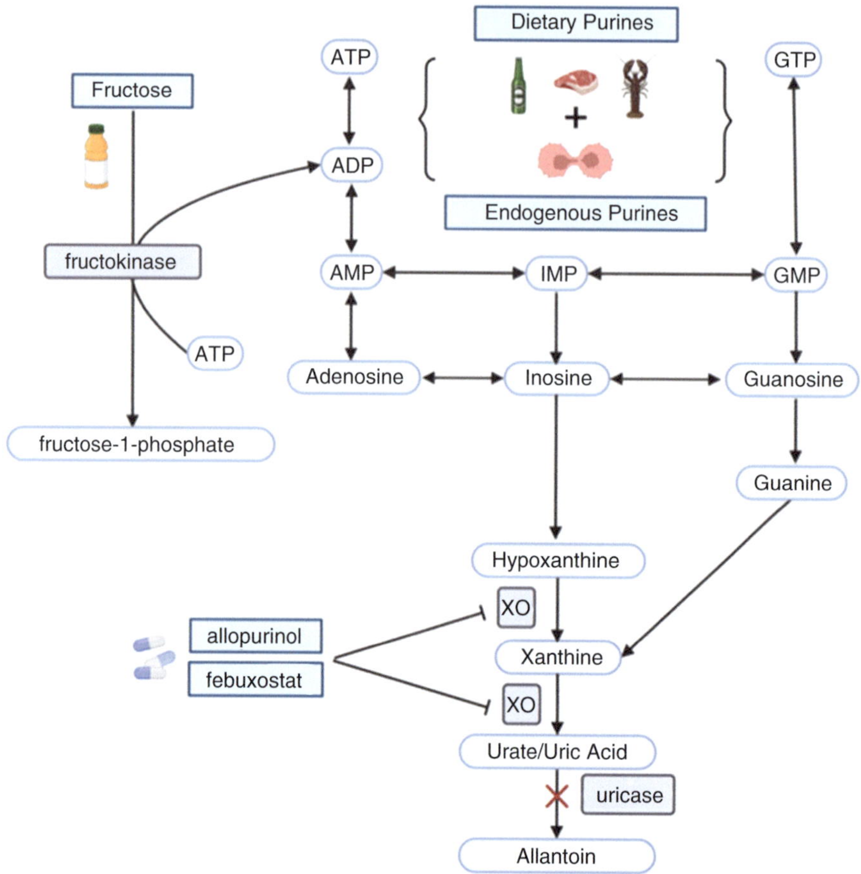

Fig. 2 Purine Catabolic Pathway. Dietary and endogenously synthesized purines are sources of purine nucleotides and purines that feed into this metabolic pathway. The nucleotides adenosine triphosphate (ATP) and guanosine triphosphate (GTP) are dephosphorylated into adenosine monophosphate (AMP) and guanosine monophosphate (GMP) respectively. Inosine monophosphate (IMP) serves as an intermediate nucleotide during the de novo purine synthesis. Nucleotides are metabolized into their respective nucleosides (i.e., adenosine, inosine, and guanosine), nucleobases (e.g., guanine), and subsequently the urate precursors hypoxanthine and xanthine. Xanthine oxidase (XO) catalyzes the oxidation of hypoxanthine to xanthine, and xanthine to uric acid. Inhibition of xanthine oxidase has been one of the main therapeutic targets in gout to lower serum urate (e.g., allopurinol, febuxostat). The left side of the figure depicts how the dietary intake of fructose rapidly depletes ATP and contributes to an excess of purine precursors. (Created with BioRender)

have lost their capacity to produce a functional final enzyme, uricase, that is still present in other mammals, who retain the ability to convert highly insoluble uric acid to the readily excretable allantoin. Thus, humans have higher levels of SU than all other mammals. The inhibition of xanthine oxidase by allopurinol or febuxostat is an effective means of lowering urate, and may also reduce oxidant burden since urate production is accompanied by oxidant generation [7].

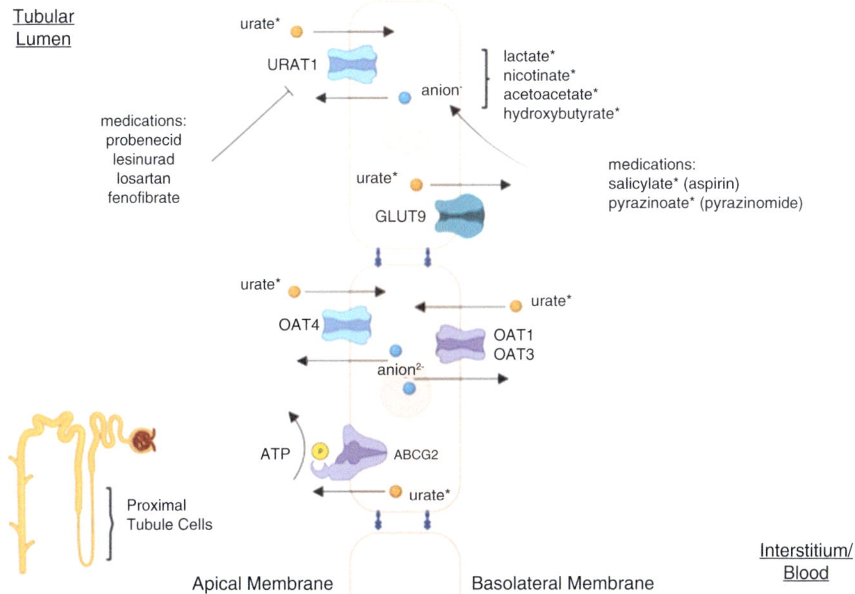

Fig. 3 Urate Handling at the Proximal Tubule, Reabsorption and Secretion. This cartoon depicts key transporters of uric acid in the proximal tubule. URAT1 is a principal anion transporter responsible for uric acid reabsorption through the apical membrane. Uric acid is exchanged with anions such as lactate and hydroxybutyrate via URAT1, which in pathophysiologic states of acidosis may lead to hyperuricemia. Low-dose aspirin and pyrazinamide are also known to contribute to hyperuricemia through facilitating urate/anion exchange. The medications probenecid and losartan competitively inhibit URAT1, thus inducing uricosuria and lowering serum urate. AGBC2, present in the gut and kidneys, is an ATP-driven urate-excreting pump; reduced activity of ABCG2 leads to hyperuricemia. Other proximal tubule urate transporters (e.g., GLUT9, OAT1, OAT3, and OAT4) are recognized to facilitate urate secretion and reabsorption at the proximal tubule. (Created with BioRender)

Underexcretion of urate is the primary driver of hyperuricemia in up to 90% of hyperuricemic individuals (Fig. 3). The kidneys secrete roughly two-thirds of the total body urate load while the gut secretes about one-third. Urate in the kidneys is freely filtered by the glomerulus (with glomerular insufficiency leading to rises in SU levels), but only a fraction of filtered urate is excreted since most is subject to proximal tubule reabsorption. Well-defined transporters that regulate uric acid transport at the proximal tubule apical membrane include URAT1 (encoded by *SLC22A12*), a urate-anion exchanger that promotes reabsorption, and ABCG2/BRCP (encoded by the *ABCG2* gene), an ATP-driven efflux pump that promotes glomerulus-independent excretion. Such transporters are influenced by pathophysiologic states and medications, leading to anti-uricosuric (e.g., lactic acidosis, ketoacidosis, pyrazinamide) and pro-uricosuric effects (e.g., probenecid, lesinurad) [8].

Genome-wide association studies (GWAS) strongly support a genetic component to hyperuricemia, with most GWAS data to date identifying genes that relate to renal urate handling rather than urate generation [9]. For example, single nucleotide polymorphisms (SNPs) in *SLC22A12*, *SLC2A9,* and *ABCG2* genes have been associated with variance in SU levels across populations in multiple countries [10]. In the gut, urate excretion is less responsive to SU than in the kidneys, but in the setting of chronic kidney disease gut excretion may play a bigger role, with the ABCG2 efflux pump again contributing significantly. Furthermore, the gut microbiota and their metabolites have been the focus of recent translational research as a contributor to SU, through intraluminal nucleotide salvage, de novo purine biosynthesis, and the catabolism of purine precursors [11].

2.3 Effects of Soluble Urate on Inflammation

Although many physicians think of gout as being entirely crystal-mediated, an extensive body of literature indicates that soluble, non-crystalline urate may have multiple effects both on the vasculature and on the mechanisms of inflammation and innate immunity. Evidence suggests that intracellular urate, whether produced endogenously within the cells, or taken up by cells via transporters, may have profound effects. Consistent with a role for soluble urate in inflammation, asymptomatic hyperuricemia, even in the absence of gout, has been shown to be an independent risk factor for CVD, albeit at a lower level than is the case for gout [12]. Asymptomatic hyperuricemia in patients with established cardiac disease therefore deserves consideration as a disease accelerant. Moreover, the ability of one soluble molecule (urate) to impact inflammation suggests the possibility that others, for example uremic toxins that are often found in patients with chronic kidney disease–and, like urate, stimulate both oxidant effects and caspase-1 activation–could do so as well [13–16].

Soluble urate acts directly on vascular cells. Exposure of endothelial cells to soluble urate—at both supersaturated and unsaturated concentrations, and in a dose-dependent manner—inhibits the ability of those endothelial cells to produce nitric oxide and other vasodilators, potentially impairing vascular function [17]. On the other hand, soluble urate promotes the proliferation of vascular smooth muscle cells [18]. Thus, exposure of the vasculature to soluble urate may result in a "muscle bound" state wherein endothelial cells have less vasodilator capacity, and the vascular smooth muscle is hyperproliferative and less responsive to vasodilator signals. In this context, recent studies suggest that urate lowering with xanthine oxidase inhibitors may restore impaired vasodilator capacity in gout patients. Specifically, patients with gout have impaired brachial artery endothelial responsiveness compared to healthy controls, but guideline-concordant treatment including allopurinol can significantly restore responsiveness toward normal levels [19, 20]. Finally, although urate is biochemically an anti-oxidant, when taken up in endothelial cells via transporters the evidence shows that it may drive pathways that lead to oxidative stress [21].

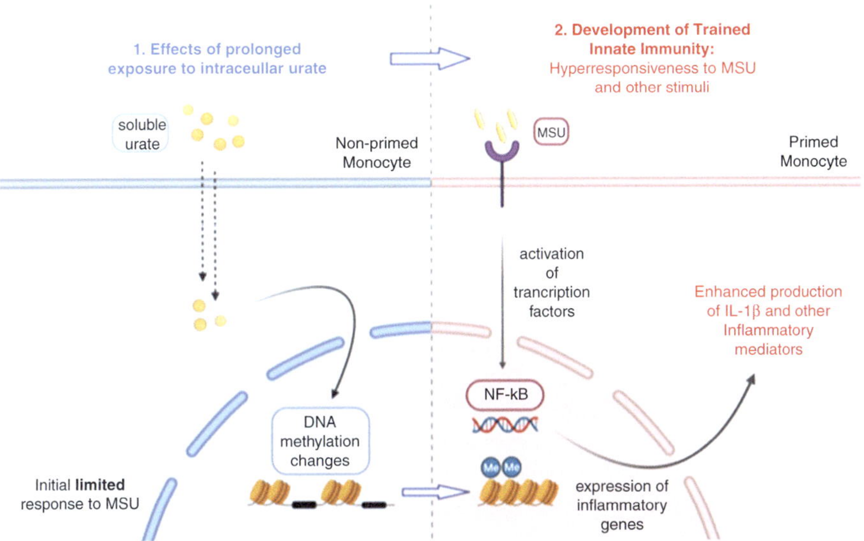

Fig. 4 Soluble Urate-induced Trained Innate Immunity. The left portion of the figure depicts a non-primed peripheral blood mononuclear cell (PBMC), which will develop a self-limited inflammatory response during its initial exposure to monosodium urate (MSU) crystals. In the setting of prolonged hyperuricemia, intracellular urate induces DNA methylation changes, thus priming the monocyte for subsequent exposure to MSU crystals. The right portion of the figure depicts trained innate immunity, where the PBMC has been epigenetically modified and becomes hyperresponsive to MSU and/or other stimuli. Upon subsequent interactions with MSU crystals, there is a more robust inflammatory response characterized by enhance secretion of IL-1β and other mediators. (Created with BioRender)

Intriguing recent work suggests an alternative and potentially important pro-inflammatory effect of soluble urate on leukocytes and endothelial cells (Fig. 4). In studies by Joosten et al., in vitro exposure of peripheral blood mononuclear cells or enriched monocytes to high concentrations of soluble urate resulted in alterations in DNA methylation, which were also seen in patients with hyperuricemia but not those with normouricemia, and the genes that undergo methylation changes include a number relevant to inflammatory signaling. Strikingly, subsequent exposure of these leukocytes to MSU crystals resulted in enhanced production of IL-1ß and other inflammatory responses [22]. Thus, persistently high levels of SU (hyperuricemia) may prime leukocytes (innate immune training) for future inflammatory responses to crystal stimulation and may provide a model for the progression and worsening of gout over time. Importantly, these cells also are primed for increased inflammatory responses to other stimuli, suggesting a possible impact of hyperuricemia on inflammation and CVD even in the absence of gout [23]. The process of epigenetic modification, while potentially reversible, creates durable changes that may be slow to resolve, and/or require longer management to undo [24]. The accrual of such changes over time suggests at least one explanation for the fact that gout severity tends to progress, and be harder to treat, if the disease is not adequately managed early.

2.4 From Asymptomatic Hyperuricemia to Gout: Factors in Crystallization

In contrast to cholesterol, the formation of MSU into graceful, diclinic needle-shaped crystals typically occurs extracellularly, and involves several factors that are well appreciated and common to all forms of crystallization. Concentration clearly plays a role in crystal formation, and the risk of gout increases with higher levels of SU. Thus, patients with asymptomatic hyperuricemia are more likely to experience MSU formation and deposition, and subsequent gout, at higher levels of SU. Recent studies by Dalbeth et al. indicate that for patients with SU levels just above the saturation point, the probability of developing gout is approximately 10% over 10 years, whereas for individuals with SU greater than 12 mg/dL, the probability rises to about 50%; still, the risk of progression to gout is never 100%, indicating that other factors must be involved [25]. Among these, as expected, are pH and temperature. As noted above, the most common first location for a gout attack is in the first metatarsal phalangeal joint of the toe, which as the structure most distal from the heart in the circulatory system, and with a large surface-to-volume ratio, is prone to lower pH and cooler temperatures [5].

Most crystallization processes occur around the formation of seed crystals. In the case of gout, the identity of such seed crystals is not known. However, the fact that MSU crystals tend to form or deposit predominantly within tissues and joints suggests that various tissue components, particularly when aberrantly expressed or exposed, may serve as nidi for crystal formation [5]. In this regard, it has long been recognized that gout and/or MSU deposition is more common in joints that are affected by osteoarthritis, particularly in the distal interphalangeal joints [26]. Some investigators have suggested that the decortication of osteoarthritic cartilage exposes the synovial fluid to deeper layers characterized by the presence of type 4 chondroitin sulfate, which provide a surface that promotes MSU crystallization [27].

It is also possible that multiple crystal types may promote each other's crystallization. In patients whose joints are aspirated during acute flares, it is not uncommon to find both MSU and calcium pyrophosphate crystals in the synovial fluid; whether one promotes the other, or vice-versa, is intriguing to consider. In the urine, where microcrystal formation may contribute to kidney stones, the presence of hyperuricemia and microscopic urinary uric acid crystals has been associated not only with uric acid stones, but also with calcium and struvite stones, suggesting that uric acid crystals may serve as nidi for other crystals. Whether similar phenomena occur in the vasculature, with cholesterol and/or calcium crystals promoting MSU crystallization, or vice-versa, is not known.

One of the more intriguing observations about the mechanisms of MSU crystal formation has come from studies suggesting that urate crystallization may be at least in part immune mediated. In vitro, supersaturated solutions urate at pH 7.4 crystallize slowly, over weeks. However, when mice were repeatedly injected with MSU crystals, fractionation of the serum revealed an immunoglobulin-rich fraction that, when added in vitro to supersaturated urate solutions, accelerated the precipitation of MSU crystals [28]. In other studies, similar results were obtained in a rabbit model, and using an immunoglobulin fraction isolated from the synovial fluid of gout patients but not non-gout controls [29]. These observations suggest that over an extended period of exposure to MSU crystals (e.g., as in longstanding gout), an immune reaction to MSU crystals may develop, wherein anti-MSU crystal antibodies might serve as a catalyst, or at least a stabilizer for further MSU crystallization. Such an observation could explain, at least in part, the fact that when not properly treated, gout over time tends to become more severe and treatment resistant, with more frequent flares and more deposition of crystals in situ. Overall, however, the process of MSU crystallization is not well understood, and aside from controlling SU levels, strategies for modulating the crystallization process have not yet been pursued, in contrast to studies intended to modulate the crystallization of cystine in kidney stones [30, 31]. Cholesterol crystal formation shares similar issues with regard to saturation, pH, and temperature and inflammatory response with NLRP3 [32, 33].

2.5 Biology of the Gout Flare: Triggering of the Acute Inflammatory Response, Role of the Inflammasome

In murine models, MSU is recognized as a danger-associated molecular signal (DAMP), provoking immune responses to dying (e.g., infected, cancerous) cells [34]. In gout, the precipitation of extracellular MSU provokes a localized, inflammatory response driven by the innate immune system and characterized by neutrophil influx and the production of pro-inflammatory cytokines, including IL-1β and IL-18 (Fig. 5). The inflammatory cascade within joints and potentially other tissues is initiated by resident macrophages, in what is currently appreciated to be a two-step process. First, MSU crystals are recognized through pathogen recognition receptors (PRRs) such as toll-like receptors on the surface of resident macrophages (Signal 1), triggering the production of pro-IL1β and pro-IL-18. Second, MSU crystals are phagocytosed and subsequently escape their phagolysosomes, causing potassium efflux and creation of reactive oxygen species via NADPH oxidase (Signal 2). These latter events trigger the assembly of the nucleotide-binding and oligomerization domain (NOD)-like receptor family pyrin domain containing 3 (NLRP3) inflammasome within macrophages. Inflammasomes are multiprotein complexes primarily found in myeloid cells that function as intracellular sensors. The oligomerization of NLRP3 triggers the aggregation and cleavage of the enzyme pro-caspase 1 into its active form, caspase-1. Caspase-1 then cleaves pro-IL-1β and pro-IL18, leading the cell to activate and secrete these cytokines. Under alternative conditions, the NLRP3 inflammasome also activates gasdermin D, inducing pyroptosis (inflammatory cell death) through the formation of plasma membrane pores, leading to cytokine and danger signal release, and cell lysis [35, 36].

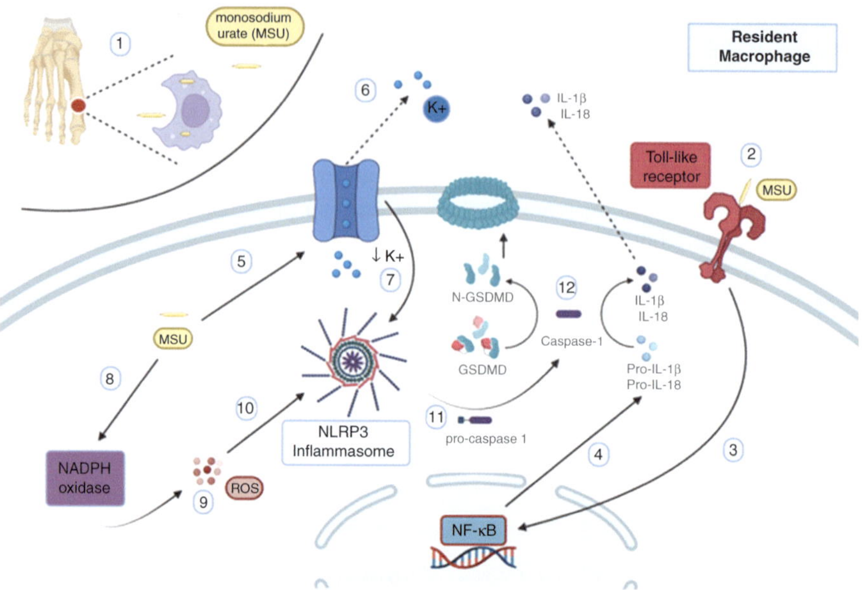

Fig. 5 Monosodium Urate and the Inflammasome. The top left of the figure depicts resident synovial macrophage phagocytosing monosodium urate (MSU) crystals at the site of a gout flare (1). Under certain circumstances toll-like receptors recognize MSU crystals as a danger signal (2), activating the NF-kB pathway (3) and triggering the production of pro-IL-1β and pro-IL-18 (4) (Signal 1). Phagocytosed MSU crystals escape from their phagolysosomes, inducing potassium efflux, resulting in decreased intracellular potassium concentrations (5–7), as well as activating the NADPH oxidase and leading to the generation of reactive oxygen species (ROS) (8, 9). These trigger the oligomerization of the NLRP3 inflammasome (10) (Signal 2). Caspase-1 becomes activated (11), and cleaves pro-IL-1β to active IL-1β, and pro-IL-18 into active IL-18 (12). Caspase-1 can also cleave and activate gasdermin (GSDMD) to release its pore-forming amino-terminal domain (N-GSDMD) (12). (Created with BioRender)

Once generated, IL-1β acts in an autocrine and paracrine manner to amplify the gouty inflammatory cascade. Key actions include inducing fever, stimulating RANK-ligand release and bone resorption, hepatic production of acute phase reactants, and activation of macrophages, neutrophils and endothelial cells to promote neutrophil adhesion and influx, trigger other cytokines and inflammatory mediators (e.g., IL-6, TNFα, prostaglandins), and drive Th17 differentiation [37, 38]. These observations place IL-1β front and center in the inflammatory response to MSU. Importantly for the current context, recent studies have similarly underlined the importance of IL-1β as a participant in CVD, as discussed further below and elsewhere in this volume.

Although MSU crystals are perhaps the most potent of crystal inflammation stimuli, their ability to activate the inflammasome is shared by a number of other crystals, including calcium pyrophosphate dihydrate [39]. These mechanisms also apply to cholesterol crystals [33] (which are known to be pro-inflammatory in olecranon bursae, pericardial and synovial fluid of patients with rheumatoid arthritis

[40]), potentially identifying yet another link between the inflammatory states of gout and CVD. Interestingly, both gout flares and myocardial infarctions are more likely to occur in the morning, although gout flares peak at 2–5 AM and myocardial infarctions peak somewhat later [41, 42]. Despite minor timing differences, these observations suggest circadian commonalities in crystal formation or exposure, or inflammatory responses that warrant further study.

2.6   Between Flares: The Role of Articular Urate Deposition in Chronic Systemic Inflammation

For centuries, gout was presumed to be exclusively an intermittent disease, and that between attacks—in the *intercritical period*—the organism returned to a state of non-inflammatory equilibrium. Indeed, during the intercritical period MSU crystals can still be found, usually at lower concentrations, in the now relatively uninflamed joint, suggesting that other factors, possibly including protein or lipid adherence, may regulate the phlogistic capacity of MSU crystals. Nonetheless, recent evidence indicates that in addition to hyperuricemia, other active processes go on intercritically. Advanced imaging has revealed that MSU deposition persists on cartilage between flares—and that MSU deposition on cartilage often occurs early, in the setting of asymptomatic hyperuricemia. Howard et al. used musculoskeletal ultrasound to compare the knee and first MTP joints of patients with intercritical gout, asymptomatic hyperuricemia, or neither, and found that whereas 50% of gout patients had evidence of MSU deposition on cartilage in these structures, 29% of asymptomatic hyperuricemics did as well [43]. Similarly, Dalbeth et al. employed dual energy CT (DECT) to assess for MSU deposition in the feet of 58 subjects, reporting that while 79–84% of gout patients demonstrated MSU deposits, so did 24% of asymptomatic hyperuricemics [44]. Since MSU deposition appears to correlate with low-level inflammation (including the fact that patients with intercritical gout tend towards mildly to moderately elevated baseline inflammatory markers), these observations suggest that MSU on cartilage serves as an engine of "quiet" inflammation, and underline the fact that inflammation must be thought of as both a local and a systemic process. In this case, MSU on cartilage, and perhaps on other tissues, may generate a chronic, low-level local inflammatory state whose effects are felt elsewhere in the body, potentially including in the cardiovascular system.

2.7   Resolution of the Gout Flare: Lessons for Controlling Inflammation

The fact that gout flares can self-resolve implies that regulatory processes exist to hold inflammation in check and may offer insight into potential novel targets for chronic inflammation in both gout and CVD. Multiple anti-inflammatory molecules, including resolvins [45], have been reported to play a role in gout flare resolution. Interestingly, animal models suggest that some of the pro-inflammatory mechanism that promote gout flares may also have anti-inflammatory capacities, underlining the importance of context and timing in inflammatory disease. For example, although prostaglandins are generally thought of as pro-inflammatory lipids, several, including PGD_2 and PGJ_2 are largely anti-inflammatory and may serve to turn inflammation off. Even PGE_2, generally recognized as pro-inflammatory, has been reported in some models to play an anti-inflammatory role once the flare has reached its peak. One possibility is that PGE_2 tends to become anti-inflammatory once intracellular inflammatory pathways (such as NF-κB) are upregulated, providing late targets for PGE_2 inhibition [46]. Bannenberg and Serhan additionally suggest that, once the process of inflammation has resulted in the co-localization of several diverse cell types (e.g., macrophages, eosinophils or neutrophils, in combination with neutrophils and platelets, and endothelial cells or platelets), these may exert a coordinated, transcellular metabolism to "hijack" cyclooxygenase 2 and allow its products to be acted on by other enzymes, to produce anti-inflammatory lipoxins rather than the typical PGE_2 produced early in inflammation [47]. Thus, at least in the acute setting, the choice and timing of anti-inflammatory therapy may be as important as the target. Interestingly, aspirin has the capacity to trigger a similar process and generate lipoxins, suggesting a possible anti-inflammatory alternative mechanism to platelet COX-1 inhibition for its cardiovascular benefit. Another example of an anti-inflammatory effect of an often-pro-inflammatory process is that of neutrophil extracellular traps (NETs). NETs are a product of highly-stimulated and/or dying neutrophils and consist of extruded chromatin decorated with neutrophil catalytic enzymes such as elastase and myeloperoxidase. The impact of NETs is complex. In infection they serve to trap and degrade microorganisms, but NETs may also contribute to autoimmunity. For example, in systemic lupus they serve as autoantigens (DNA), drive cytokine production, and induce renal cell death [48]. In gout on the other hand, the generation of large aggregated NETs by activated neutrophils has been shown to promote flare abrogation, mainly through the degradation of cytokines by NET-associated serine proteases [49]. The role of NETs in CVD is less clear, but NETs accumulate in the vulnerable regions of human carotid erosion-like and rupture-prone (but not stable) plaque [50]. Although the role of NETs in acute myocardial infarction remains incompletely elucidated, luminal NETs appear to adhere to damaged endothelium, other leukocytes and platelets, causing endothelial dysfunction, increased inflammatory activity, and thrombus formation [51, 52]. Indeed, NET burden is significantly elevated in thrombi aspirated from patients with AMI, and thrombus NET burden correlates with infarct [52]. Thus, in contrast to gout, in CVD NETs may represent a novel therapeutic target.

2.8   Tophi as a Special Case: The Effect of Massive MSU Deposition on Chronic Inflammation

A tophus is a collection of MSU crystals surrounded by a granuloma-like inflammatory response by the immune system, similar to a chronic foreign body [53]. Tophi are a hallmark of more advanced, chronic gout, and can be found periarticularly, adjacent to tendons, in bursae (e.g., the olecranon bursa), in the pulps of the fingertips, in the earlobe and rarely in other locations (see below) [54]. Their morphology would seem to mimic the composition of an atheromatous plaque, with cholesterol crystals forming within the plaque core and inflammatory cell infiltration, including macrophages and lymphocytes that may lead to plaque instability [55].

Tophi are composed of three distinct zones [56]. In the center, a core of MSU crystals is interspersed sparsely with inflammatory cells. Surrounding the MSU core is a hypercellular corona zone, which in turn is surrounded by a fibrovascular zone. Both outer zones contain a variety of inflammatory cells, predominantly macrophages, neutrophils, histiocytes, plasma cells, and T and B lymphocytes [57]. These cells release various pro-inflammatory cytokines including IL-1β, IL-6, and TNFα, as well as anti-inflammatory/pro-fibrotic cytokines such as transforming growth factor-β [57, 58]. Thus, the tophus effectively functions as a granuloma, with similar although non-identical clinical impact to other granulomatous diseases. When present adjacent to bone, tophi drive both mechanical damage and enzymatic erosion, leading to the classic punched-out lesions seen on X-rays of patients with advanced gout. In particular, elucidation of RANK-ligand by tophi activates osteoclasts to resorb bone matrix.

In addition to local inflammatory changes, there is evidence of increased elevation of systemic inflammation in tophaceous gout. Cavalcanti and colleagues found an association between the presence of tophi and serum IL-6 levels and in a group of gout patients, compared with control patients without gout [59]. IL-6 is a pro-inflammatory cytokine released by macrophages and monocytes that stimulates hepatic production of acute phase reactants including C-reactive protein (CRP), serum amyloid A (SAA), fibrinogen, and haptoglobin [60], which in turn promote further systemic inflammation. (IL-6 has also been shown to have a potentially pro-atherogenic role in CVD [61]). In the Canakinumab Anti-inflammatory Thrombosis Outcome Study (CANTOS) trial, risk reduction using canakinumab was directly related to the amount of IL-6 reduction achieved [62]. Another study comparing cytokine levels among gout patients found significant elevations in serum IL-1β, IL-6, IL-18, and IL-37 levels in gout patients with versus without tophi. These elevated cytokine levels correlated with elevations in CRP and ESR [63].

2.9 Beyond the Joint: MSU Is in More Places Than We Thought It Was

A common misconception is that MSU crystals deposit exclusively within and around peripheral articular joints as well as other cartilaginous and musculoskeletal structures [64]. In fact, multiple case reports and series indicate that the geography of MSU deposition varies widely. For example, increasing evidence now points to the deposition of MSU within the axial skeleton, including sacroiliac joints and along various levels of the spine. Typically, spinal MSU deposition has been discovered when patients presenting with back pain or cord compression symptoms were incidentally found to have a compressing or erosive tophus on surgical excision or biopsy of a mass discovered on imaging [65]. With the increasing use of dual energy CT (DECT) to identify MSU deposits noninvasively, MSU appears to be deposited more diffusely within the spines of as many as 40% of gout patients, although the definitive confirmation and impact of this putative non-tophaceous MSU spinal depositions are still ongoing [66] .

Given the role of the kidneys in filtering urate, it is not surprising to find urate and/or uric acid in the kidneys, particularly in the form of uric acid kidney stones, which constitute 4–10% of all renal calculi. DECT has played a significant role in the imaging of kidney stones, given its ability to not only image the stones but to differentiate between calcium and uric acid containing stones with a specificity of 98.1% [67]. However, MSU deposition has also been documented within the renal parenchyma, including the medulla, the collecting ducts and the interstitium [68]. For example, Ayoub et al. found that among a cohort of 7409 native kidney biopsies, 36 patients had medullary tophi, 35 of whom had CKD. The authors postulated that based upon the location and bulk of these tophi, they may have played a role in the contribution of CKD by upstream damage to the nephrons [69].

MSU has also been found within other organ systems. Birefringent crystals were found in almost half of all prostate specimens resected during cancer surgery [70]. Cases have been reported of patients with severe tophaceous gout who developed symptoms of blockage or perforation of the intestines secondary to intra-intestinal tophi [71, 72]. MSU deposition has been found in different parts of the eye manifesting as scleritis, episcleritis, and uveitis [68, 73]. Urate crystals have even been documented within breast tissue in five published cases, initially seen on mammography, before a biopsy of the mass revealed tophi [74].

In sum, although MSU crystals are typically found within and around joints where they can cause gout flares, they may deposit in virtually any organ in the body, where they may cause a variety of symptoms, including mechanical damage to surrounding tissue, and local as well as systemic inflammation. These widely disbursed deposits complicate the case of already sick gout patients, and contribute to the total body burden of urate, potentially contributing to resistance to standard doses of urate lowering therapy.

3　GOUT and CVD: A Complex Relationship

Though patients with gout often have concomitant traditional cardiovascular risk factors (male sex, hypertension, dyslipidemia, chronic kidney disease), both hyperuricemia and gout are recognized as independent, non-traditional cardiovascular risk factors [75]. A subgroup analysis of 6912 patients from the first National Health and Nutrition Examination Survey showed that increasing SU level was an independent predictor of cardiovascular mortality in both men and women [76]. A meta-analysis of 12 cohort studies comprised of a total of 457,915 participants without CVD found that SU concentrations greater than 7.0 mg/dL significantly increased the risk of coronary artery disease [77]. In a 12-year follow-up study of 51,297 patients, men with history of gout had higher death from all causes, particularly cardiovascular death [78]. Another study reported that gout was independently associated with increased coronary artery calcium scores and increased incidence of major adverse cardiovascular events [79].

3.1　Gout as a Metabolic Disease

Unpacking the independent association between gout and CVD was initially challenging, since gout is also associated with multiple other conditions that themselves are associated with cardiovascular risk. In general, gout patients have significantly higher rates of chronic kidney disease, diabetes, hypertension, hyperlipidemia, non-alcoholic fatty liver and obesity, all of which contribute to cardiovascular risk [80, 81]. In fact, gout patients are at markedly increased risk for metabolic syndrome, confirming that these conditions form a web of associations of which gout is an integral strand [82]. The initial presumption that gout (and more specifically hyperuricemia) is a consequence of some of these other conditions (e.g., kidney disease leading to hyperuricemia), while broadly true, has given way to a more nuanced view in which hyperuricemia and/or gout may themselves predispose to some of these conditions, thus indirectly promoting cardiovascular risk. How these relationships operate, however, remains incompletely elucidated. An evolving body of literature suggests that proper gout treatment may help ameliorate several of these comorbidities, suggesting that gout treatment may have indirect benefits on CVD.

One area that is increasingly being recognized is intracellular urate's ability to regulate the enzyme adenosine monophosphate kinase (AMPK). In the liver, AMPK serves as a master down regulator of multiple metabolic-syndrome-interrelated pathways, inhibiting gluconeogenesis and promoting glycogenolysis, inhibiting lipid production and reducing the development of fatty liver. Within hepatic cells, urate has been shown to inhibit AMPK, thus reversing its activity and promoting these cardiac-related comorbidities. Moreover, in animal models the application of allopurinol, which blocks intracellular production of urate, reverses the effects of urate and reduces adverse metabolic activities. It is likely that AMPK inhibition therefore provides a point of intersection between gout and cholesterol crystal deposition in CVD. AMPK activity also appears to downregulate inflammation. In macrophages, Wang et al. have reported that exposure to MSU crystals results in AMPK downregulation which mediates the inflammatory response (including inflammasome activation), and that these inflammatory effects can be blocked by treatment with an AMPK activator [83]. Strategies to maintain AMPK activation may thus hold promise for suppressing both gouty and other inflammation, and gout-related cardiovascular comorbidities.

Gout has long been associated with hypertension, and although the direction of causality remains somewhat murky, recent clinical evidence suggests that urate may adversely impact blood pressure [84, 85]. In a study of adolescents with new-onset essential hypertension and asymptomatic hyperuricemia, treatment with the urate lowering drug allopurinol reduced or normalized both systolic and diastolic blood pressure [86]. It has been harder to document similar findings in adults, perhaps because aging blood vessels may be characterized by additional disease (e.g., arterial rigidity) that is not remediable to SU lowering [87]. However, in at least two studies with the very potent urate lowering agent pegloticase, reduction and in some cases normalization of blood pressure was observed [88, 89]. Consistent with these observations, in one study in which gout treatment resulted in improved endothelial function with potential implication for blood pressure, the allopurinol response was significantly greater in patients with fewer comorbidities [20]. Collectively, these data underline that early gout treatment may be an important strategy to limit CVD-related comorbidities.

3.2 MSU Deposition in the Vasculature

As early as 1933, reports identified MSU crystals found posthumously in the cardiovascular system [90]. With the advent of advanced imaging including DECT, reports of MSU in cardiac and vascular tissues have become more common. In one study, a group of cadavers were examined by DECT to identify the presence of MSU deposits in the thoracic aorta and coronary arteries. Subsequently, the identified tissues were resected, and MSU deposition was histologically confirmed by polarized microscopy [91]. Several other autopsies have been done that have revealed MSU deposition in various parts of the heart, including the myocardium [92].

Vascular MSU deposition has been identified during surgical vascular procedures including carotid endarterectomies [93] and aortic aneurysm repairs [94]. In both cases, the MSU was found adjacent to cholesterol deposition of atherosclerotic plaques, themselves inflammatory lesions, as previously mentioned. It is unclear from these studies whether the MSU deposition is primary or secondary to the inflammatory atherosclerotic process, but it is possible that MSU deposition in these areas serves as either a nidus, or a response to a nidus of other crystals including cholesterol and calcium. Most recently, plaques collected during carotid endarterec-tomy were found to contain MSU crystals, and these were more commonly detected, and greater in concentration, in patients with ischemic cerebrovascular symptoms compared with asymptomatic disease [95]. The presence of MSU crystals in the carotid plaque also correlated with greater long-term risk for MACE. While further study is needed, these observations suggest that in some cases, the deposition and/or formation of MSU crystals in the vasculature could directly participate in local inflammation and contribute to cardiovascular risk.

Consistent with the above observations, Feuchtner et al. applied DECT imaging to 37 gout patients, 33 hyperuricemic patients without gout, and 26 controls. MSU-containing plaques were found in 91.9% of gout patients, 2.9% of hyperuricemic patients without gout, and only 0.38% of controls ($P < 0.0001$) [96]. Interestingly, most plaques were a mixture of MSU and calcium (74.2%), with only 26.7% being solely MSU. Gout patients also had a higher coronary artery calcium score than the other two groups. Although these data are striking, one limiting factor is the accuracy of DECT scans in differentiating non-massive MSU (for which DECT is less specific than for tophi) from calcium or artifact (such as image noise in smaller pixel images, beam hardening, streak or motion artifacts, or dehydrated cartilage). The recent development of multi-energy energy photon detectors should improve the accuracy of detecting low concentration MSU and may permit the validation of the current DECT findings.

Other reports suggest that gout and/or MSU may also impact valvular structures, including case reports of MSU deposition involving all of the cardiac valves in tophaceous gout patients [68]. These cases were often discovered after the patients presented with valvular dysfunction and/or cardiac murmurs, indicating that the deposition was a pathologic rather than an incidental finding. Independent of these rare events of tophus formation, recent reports suggest that gout is more common among patients with aortic stenosis, and that patients with gout experience more rapid progression of aortic stenosis than those without [97, 98]. Given the associa-tion between gout, cardiovascular risk factors and the presence of cholesterol-driven inflammation, there are also likely co-infiltration of cholesterol crystals in cardiac valves, with a larger burden observed in the aortic valve in rabbit models [99]. These data serve as a reminder that the vasculature consists of multiple components, all of which may be affected by gout and/or inflammation.

4 Lessons from Treatment: Impact of Colchicine on CVD in Patients with and Without Gout

Colchicine has been used for millennia to treat gout. The first reference to the thera-peutic use of *Colchicum* appeared in the Egyptian Papyrus Ebers, circa 1500 BC, and nearly a millennium later, Aetius of Amida and Alexander of Tralles described its anti-inflammatory properties [100, 101]. The inflammatory pathway plays a prominent role in CVD. Colchicine has long been used for pericarditis, and emerging data demonstrating value for atherosclerotic heart disease has recently led the FDA to approve colchicine use for the prevention of acute cardiovascular events in high-risk patients. The translation of colchicine to cardiac disease, in both patients with and without gout, underlines the insights discussed above.

4.1 Mechanisms of Action of Potential Benefit in the Cardiovascular Setting

Due to a deficiency of the P-glycoprotein efflux pump, colchicine concentrates in neutrophils, but also exerts anti-inflammatory effects on macrophages and endothelia [102]. Colchicine predominantly acts by binding to soluble tubulin monomers. Colchicine/tubulin complexes incorporate into elongating microtubule structures, limiting their extension [103]. Colchicine also effects signal transduction, subcellular trafficking, adhesion of leukocytes to endothelium (by altering quantitative L-selectin and qualitative E-selectin expression), and chemotaxis-directed migration into inflamed tissues [104, 105]. Importantly, colchicine suppresses the NLRP3 inflammasome, decreasing production of interleukin (IL)-1β and IL-18, which in turn decreases IL-6 and C-reactive protein, a pathway implicated in cardiovascular inflammation [33, 106]. Colchicine also inhibits neutrophil release of α-defensin, a peptide associated with large thrombus burdens [107]. All of these actions hold relevance for both gout and cardiac disease. Finally, at clinically used doses, colchicine does not suppress platelet-platelet aggregation but does decrease neutrophil-platelet aggregation, suggesting a preferential impact at the inflammatory-thrombosis interface [108].

4.2 Targeting IL-1β in Coronary Artery Disease

Atherosclerosis is an inflammatory disease prevalent in patients with gout, acting through both low-density lipoprotein (LDL)-mediated inflammation and an independent IL-β/IL-6/CRP pathway [109, 110]. In the early stages of atherosclerosis, oxidized lipids promote recruitment and activation of leukocytes, uptake of lipids into macrophages, and subsequent conversion of macrophages into pro-inflammatory foam cells. As noted earlier, cholesterol crystals share with MSU the capacity to activate the NLRP3 inflammasome and further amplify the inflammatory process [33]. Multiple observational studies demonstrated an increase in cardiovascular risk in patients with LDL at goal but elevated CRP, and CANTOS established that specific targeting of IL-1β, using the anti-IL-1β-directed biologic canakinumab, reduces major adverse cardiovascular events (MACE) in high-risk patients [106, 111]. In CANTOS, patients in the canakinumab arm also experienced significant reductions in incident gout [112]. While colchicine does not affect the LDL-mediated inflammatory pathway, it inhibits the IL-β/IL-6/CRP pathway by inhibiting assembly of the inflammasome, as well as inhibiting leukocyte activation, adhesion, and migration. Importantly, colchicine reduces CRP concentration in patients with CAD even in the setting of aspirin and high-intensity statin [113]. In gout patients, reduction in CRP is seen upon colchicine treatment initiation, with further reduction after urate lowering [20].

4.3 Colchicine in Coronary Artery Disease

Incident Coronary Artery Disease--Observational data suggest colchicine may reduce the development of new-onset CAD, at least in patients with rheumatic disease. A case-control series of patients with familial Mediterranean fever (another disease for which colchicine is a first-line treatment agent) suggested that long-term prophylactic colchicine was associated with a lower incidence of CAD compared to those not on colchicine therapy [114]. Similarly, a retrospective study of patients with gout without known CAD were followed for 96 months and showed an association between use of colchicine and lower rate of development of incident CAD in patients without chronic kidney disease [115].

Established CAD—Studies have also shown a reduction in acute cardiovascular events in patients at high risk for, or with known CAD, including patients with gout. One retrospective study in a gout cohort reported a 54% lower rate of MI in patients on colchicine versus those not on colchicine, while another observational study in a gout cohort demonstrated a 49% relative risk reduction in the composite of MI, stroke, or transient ischemic attack, and a 73% relative risk reduction in all-cause mortality compared with untreated patients [116, 117]. Beyond the gout population, an open-label randomized study of patients with angiographically-proven CAD on optimal medical therapy showed a lower composite rate of MACE at 3 years follow-up [118]. This was followed by the large, multicenter, placebo-controlled Low Dose Colchicine 2 (LoDoCo2) trial in which colchicine reduced the risk of MACE by 31% at 29 months follow-up [119]. As-yet unpublished data from our own group, examining 239 gout patients with established CAD, indicated that those who used colchicine consistently had significantly fewer MACE events, over a 10-year observation period, compared with those who used colchicine less than 50% of the time (manuscript in preparation).

During and post-MI—The role and timing of colchicine in the setting of acute coronary syndrome is an area of ongoing investigation. Although in vivo data suggested that colchicine could reduce infarct size when administered early post-MI, this area remains a matter of further research given paucity of data from small trials [120, 121].

Several relatively small, randomized studies in the setting of acute MI demonstrated no difference in CRP concentrations, infarct size on cardiac magnetic resonance imaging, and left ventricle remodeling with 30 days of low-dose colchicine treatment in patients with acute MI [122, 123]. Similarly, the Colchicine in Patients With Acute Coronary Syndromes (COPS, $n = 795$), a study of low-dose colchicine versus placebo during index hospitalization, failed to demonstrate a difference in MACE [124]. However, the much larger, double-blind, placebo-controlled, randomized Colchicine Cardiovascular Outcomes Trial (COLCOT, $n = 4745$) trial of patients within 30 days after MI (median time for initiation 14 days) reported a 23% reduction in MACE [125]. This reduction, unlike in the gout cohort studies and LoDoCo2, was driven by a reduction in stroke (not MI) and the "soft" endpoint of urgent coronary revascularization. The ongoing international, double-blind, placebo-controlled, 7000 patient colchicine and spironolactone in patients with MI (CLEAR, NCT03048825) trial randomizes patients with a large MI to therapy within 72 h of percutaneous coronary intervention and planned to follow-up for extended period of 5 years will hopefully provide some more clarity on the impact of colchicine on individual cardiovascular endpoints, optimal timing of starting colchicine therapy, and any potential impact on non-cardiovascular mortality. Nonetheless, based on the totality of the currently available data, the 2021 European Society of Cardiology guidelines on the prevention of CVD recommend colchicine be considered for the secondary prevention of CVD, especially in patients at higher risk of recurrent events [126]. Whether more aggressive colchicine therapy should be recommended for patients with gout, with or without active cardiovascular disease, remains unknown. Current recommendations for gout treatment from the American College of Rheumatology recommend colchicine exclusively for treating gout flares and/or prophylaxis against flares during initiation of urate lowering therapy (a period of several months), with no consideration given for cardiovascular risk [127].

5 Conclusion and Final Thoughts

Gout, the archetypal inflammatory arthritis, drives inflammation via both metabolic and crystal-driven pathways. Beyond arthritis, gout has implications for multiple other conditions, including cardiovascular disease. The mechanisms by which MSU crystals trigger both local and systemic inflammation, as well as the toxic and pro-inflammatory effects of soluble urate on the vasculature, contribute to cardiovascular disease in gout, and offer molecular and cellular clues into the mechanisms through which cardiovascular disease progresses even in the absence of gout. In particular, the manner in which MSU crystals form, and how they activate myeloid lineage and other inflammatory cells, may provide a window into the mechanisms through which cholesterol and cholesterol crystals drive similar effects. Within the vasculature, the ways in which these crystals interact and synergize with each other may promote more cardiovascular risk than either crystal alone.

References

1. Yu W, Cheng JD. Uric acid and cardiovascular disease: an update from molecular mechanism to clinical perspective. Front Pharmacol. 2020;11:582680. https://doi.org/10.3389/fphar.2020.582680. Epub 2020/12/12. PubMed PMID: 33304270; PubMed Central PMCID: PMCPMC7701250.
2. Bardin T, Richette P. Impact of comorbidities on gout and hyperuricaemia: an update on prevalence and treatment options. BMC Med. 2017;15(1):123. https://doi.org/10.1186/s12916-017-0890-9. Epub 2017/07/04. PubMed PMID: 28669352; PubMed Central PMCID: PMCPMC5494879.
3. Abeles AM. Hyperuricemia, gout, and cardiovascular disease: an update. Curr Rheumatol Rep. 2015;17(3):13. Epub 2015/03/06. PubMed PMID: 25740704. https://doi.org/10.1007/s11926-015-0495-2.
4. Chen-Xu M, Yokose C, Rai SK, Pillinger MH, Choi HK. Contemporary prevalence of gout and hyperuricemia in the united states and decadal trends: the National Health and Nutrition Examination Survey, 2007–2016. Arthritis Rheumatol (Hoboken, NJ). 2019;71(6):991–9. https://doi.org/10.1002/art.40807. Epub 2019/01/09. PubMed PMID: 30618180; PubMed Central PMCID: PMCPMC6536335.
5. Martillo MA, Nazzal L, Crittenden DB. The crystallization of monosodium urate. Curr Rheumatol Rep. 2014;16(2):400. https://doi.org/10.1007/s11926-013-0400-9. PubMed PMID: 24357445.
6. Singh G, Lingala B, Mithal A. Gout and hyperuricaemia in the USA: prevalence and trends. Rheumatology. 2019;58(12):2177–80. https://doi.org/10.1093/rheumatology/kez196.
7. Keenan RT. The biology of urate. Semin Arthritis Rheum. 2020;50(3s):S2–S10. Epub 2020/07/06. PubMed PMID: 32620198. https://doi.org/10.1016/j.semarthrit.2020.04.007.
8. Mandal AK, Mount DB. The molecular physiology of uric acid homeostasis. Annu Rev Physiol. 2015;77:323–45. Epub 2014/11/26. PubMed PMID: 25422986. https://doi.org/10.1146/annurev-physiol-021113-170343.
9. Krishnan E, Lessov-Schlaggar CN, Krasnow RE, Swan GE. Nature versus nurture in gout: a twin study. Am J Med. 2012;125(5):499–504. Epub 2012/03/01. PubMed PMID: 22365026. https://doi.org/10.1016/j.amjmed.2011.11.010.
10. Major TJ, Dalbeth N, Stahl EA, Merriman TR. An update on the genetics of hyperuricaemia and gout. Nat Rev Rheumatol. 2018;14(6):341–53. Epub 2018/05/10. PubMed PMID: 29740155. https://doi.org/10.1038/s41584-018-0004-x.
11. Méndez-Salazar EO, Martínez-Nava GA. Uric acid extrarenal excretion: the gut microbiome as an evident yet understated factor in gout development. Rheumatol Int. 2022;42(3):403–12. Epub 2021/09/30. PubMed PMID: 34586473. https://doi.org/10.1007/s00296-021-05007-x.
12. Kuwabara M, Niwa K, Hisatome I, Nakagawa T, Roncal-Jimenez CA, Andres-Hernando A, et al. Asymptomatic hyperuricemia without comorbidities predicts cardiometabolic diseases: five-year japanese cohort study. Hypertension. 2017;69(6):1036–44. https://doi.org/10.1161/hypertensionaha.116.08998. Epub 2017/04/12.PubMed PMID: 28396536; PubMed Central PMCID: PMCPMC5426964.
13. Treviño-Becerra A. Uric acid: the unknown uremic toxin. Contrib Nephrol. 2018;192:25–33. Epub 2018/02/03. PubMed PMID: 29393086. https://doi.org/10.1159/000484275.
14. Meijers B, Lowenstein J. The evolving view of uremic toxicity. Toxins (Basel). 2022;14(4):274. Epub 2022/04/22. PubMed PMID: 35448883; PubMed Central PMCID: PMCPMC9031373. https://doi.org/10.3390/toxins14040274.
15. Gao H, Liu S. Role of uremic toxin indoxyl sulfate in the progression of cardiovascular disease. Life Sci. 2017;185:23–9. Epub 2017/07/30. PubMed PMID: 28754616. https://doi.org/10.1016/j.lfs.2017.07.027.

16. Sun Y, Johnson C, Zhou J, Wang L, Li YF, Lu Y, et al. Uremic toxins are conditional danger- or homeostasis-associated molecular patterns. Front Biosci (Landmark Ed). 2018;23(2):348–87. https://doi.org/10.2741/4595. Epub 2017/09/21. PubMed PMID: 28930551; PubMed Central PMCID: PMCPMC5627515.

17. Kang DH, Park SK, Lee IK, Johnson RJ. Uric acid-induced C-reactive protein expression: implication on cell proliferation and nitric oxide production of human vascular cells. J Am Soc Nephrol. 2005;16(12):3553–62. Epub 2005/10/28. PubMed PMID: 16251237. https://doi.org/10.1681/asn.2005050572.

18. Kang DH, Han L, Ouyang X, Kahn AM, Kanellis J, Li P, et al. Uric acid causes vascular smooth muscle cell proliferation by entering cells via a functional urate transporter. Am J Nephrol. 2005;25(5):425–33. Epub 2005/08/23. PubMed PMID: 16113518. https://doi.org/10.1159/000087713.

19. Krasnokutsky S, Romero AG, Bang D, Pike VC, Shah B, Igel TF, et al. Impaired arterial responsiveness in untreated gout patients compared with healthy non-gout controls: association with serum urate and C-reactive protein. Clin Rheumatol. 2018;37(7):1903–11. https://doi.org/10.1007/s10067-018-4029-y. Epub 2018/02/17. PubMed PMID: 29450849; PubMed Central PMCID: PMCPMC8476227.

20. Toprover M, Shah B, Oh C, Igel TF, Romero AG, Pike VC, et al. Initiating guideline-concordant gout treatment improves arterial endothelial function and reduces intercritical inflammation: a prospective observational study. Arthritis Res Ther. 2020;22(1):169. https://doi.org/10.1186/s13075-020-02260-6. Epub 2020/07/13. PubMed PMID: 32653044; PubMed Central PMCID: PMCPMC7353742.

21. Sautin YY, Nakagawa T, Zharikov S, Johnson RJ. Adverse effects of the classic antioxidant uric acid in adipocytes: NADPH oxidase-mediated oxidative/nitrosative stress. Am J Physiol Cell Physiol. 2007;293(2):C584–96. Epub 2007/04/13. PubMed PMID: 17428837. https://doi.org/10.1152/ajpcell.00600.2006.

22. Badii M, Gaal OI, Cleophas MC, Klück V, Davar R, Habibi E, et al. Urate-induced epigenetic modifications in myeloid cells. Arthritis Res Ther. 2021;23(1):202. https://doi.org/10.1186/s13075-021-02580-1. Epub 2021/07/30. PubMed PMID: 34321071; PubMed Central PMCID: PMCPMC8317351.

23. Joosten LAB, Crişan TO, Bjornstad P, Johnson RJ. Asymptomatic hyperuricaemia: a silent activator of the innate immune system. Nat Rev Rheumatol. 2020;16(2):75–86. https://doi.org/10.1038/s41584-019-0334-3. Epub 2019/12/12. PubMed PMID: 31822862; PubMed Central PMCID: PMCPMC7075706.

24. Tercan H, Riksen NP, Joosten LAB, Netea MG, Bekkering S. Trained immunity: long-term adaptation in innate immune responses. Arterioscler Thromb Vasc Biol. 2021;41(1):55–61. Epub 2020/10/23. PubMed PMID: 33086868. https://doi.org/10.1161/atvbaha.120.314212.

25. Dalbeth N, Phipps-Green A, Frampton C, Neogi T, Taylor WJ, Merriman TR. Relationship between serum urate concentration and clinically evident incident gout: an individual participant data analysis. Ann Rheum Dis. 2018;77(7):1048–52. Epub 2018/02/22. PubMed PMID: 29463518. https://doi.org/10.1136/annrheumdis-2017-212288.

26. Yokose C, Chen M, Berhanu A, Pillinger MH, Krasnokutsky S. Gout and osteoarthritis: associations, pathophysiology, and therapeutic implications. Curr Rheumatol Rep. 2016;18(10):65. Epub 2016/10/01. PubMed PMID: 27686950. https://doi.org/10.1007/s11926-016-0613-9.

27. Neogi T, Krasnokutsky S, Pillinger MH. Urate and osteoarthritis: evidence for a reciprocal relationship. Joint Bone Spine. 2019;86(5):576–82. https://doi.org/10.1016/j.jbspin.2018.11.002. Epub 2018/11/25. PubMed PMID: 30471419; PubMed Central PMCID: PMCPMC6531371.

28. Kanevets U, Sharma K, Dresser K, Shi Y. A role of IgM antibodies in monosodium urate crystal formation and associated adjuvanticity. J Immunol. 2009;182(4):1912–8. https://doi.org/10.4049/jimmunol.0803777. Epub 2009/02/10. PubMed PMID: 19201844; PubMed Central PMCID: PMCPMC2663336.

29. Kam M, Perl-Treves D, Caspi D, Addadi L. Antibodies against crystals. FASEB J. 1992;6(8):2608–13. Epub 1992/05/01. PubMed PMID: 1592211. https://doi.org/10.1096/fasebj.6.8.1592211.

30. Rimer JD, An Z, Zhu Z, Lee MH, Goldfarb DS, Wesson JA, et al. Crystal growth inhibitors for the prevention of L-cystine kidney stones through molecular design. Science. 2010;330(6002):337–41. https://doi.org/10.1126/science.1191968. Epub 2010/10/16. PubMed PMID: 20947757; PubMed Central PMCID: PMCPMC5166609.

31. Lee MH, Sahota A, Ward MD, Goldfarb DS. Cystine growth inhibition through molecular mimicry: a new paradigm for the prevention of crystal diseases. Curr Rheumatol Rep. 2015;17(5):33. https://doi.org/10.1007/s11926-015-0510-7. Epub 2015/04/16. PubMed PMID: 25874348; PubMed Central PMCID: PMCPMC4518543.

32. Vedre A, Pathak DR, Crimp M, Lum C, Koochesfahani M, Abela GS. Physical factors that trigger cholesterol crystallization leading to plaque rupture. Atherosclerosis. 2009;203(1):89–96. Epub 2008/08/16. PubMed PMID: 18703195. https://doi.org/10.1016/j.atherosclerosis.2008.06.027.

33. Duewell P, Kono H, Rayner KJ, Sirois CM, Vladimer G, Bauernfeind FG, et al. NLRP3 inflammasomes are required for atherogenesis and activated by cholesterol crystals. Nature. 2010;464(7293):1357–61. https://doi.org/10.1038/nature08938. Epub 2010/04/30. PubMed PMID: 20428172; PubMed Central PMCID: PMCPMC2946640.

34. Rock KL, Kataoka H, Lai JJ. Uric acid as a danger signal in gout and its comorbidities. Nat Rev Rheumatol. 2013;9(1):13–23. https://doi.org/10.1038/nrrheum.2012.143. Epub 2012/09/05. PubMed PMID: 22945591; PubMed Central PMCID: PMCPMC3648987.

35. Kingsbury SR, Conaghan PG, McDermott MF. The role of the NLRP3 inflammasome in gout. J Inflamm Res. 2011;4:39–49. https://doi.org/10.2147/jir.S11330. Epub 2011/11/19. PubMed PMID: 22096368; PubMed Central PMCID: PMCPMC3218743.

36. Swanson KV, Deng M, Ting JP. The NLRP3 inflammasome: molecular activation and regulation to therapeutics. Nat Rev Immunol. 2019;19(8):477–89. https://doi.org/10.1038/s41577-019-0165-0. Epub 2019/05/01. PubMed PMID: 31036962; PubMed Central PMCID: PMCPMC7807242.

37. Kaneko N, Kurata M, Yamamoto T, Morikawa S, Masumoto J. The role of interleukin-1 in general pathology. Inflamm Regen. 2019;39:12. https://doi.org/10.1186/s41232-019-0101-5. Epub 2019/06/12. PubMed PMID: 31182982; PubMed Central PMCID: PMCPMC6551897.

38. LA Abbas DK, Pillai S. Basic immunology. 5th ed. Amsterdam: Elsevier; 2016.

39. Martinon F, Pétrilli V, Mayor A, Tardivel A, Tschopp J. Gout-associated uric acid crystals activate the NALP3 inflammasome. Nature. 2006;440(7081):237–41. Epub 2006/01/13. PubMed PMID: 16407889. https://doi.org/10.1038/nature04516.

40. Zhu J, Chu CQ. Cholesterol crystals in rheumatoid bursal fluid. Rheumatology (Oxford). 2022;61(5):e132. Epub 2021/07/16. PubMed PMID: 34264345. https://doi.org/10.1093/rheumatology/keab561.

41. Choi HK, Niu J, Neogi T, Chen CA, Chaisson C, Hunter D, et al. Nocturnal risk of gout attacks. Arthritis Rheumatol (Hoboken, NJ). 2015;67(2):555–62. https://doi.org/10.1002/art.38917. Epub 2014/12/17. PubMed PMID: 25504842; PubMed Central PMCID: PMCPMC4360969.

42. Muller JE, Tofler GH, Stone PH. Circadian variation and triggers of onset of acute cardiovascular disease. Circulation. 1989;79(4):733–43. Epub 1989/04/01. PubMed PMID: 2647318. https://doi.org/10.1161/01.cir.79.4.733.

43. Howard RG, Pillinger MH, Gyftopoulos S, Thiele RG, Swearingen CJ, Samuels J. Reproducibility of musculoskeletal ultrasound for determining monosodium urate deposition: concordance between readers. Arthritis Care Res (Hoboken). 2011;63(10):1456–62. https://doi.org/10.1002/acr.20527. Epub 2011/06/28. PubMed PMID: 21702086; PubMed Central PMCID: PMCPMC3183112.

44. Dalbeth N, House ME, Aati O, Tan P, Franklin C, Horne A, et al. Urate crystal deposition in asymptomatic hyperuricaemia and symptomatic gout: a dual energy CT study. Ann Rheum

Dis. 2015;74(5):908–11. https://doi.org/10.1136/annrheumdis-2014-206397. PubMed PMID: 25637002.

45. Zaninelli TH, Fattori V, Saraiva-Santos T, Badaro-Garcia S, Staurengo-Ferrari L, Andrade KC, et al. RvD1 disrupts nociceptor neuron and macrophage activation and neuroimmune communication, reducing pain and inflammation in gouty arthritis in mice. Br J Pharmacol. 2022;179:4500. https://doi.org/10.1111/bph.15897. Epub 2022/06/19. PubMed PMID: 35716378.

46. Scher JU, Pillinger MH. The anti-inflammatory effects of prostaglandins. J Investig Med. 2009;57(6):703–8. Epub 2009/02/26. PubMed PMID: 19240648. https://doi.org/10.2310/JIM.0b013e31819aaa76.

47. Bannenberg G, Serhan CN. Specialized pro-resolving lipid mediators in the inflammatory response: an update. Biochim Biophys Acta. 2010;1801(12):1260–73. https://doi.org/10.1016/j.bbalip.2010.08.002. Epub 2010/08/17. PubMed PMID: 20708099; PubMed Central PMCID: PMCPMC2994245.

48. Wang M, Ishikawa T, Lai Y, Nallapothula D, Singh RR. Diverse roles of NETosis in the pathogenesis of lupus. Front Immunol. 2022;13:895216. https://doi.org/10.3389/fimmu.2022.895216. Epub 2022/06/11. PubMed PMID: 35686129; PubMed Central PMCID: PMCPMC9170953.

49. Schauer C, Janko C, Munoz LE, Zhao Y, Kienhöfer D, Frey B, et al. Aggregated neutrophil extracellular traps limit inflammation by degrading cytokines and chemokines. Nat Med. 2014;20(5):511–7. Epub 2014/05/03. PubMed PMID: 24784231. https://doi.org/10.1038/nm.3547.

50. Quillard T, Araújo HA, Franck G, Shvartz E, Sukhova G, Libby P. TLR2 and neutrophils potentiate endothelial stress, apoptosis and detachment: implications for superficial erosion. Eur Heart J. 2015;36(22):1394–404. https://doi.org/10.1093/eurheartj/ehv044. Epub 2015/03/11. PubMed PMID: 25755115; PubMed Central PMCID: PMCPMC4458287.

51. Döring Y, Soehnlein O, Weber C. Neutrophils cast NETs in atherosclerosis: employing peptidylarginine deiminase as a therapeutic target. Circ Res. 2014;114(6):931–4. Epub 2014/03/15. PubMed PMID: 24625721. https://doi.org/10.1161/circresaha.114.303479.

52. Mangold A, Alias S, Scherz T, Hofbauer M, Jakowitsch J, Panzenböck A, et al. Coronary neutrophil extracellular trap burden and deoxyribonuclease activity in ST-elevation acute coronary syndrome are predictors of ST-segment resolution and infarct size. Circ Res. 2015;116(7):1182–92. Epub 2014/12/31. PubMed PMID: 25547404. https://doi.org/10.1161/circresaha.116.304944.

53. Chhana A, Dalbeth N. The gouty tophus: a review. Curr Rheumatol Rep. 2015;17(3):19. https://doi.org/10.1007/s11926-014-0492-x. PubMed PMID: 25761926.

54. Narang RK, Dalbeth N. Pathophysiology of gout. Semin Nephrol. 2020;40(6):550–63. https://doi.org/10.1016/j.semnephrol.2020.12.001.

55. Janoudi A, Shamoun FE, Kalavakunta JK, Abela GS. Cholesterol crystal induced arterial inflammation and destabilization of atherosclerotic plaque. Eur Heart J. 2016;37(25):1959–67. Epub 2015/12/26. PubMed PMID: 26705388. https://doi.org/10.1093/eurheartj/ehv653.

56. Palmer DG, Hogg N, Denholm I, Allen CA, Highton J, Hessian PA. Comparison of phenotype expression by mononuclear phagocytes within subcutaneous gouty tophi and rheumatoid nodules. Rheumatol Int. 1987;7(5):187–93. Epub 1987/01/01. PubMed PMID: 3321380. https://doi.org/10.1007/bf00541376.

57. Dalbeth N, Pool B, Gamble GD, Smith T, Callon KE, McQueen FM, et al. Cellular characterization of the gouty tophus: a quantitative analysis. Arthritis Rheum. 2010;62(5):1549–56. Epub 2010/02/05. PubMed PMID: 20131281. https://doi.org/10.1002/art.27356.

58. Lee SJ, Nam KI, Jin HM, Cho YN, Lee SE, Kim TJ, et al. Bone destruction by receptor activator of nuclear factor κB ligand-expressing T cells in chronic gouty arthritis. Arthritis Res Ther. 2011;13(5):R164. https://doi.org/10.1186/ar3483. Epub 2011/10/14. PubMed PMID: 21992185; PubMed Central PMCID: PMCPMC3308097.

59. Cavalcanti NG, Marques CD, Lins ELTU, Pereira MC, Rêgo MJ, Duarte AL, et al. Cytokine profile in gout: inflammation driven by IL-6 and IL-18? Immunol Investig. 2016;45(5):383–95. Epub 2016/05/25. PubMed PMID: 27219123. https://doi.org/10.310 9/08820139.2016.1153651.

60. Heinrich PC, Castell JV, Andus T. Interleukin-6 and the acute phase response. Biochem J. 1990;265(3):621–36. https://doi.org/10.1042/bj2650621. Epub 1990/02/01. PubMed PMID: 1689567; PubMed Central PMCID: PMCPMC1133681.

61. Ridker PM, Rane M. Interleukin-6 signaling and anti-Interleukin-6 therapeutics in cardiovascular disease. Circ Res. 2021;128(11):1728–46. Epub 2021/05/18. PubMed PMID: 33998272. https://doi.org/10.1161/circresaha.121.319077.

62. Ridker PM, Libby P, MacFadyen JG, Thuren T, Ballantyne C, Fonseca F, et al. Modulation of the interleukin-6 signalling pathway and incidence rates of atherosclerotic events and all-cause mortality: analyses from the Canakinumab Anti-Inflammatory Thrombosis Outcomes Study (CANTOS). Eur Heart J. 2018;39(38):3499–507. https://doi.org/10.1093/eurheartj/ehy310.

63. Ding L, Li H, Sun B, Wang T, Meng S, Huang Q, et al. Elevated interleukin-37 associated with tophus and pro-inflammatory mediators in Chinese gout patients. Cytokine. 2021;141:155468. Epub 2021/03/02. PubMed PMID: 33647713. https://doi.org/10.1016/j.cyto.2021.155468.

64. Dalbeth N, Gosling AL, Gaffo A, Abhishek A. Gout. Lancet (London, England). 2021;397(10287):1843–55. Epub 2021/04/03. PubMed PMID: 33798500. https://doi.org/10.1016/s0140-6736(21)00569-9.

65. Toprover M, Krasnokutsky S, Pillinger MH. Gout in the spine: imaging, diagnosis, and outcomes. Curr Rheumatol Rep. 2015;17(12):70. Epub 2015/10/23. PubMed PMID: 26490179. https://doi.org/10.1007/s11926-015-0547-7.

66. Toprover M, Mechlin M, Slobodnick A, Pike VC, Oh C, Davis C, et al. Gout and serum urate levels are associated with lumbar spine monosodium urate deposition and chronic low back pain: a dual-energy CT study [Abstract]. Arthritis Rheum. 2020;2020.

67. Spek A, Strittmatter F, Graser A, Kufer P, Stief C, Staehler M. Dual energy can accurately differentiate uric acid-containing urinary calculi from calcium stones. World J Urol. 2016;34(9):1297–302. Epub 2016/01/11. PubMed PMID: 26749082. https://doi.org/10.1007/s00345-015-1756-4.

68. Khanna P, Johnson RJ, Marder B, LaMoreaux B, Kumar A. Systemic urate deposition: an unrecognized complication of gout? J Clin Med. 2020;9(10):3204. https://doi.org/10.3390/jcm9103204. Epub 2020/10/08. PubMed PMID: 33023045; PubMed Central PMCID: PMCPMC7600842.

69. Ayoub I, Almaani S, Brodsky S, Nadasdy T, Prosek J, Hebert L, et al. Revisiting medullary tophi: a link between uric acid and progressive chronic kidney disease? Clin Nephrol. 2016;85(2):109–13. Epub 2015/12/29. Epub 2020/10/08. https://doi.org/10.5414/cn108663.x.

70. Park JJ, Roudier MP, Soman D, Mokadam NA, Simkin PA. Prevalence of birefringent crystals in cardiac and prostatic tissues, an observational study. BMJ Open. 2014;4(7):e005308. https://doi.org/10.1136/bmjopen-2014-005308. Epub 2014/07/18. PubMed PMID: 25031195; PubMed Central PMCID: PMCPMC4120371.

71. Katoch P, Trier-Mørch S, Vyberg M. Small intestinal tophus mimicking tumor. Hum Pathol Case Rep. 2014;1(1):2–5. https://doi.org/10.1016/j.ehpc.2014.05.001.

72. Moiseev V, Shavarov A, Varshavsky V, Reshetin V. Multiple pseudotumorous crystalline deposits in small intestine, mesentery and lungs in terminal heart failure patent without gouty arthritis. Eur J Heart Fail. 2016.

73. Sharon Y, Schlesinger N. Beyond joints: a review of ocular abnormalities in gout and hyperuricemia. Curr Rheumatol Rep. 2016;18(6):37. Epub 2016/05/04. PubMed PMID: 27138165. https://doi.org/10.1007/s11926-016-0586-8.

74. Sharifabad MA, Tzeng J, Gharibshahi S. Mammary gouty tophus: a case report and review of the literature. Breast J. 2006;12(3):263–5. Epub 2006/05/11. PubMed PMID: 16684326. https://doi.org/10.1111/j.1075-122X.2006.00252.x.

75. Disveld IJM, Fransen J, Rongen GA, Kienhorst LBE, Zoakman S, Janssens H, et al. Crystal-proven gout and characteristic gout severity factors are associated with cardiovascular disease. J Rheumatol. 2018;45(6):858–63. Epub 2018/04/17. PubMed PMID: 29657151. https://doi.org/10.3899/jrheum.170555.
76. Freedman DS, Williamson DF, Gunter EW, Byers T. Relation of serum uric acid to mortality and ischemic heart disease. The NHANES I Epidemiologic Follow-up Study. Am J Epidemiol. 1995;141(7):637–44. Epub 1995/04/01. PubMed PMID: 7702038. https://doi.org/10.1093/oxfordjournals.aje.a117479.
77. Braga F, Pasqualetti S, Ferraro S, Panteghini M. Hyperuricemia as risk factor for coronary heart disease incidence and mortality in the general population: a systematic review and meta-analysis. Clin Chem Lab Med. 2016;54(1):7–15. Epub 2015/09/10. PubMed PMID: 26351943. https://doi.org/10.1515/cclm-2015-0523.
78. Choi HK, Curhan G. Independent impact of gout on mortality and risk for coronary heart disease. Circulation. 2007;116(8):894–900. Epub 2007/08/19. PubMed PMID: 17698728. https://doi.org/10.1161/circulationaha.107.703389.
79. Christensen JL, Yu W, Tan S, Chu A, Vargas F, Assali M, et al. Gout is associated with increased coronary artery calcification and adverse cardiovascular outcomes. JACC Cardiovasc Imaging. 2019. Epub 2019/12/23. PubMed PMID: 31864984;13:884. https://doi.org/10.1016/j.jcmg.2019.10.019.
80. Keenan RT, O'Brien WR, Lee KH, Crittenden DB, Fisher MC, Goldfarb DS, et al. Prevalence of contraindications and prescription of pharmacologic therapies for gout. Am J Med. 2011;124(2):155–63. Epub 2011/02/08. PubMed PMID: 21295195. https://doi.org/10.1016/j.amjmed.2010.09.012.
81. Zhu Y, Pandya BJ, Choi HK. Comorbidities of gout and hyperuricemia in the US general population: NHANES 2007-2008. Am J Med. 2012;125(7):679–87.e1. Epub 2012/05/26. PubMed PMID: 22626509. https://doi.org/10.1016/j.amjmed.2011.09.033.
82. Yoo HG, Lee SI, Chae HJ, Park SJ, Lee YC, Yoo WH. Prevalence of insulin resistance and metabolic syndrome in patients with gouty arthritis. Rheumatol Int. 2011;31(4):485–91. Epub 2010/01/22. PubMed PMID: 20091036. https://doi.org/10.1007/s00296-009-1304-x.
83. Wang Y, Viollet B, Terkeltaub R, Liu-Bryan R. AMP-activated protein kinase suppresses urate crystal-induced inflammation and transduces colchicine effects in macrophages. Ann Rheum Dis. 2016;75(1):286–94. https://doi.org/10.1136/annrheumdis-2014-206074. Epub 2014/11/02. PubMed PMID: 25362043; PubMed Central PMCID: PMCPMC4417082.
84. Sun HL, Pei D, Lue KH, Chen YL. Uric acid levels can predict metabolic syndrome and hypertension in adolescents: a 10-year longitudinal study. PLoS One. 2015;10(11):e0143786. https://doi.org/10.1371/journal.pone.0143786. Epub 2015/12/01. PubMed PMID: 26618358; PubMed Central PMCID: PMCPMC4664290.
85. Grayson PC, Kim SY, LaValley M, Choi HK. Hyperuricemia and incident hypertension: a systematic review and meta-analysis. Arthritis Care Res (Hoboken). 2011;63(1):102–10. https://doi.org/10.1002/acr.20344. Epub 2010/09/09. PubMed PMID: 20824805; PubMed Central PMCID: PMCPMC3016454.
86. Feig DI, Soletsky B, Johnson RJ. Effect of allopurinol on blood pressure of adolescents with newly diagnosed essential hypertension: a randomized trial. JAMA. 2008;300(8):924–32. https://doi.org/10.1001/jama.300.8.924. Epub 2008/08/30. PubMed PMID: 18728266; PubMed Central PMCID: PMCPMC2684336.
87. Gaffo AL, Calhoun DA, Rahn EJ, Oparil S, Li P, Dudenbostel T, et al. Effect of serum urate lowering with allopurinol on blood pressure in young adults: a randomized, controlled, crossover trial. Arthritis Rheumatol (Hoboken, NJ). 2021;73(8):1514–22. Epub 2021/03/30. PubMed PMID: 33779064. https://doi.org/10.1002/art.41749.
88. Johnson RJ, Choi HK, Yeo AE, Lipsky PE. Pegloticase treatment significantly decreases blood pressure in patients with chronic gout. Hypertension. 2019;74(1):95–101. Epub 2019/05/14. PubMed PMID: 31079535. https://doi.org/10.1161/hypertensionaha.119.12727.

89. Abdellatif A, Zhao L, Cherny K, Marder B, Scandling J, Saag K. POS1160 protect: PEGLOTICASE treatment for uncontrolled gout in kidney transplanted patients; results from a phase 4 trial. Ann Rheum Dis. 2022;81(Suppl 1):908–9. https://doi.org/10.1136/annrheumdis-2022-eular.2175.

90. Hench P, Darnall C. A clinic on acute, old-fashioned gout; with special reference to its inciting factors. Med Clin North Am. 1933;16:1371–400.

91. Klauser AS, Halpern EJ, Strobl S, Gruber J, Feuchtner G, Bellmann-Weiler R, et al. Dual-energy computed tomography detection of cardiovascular monosodium urate deposits in patients with gout. JAMA Cardiol. 2019;4(10):1019–28. https://doi.org/10.1001/jamacardio.2019.3201. PubMed PMID: 31509156.

92. Pund EE Jr, Hawley RL, Mc GH, Blount SG Jr. Gouty heart. N Engl J Med. 1960;263:835–8. Epub 1960/10/27. PubMed PMID: 13738492. https://doi.org/10.1056/nejm196010272631705.

93. Patetsios P, Song M, Shutze WP, Pappas C, Rodino W, Ramirez JA, et al. Identification of uric acid and xanthine oxidase in atherosclerotic plaque. Am J Cardiol. 2001;88(2):188–91, , a6. Epub 2001/07/13. PubMed PMID: 11448423. https://doi.org/10.1016/s0002-9149(01)01621-6.

94. Patetsios P, Rodino W, Wisselink W, Bryan D, Kirwin JD, Panetta TF. Identification of uric acid in aortic aneurysms and atherosclerotic artery. Ann N Y Acad Sci. 1996;800:243–5. Epub 1996/11/18. PubMed PMID: 8959001. https://doi.org/10.1111/j.1749-6632.1996.tb33318.x.

95. Nardi V, Franchi F, Prasad M, Fatica EM, Alexander MP, Bois MC, et al. Uric acid expression in carotid atherosclerotic plaque and serum uric acid are associated with cerebrovascular events. Hypertension. 2022;79(8):1814–23. Epub 2022/06/04. PubMed PMID: 35656807. https://doi.org/10.1161/hypertensionaha.122.19247.

96. Feuchtner GM, Plank F, Beyer C, Schwabl C, Held J, Bellmann-Weiler R, et al. Monosodium urate crystal deposition in coronary artery plaque by 128-slice dual-energy computed tomography: an ex vivo phantom and in vivo study. J Comput Assist Tomogr. 2021;45(6):856–62. Epub 2021/09/02. PubMed PMID: 34469909. https://doi.org/10.1097/rct.0000000000001222.

97. Chang K, Yokose C, Tenner C, Oh C, Donnino R, Choy-Shan A, et al. Association between gout and aortic stenosis. Am J Med. 2017;130(2):230.e1–8. https://doi.org/10.1016/j.amjmed.2016.09.005. Epub 2016/10/11. PubMed PMID: 27720853; PubMed Central PMCID: PMCPMC5357081.

98. Adelsheimer A, Shah B, Choy-Shan A, Tenner CT, Lorin JD, Smilowitz NR, et al. Gout and progression of aortic stenosis. Am J Med. 2020;133(9):1095–1100.e1. https://doi.org/10.1016/j.amjmed.2020.01.019. Epub 2020/02/23. PubMed PMID: 32081657; PubMed Central PMCID: PMCPMC7429243.

99. El-Khatib LA, De Feijter-Rupp H, Janoudi A, Fry L, Kehdi M, Abela GS. Cholesterol induced heart valve inflammation and injury: efficacy of cholesterol lowering treatment. Open Heart. 2020;7(2):e001274. https://doi.org/10.1136/openhrt-2020-001274. Epub 2020/08/05. PubMed PMID: 32747455; PubMed Central PMCID: PMCPMC7402193.

100. Dasgeb B, Kornreich D, McGuinn K, Okon L, Brownell I, Sackett DL. Colchicine: an ancient drug with novel applications. Br J Dermatol. 2018;178(2):350–6. https://doi.org/10.1111/bjd.15896. Epub 2017/08/24. PubMed PMID: 28832953; PubMed Central PMCID: PMCPMC5812812.

101. Wallace SL. In: Copeman, WSC, editor. A short history of the gout and the rheumatic diseases. Berkeley: University of California Press; 1964, 236 pp. Arthritis Rheumatism. 1964;7(6):722–3. https://doi.org/10.1002/art.1780070613.

102. Bauriedel G, Heimerl J, Beinert T, Welsch U, Höfling B. Colchicine antagonizes the activity of human smooth muscle cells cultivated from arteriosclerotic lesions after atherectomy. Coron Artery Dis. 1994;5(6):531–9. Epub 1994/06/01. PubMed PMID: 7952413.

103. Nuki G. Colchicine: its mechanism of action and efficacy in crystal-induced inflammation. Curr Rheumatol Rep. 2008;10(3):218–27. Epub 2008/07/22. PubMed PMID: 18638431. https://doi.org/10.1007/s11926-008-0036-3.

104. Caner JE. Colchicine inhibition of chemotaxis. Arthritis Rheum. 1965;8(5):757–64. Epub 1965/10/01. PubMed PMID: 5859551. https://doi.org/10.1002/art.1780080438.

105. Cronstein BN, Molad Y, Reibman J, Balakhane E, Levin RI, Weissmann G. Colchicine alters the quantitative and qualitative display of selectins on endothelial cells and neutrophils. J Clin Invest. 1995;96(2):994–1002. https://doi.org/10.1172/jci118147. Epub 1995/08/01. PubMed PMID: 7543498; PubMed Central PMCID: PMCPMC185287.

106. Ridker PM, Everett BM, Thuren T, MacFadyen JG, Chang WH, Ballantyne C, et al. Antiinflammatory therapy with canakinumab for atherosclerotic disease. N Engl J Med. 2017;377(12):1119–31. Epub 2017/08/29. PubMed PMID: 28845751. https://doi.org/10.1056/NEJMoa1707914.

107. Abu-Fanne R, Stepanova V, Litvinov RI, Abdeen S, Bdeir K, Higazi M, et al. Neutrophil α-defensins promote thrombosis in vivo by altering fibrin formation, structure, and stability. Blood. 2019;133(5):481–93. https://doi.org/10.1182/blood-2018-07-861237. Epub 2018/11/18. PubMed PMID: 30442678; PubMed Central PMCID: PMCPMC6356988 interests.

108. Shah B, Allen N, Harchandani B, Pillinger M, Katz S, Sedlis SP, et al. Effect of colchicine on platelet-platelet and platelet-leukocyte interactions: a pilot study in healthy subjects. Inflammation. 2016;39(1):182–9. https://doi.org/10.1007/s10753-015-0237-7. Epub 2015/09/01. PubMed PMID: 26318864; PubMed Central PMCID: PMCPMC4753094.

109. Nidorf SM, Fiolet A, Abela GS. Viewing atherosclerosis through a crystal lens: how the evolving structure of cholesterol crystals in atherosclerotic plaque alters its stability. J Clin Lipidol. 2020;14(5):619–30. Epub 2020/08/15. PubMed PMID: 32792218. https://doi.org/10.1016/j.jacl.2020.07.003.

110. Strandberg TE, Kovanen PT. Coronary artery disease: 'gout' in the artery? Eur Heart J. 2021;42(28):2761–4. https://doi.org/10.1093/eurheartj/ehab276. Epub 2021/05/30. PubMed PMID: 34050656; PubMed Central PMCID: PMCPMC8845033.

111. Ridker PM, MacFadyen JG, Everett BM, Libby P, Thuren T, Glynn RJ. Relationship of C-reactive protein reduction to cardiovascular event reduction following treatment with canakinumab: a secondary analysis from the CANTOS randomised controlled trial. Lancet (London, England). 2018;391(10118):319–28. Epub 2017/11/18. PubMed PMID: 29146124. https://doi.org/10.1016/s0140-6736(17)32814-3.

112. Solomon DH, Glynn RJ, MacFadyen JG, Libby P, Thuren T, Everett BM, et al. Relationship of interleukin-1β blockade with incident gout and serum uric acid levels: exploratory analysis of a randomized controlled trial. Ann Intern Med. 2018;169(8):535–42. Epub 2018/09/23. PubMed PMID: 30242335. https://doi.org/10.7326/m18-1167.

113. Nidorf M, Thompson PL. Effect of colchicine (0.5 mg twice daily) on high-sensitivity C-reactive protein independent of aspirin and atorvastatin in patients with stable coronary artery disease. Am J Cardiol. 2007;99(6):805–7. Epub 2007/03/14. PubMed PMID: 17350370. https://doi.org/10.1016/j.amjcard.2006.10.039.

114. Langevitz P, Livneh A, Neumann L, Buskila D, Shemer J, Amolsky D, et al. Prevalence of ischemic heart disease in patients with familial Mediterranean fever. Isr Med Assoc J. 2001;3(1):9–12. Epub 2001/05/10. PubMed PMID: 11344818.

115. Shah B, Toprover M, Crittenden DB, Jeurling S, Pike VC, Krasnokutsky S, et al. Colchicine use and incident coronary artery disease in male patients with gout. Can J Cardiol. 2020;36(11):1722–8. https://doi.org/10.1016/j.cjca.2020.05.026. Epub 2020/05/27. PubMed PMID: 32454073; PubMed Central PMCID: PMCPMC8464652.

116. Crittenden DB, Lehmann RA, Schneck L, Keenan RT, Shah B, Greenberg JD, et al. Colchicine use is associated with decreased prevalence of myocardial infarction in patients with gout. J Rheumatol. 2012;39(7):1458–64. https://doi.org/10.3899/jrheum.111533. Epub 2012/06/05. PubMed PMID: 22660810; PubMed Central PMCID: PMCPMC3733459.

117. Solomon DH, Liu CC, Kuo IH, Zak A, Kim SC. Effects of colchicine on risk of cardio-vascular events and mortality among patients with gout: a cohort study using electronic medical records linked with Medicare claims. Ann Rheum Dis. 2016;75(9):1674–9. https://doi.org/10.1136/annrheumdis-2015-207984. Epub 2015/11/20. PubMed PMID: 26582823; PubMed Central PMCID: PMCPMC5049504.
118. Nidorf SM, Eikelboom JW, Budgeon CA, Thompson PL. Low-dose colchicine for secondary prevention of cardiovascular disease. J Am Coll Cardiol. 2013;61(4):404–10. Epub 2012/12/26. PubMed PMID: 23265346. https://doi.org/10.1016/j.jacc.2012.10.027.
119. Nidorf SM, Fiolet ATL, Mosterd A, Eikelboom JW, Schut A, Opstal TSJ, et al. Colchicine in patients with chronic coronary disease. N Engl J Med. 2020;383(19):1838–47. Epub 2020/09/01. PubMed PMID: 32865380. https://doi.org/10.1056/NEJMoa2021372.
120. Mastrocola R, Penna C, Tullio F, Femminò S, Nigro D, Chiazza F, et al. Pharmacological inhibition of NLRP3 inflammasome attenuates myocardial ischemia/reperfusion injury by activation of RISK and mitochondrial pathways. Oxid Med Cell Longev. 2016;2016:5271251. https://doi.org/10.1155/2016/5271251. Epub 2017/01/06. PubMed PMID: 28053692; PubMed Central PMCID: PMCPMC5178375.
121. Deftereos S, Giannopoulos G, Angelidis C, Alexopoulos N, Filippatos G, Papoutsidakis N, et al. Anti-inflammatory treatment with colchicine in acute myocardial infarction: a pilot study. Circulation. 2015;132(15):1395–403. Epub 2015/08/13. PubMed PMID: 26265659. https://doi.org/10.1161/circulationaha.115.017611.
122. Hennessy T, Soh L, Bowman M, Kurup R, Schultz C, Patel S, et al. The low dose colchicine after myocardial infarction (LoDoCo-MI) study: a pilot randomized placebo controlled trial of colchicine following acute myocardial infarction. Am Heart J. 2019;215:62–9. Epub 2019/07/10. PubMed PMID: 26265659. https://doi.org/10.1016/j.ahj.2019.06.003.x.
123. Mewton N, Roubille F, Bresson D, Prieur C, Bouleti C, Bochaton T, et al. Effect of colchicine on myocardial injury in acute myocardial infarction. Circulation. 2021;144(11):859–69. https://doi.org/10.1161/circulationaha.121.056177. Epub 2021/08/24. PubMed PMID: 34420373; PubMed Central PMCID: PMCPMC8462445.
124. Tong DC, Quinn S, Nasis A, Hiew C, Roberts-Thomson P, Adams H, et al. Colchicine in patients with acute coronary syndrome: the Australian COPS Randomized Clinical Trial. Circulation. 2020;142(20):1890–900. Epub 2020/08/31. PubMed PMID: 32862667. https://doi.org/10.1161/circulationaha.120.050771.
125. Tardif JC, Kouz S, Waters DD, Bertrand OF, Diaz R, Maggioni AP, et al. Efficacy and safety of low-dose colchicine after myocardial infarction. N Engl J Med. 2019;381(26):2497–505. Epub 2019/11/17. PubMed PMID: 31733140. https://doi.org/10.1056/NEJMoa1912388.
126. Visseren FLJ, Mach F, Smulders YM, Carballo D, Koskinas KC, Bäck M, et al. 2021 ESC Guidelines on cardiovascular disease prevention in clinical practice. Eur Heart J. 2021;42(34):3227–337. Epub 2021/08/31. PubMed PMID: 34458905. https://doi.org/10.1093/eurheartj/ehab484.
127. FitzGerald JD, Dalbeth N, Mikuls T, Brignardello-Petersen R, Guyatt G, Abeles AM, et al. 2020 American College of Rheumatology Guideline for the Management of Gout. Arthritis Care Res (Hoboken). 2020;72(6):744–60. Epub 2020/05/12. PubMed PMID: 32391934. https://doi.org/10.1002/acr.24180.

Calcium Crystals in Arterial Disease

Sandeep Banga, Jagadeesh K. Kalavakunta, Oliver Abela, and On Topaz

1 Introduction

The appearance of detectable amounts of coronary artery calcium (CAC) by CT scanning marks an inflection point in the natural history of coronary disease as the risk of atherothrombotic event increases exponentially once calcification becomes evident in the atherosclerotic bed of the coronary vessels. CAC is associated with the presence of advanced atherosclerosis in coronary artery disease [1]. The calcium detected in the vasculature for the most part results from the development of calcium phosphate (hydroxyapatite) crystals that form into larger aggregates and sheet-like lattices onto which free calcium continues to accrete. Calcium crystals may begin to form either within and adjacent to the necrotic core of atherosclerotic plaque or within the media of the vessel wall. Although the processes that lead to calcium deposition in these sites are separate and distinct, when extensive, calcification in either site may be associated with reduced vascular compliance, impaired

S. Banga (✉)
Department of Cardiology, Michigan State University/Sparrow Hospital, Lansing, MI, USA

J. K. Kalavakunta
Department of Cardiology, Ascension Borgess Center, Michigan State University/Western Michigan University Homer Stryker M.D. School of Medicine, Kalamazoo, MI, USA

O. Abela
Department of Medicine, Cardiology Section, Advent Health, Tampa, FL, USA

O. Topaz
Duke University School of Medicine, Durham, NC, USA

© The Author(s), under exclusive license to Springer Nature Switzerland AG 2023
G. S. Abela, S. M. Nidorf (eds.), *Cholesterol Crystals in Atherosclerosis and Other Related Diseases*, Contemporary Cardiology,
https://doi.org/10.1007/978-3-031-41192-2_19

vasomotor tone and in some circumstances a reduction in luminal diameter [2, 3]. However, since calcium crystals rarely develop or deposit in the media of coronary arteries it is self-evident that the detection of CAC is specific for atherosclerosis and explains why it has proven to be a strong independent marker of prognosis and predictor of future cardiac events in patients with coronary artery disease [4, 5].

This chapter summarizes how calcium crystals develop in atherosclerotic plaque and the media of peripheral arteries, examines how and why identification of coronary calcium affects assessment of prognosis of patients with coronary disease, and summaries the clinical effects of efforts to modify the process of vascular calcification.

2 Formation of Calcium Crystals in the Atherosclerotic Arteries

Crystalline calcium in atherosclerotic plaque most commonly forms when free calcium and phosphate molecules associate and form micro-calcific crystal deposits. Like the lipid in the atherosclerotic core, these elements are believed to originate from apoptotic smooth muscle cells and macrophage-derived matrix vesicles [6–9]. Whereas apoptosis of smooth muscle cells has been demonstrated to results in the formation of fine (small) deposits of calcium crystals, apoptosis of macrophages appears to lead to the formation of (larger) "punctate" deposits of calcium crystals (Fig. 1b, c) [10].

Microscopic calcium crystal deposits measuring 0.5–15 µm are visible at microscopy in atherosclerotic plaque, and are commonly seen deep in the necrotic core adjacent to the internal elastic lamina (Fig. 1d, e) [10]. As they aggregate, they become increasingly evident in the matrix surrounding the necrotic core where they have a speckled appearance (Fig. 1f) [10]. As these deposits grow, they develop into sheet-like structures (>3 mm) that appear deeper in the vessel wall adjacent to smooth muscle cells and within the collagenous matrix (Fig. 1g, h) [10]. Thus, the different patterns of calcification provide some insight into the age and potential stability of the plaque.

In the presence of sufficient free calcium, these calcified structures continue to grow. Once they enlarge >2 mm they become detectable by CT imaging, and in some instances, large nodular aggregates of calcium crystalline deposits may be visible to the naked eye (Fig. 1l).

On occasions, very large-calcified nodules form that may extend into the vessel lumen and limit coronary flow or cause erosion of the vascular endothelium resulting in atherothrombosis. In angiographic studies in patients presenting with an acute coronary syndrome, calcified nodules were identified and believed to be primary cause of atherothrombosis in 2% to 7% of patients [11].

The relationship between free calcium and free cholesterol in the plaque core is interesting. While free calcium may enhance the formation of cholesterol crystals

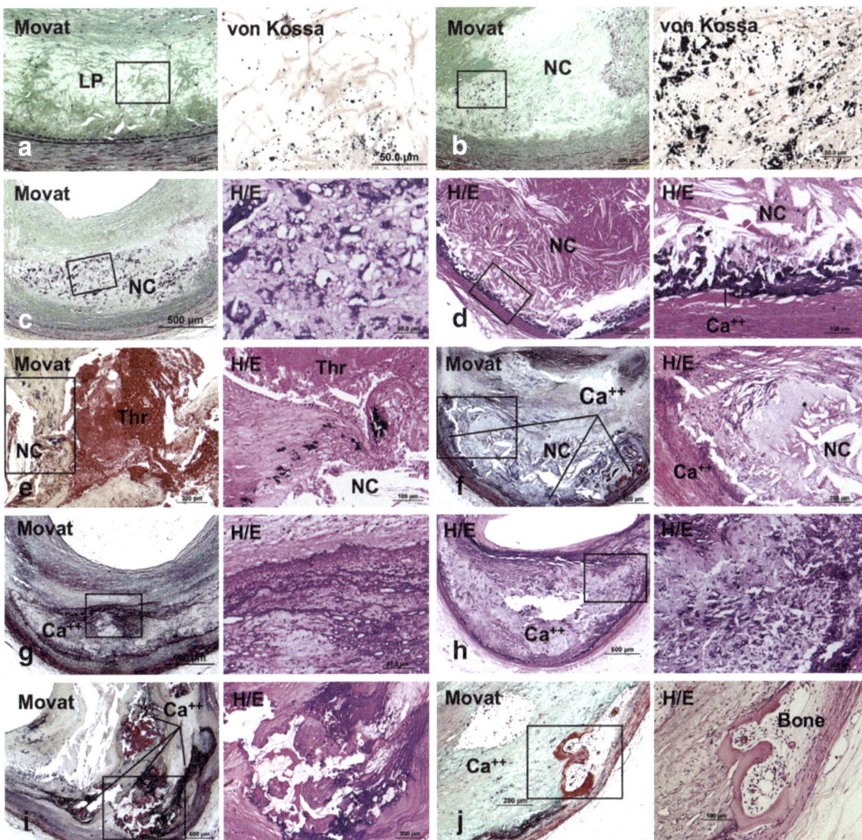

Fig. 1 Various forms of arterial calcification. Non-decalcified arterial segments (**a** and **b**) and decalcified segments (**c**–**j**) were serially cut for microscopic assessment. (**a**) Pathologic intimal thickening (PIT) is shown characterized by lipid pool (LP) that lacks smooth muscle cells (SMCs). Early microcalcification (≥0.5 mm, typically <15 mm in diameter) likely results from SMC apoptosis and calcification is detected by von Kossa staining within the LP (high-power image of boxed area in the Movat pentachrome-stained image). Early necrotic core (NC) (**b**) not only lacks SMCs but also is infiltrated by macrophages which eventually undergo apoptosis and calcification, which is observed as punctate (≥15 µm) areas of calcification. Von Kossa staining clearly shows relatively larger punctate areas of calcification resulting from macrophage cell death within the NC as compared to microcalcification of dying SMCs. A substantial amount of macrophage calcification can be observed in early NC (**c**), but the degree of calcification in NC is typically located close to the medial wall where fragmented calcifications can be seen (**d**). Microcalcification resulting from macrophage and/or SMC death can also be detected within a thin fibrous cap and has been associated with plaque rupture. Calcification generally progresses into the surrounding area of the NC (**f**), which leads to the development of sheets of calcification where both collagen matrix (**g**) and NC itself are calcified (**h**). Nodular calcification may occur within the plaque in the absence of luminal thrombus and is characterized by breaks in calcified plates with fragments of calcium separated by fibrin (**i**). Ossification may occur at the edge of an area of sheet calcification (**j**). (Reproduced with permission from Otsuka et al. [1]). Ca^{+2} calcium, *H/E* hematoxylin-eosin stain, *Thr* thrombus. (Reproduced with permission [10])

(CCs), CCs may in turn act as a nidus for the formation of calcium crystals [12–17]. Thus, as the plaque matures, the necrotic core contains increasing amounts of both cholesterol and calcium crystals. Indeed, both are often found alongside the other in aspirates of ruptured atherosclerotic plaques following acute myocardial infarction [18] (see Chap. "Crystals in Atherosclerosis: Crystal Cholesterol Structures, Morphologies, Formation and Dissolution. What Do We Know?", Fig. 8). Various forms of coronary artery calcification have been described (Fig. 2).

Aside from the potentially erosive effect of large-calcified nodules on the vascular endothelium, there is now increasing evidence that calcium crystals may act synergistically with CCs to increase the risk of plaque instability by enhancing innate inflammation in the atherosclerotic bed, where they activate proinflammatory

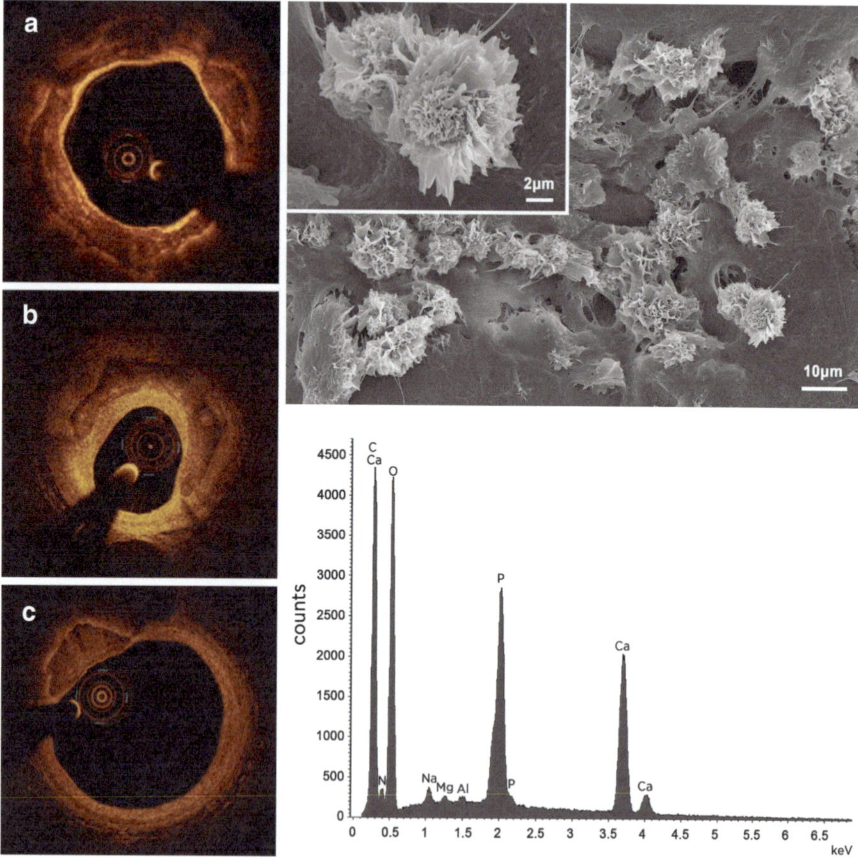

Fig. 2 Calcium phosphate crystals in coronary arteries. Optical coherence tomography of calcification in coronary arteries depicting (**a**) superficial, (**b**) deep calcification, and (**c**) a calcium nodule. Calcium phosphate crystals are noted by scanning electron microscopy obtained from coronary atherosclerotic plaques. Graph of the plaque composition is illustrated by energy-dispersive X-ray spectroscopy (EDS). Calcium and phosphate is the predominant species. *Al* aluminum, *C* carbon, *Ca* calcium, *N* nitrogen, *Na* sodium, *Mg* magnesium, *O* oxygen, *P* phosphate. (Courtesy of Eric Schiedel, CNMT, RCIS (OCT) and Dr. George Abela (SEM and EDS))

cytokines including interleukin 1β (IL-1β) and IL-8 that promote the recruitment of leukocytes into the vascular bed [19–23], and increase the expression of tumor necrosis factor, myeloperoxidase, and other proinflammatory factors. Thus, as the crystalline environment of the plaque becomes more complex, the disease progresses more rapidly, and the risk of plaque instability increases accordingly.

3 Calcification of the Vascular Media

The processes that lead to the development and growth of calcium crystals in the vascular media involves distinct and independent processes responsible for the formation in the atherosclerotic core, as it closely resembles the processes active in bone [24]. Osteoblasts derived from the mesenchymal vascular smooth muscle cell (VSMC) precursors in the media may develop bone like structures over templates formed by mesenchymal cells that begin to resemble and act as chondrocytes. The osteoclasts derived from hematopoietic mononuclear phagocyte progenitor cells in the media may resorb the mineral bone [25] (Fig. 3).

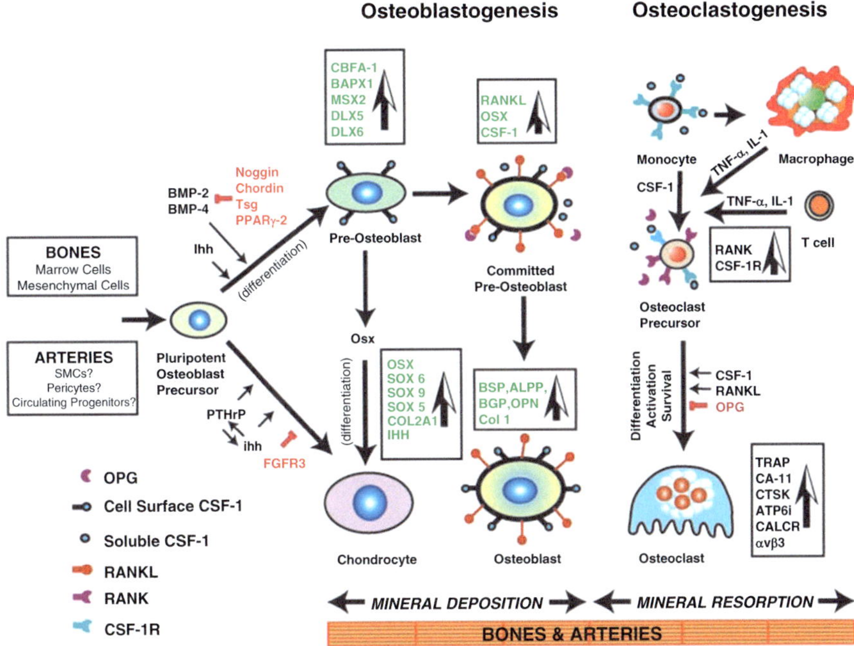

Fig. 3 Mechanism of Osteogenesis. The major genes, growth factors, and signaling pathways culminating in fully mature chondrocytes, osteoblasts, and osteoclasts. Inhibitory influences are shown in red. Considerable ontogenetic plasticity is retained at each step but appears to diminish as terminally differentiated cellular phenotypes are approached. The proposed mechanism of arterial calcification appears to involve many of the same components. (Reproduced with permission: Copyright (2003) National Academy of Sciences, U.S.A [25])

Osteogenic transformation of VSMCs enables them to secrete an osteoid-like extracellular matrix that promotes the formation of calcium deposits in the media [26]. Various proteins involved in osteogenesis have been detected in VSMCs (and in some models in atherosclerotic lesions) including osteopontin, bone morphogenetic protein-2, matrix Gla protein (MGP), fetuin-A, osteoprotegerin, and receptor activator of NF-κB ligand. These proteins can have either a stimulatory or an inhibitory role in the calcification process [27]. In the media therefore, calcium deposition is affected by factors that inhibit or enhance calcium flux at a cellular level [28]. Thus, mineralization is enhanced in patients with metabolic disorders including primary and secondary hyperparathyroidism as seen in chronic kidney disease and diabetes.

Genetic factors may also affect this process as evidence by calcification of the media in patients with Mönckeberg's sclerosis, and in phenotypically distinct forms of genetically altered mice that form calcium deposits in the vascular media after administration of vitamin D1, D3, and nicotine [16], and in the vascular media of rats after injections of warfarin and vitamin K [17]. MGP expressed by chondrocytes in normal and atherosclerotic arteries can inhibit calcification in the media [21, 22]. In mice models the deletion of the gene encoding MGP results in extensive calcification of cartilage and the medial layer of arteries [23]. These findings suggest that MGP may function in cartilage and healthy arteries to inhibit mineralization [12].

4 The Effect of Magnesium and Vitamin D on Calcification in the Media

The process of transdifferentiation of VSMCs initiated by reduced levels of circulating inhibitors of vascular calcification, elevated levels of inorganic phosphate, and formation of amorphous calcium phosphate particles in the circulation; is accelerated by the expression of osteogenic genes and amplified by the release of exosomes and apoptotic bodies from VSMCs. Intra- and extracellular magnesium and vitamin D may affect these processes in different ways [28] (Fig. 4).

Magnesium has been shown in some animal models to actively slow the formation of calcium crystals in the media [29–31] possibly due to its ability to form stronger bonds with phosphate than calcium [32], however, magnesium has several additional actions that may affect calcification in the media (Table 1). Notably, in patients on hemodialysis, magnesium has been reported to slow the rate of medial calcification [33].

Thus far, the data on the role of vitamin D in vascular calcification has been conflicting. While in vitro multiple effects of vitamin D have been found to have protective effects on medial calcification in the presence of high phosphate medium [34–39], the results of clinical studies have been mixed. In some studies, in patients with chronic kidney disease (CKD), an inverse relationship was found between serum vitamin D and medial as well as coronary artery calcification [40–42] whereas

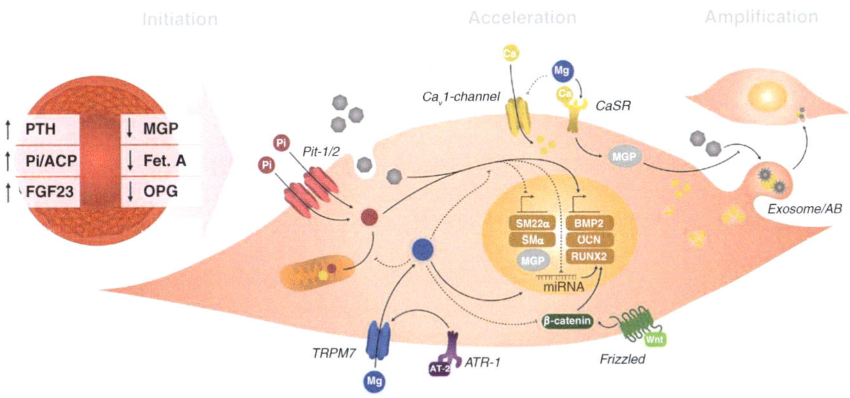

Fig. 4 Active modulation of vascular calcification by magnesium. Mg^{+2} inhibits vascular smooth muscle cell transdifferentiation. Diminished levels of circulating inhibitors of vascular calcification, elevated levels of inorganic phosphate (Pi), and formation of amorphous Ca2 + -Pi particle (ACP) in the circulation initiate the transdifferentiation of vascular smooth muscle cell (VSMC). VSMC transdifferentiation is accelerated by the expression of osteogenic genes and amplified by the VSMCs through the release of exosomes and apoptotic bodies. Mg^{2+} potentially prevents this process via different pathways both on the level of initiation and acceleration of VSMC calcification. *AB* apoptotic body, *AT2* angiotensin type 2, *ATR-1* angiotensin 2 type 1 receptor, *BMP-2* bone morphogenetic protein 2, *Cav1 channel* L-Type calcium channel, *CaSR* calcium- sensing receptor, *Fet. A* fetuin-A, *FGF23* fibroblast growth factor 23, *MGP* matrix Gla protein, *OCN* osteocalcin, *OPG* osteoprotegerin, *PiT* sodium-dependent inorganic phosphate transporter, *PTH* parathyroid hormone, *SM22%* transgelin, *%-SMA* %–smooth muscle actin, *RUNX2* runt-related transcription factor 2, *TRPM7* transient receptor potential melastatin 7. (Reproduced with permission [28])

Table 1 Role of magnesium on coronary artery calcification

1. Prevents the loss of calcification inhibitors (BMP-7, MGP, osteopontin) that protect against osteogenic conversion [28]

2. Stabilizing amorphous calcium phosphate (ACP) by forming stronger complexes of Mg^{+2} with Pi than Ca^{+2} [32]

3. Delays maturation of primary calciprotein particle (CPP) to secondary CPP which has been shown to induce in vitro calcification [33]

4. Prevents transcriptional changes in VSMC trans-differentiation and apoptosis [99]

5. Inhibits expression of genes associated with secretion of osteocalcin and alkaline phosphatase that promote matrix mineralization [100, 101]

6. Abolishes phosphate induced Wnt/β-catenin signaling, involved in osteoblast maturation and increases RUNX2 expression, which is osteogenic [102, 103]

7. Regulates miRNAs involved in vascular homeostasis [104, 105]. Modulates VSMC calcium handling and the activation of the Ca^{+2} sensing receptor (CaSR) important for MGP function [106]

8. Blocks Ca^{+2} channels in VSMCs thus preventing Ca^{+2} overload [107, 108] that leads VSMC death

9. VSMC death following blockage of Ca^{+2} channels leads to release of apoptotic bodies which provides ACP nucleation sites for matrix calcification [109–111]

(continued)

Table 1 (continued)

10. Stabilizes extracellular ATP (adenosine triphosphate) from breakdown, which leads to hydroxyapatite formation [112]
11. Promotes whitlockite (Ca9Mg (HPO4) (PO46) formation instead of hydroxyapatite [113]
12. Prevents intracellular Ca^{+2} bursts that cause apoptosis and VSMC calcification [114]. In VSMCs, Ca^{+2} channel blocking by Mg^{+2} has been implicated in CaSR receptor activation which regulates PTH secretion affecting mineral-bone hemostasis [115]
13. Mg^{+2} acts as a partial agonist that activates the CaSR 2 to 3 times less potently than Ca^{+2} [115–117]. Lower PTH after CaSR activation results in decreased bone turnover and intestinal Ca^{+2} absorption and promotes renal Pi reabsorption
14. Higher Mg^{+2} concentrations correlate with decreased PTH levels as seen in dialysis patients [118]. Studies have shown that Mg^{+2} supplementation in VSMCs resulted in reduced Pi- and hydroxyapatite induced calcification through restoring CaSR mRNA and protein levels [119]
15. Mg^{+2} did not show the effect in human calcifying vascular smooth muscle cells on cellular apatite architecture or whitlockite formation [120]

in other studies in patients with CKD, a significant positive correlation between the extent of vascular calcification and vitamin D levels was observed [43–46]. These divergent results may reflect the complex vascular-renal-endocrine-bone axis which is implicated in this process in CKD that affect the levels of phosphorus, calcium, parathormone, and other potential uremic toxins that may influence the transformation of VSMCs into osteoblast-like cells, and also reflects differences in the experimental model or the dose or type of active vitamin D used [47]. Notwithstanding these results, there is an evidence that vitamin D may shift the immune response toward a Th2 profile, thus promoting an antiatherogenic immune profile [48, 49] (Fig. 5). Thus, the protective or harmful effect of vitamin D on vascular calcification in general and atherosclerosis, in particular remains controversial (Table 2).

In vitro studies of the effect of calciferol (Vitamin D3) on cholesterol crystallization demonstrated a bimodal response that may help explain the clinical observations. Calciferol reduced cholesterol crystallization, but the effect was not linear and varied with the concentration of calciferol and the initial concentration of cholesterol in solution. The results indicated that calciferol can interfere with cholesterol crystal formation and volume expansion but an excess of calciferol can condense cholesterol and promote crystal formation [50] (Fig. 6).

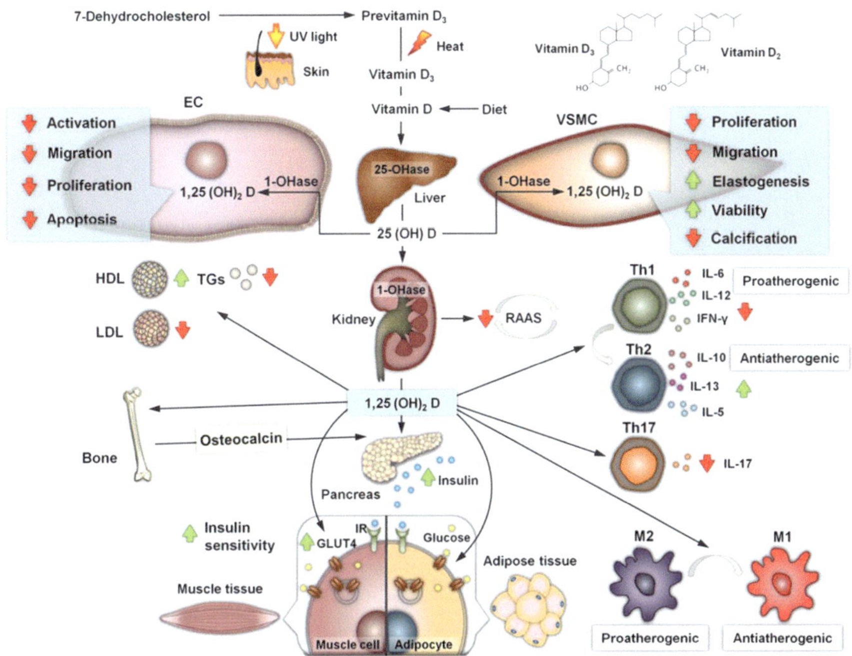

Fig. 5 Role of vitamin D in Atherosclerosis. Schematic representation illustrating synoptically the metabolism and actions of vitamin D in cells and tissues that are implicated directly and indirectly in the atherogenic process. *EC* endothelial cell, *Glut-4* glucose transporter 4, *HDL* high-density lipoprotein, *IL* interleukin, *IR* insulin receptor, *LDL* low-density lipoprotein, *M1* macrophage/monocyte 1, *M2* macrophage/monocyte 2, *RAAS* renin-angiotensin-aldosterone system, *TGs* triglycerides, *Th* T helper, *VSMC* vascular smooth muscle cell. (Reproduced with permission [49])

Table 2 Effects of vitamin D on vascular smooth muscle cells and immune response

1. Vitamin D has antiatherogenic effects on the vascular smooth muscle cells (VSMCs) that ordinarily contribute to atherosclerosis by proliferation and migration [121–123]
2. 1 alfa,25(OH)2D3 inhibits the proliferative effects of both epidermal growth factor and endothelin on VSMCs [124–127]
3. Calcitriol inhibits proliferation by an acute influx of Ca^{2+} into the VSMCs [128]
4. Effects of vitamin D on immune response has been seen that both innate and adaptive immunity1,25(OH) 2 D has been shown to shift the immune response toward a Th2 profile, thus, promoting an antiatherogenic immune profile [48, 129]
5. Either a positive or an inverse relationship between vitamin D levels and vascular calcification has been observed [40, 130]. These contradictory data reflect the complex, vascular-renal-endocrine-bone axis which is implicated in this process

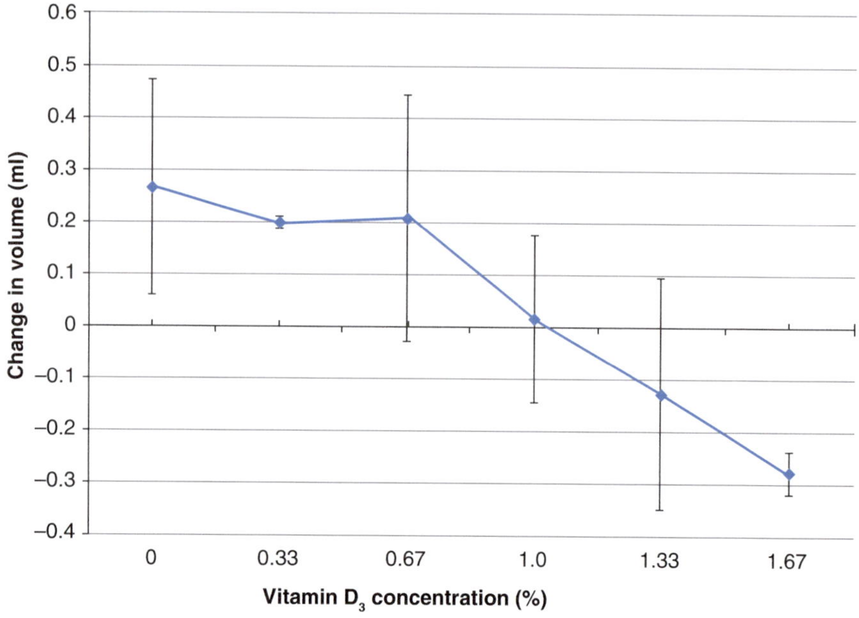

Fig. 6 Effect of vitamin D3 on cholesterol volume expansion during cholesterol crystallization. This illustrates the dual effect of vitamin D on cholesterol crystallization. Low doses inhibit while high doses accelerate crystallization. (Reproduced with permission [50])

5 Effects of Strategies to Reduce Coronary Artery Calcification

Like other crystals that deposit elsewhere in the body, once calcification appears in the vasculature it cannot be removed or dissolved. Despite attempts to reduce the rate of progressive vascular calcification in the hope that it might improve cardiovascular prognosis over and above current secondary prevention measures which do not appear to affect this process.

Chelation: Chelation therapy employs the use of disodium edetate (EDTA) in the expectation that it might remove heavy metals including ionized calcium from the vasculature. The hypothesis is that EDTA would stimulate secretion of parathyroid hormone by reducing serum calcium and thus enhanced bone mineralization that would lead to reverse calcium transport from the vasculature back to the bones [51, 52]. In the only double blind multicenter study, the Trial to Assess Chelation Therapy trial (TACT) that included 1708 individuals age > 50 with known history of coronary artery disease that were randomized to intravenous chelation with EDTA or placebo, the primary composite endpoint of MACE or coronary revascularization or hospitalization for angina was only mildly reduced (26% vs. 30%; $p = 0.035$) but not individually [53]. Because EDTA can cause severe hypocalcemia, allergic reactions, leukopenia, thrombocytopenia, vasculitis, dermatitis, seizures, and even death it is not FDA approved for routine use [54–57]. Currently TACT2 is underway [57]. TACT2 is an NIH-sponsored, randomized, 2 × 2 factorial, double blind, placebo-controlled, multicenter clinical trial testing 40 weekly infusions of a multi-component EDTA-based chelation solution and twice daily oral, high-dose multivitamin and mineral supplements in patients with diabetes and a prior myocardial infarction (MI). TACT2 completed enrollment of 1000 subjects in December 2020 and is expected to report in 2024 [58].

Phosphate Binders: Two studies that employed phosphate binders to interrupt the formation of calcium phosphate crystals by reduced availability of phosphate have failed to demonstrate this strategy to be effective [59, 60].

Magnesium: Magnesium has been demonstrated to have multiple effects on calcification in the vascular media (Table 1). In addition, hypomagnesemia has been associated with higher cardiovascular risk both in the general population and in patients with CKD [61, 62]. Despite this, there is currently no robust clinical trial to support its routine use for secondary prevention in patients with coronary disease. Much of the magnesium effect is also by a passive reduction in the interference of absorption in the gastrointestinal tract (Fig. 7) [28].

Lipid lowering agents: Numerous studies have demonstrated that effective lipid lowering therapy with ezetimibe, statins, and PCSK-9 inhibitors can reduce plaque

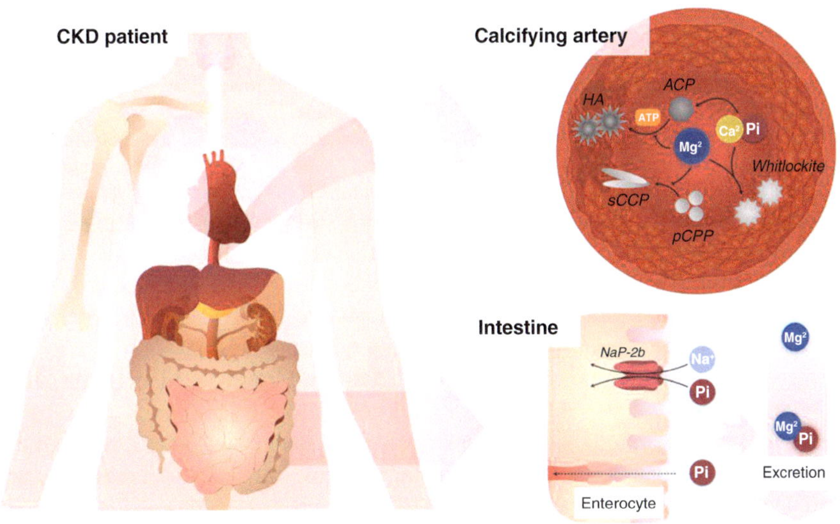

Fig. 7 Passive interference by magnesium on vascular calcification. Phosphate binding and crystal inhibition by Mg^{+2}. Elevated blood Mg^{+2} interferes with both amorphous calcium phosphate (ACP) and primary calciprotein particle (CPP) maturation into hydroxyapatite (HA) crystals and secondary CPP (sCPP). Mg^{+2} promotes the formation of the more soluble and smaller whitlockite crystal. In the intestine, Mg^{+2}-based inorganic phosphate (Pi) binders promote fecal Pi excretion, reducing Pi uptake via sodium phosphate cotransporter IIb (NaPi-2b) in enterocytes. *CKD* chronic kidney disease, *pCPP* primary CPP. (Reproduced with permission [28])

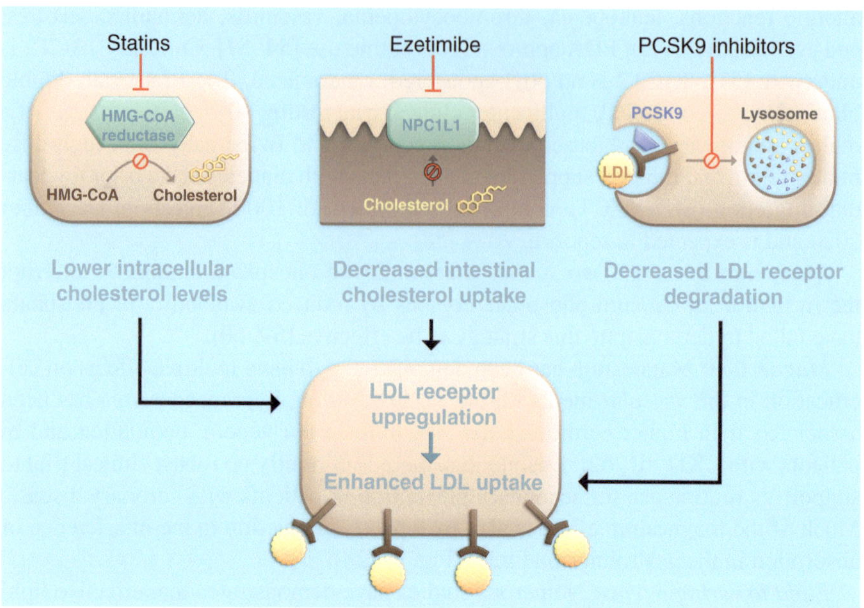

Fig. 8 Pharmacologic approaches to lower LDL cholesterol. Statins inhibit the rate-limiting enzyme of cholesterol biosynthesis, HMG-CoA reductase, leading to decreased hepatic cholesterol production. Ezetimibe is an inhibitor of NPC1L1 which facilitates the absorption of intestinal cholesterol and therefore selectively decreases dietary cholesterol uptake and hepatic cholesterol supply. The inhibition of cholesterol synthesis or intestinal absorption both lead to an upregulation of the LDL receptor and subsequently, enhance LDL uptake and lower LDL cholesterol serum concentrations. Therapeutic inhibition of PCSK9 also leads to a higher density of LDL receptors on the hepatocyte surface, but not primarily through targeting cholesterol metabolism, but by affecting LDL receptor degradation and recycling pathways. *HMG-CoA* 3-hydroxy-3-methylglutaryl-coenzyme A, *LDL* low-density lipoprotein, *PCSK9* proprotein convertase subtilisin/kexin type9, *NPC1L1* Niemann-Pick C1-like protein 1. (Reproduced with permission [64])

volume and the risk of MACE events in patients with proven atherosclerosis [63, 64] (Fig. 8). Despite these benefits, these agents are associated with accelerated increase in vascular calcification as assessed by CT scanning [65–67].

Interestingly, there is now some evidence that lipid lowering therapy may alter the morphology of calcium deposits [68]. In a study using Aged *Apoe*$^{-/-}$ mice, treatment with pravastatin reduced ^{18}F uptake in plaques, suggesting that it reduced the surface area of actively mineralizing calcium deposits, (albeit this decrease was not sustained). In addition, pravastatin increased the number of micro-calcium deposits (<50 μm in diameter), and the number of vascular cells positive for alkaline phosphatase activity compared with control mice. The amount of collagen and osteopontin, used as additional osteoblastic markers, were not significantly different between the two groups [68].

The observation that pravastatin could change the microarchitecture of the calcium deposits is of interest as speckled calcium in plaque has typically been associated with an increased risk of plaque rupture. Importantly the results suggest that while statins may not affect total calcium scores that are predominantly affected by the progression of larger sheet-like calcium deposits, they may modify the morphology of calcium crystals at an early phase, when calcium deposits impose their greatest risk to the integrity of the plaque. *Thus, statins might reduce the risk of plaque rupture not just by virtue of their effects on cholesterol crystallization, but also by virtue of their ability to modify the growth and morphology of calcium deposits in plaque* [68].

6 Detecting Coronary Calcification *in vivo*

Multiple imaging methods can detect vascular calcification (Table 3) [69]. Although computer tomography (CT) scanning is not the most sensitive means of detecting coronary calcification *in vivo*, it is the most widely accessible and most frequently

Table 3 Current imaging techniques for vascular calcification

Technique	Advantages	Disadvantages	Macrocalcification	Microcalcification
IVUS	Direct image of calcified plaque in arterial wall	Limited axial resolution and limited assessment of plaque composition and microcalcification	+	
CACS	Simple and reliable quantification of macroscopic calcium and coronary calcification burden	Low resolution and tissue contrast and plaque morphology	+	
CCTA	High spatial and temporal resolution of severity of coronary stenosis and detailed plaque morphology	Requires contrast agent. Difficult to identify and quantify calcium due to contrast agent	+	
MRI	Superior soft-tissue resolution. Localizes and detects volume of arterial calcification	Prolonged acquisition. Due to motion artifacts, cardiac contractions and respiration, it cannot detect microcalcification	+	

(continued)

Table 3 (continued)

Technique	Advantages	Disadvantages	Macrocalcification	Microcalcification
OCT	High spatial resolution. Assesses fibrous cap thickness, macrophage infiltration and border of arterial calcification	Difficult to differentiate calcium from lipid pool. Limited tissue penetration	+	
Invasive angiography	Superior spatial and temporal resolution	Inability to directly image calcification or the plaque	+	
18F-NaF PET	High sensitivity. Able to detect microcalcification in atherosclerotic plaque	Low special resolution. Limited by cardiac motion to quantify coronary artery microcalcification		+
18F-FDG PET/CT	Attenuated -CT can visualize macrocalcification	Background myocardial uptake limits coronary artery assessment	+	

CACS coronary artery calcium score, *CCTA* coronary computed tomographic angiography, *CT* computed tomography, *FDG* 2-deoxy-2-fluoro-d-glucose, *IVUS* intravascular ultrasound, *MRI* magnetic resonance imaging, *OCT* optical coherence tomography, *PET* positron emission tomography. (Modified from Wang Y et al. [69])

used in routine clinical practice. *More importantly, its major advantage relates to its able to detect calcification in the coronary arteries at a time when the risk of plaque instability begins to rise*, as evidenced by the relationship between quantification of CAC by CT scanning using the Agatston Score and estimates of cardiovascular risk over 10 years [70–76].

Numerous studies have confirmed that coronary calcium is rarely detected by CT scanning in men <40 years and women <50 years of age. Thus, CAC screening with CT scans in patients <40 years of age is of limited value in the absence of significant risk factors including a family history of premature coronary disease [77].

Furthermore, patients with a CAC score of 0 have been shown to have a benign prognosis over 10–12 years [70–75]. Thus, in these patients, many of whom likely have soft atheromatous plaques in their coronary arteries, the benefit of secondary prevention therapies including anti-platelet and lipid lowering agents and low-dose colchicine have not been demonstrated.

In contrast, patients with a CACs >100 have been demonstrated to receive a prognostic benefit from aspirin and lipid lowering therapy for secondary prevention [73, 77–79], and patients with scores >400 Agatston units who have more extensive coronary atherosclerosis often associated with obstructive coronary disease have been demonstrated to benefit from the addition of low-dose colchicine [80].

Although each of these therapies has been demonstrated to improve prognosis, none have been demonstrated to reduce CAC scores over time. Thus, while these strategies alter the risk of plaque growth and instability, they do not appear to affect the processes that lead to calcification in the coronary or peripheral circulations as assessed by CT scanning.

Contemporary guidelines now endorses CAC scoring using the Agatston method as an established adjunct to traditional risk factors for enhanced risk assessment to guide management in asymptomatic individuals [81–83].

In animal models, statins modestly accelerate calcification of plaques leading to more stable and lower-risk compositions. This phenomenon is also seen in human studies with coronary CT angiography and IVUS [84], leading to the suggestion by some, that statins might *promote* coronary calcification while at the same time slowing the progression of non-calcified coronary plaque, perhaps contributing to plaque stabilization [85–90]. As indicated above, statins may modify the growth and morphology of early microscopic calcium crystals when they present to the greatest risk to the plaque structure, an observation that could not be made by CT imaging.

Although the 2018 AHA/ACC Cholesterol Management Guidelines stated that there is no clinical utility for CAC scoring among statin users, as it does not change treatment strategies, there is evidence that CAC among statin users still remains highly predictive of cardiovascular mortality. This suggests that once the costs of Proprotein Convertase Subtilisin/ Kexin type 9 (PCSK-9) inhibitors lowers down, CAC scanning might be useful option to select patients who might receive benefits of lipid lowering beyond stain therapy. PCSK-9 inhibitors have shown to reduce the atheroma and improve clinical outcome when added to statin therapy [91–93].

7 The Challenge of Revascularization in the Presence of Extensive Vascular calcification

The constituents of atherosclerotic plaques carry critical impact on revascularization attempts. Among the major intraplaque components involved in the development of resistant plaques are the cholesterol crystals, calcifications and thrombus [93]. Extensive vascular calcification is not only associated with an increased risk of spontaneous plaque rupture but is also associated with an increased risk of procedural complications during coronary stenting including dissection, perforation, and abrupt vessel closure, myocardial infarction, and restenosis [94–96] which arise due to the need to apply high levels of non-uniform force across the length of the lesion being manipulated. Unfortunately, the procedural risks remain high despite the use of devices designed to reduce the risk of under-expansion and mal positioning of stents, including cutting/scoring balloons, double layered high pressure non-compliant balloons, lasers, intravascular lithotripsy balloons, and atherectomy devices.

Similarly, the presence of severe coronary calcification has been demonstrated to be associated with worse outcomes after coronary bypass surgery, including an increased risk of perioperative death, as well as MACE events in the first year following surgery [97, 98].

8 Summary

The appearance of calcium in atheromatous plaque in the coronary circulation by CT scanning is invariably due to the presence of atherosclerosis rather than calcification in the media, which occurs via different mechanisms and is most marked in the peripheral vasculature.

Detection of coronary calcium by CT imaging marks an inflection point in the natural history of coronary artery disease, most likely because the formation of calcium crystals in the plaque act synergistically with cholesterol crystals to cause local traumatic and inflammatory injury. Although secondary prevention therapies reduce cardiovascular risk, they do not slow, and may even accelerate the process of coronary calcification as assessed by CT scanning, however, there is evidence to suggest that statins may modify the growth and morphology of smaller calcium crystal deposits in plaque that have been associated with increased cardiovascular risk. Thus, while there is no compelling evidence that reducing vascular calcification impacts the natural history of patients with coronary atherosclerosis or peripheral vascular disease, it is possible that the assessment of total coronary calcium scores are too blunt to measure the benefits of therapies that can modify early formation of calcium crystals in the atherosclerotic bed.

References

1. Otsuka F, Sakakura K, Yahagi K, Joner M, Virmani R. Has our understanding of calcification in human coronary atherosclerosis progressed? Arterioscler Thromb Vasc Biol. 2014;34:724–36.
2. Wang L, Jerosch-Herold M, Jacobs DR Jr, Shahar E, Detrano R, Folsom AR, MESA Study Investigators. Coronary artery calcification and myocardial perfusion in asymptomatic adults: the MESA (multi-ethnic study of atherosclerosis). J Am Coll Cardiol. 2006;48:1018–26.
3. Kalra SS, Shanahan CM. Vascular calcification and hypertension: cause and effect. Ann Med. 2012;44(Suppl 1):S85–92.
4. Greenland P, LaBree L, Azen SP, Doherty TM, Detrano RC. Coronary artery calcium score combined with Framingham score for risk prediction in asymptomatic individuals. JAMA. 2004;291:210–5.
5. Criqui MH, Denenberg JO, Ix JH, et al. Calcium density of coronary artery plaque and risk of incident cardiovascular events. JAMA. 2014;311:271–8.
6. Kockx MM, De Meyer GR, Muhring J, Jacob W, Bult H, Herman AG. Apoptosis and related proteins in different stages of human atherosclerotic plaques. Circulation. 1998;97:2307–15.

7. Vengrenyuk Y, Carlier S, Xanthos S, et al. A hypothesis for vulnerable plaque rupture due to stress-induced debonding around cellular microcalcifications in thin fibrous caps. Proc Natl Acad Sci U S A. 2006;103:14678–83.

8. Kelly-Arnold A, Maldonado N, Laudier D, Aikawa E, Cardoso L, Weinbaum S. Revised microcalcification hypothesis for fibrous cap rupture in human coronary arteries. Proc Natl Acad Sci U S A. 2013;110:10741–6.

9. New SE, Goettsch C, Aikawa M, et al. Macrophage-derived matrix vesicles: an alternative novel mechanism for microcalcification in atherosclerotic plaques. Circ Res. 2013;113:72–7.

10. Mori H, Torii S, KutynaM SA, Finn AV, Virmani R. Coronary artery calcification and its progression: what does it really mean. JACC Cardiovasc Imaging. 2018;11:127–42.

11. Virmani R, Kolodgie FD, Burke AP, Farb A, Schwartz SM. Lessons from sudden coronary death: a comprehensive morphological classification scheme for atherosclerotic lesions. Arterioscler Thromb Vasc Biol. 2000;20:1262–75.

12. Dorozhkina E, Dorozhkin S. In vitro crystallization of carbonateapatite on cholesterol from a modified simulated body fluid. Colloids Surf. 2003;223:231–7. https://doi.org/10.1016/S0927-7757(03)00221-8.

13. Laird DF, Mucalo MR, Yokogawa Y. Growth of calcium hydroxyapatite (ca-HAp) on cholesterol and cholestanol crystals from a simulated body fluid: a possible insight into the pathological calcifications associated with atherosclerosis. J Colloid Interface Sci. 2006;295:348–63. https://doi.org/10.1016/j.jcis.2005.09.013.

14. Abedin M, Tintut Y, Demer LL. Vascular calcification: mechanisms and clinical ramifications. Arterioscler Thromb Vasc Biol. 2004;24:1161–70. https://doi.org/10.1161/01.ATV.0000133194.94939.42.

15. Johnson RC, Leopold JA, Loscalzo J. Vascular calcification: pathobiological mechanisms and clinical implications. Circ Res. 2006;99:1044–59. https://doi.org/10.1161/01.RES.0000249379.55535.21.

16. Fishbein GA, Micheletti RG, Currier JS, Singer E, Fishbein MC. Atherosclerotic oxalosis in coronary arteries. Cardiovasc Pathol. 2008;17:117–23. https://doi.org/10.1016/j.carpath.2007.07.002.

17. Khan SR, Pearle MS, Robertson WG, Gambaro G, Canles BK, Doizi S, Traxer O, Tiselius H-G. Kidney stones. Nat Rev Dis Primers. 2016;2:16008. https://doi.org/10.1038/nrdp.2016.8.

18. Abela GS, Kalavakunta JK, Janoudi A, Leffler D, Dhar G, Salehi N, Cohn J, Shah I, Karve M, Kotaru VPK, Gupta V, David S, Narisetty KK, Rich M, Vanderberg A, Pathak DR, Shamoun FE. Frequency of cholesterol crystals in culprit coronary artery aspirate during acute myocardial infarction and their relation to inflammation and myocardial injury. Am J Cardiol. 2017;120:1699–707. https://doi.org/10.1016/j.amjcard.2017.07.075.

19. Nadra I, Mason JC, Philippidis P, Florey O, Smythe CDW, McCarthy GM, Landis RC, Haskard DO. Proinflammatory activation of macrophages by basic calcium phosphate crystals via protein kinase C and MAP kinase pathways: a vicious cycle of inflammation and arterial calcification? Circ Res. 2005;96:1248–56. https://doi.org/10.1161/01.RES.0000171451.88616.c2.

20. Düewell P, Kono H, Rayner KJ, Sirois CM, Vladimer G, Bauernfeind FG, Abela GS, Franchi L, Nuñez G, Schnurr M, Espevik T, Lien E, Fitzgerald KA, Rock KL, Moore KJ, Wright SD, Hornung V, Latz E. NLRP3 inflammasomes are required for atherogenesis and activated by cholesterol crystals. Nature. 2010;464:1357–61. https://doi.org/10.1038/nature08938.

21. Rajamaki K, Lappalainen J, Oorni K, Valimaki E, Matikainen S, Kovanen PT, Eklund KK. Cholesterol crystals activate the NLRP3 inflammasome in human macrophages: a novel link between cholesterol metabolism and inflammation. PLoS One. 2010;5(7):e11765.

22. Patel R, Janoudi A, Vedre A, Aziz K, Tamhane U, Rubinstein J, Abela OG, Berger K, Abela GS. Plaque rupture and thrombosis is reduced by lowering cholesterol levels and crystallization with ezetimibe and is correlated with FDG-PET. Arterioscler Thromb Vasc Biol. 2011;31:2007–14. https://doi.org/10.1161/ATVBAHA.111.226167.

23. Martinon F, Pétrilli V, Mayor A, Tardivel A, Tschopp J. Gout-associated uric acid crystals activate the NALP3 inflammasome. Nature. 2006;440(7081):237–41. https://doi.org/10.1038/nature04516.

24. McCullough PA, Chinnaiyan KM, Agrawal V, Danielewicz E, Abela GS. Amplification of atherosclerotic calcification and Mönckeberg's sclerosis: a spectrum of the same disease process. Adv Chronic Kidney Dis. 2008;4:396–412.

25. Doherty TM, Asotra K, Fitzpatrick LA, Qiao J-H, Wilkin DJ, Detrano RC, Dunstan CR, Shah PK, Rajavashisth TB. Calcification in atherosclerosis: bone biology and chronic inflammation at the arterial crossroads. PNAS. 2003;100:11201–6. https://doi.org/10.1073/pnas.1932554100.

26. Speer MY, Yang HY, Brabb T, Leaf E, Look A, Lin WL, Frutkin A, Dichek D, Giachelli CM. Smooth muscle cells give rise to osteochondrogenic precursors and chondrocytes in calcifying arteries. Circ Res. 2009;104:733–41.

27. Hsu JJ, Tintut Y, Demer LL. Vitamin D and osteogenic differentiation in the artery wall. Clin J Am Soc Nephrol. 2008;3:1542–7.

28. Ter Btaake AD, Shahahan CM, de Baaij JHF. Magnesium counteracts vascular calcification; passive interference or active modulation? Atheroscler Thromb Vasc Biol. 2017;37:1431–45. https://doi.org/10.1161/ATVBAHA.117.309182.

29. Boistelle R, Lopez-Valero I, Abbona F. Crystallization of calcium phosphate in the presence of magnesium. Nephrologie. 1993;14:265–9.

30. Eanes ED, Posner AS. Kinetics and mechanism of conversion of noncrystalline calcium phosphate to hydroxyapatite. Trans N Y Acad Sci. 1965;28:233–41.

31. Termine JD, Peckauskas RA, Posner AS. Calcium phosphate formation in vitro. II. Effects of environment on amorphous-crystalline transformation. Arch Biochem Biophys. 1970;140:318–25.

32. Boskey AL, Posner AS. Magnesium stabilization of amorphous calcium phosphate: a kinetic study. Mater Res Bull. 1974;9:907–16.

33. Aghagolzadeh P, Bachtler M, Bijarnia R, Jackson C, Smith ER, Odermatt A, Radpour R, Pasch A. Calcification of vascular smooth muscle cells is induced by secondary calciprotein particles and enhanced by tumor necrosis factor-α. Atherosclerosis. 2016;251:404–14. https://doi.org/10.1016/j.atherosclerosis.2016.05.044.

34. Inoue T, Kawashima H. 1,25-Dihydroxyvitamin D3 stimulates 45Ca2+−uptake by cultured vascular smooth muscle cells derived from rat aorta. Biochem Biophys Res Commun. 1988;152:1388–94.

35. Jono S, Nishizawa Y, Shioi A, Morii H. 1,25-Dihydroxyvitamin D3 increases in vitro vascular calcification by modulating secretion of endogenous parathyroid hormone-related peptide. Circulation. 1998;98:1302–6.

36. Ix JH, Barrett-Connor E, Wassel CL, Cummins K, Bergstrom J, Daniels LB, Laughlin GA. The associations of fetuin-A with subclinical cardiovascular disease in community-dwelling persons: the rancho Bernardo study. J Am Coll Cardiol. 2011;58:2372–9.

37. Shalhoub V, Shatzen EM, Ward SC, Young JI, Boedigheimer M, Twehues L, McNinch J, Scully S, Twomey B, Baker D, Kiaei P, Damore MA, Pan Z, Haas K, Martin D. Chondro/osteoblastic and cardiovascular gene modulation in human artery smooth muscle cells that calcify in the presence of phosphate and calcitriol or paricalcitol. J Cell Biochem. 2010;111:911–21.

38. Zittermann A, Schleithoff SS, Koerfer R. Putting cardiovascular disease and vitamin D insufficiency into perspective. Br J Nutr. 2005;94:483–92.

39. Aoshima Y, Mizobuchi M, Ogata H, Kumata C, Nakazawa A, Kondo F, Ono N, Koiwa F, Kinugasa E, Akizawa T. Vitamin D receptor activators inhibit vascular smooth muscle cell mineralization induced by phosphate and TNF-α. Nephrol Dial Transplant. 2012;27:1800–6.

40. Watson KE, Abrolat ML, Malone LL, Hoeg JM, Doherty T, Detrano R, Demer LL. Active serum vitamin D levels are inversely correlated with coronary calcification. Circulation. 1997;96:1755–60.

41. Braam LA, Hoeks AP, Brouns F, Hamulyák K, Gerichhausen MJ, Vermeer C. Beneficial effects of vitamins D and K on the elastic properties of the vessel wall in postmenopausal women: a follow-up study. Thromb Haemost. 2004;91:373–80.

42. Doherty TM, Tang W, Dascalos S, Watson KE, Demer LL, Shavelle RM, Detrano RC. Ethnic origin and serum levels of 1alpha,25- Dihydroxyvitamin D3 are independent predictors of coronary calcium mass measured by electron-beam computed tomography. Circulation. 1997;96:1477–81.

43. McCullough PA, Sandberg KR, Dumler F, Yanez JE. Determinants of coronary vascular calcification in patients with chronic kidney disease and end-stage renal disease: a systematic review. J Nephrol. 2004;17:205–15.

44. Memon F, El-Abbadi M, Nakatani T, Taguchi T, Lanske B, Razzaque MS. Does Fgf23-klotho activity influence vascular and soft tissue calcification through regulating mineral ion metabolism? Kidney Int. 2008;74:566–70.

45. Razzaque MS, Lanske B. Hypervitaminosis D and premature aging: lessons learned from Fgf23 and klotho mutant mice. Trends Mol Med. 2006;12:298–305.

46. Schoppet M, Shroff RC, Hofbauer LC, Shanahan CM. Exploring the biology of vascular calcification in chronic kidney disease: what's circulating? Kidney Int. 2008;73:384–90.

47. Zittermann A, Schleithoff SS, Koerfer R. Vitamin D and vascular calcification. Curr Opin Lipidol. 2007;18:41–6.

48. Hewison M. Vitamin D and the immune system: new perspectives on an old theme. Rheum Dis Clin N Am. 2012;38:125–39.

49. Kassi E, Adamopoulous C, Basdra EK, Papavassiliou AG. Role of vitamin D in atherosclerosis. Circulation. 2013;128:2517–31.

50. Jildeh TR, Janoudi A, Abela GS. Vitamin D3 alters the crystallization and volume expansion of cholesterol. J Clin Lipidol. 2012;6 Suppl A:154.

51. Sultan S, Murarka S, Jahanfir A, Mookadam F, Tajik AJ, Jahangir A. Chelation therapy in cardiovascular disease: an update. Expert Rev Clin Pharmacol. 2017;10:843–54.

52. Singh D, Das K, Sheth R, Abela GS. Perspectives on the role of chelation therapy in the treatment of atherosclerosis: principles of application, clinical results, and practical implications. In: Topaz O, editor. Debulking in cardiovascular interventions and revascularization strategies-between the rock and the heart. London: Elsevier; 2022. p. 795–804.

53. Lamas GA, Goertz C, Boineau R, et al. Effect of disodium EDTA chelation regimen on cardiovascular events in patients with previous myocardial infarction: the TACT randomized trial. JAMA. 2013;309:1241–50.

54. Mark DB, Anstrom KJ, Clapp-Channing NE, et al. Quality-of-life outcomes with a disodium EDTA chelation regimen for coronary disease: results from the trial to assess chelation therapy rando- mized trial. Circ Cardiovasc Qual Outcomes. 2014;7:508–16.

55. Centers for Disease Control and Prevention (CDC). Deaths associated with hypocalcemia from chelation therapy—Texas, Pennsylvania, and Oregon, 2003-2005. MMWR Morb Mortal Wkly Rep. 2006;55:204–7.

56. Whayne TF Jr. What should medical practitioners know about the role of alternative medicines in cardiovascular disease management? Cardiovasc Ther. 2010;28:106–23.

57. Fihn SD, Gardin JM, Abrams J, et al. 2012 ACCF/AHA/ACP/AATS/ PCNA/SCAI/STS guideline for the diagnosis and management of patients with stable ischemic heart disease: executive summary: a report of the American College of Cardiology Foundation/American Heart Association task force on practice guidelines, and the American College of Physicians, American Association for Thoracic Surgery, Preventive Cardiovascular Nurses Association, Society for Cardiovascular Angiography and Interventions, and Society of Thoracic Surgeons. Circulation. 2012;126(25):3097–137; Erratum in: Circulation. 2014;129(16):e462.

58. Lamas GA, Anstrom KJ, Navas-Acien A, et al. The trial to assess chelation therapy 2 [RACT 2]: rationale and design. Am Heart J. 2022;252:1–11. https://doi.org/10.1016/j.ahj.2022.05.013.

59. Qunibi W, Moustafa M, Muenz LR, et al. A 1-year randomized trial of calcium acetate versus sevelamer on progression of coronary artery calcification in hemodialysis patients with comparable lipid control: the calcium acetate renagel evaluation-2 (CARE-2) study. Am J Kidney Dis. 2008;51:952–65.

60. Madhavan MV, Tarigopula M, Mintz GS, Maehara A, Stone GW, Généreux P. Coronary artery calcification pathogenesis and prognostic implications. J Am Coll Cardiol. 2014;63:1703–14. https://doi.org/10.1016/j.jacc.2014.01.017.

61. Sakaguchi Y, Fujii N, Shoji T, Hayashi T, Rakugi H, Isaka Y. Hypomagnesemia is a significant predictor of cardiovascular and non-cardiovascular mortality in patients undergoing hemodialysis. Kidney Int. 2014;85(1):174–81. https://doi.org/10.1038/ki.2013.327; Epub 2013 Aug 28.

62. DiNicolantonio JJ, Liu J, O'Keefe JH. Magnesium for the prevention and treatment of cardiovascular disease. Open Heart. 2018;5:e000775. https://doi.org/10.1136/openhrt-2018-000775.

63. Nissen SE, Nicholls SJ, Sipahi I, Libby P, Raichlen JS, Ballantyne CM, Davignon J, Erbel R, Fruchart JC, Tardif J-C, Schoenhagen P, Crowe T, Cain V, Wolski K, Goormastic M, Tuzcu EM, ASTEROID Investigators. Effect of very high-intensity statin therapy on regression of coronary atherosclerosis: the ASTEROID trial. JAMA. 2006;295:1556–65. https://doi.org/10.1001/jama.295.13.jpc60002.

64. Katzmann JL, Gouni-Berthhold I, Laufs U. PCSK9 inhibition:insight from clinical trials and future prospects. Front Physiol. 2020;11:595819. https://doi.org/10.3389/fphys.2020.595819.

65. Henein M, Granåsen G, Wiklund U, Schmermund A, Guerci A, Erbel R, Raggi P. High dose and long-term statin therapy accelerate coronary artery calcification. Int J Cardiol. 2015;184:581–6.

66. Dykun I, Lehmann N, Kälsch H, Möhlenkamp S, Moebus S, Budde T, Seibel R, Grönemeyer D, Jöckel KH, Erbel R, et al. Statin medication enhances progression of coronary artery calcification: the Heinz Nixdorf recall study. J Am Coll Cardiol. 2016;68:2123–5.

67. Saremi A, Bahn G, Reaven PD, VADT Investigators. Progression of vascular calcification is increased with statin use in the veterans affairs diabetes trial (VADT). Diabetes Care. 2012;35:2390–2.

68. Xian JZ, Lu M, Fong F, Qiao R, Patel NR, Abeydeera D, Iriana S, Demer LL, Tintut Y. Statin effects on vascular calcification: microarchitectural changes in aortic calcium deposits in aged hyperlipidemic mice. Arterioscler Thromb Vasc Biol. 2021;41(4):e185–92.

69. Wang Y, Osborne MT, Tung B, Li M, Li Y. Imaging cardiovascular calcification. J Am Heart Assoc. 2018;7(13):e008564. https://doi.org/10.1161/JAHA.118.008564.

70. Agatston AS, Janowitz WR, Hildner FJ, Zusmer NR, Viamonte M Jr, Detrao R. Quantification of coronary artery calcium using ultrafast computed tomography. J Am Coll Cardiol. 1990;15:827–32.

71. Detrano R, Guerci AD, Carr JJ, et al. Coronary calcium as a predictor of coronary events in four racial or ethnic groups. N Engl J Med. 2008;358:1336–45.

72. Kavousi M, Elias-Smale S, Rutten JHW, et al. Evaluation of newer risk markers for coronary heart disease risk classification: a cohort study. Ann Intern Med. 2012;156:438–44.

73. Erbel R, Möhlenkamp S, Moebus S, et al. Coronary risk stratification, discrimination, and reclassification improvement based on quantification of subclinical coronary atherosclerosis: the Heinz Nixdorf recall study. J Am Coll Cardiol. 2010;56:1397–406.

74. Carr JJ, Jacobs DR Jr, Terry JG, et al. Association of coronary artery calcium in adults aged 32 to 46 years with incident coronary heart disease and death. JAMA Cardiol. 2017;2:391–9.

75. Budoff MJ, Young R, Burke G, et al. Ten-year association of coronary artery calcium with atherosclerotic cardiovascular disease (ASCVD) events: the multi-ethnic study of atherosclerosis (MESA). Eur Heart J. 2018;39:2401–8.

76. Agatston AS, Janowitz WR, Hildner FJ, et al. Quantification of coronary artery calcium using ultrafast computed tomography. J Am Coll Cardiol. 1990;15:827–32. https://doi.org/10.1016/0735-1097(90)90282-t.

77. Gupta A, Lau E, Varshney R, et al. The identification of calcified coronary plaque is associated with initiation and continuation of pharmacological and lifestyle preventive therapies: a systematic review and meta-analysis. JACC Cardiovasc Imaging. 2017;10:833–42. https://doi.org/10.1016/j.jcmg.2017.01.030.

78. Cainzos-Achirica M, Miedema MD, McEvoy JW, et al. Coronary artery calcium for personalized allocation of aspirin in primary prevention of cardiovascular disease in 2019: the MESA study (multi-ethnic study of atherosclerosis). Circulation. 2020;141:1541–53. https://doi.org/10.1161/CIRCULATIONAHA.119.045010.

79. Kim J, McEvoy JW, Nasir K, et al. Critical review of high-sensitivity C-reactive protein and coronary artery calcium for the guidance of statin allocation: head-to-head comparison of the JUPITER and St. Francis heart trials. Circ Cardiovasc Qual Outcomes. 2014;7:315–22. https://doi.org/10.1161/CIRCOUTCOMES.113.000519.

80. Kofler T, Kurmann R, Lehnick D, Cioffi GM, Chandran S, Attinger-Toller A, Toggweiler S, Kobza R, Moccetti F, Cuculi F, Jolly SS, Bossard M. Colchicine in patients with coronary artery disease: a systematic review and meta-analysis of randomized trials. J Am Heart Assoc. 2021;10(16):e021198. https://doi.org/10.1161/JAHA.121.021198.

81. Greenland P, Blaha MJ, Budoff MJ, Erbel R, Watson KE. Coronary calcium score and cardiovascular risk. J Am Coll Cardiol. 2018;72:434–47.

82. Grundy SM, Stone NJ, Bailey AL, et al. 2018 AHA/ACC/AACVPR/AAPA/ABC/ACPM/ADA/AGS/APhA/ASPC/NLA/PCNA guideline on the management of blood cholesterol: executive summary. J Am Coll Cardiol. 2019;73:3168–209.

83. Arnett DK, Blumenthal RS, Albert MA, et al. 2019 ACC/AHA guideline on the primary prevention of cardiovascular disease: a report of the American College of Cardiology/American Heart Association task force on clinical practice guidelines. J Am Coll Cardiol. 2019;74:e177–232.

84. Osei AD, Mirbolouk M, Berman D, Budoff MJ, Miedema MD, Rozanski A, Rumberger JA, Shaw L, Al Rifai M, Dzaye O, Graham GN, Banach M, Blumenthal RS, Dardari ZA, Nasir K, Blaha MJ. Prognostic value of coronary artery calcium score, area, and density among individuals on statin therapy vs. non-users: the coronary artery calcium consortium. Atherosclerosis. 2021;316:79–83. https://doi.org/10.1016/j.atherosclerosis.2020.10.009.

85. Lee S-E, Chang H-J, Sung JM, et al. Effects of statins on coronary atherosclerotic plaques: the PARADIGM study. JACC Cardiovasc Imaging. 2018;11:1475–84.

86. Achenbach S, Ropers D, Pohle K, et al. Influence of lipid-lowering therapy on the progression of coronary artery calcification: a prospective evaluation. Circulation. 2002;106:1077–82.

87. Nakazato R, Gransar H, Berman DS, et al. Statins use and coronary artery plaque composition: results from the international multicenter CONFIRM registry. Atherosclerosis. 2012;225:148–53.

88. Shemesh J, Apter S, Itzchak Y, Motro M. Coronary calcification compared in patients with acute versus in those with chronic coronary events by using dual-sector spiral CT. Radiology. 2003;226:483–8.

89. Henein M, Granåsen G, Wiklund U, et al. High dose and long-term statin therapy accelerate coronary artery calcification. Int J Cardiol. 2015;184:581–6.

90. Puri R, Nicholls SJ, Shao M, et al. Impact of statins on serial coronary calcification during atheroma progression and regression. J Am Coll Cardiol. 2015;65:1273–82.

91. Gonzalo N, et al. Coronary plaque composition as assessed by greyscale intravascular ultrasound and radiofrequency spectral data analysis. Int J Cardiovasc Imaging. 2008;24:811–8. https://doi.org/10.1007/s10554-008-9324-2.

92. Li S, et al. Proprotein convertase subtilisin-kexin type 9 as a biomarker for the severity of coronary artery disease. Ann Med. 2015;47:386–93. https://doi.org/10.3109/07853890.2015.1042908.

93. Li JJ, et al. Proprotein convertase subtilisin/kexin type 9, C-reactive protein, coronary severity, and outcomes in patients with stable coronary artery disease: a prospective observational cohort study. Medicine. 2015;94:52–60.

94. Abela OG, Singh D, Abela GS. The resistant atherosclerotic plaques: pathologic features and their impact on revascularization. In: Topaz O, editor. Debulking in cardiovascular interventions and revascularization strategies-between the rock and the heart. London: Elsevier; 2022. p. 29–59.

95. Fitzgerald PJ, Ports TA, Yock PG. Contribution of localized calcium deposits to dissection after angioplasty. An observational study using intravascular ultrasound. Circulation. 1992;86:64–70.

96. Díaz JF, Gómez-Menchero A, Cardenal R, et al. Extremely high-pressure dilation with a new noncompliant balloon. Tex Heart Inst J. 2012;39:635–8.

97. Ertelt K, Généreux P, Mintz GS, Reiss GR, Kirtane AJ, Madhavan MV, Fahy M, Williams MR, Brener SJ, Mehran R, Stone GW. Impact of the severity of coronary artery calcification on clinical events in patients undergoing coronary artery bypass grafting (from the acute catheterization and urgent intervention triage strategy trial). Am J Cardiol. 2013;2013(112):1730–7. https://doi.org/10.1016/j.amjcard.2013.07.038.

98. Gonzalez JN, Macias AE, Salerno TA, Magarakis M. Coronary calcifications: effect on coronary artery bypass surgery. In: Topaz O, editor. Debulking in cardiovascular interventions and revascularization strategies-between the rock and the heart. London: Elsevier; 2022. p. 361–76.

99. Kircelli F, Peter ME, Sevinc Ok E, Celenk FG, Yilmaz M, Steppan S, Asci G, Ok E, Passlick-Deetjen J. Magnesium reduces calcification in bovine vascular smooth muscle cells in a dose-dependent manner. Nephrol Dial Transplant. 2012;27:514–21. https://doi.org/10.1093/ndt/gfr321.

100. Montezano AC, Zimmerman D, Yusuf H, Burger D, Chignalia AZ, Wadhera V, van Leeuwen FN, Touyz RM. Vascular smooth muscle cell differentiation to an osteogenic phenotype involves TRPM7 modulation by magnesium. Hypertension. 2010;56:453–62.

101. Louvet L, Büchel J, Steppan S, Passlick-Deetjen J, Massy ZA. Magnesium prevents phosphate-induced calcification in human aortic vascular smooth muscle cells. Nephrol Dial Transplant. 2013;28:869–78. https://doi.org/10.1093/ndt/gfs520.

102. Shao JS, Cheng SL, Pingsterhaus JM, Charlton-Kachigian N, Loewy AP, Towler DA. Msx2 promotes cardiovascular calcification by activating paracrine Wnt signals. J Clin Invest. 2005;115:1210–20. https://doi.org/10.1172/JCI24140.

103. Montes de Oca A, Guerrero F, Martinez-Moreno JM, Madueño JA, Herencia C, Peralta A, Almaden Y, Lopez I, Aguilera-Tejero E, Gundlach K, Büchel J, Peter ME, Passlick-Deetjen J, Rodriguez M, MuñozCastañeda JR. Magnesium inhibits Wnt/β-catenin activity and reverses the osteogenic transformation of vascular smooth muscle cells. PLoS One. 2014;9:e89525. https://doi.org/10.1371/journal.pone.0089525.

104. Brigant B, Metzinger-Le Meuth V, Massy ZA, et al. Serum microRNAs are altered in various stages of chronic kidney disease: a preliminary study. Clin Kidney J. 2017;10:30–7.

105. Cui RR, Li SJ, Liu LJ, Yi L, Liang QH, Zhu X, Liu GY, Liu Y, Wu SS, Liao XB, Yuan LQ, Mao DA, Liao EY. MicroRNA-204 regulates vascular smooth muscle cell calcification in vitro and in vivo. Cardiovasc Res. 2012;96:320–9. https://doi.org/10.1093/cvr/cvs258.

106. Louvet L, Metzinger L, Büchel J, Steppan S, Massy ZA. Magnesium attenuates phosphate-induced deregulation of a microRNA signature and prevents modulation of Smad1 and osterix during the course of vascular calcification. Biomed Res Int. 2016;2016:7419524. https://doi.org/10.1155/2016/7419524.

107. Altura BM, Altura BT, Carella A, Gebrewold A, Murakawa T, Nishio A. Mg2+-Ca2+ interaction in contractility of vascular smooth muscle: Mg2+ versus organic calcium channel blockers on myogenic tone and agonist-induced responsiveness of blood vessels. Can J Physiol Pharmacol. 1987;65:729–45.

108. Iseri LT, French JH. Magnesium: nature's physiologic calcium blocker. Am Heart J. 1984;108:188–93.

109. Shanahan CM, Crouthamel MH, Kapustin A, Giachelli CM. Arterial calcification in chronic kidney disease: key roles for calcium and phosphate. Circ Res. 2011;109:697–711. https://doi.org/10.1161/CIRCRESAHA.110.234914.

110. Proudfoot D, Skepper JN, Hegyi L, Bennett MR, Shanahan CM, Weissberg PL. Apoptosis regulates human vascular calcification in vitro: evidence for initiation of vascular calcification by apoptotic bodies. Circ Res. 2000;87:1055–62.

111. Rodenbeck SD, Zarse CA, McKenney-Drake ML, et al. Intracellular calcium increases in vascular smooth muscle cells with progression of chronic kidney disease in a rat model. Nephrol Dial Transplant. 2017;32:450–8.

112. Blumenthal NC, Betts F, Posner AS. Stabilization of amorphous calcium phosphate by mg and ATP. Calcif Tissue Res. 1977;23:245–50.

113. LeGeros RZ, Contiguglia SR, Alfrey AC. Pathological calcifications associated with uremia: two types of calcium phosphate deposits. Calcif Tissue Res. 1973;13:173–85.

114. Massy ZA, Drüeke TB. Magnesium and outcomes in patients with chronic kidney disease: focus on vascular calcification, atherosclerosis and survival. Clin Kidney J. 2012;5(suppl 1):i52–61. https://doi.org/10.1093/ndtplus/sfr167.

115. Brown EM, Gamba G, Riccardi D, Lombardi M, Butters R, Kifor O, Sun A, Hediger MA, Lytton J, Hebert SC. Cloning and characterization of an extracellular ca(2+)-sensing receptor from bovine parathyroid. Nature. 1993;366:575–80. https://doi.org/10.1038/366575a0.

116. Riccardi D. Cell surface, Ca2+(cation)-sensing receptor(s): one or many? Cell Calcium. 1999;26:77–83. https://doi.org/10.1054/ceca.1999.0066.

117. Ruat M, Snowman AM, Hester LD, Snyder SH. Cloned and expressed rat Ca2+−sensing receptor. J Biol Chem. 1996;271:5972–5.

118. Rodríguez-Ortiz ME, Canalejo A, Herencia C, Martínez-Moreno JM, Peralta-Ramírez A, Perez-Martinez P, Navarro-González JF, Rodríguez M, Peter M, Gundlach K, Steppan S, Passlick-Deetjen J, MuñozCastañeda JR, Almaden Y. Magnesium modulates parathyroid hormone secretion and upregulates parathyroid receptor expression at moderately low calcium concentration. Nephrol Dial Transplant. 2014;29:282–9. https://doi.org/10.1093/ndt/gft400.

119. Alesutan I, Tuffaha R, Auer T, et al. Inhibition of osteo/chondrogenic transformation of vascular smooth muscle cells by MgCl2 via calcium sensing receptor. J Hypertens. 2016;35:523–32.

120. Louvet L, Bazin D, Büchel J, Steppan S, Passlick-Deetjen J, Massy ZA. Characterization of calcium phosphate crystals on calcified human aortic vascular smooth muscle cells and potential role of magnesium. PLoS One. 2015;10:e0115342. https://doi.org/10.1371/journal.pone.0115342.

121. Doran AC, Meller N, McNamara CA. Role of smooth muscle cells in the initiation and early progression of atherosclerosis. Arterioscler Thromb Vasc Biol. 2008;28:812–9.

122. Kawashima H. Receptor for 1,25-dihydroxyvitamin D in a vascular smooth muscle cell line derived from rat aorta. Biochem Biophys Res Commun. 1987;146:1–6.

123. Somjen D, Weisman Y, Kohen F, Gayer B, Limor R, Sharon O, Jaccard N, Knoll E, Stern N. 25-hydroxyvitamin D3-1alpha-hydroxylase is expressed in human vascular smooth muscle cells and is upregulated by parathyroid hormone and estrogenic compounds. Circulation. 2005;111:1666–71.

124. Carthy EP, Yamashita W, Hsu A, Ooi BS. 1,25-Dihydroxyvitamin D3 and rat vascular smooth muscle cell growth. Hypertension. 1989;13(2):954–9.

125. Wu-Wong JR, Nakane M, Ma J. Effects of vitamin D analogs on the expression of plasminogen activator inhibitor-1 in human vascular cells. Thromb Res. 2006;118:709–14.

126. Mitsuhashi T, Morris RC, Ives HE. 1,25-Dihydroxyvitamin D3 modulates growth of vascular smooth muscle cells. J Clin Invest. 1991;87:1889–95.

127. Chen S, Law CS, Gardner DG. Vitamin D-dependent suppression of endothelin-induced vascular smooth muscle cell proliferation through inhibition of CDK2 activity. J Steroid Biochem Mol Biol. 2010;118:135–41.

128. Davies MR, Hruska KA. Pathophysiological mechanisms of vascular calcification in end-stage renal disease. Kidney Int. 2001;60:472–9.
129. Holick MF, Binkley NC, Bischoff-Ferrari HA, Gordon CM, Hanley DA, Heaney RP, Murad MH, Weaver CM, Endocrine Society. Evaluation, treatment, and prevention of vitamin D deficiency: an Endocrine Society clinical practice guideline. J Clin Endocrinol Metab. 2011;96:1911–30.
130. Arad Y, Spadaro LA, Roth M, Scordo J, Goodman K, Sherman S, Lerner G, Newstein D, Guerci AD. Serum concentration of calcium, 1,25 vitamin D and parathyroid hormone are not correlated with coronary calcifications: an electron beam computed tomography study. Coron Artery Dis. 1998;9:513–8.

Cholesterol Crystals in Diabetic Retinopathy

Yazen A. Shihab, Yvonne Adu Agyeiwaah, Tim F. Dorweiler, Irina Pikuleva, Julia V. Busik, and Maria B. Grant

1 Introduction

Cholesterol is an important structural component of plasma membranes and crucial for normal cellular and organ function. Its unique planar and rigid structure comprised of 27 carbon atoms determine the physicochemical properties of plasma membranes such as membrane fluidity, thickness, compressibility, water penetration, and intrinsic curvature [1]. In addition, cholesterol is used for the synthesis of oxysterols, steroid hormones, vitamin D, and bile acids and thereby regulates cellular and organ function [1, 2].

Every nucleated cell in mammals can produce cholesterol via a complex cascade of *de-novo* synthesis that accounts for approximately 80% of its daily need; the remaining 20% is derived from diet [3, 4]. The cholesterol molecule is hydrophobic. After the absorption by enterocyte and esterification, dietary cholesterol is transported within the bloodstream on different apolipoprotein particles—chylomicrons, very low-density lipoproteins (VLDL), and low-density lipoproteins (LDL) that are

Y. A. Shihab · Y. A. Agyeiwaah · M. B. Grant (✉)
Department of Ophthalmology and Visual Sciences, University of Alabama,
Birmingham, AL, USA
e-mail: yazen@uab.edu; yvonnad@uab.edu; mariagrant@uabmc.edu

T. F. Dorweiler · J. V. Busik
Department of Physiology, Michigan State University, East Lansing, MI, USA
e-mail: dorweile@msu.edu; busik@msu.edu

I. Pikuleva
Department of Translational Research, Western University of Health Sciences,
Pomona, CA, USA
e-mail: iap8@case.edu

© The Author(s), under exclusive license to Springer Nature
Switzerland AG 2023
G. S. Abela, S. M. Nidorf (eds.), *Cholesterol Crystals in Atherosclerosis and
Other Related Diseases*, Contemporary Cardiology,
https://doi.org/10.1007/978-3-031-41192-2_20

taken up by peripheral tissues upon binding to LDL receptors. Once lipids are utilized by the tissues, protein-rich lipoprotein remnants are remodeled into high-density lipoproteins (HDL) that remove excess cholesterol from peripheral tissues by reverse cholesterol transport back to the liver.

Accordingly, tight regulation of cholesterol levels within the body is imperative for normal function as insufficient or excessive cholesterol levels expose the body to risk of pathological states, of which atherosclerosis is a prime example. Elevated levels of circulating LDL pose a risk of being deposited within arterial walls, where their uptake by macrophages leads to the formation of "foam" cells. As cholesterol continues to accumulate in the arterial wall it predisposes to the formation of intra- and extracellular cholesterol crystals (CCs) that promote the development and progression of atherosclerotic plaques and contribute to plaque instability that leads to acute atherosclerotic events [5, 6].

There is now increasing evidence that cholesterol may also accumulate in the retina and promote retinal injury as it does in the arterial wall. Herein, we summarize the evidence that supports this thesis.

2 Basics of Cholesterol Delivery and Removal from the Retina

Retinal synthesis of cholesterol; as in other tissues, there are mechanisms in the retina that reduce its dependence on cholesterol in the systemic circulation and thus balance the input and output within the retina [7–10]. Specifically, retinal cells, like other cells in the body, can supply themselves with cholesterol by means of local synthesis, thus decreasing retinal reliance on systemic lipid supply [11, 12]. In fact, greater than 70% of retinal sterol are derived from *de-novo* synthesis, as indicated by studies in mice, with cholesterol biosynthesis being the most pronounced in Muller cells and photoreceptor inner segments [7, 13].

Systemic uptake of cholesterol by the retina: Beyond local biosynthesis, cholesterol may be taken up from the systemic circulation through the highly specialized transport mechanisms found in the outer blood–retina barrier (oBRB). The oBRB is formed by the tight junctions between the Retinal Pigment Epithelium (RPE) and functions to prevent unwanted materials in the systemic circulation (the fenestrated choriocapillaris) from entering the retina, by allowing highly selective uptake of different molecules, including cholesterol [14, 15]. In addition, the retina has an inner blood–retina barrier (iBRB) formed by the endothelium of the inner retinal vasculature. Normally, cholesterol supply to the retina via the iBRB is limited, but in some pathologic conditions including diabetic retinopathy it may be dramatically increased [9, 16].

Cholesterol delivery to the retina from the systemic circulation is achieved through numerous receptors present on the basal surface of the RPE, including LDL receptors, scavenger receptors class B (SR-B) type 1, type 3 and CD36 [17, 18].

Following sequestration from the circulation, the RPE is proposed to process the LDL and HDL and repackage the released cholesterol into HDL-like particles, which are secreted into the interphotoreceptor matrix via the ABCA1 transporter [17]. These HDL-like particles then move from the RPE to different retinal cells and back to the RPE, thus delivering cholesterol for utilization and removing cholesterol excess in the retina for subsequent transport to the systemic circulation [17].

Elimination of cholesterol from the retina: At least three different pathways mediate cholesterol elimination from the retina to maintain lipid homeostasis including photoreceptor phagocytosis, reverse cholesterol transport, and metabolism of cholesterol into oxysterols. The relative contribution of each of these pathways to the total retinal cholesterol output is currently unknown.

While photoreceptor phagocytosis is a retina-specific pathway, the retinal pathway of reverse cholesterol transport is like that from other tissues, in that it includes cholesterol efflux from different retinal cells and integration with different apolipoproteins that form particles, which are delivered to the systemic circulation. The only difference is that in order to pass the RPE during its transit from the retina to the choroidal circulation, the HDL-like particle cholesterol has to be re-packaged in the RPE into the so-called Bruch's membrane lipoprotein particles (differ in density and protein composition from chylomicrons, VLDL, LDL, and HDL), which are secreted into the circulation [19].

The third pathway relates to the ability of the retina to metabolize cholesterol into more soluble oxysterols which then diffuse into the systemic circulation to ultimately contribute to the production of bile acids in the liver [20, 21]. Retinal oxysterols are generated by the cytochrome P450 enzymes 27A1 and 46A1 (CYP27A1 and CYP46A1, respectively), which convert cholesterol into 27-hydroxycholesterol and other C27-oxygeneated sterols (CYP27A1) and 24-hydroxycholesterol (CYP46A1) [9, 22]. Importantly, these oxysterols are activating ligands for liver X receptors (LXR), which are transcription factors [23].

3 Cholesterol Dysregulation in Diabetic Retinopathy

Certain pathological states have been found to influence cholesterol regulation in the retina. Prime among these pathologies is diabetic retinopathy (DR) which results from progressive microvascular damage to the retina. Recently, the association between DR and abnormal lipid metabolism has been described, however, the mechanisms by which cholesterol dysregulation leads to DR is not certain.

One potential mechanism is the effect of diabetes on the downregulation of liver X receptors (LXRs) [24]. The role of LXRs has been well established in the regulation of genes related to reverse cholesterol transport and thus cholesterol homeostasis. It has also been found that LXRs influence glucose homeostasis by modulating insulin sensitivity amongst other tissue specific and hormonal mechanisms [25, 26]. It has been postulated that LXRs act to curtail gluconeogenesis while inducing hepatic glucokinase and GLUT4 expression in adipose; the collective effects of proper LXR functioning promotes glucose uptake in the periphery. Additionally, LXRs indirectly regulate inflammatory responses [27–31]. In diabetes, LXRs are downregulated, resulting in disrupted cholesterol metabolism and amplified pro-inflammatory signaling. In addition, there could be diminished synthesis of oxysterols by cytochrome P450 27A1 and 46A1, which further hampers LXR activity.

CYP46A1 is the principal enzyme controlling cholesterol elimination from the brain [32, 33]. In addition, CYP46A1, along with CYP27A1, participate in cholesterol removal from the retina [34–36]. Importantly, as the oxysterol products of CYP46A1 and CYP27A1 are the ligands for LXRs, these oxysterols were shown to affect the expression of the LXR target gene in retinal macrophage/microglia as well as bone marrow-derived macrophages (to a lesser extent) [36]. The effect was on both genes involved in reverse cholesterol transport and inflammatory response as indicated by studies in macrophages from *Cyp46a1$^{-/-}$*, *Cyp27a1$^{-/-}$*, and *Cyp46a1$^{-/-}$Cyp27a1$^{-/-}$* mice [36]. Furthermore, *Cyp46a1$^-$* and *Cyp27a1$^{-/-}$* were shown to be expressed in human retinal endothelial cells, and the diabetic environment was found to modulate the *Cyp46a1$^{-/-}$* and *Cyp27a1* expression in bovine retinal endothelial cells and the RPE. Studies by immunohistochemistry confirmed CYP46A1 expression in retinal vascular endothelial cells [36].

Thus, either LXR downregulation in diabetes or reduced production of the LXR activating oxysterols will impair the efficiency of cholesterol removal from the retina. In diabetic animal models, activation of LXRs normalizes cholesterol efflux [24, 37–39].

4 The Pathogenic Role of Cholesterol Crystals in Diabetic Retinopathy

Both disruption of the blood–retinal barrier leads to leakage of circulating lipids into the retina and aberrant cholesterol retinal homeostasis contributes to cholesterol accumulation. Over time, as elsewhere, the accumulation of sufficient free cholesterol may promote the formation of intra- and extracellular cholesterol crystals (CCs). CCs are hyperreflective structures and are seen in numerous pathological ocular diseases, including diabetic retinopathy (DR) and age-related macular degeneration [40, 41].

Although CCs have been known to exists in vivo for over a century, sampling techniques used to fix tissue inadvertently hid them from direct detection [42]. Scanning and transmission electron microscopy used to study atherosclerosis progression requires ethanol to dehydrate free water, causing tissue specimen proteins to fixate [43]. Consequently, tissue morphology is altered, and CCs are readily dissolved, thus underestimating their presence [44]. Because of this, studies of atherosclerotic specimens demonstrated the presence of "clefts" or empty spaces occupying advanced atherosclerotic lesions and thus failed to directly visualize CCs. It is only when ethanol was avoided when preparing atherosclerotic specimens that their presence became clear [42].

Advances in non-invasive imaging with optical coherence tomography (OCT) has confirmed the presence of monohydrate CCs in vivo, as a component within the necrotic core of atherosclerotic lesions [45, 46]. Similarly, spectral-domain OCT has demonstrated the presence of hyperreflective CC deposits within the retina of patients with diabetes, age-related macular degeneration, and Coats disease [47, 48].

The presence of CCs has now been implicated in the progression of DR [49, 50]. In the retina, CCs exist in two forms: monohydrate and pure. Monohydrate forms of CCs exhibit a flat "knife-like" shape, while pure CCs are sharper and more "needle-like" morphology [51]. The firm, insoluble nature of CCs makes them recognizable as foreign bodies. Thus, it is believed that their presence may contribute to chronic inflammation and cell death through various pathways [49, 52, 53].

Inflammation is a key driver of DR progression that includes the upregulation of cytokines, chemokines, and growth factors, all of which contribute to BRB break-down and poor visual outcomes [54]. The innate immune system is among the various immunologic mechanisms that react to CC deposits. NLRP3 inflammasomes are synthesized within macrophages in response to exposure of cholesterol aggregates. Downstream, pro-inflammatory IL-1β cytokines are released [55]. IL-1β has been found to influence retinal damage and to be significantly elevated in patients with DR [55, 56]. Moreover, this pro-inflammatory mediator promotes the release of additional cytokines, subsequently activating microglial cells (Fig. 1). The now enabled microglial further stimulate a cascade of inflammation resulting in vascular breakdown and progression of DR [57]. CCs also initiate a robust activation of classical, alternative, and lectin complement pathways [56, 58]. These three

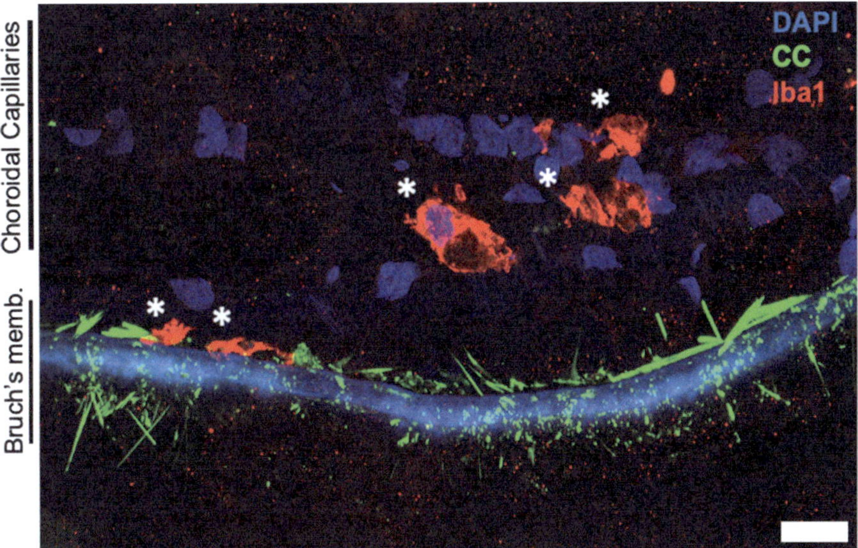

Fig. 1 Crystalized cholesterol in the human retinal microstructure. Cholesterol crystals in Bruch's membrane in the retina with proliferative diabetic retinopathy. 10 μm thick sections of a human eye have been stained for nuclei (DAPI), cholesterol crystals (CC), and microglia (Iba1). * indicate activated micro-glia. Scale bar = 10 μm

pathways enable complement fragments to arrive at a common endpoint: the membrane attack complex (MAC); a cytotoxic pore that lyses foreign microbes. Overabundant MAC deposition has been demonstrated in the DR-laden retinal epithelium which may be contributory to apoptosis of RPE [59].

Aside from the ability to induce inflammation, it is possible, albeit not proven, that CC growth may trigger direct microvascular trauma, and this predispose to retinal hemorrhage as has been observed with vasa vasorum in atherosclerotic plaque (See Fig. 4 in Chap. 16 "Molecular Pathomechanisms of Crystal-Induced Disorders") [60].

Individuals with diabetes, especially those with diabetes-related microvascular complications including DR, typically have abnormal lipid profiles that are thought to contribute to the formation of CCs in the retina. Among the changes in serum lipids is a reduction in circulating HDL. The primary purpose of HDL is to scavenge free cholesterol from tissues and transport them to the liver for redistribution to other tissues for eventual elimination [61]. It also known that it can dissolve CCs [62]. This raises the intriguing possibility that reduced systemic levels of HDL, and possibly reduced ability to form HDL-like proteins in the retina, may diminish the ability to clear CCs and thus promote DR [63–65].

5 Potential Benefit of Lipid-Lowering Therapy in Diabetic Retinopathy

Based upon the evidence supporting the role of CCs in DR progression, attempts to reduce the formation of CCs to prevent the development or retard the process of DR has sparked interest. To date, however, evidence that this strategy may be of value in DR as it is in atherosclerosis [66, 67] is still sparse.

Studies that have analyzed the association between lipid-lowering therapy and DR are conflicting, possibly reflecting the complex nature of DR, however, interpretation of these studies is also affected by their differing endpoints and their variable design. These issues also limit the ability to make sense of meta-analyses of these studies which are further limited by the variance of inclusion criteria, sample size, blood lipids evaluated, and severity or presence of DR [68]. Moreover, it is not clear that findings from basic science studies that use animal models can be translated into human disease. Despite these limitations, there is some evidence that lipid-lowering therapies may reduce the risk and consequences of DR.

6 Fibrates

Sub-studies conducted within two large, randomized control trials, including the Fenofibrate Intervention and Event Lowering in Diabetes (FIELD) trial and Action to Control Cardiovascular Risk in Diabetes (ACCORD) Lipid Eye Trial, suggest that fenofibrate may improve DR-related outcomes [69, 70].

The FIELD trial ($n = 9795$) was designed to evaluate the effect of fenofibrate 200 mg once daily for 5 years compared to placebo on cardiovascular (CV) outcomes in diabetic patients. While therapy did not reduce the risk of CV events, in a sub-study of 1012 patients conducted to assess the effect of therapy on retinal disease. Therapy was associated with a 31% reduction in the incidence of sight-threatening DR requiring laser photocoagulation. Unfortunately, retinal CT scans were performed in very few participants.

In the ACCORD trial ($n - 1593$), which examined the effect of daily simvastatin and fenofibrate use at a dose of 160 mg for 4 years, the need for laser therapy for DR was reduced compared to placebo. This endpoint was determined by a difference of ≥ 3 early treatment diabetic retinopathy study (ETDRS) scale steps based on imaging or need for laser therapy.

Comparable to fenofibrate, clofibrate has also been found to reduce retinal exudates in patients with DR, however, albeit it was not associated with an improvement in visual acuity or retinal vascular lesions [71]. Recent systemic and meta-analysis reviews of fibrate therapy demonstrated a 45% risk reduction in diabetic macular edema in 1309 participants [72]. Thus, current evidence suggests that fenofibrates may provide benefits in DR, independent of lipid profile, however, further dedicated controlled trials are required to confirm these effects.

7 Omega-3 Fatty Acids Supplements, Diet and Statins

Omega-3 fatty acids found in fish and poultry meat have demonstrated efficacy in lowering triglycerides (TGs) [73]. To date most evidences suggest that standard dose therapy does not affect CV outcome, and little research has analyzed its effect in DR.

The Prevención con Dieta Mediterránea (PREDIMED) study ($n = 3482$) evaluated the effect of a Mediterranean diet bolstered with extra virgin olive oil and nuts on CV outcomes in patients with type 2 diabetes. Although no CV benefit was found, in the study population who met the long chain ω-3 polyunsaturated fatty acids (LCω3PUFA) dietary recommendation (≥ 500 mg/day), there was a 48% reduction in the incidence of sight-threatening DR compared to control diets [74]. Thus, these post hoc observations support the need for clinical trials to determine the effect of omega-3 fatty acid supplements on diabetic retinopathy.

Several studies have explored the effects of statins on DR. Although large observational studies do not suggest that they offer a benefit, they lack the fidelity to answer this question. Thus, dedicated controlled trials are required to determine whether their pleiotropic effects that include anti-inflammatory, antioxidant, vasodilatory, and anti-clotting effects offer benefits in alleviating sight-threatening outcomes in DR.

8   Cyclodextrins

Cyclodextrins (CDs) are macrocyclic oligosaccharides that form complexes with crystalline cholesterol for breakdown and elimination. In nature, they are formed from digestion of glucose by bacteria and can also be produced by enzymatic conversion using glucosyltransferase. The most abundant types of cyclodextrins are α-, β-, and γ-CDs with six, seven, and eight glucopyranose monomers, respectively.

Cyclodextrins have been found to alter various cellular functions, including lipid composition and removal of cellular cholesterol. In animal models intravenous administration of hydroxypropyl-β-cyclodextrin led to a transient decrease in plasma cholesterol in a dose-dependent manner. A phase 1 randomized, double-blind, parallel group study has been conducted in adults with Niemann-Pick Disease Type C1 (NPC1), a disorder of intracellular cholesterol and lipid trafficking, in which subjects received 2-hydroxypropyl-β-cyclodextrin (HPβCD; Trappsol® Cyclo™) intravenously. The study demonstrated a reduction in the synthesis of serum biomarkers of cholesterol. HPβCD also improved cholesterol clearance from the liver and improved cholesterol homeostasis. No studies have examined its effects on DR in humans.

In our lab we detected CCs, increased inflammation and macroglia activation in the retina of diabetic mice associated with an increase in leukocyte recruitment into the retina. In an ongoing study we employed cyclodextrins in an effort to eliminate CCs from the retina in this model. Interestingly, compared to untreated mice, we found that treatment with oral alpha-cyclodextrin for 4 months decreased both inflammation and leukostasis in the retina (Figs. 2 and 3), thus providing evidence of that the ability of cyclodextrins to dissolve retinal CCs may act to reverse CC-induced inflammation in diabetic retinopathy.

Thus, the identification of CCs within the retina of in diabetic with DR and diabetic mice offers insight into a novel (CC induced) inflammatory mechanisms that

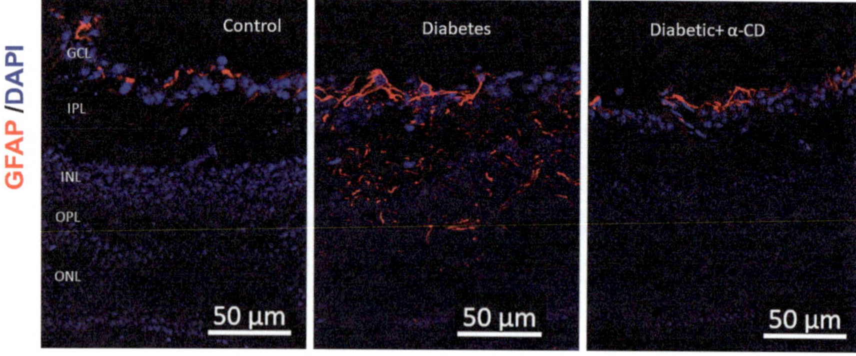

Fig. 2 Diabetic retina GFAP Response to α-Cyclodextrin. Glial Fibrillary Acidic Protein (GFAP) staining in the retina of control mice, diabetic mice, and diabetic mice with the oral alpha-cyclodextrin treatment. Scale bar = 50 µm

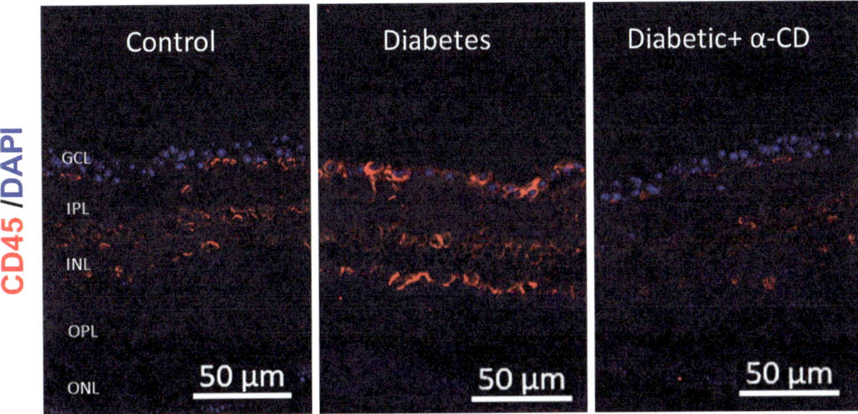

Fig. 3 α-Cyclodextrin alters CD45 Expression. CD45 staining in the retina of control mice, diabetic mice, and diabetic mice with the oral alpha-cyclodextrin treatment. Scale bar = 50 µm

may predispose to and promote DR which in turn may aid in the development of therapies to prevent and treat DR and other retinal diseases in which CCs have been found including age-related macular degeneration.

9 Conclusion

CCs have been found in the retina of patients with DR and age-related macular degeneration, and there is now strong evidence in an animal model that they may play a role in the progression of diabetic retinopathy and possibly cause direct trauma that might predispose to retinal hemorrhage. This suggests that further efforts to develop therapies that prevent CC formation, dissolve them or to inhibit the inflammatory process they induce may act to alleviate their pernicious effects on the retina in diabetes and people suffering from age-related macular degeneration which together are the most common causes of blindness in the world today.

References

1. Yang S-T, Kreutzberger AJB, Lee J, et al. The role of cholesterol in membrane fusion. Chem Phys Lipids. 2016;199:136–43.
2. Craig M, Yarrarapu SNS, Dimri M. Biochemistry, cholesterol. In: Stat pearls. Treasure Island (FL): Stat Pearls Publishing; 2022.
3. Bloch K. The biological synthesis of cholesterol. Science. 1965;150:19–28.
4. Harvard Health (2017) How it's made: cholesterol production in your body; Retrieved 13 Jan 2023. https://www.health.harvard.edu/heart-health/how-its-made-cholesterol-production-in-your-body.

5. Mc Namara K, Alzubaidi H, Jackson JK. Cardiovascular disease as a leading cause of death: how are pharmacists getting involved? Integr Pharm Res Pract. 2019;8:1–11. https://doi.org/10.2147/IPRP.S133088.

6. Brown JC, Gerhardt TE, Kwon E. Risk factors for coronary artery disease. In: Stat pearls. Treasure Island (FL): Stat Pearls Publishing; 2022.

7. Fliesler SJ, Bretillon L. The ins and outs of cholesterol in the vertebrate retina. J Lipid Res. 2010;51:3399–413.

8. Zheng W, Reem RE, Omarova S, Huang S, DiPatre PL, Charvet CD, Curcio CA, Pikuleva IA. Spatial distribution of the pathways of cholesterol homeostasis in human retina. PLoS One. 2012;7:e37926.

9. Pikuleva IA, Curcio CA. Cholesterol in the retina: the best is yet to come. Prog Retin Eye Res. 2014;41:64–89.

10. Zheng W, Mast N, Saadane A, Pikuleva IA. Pathways of cholesterol homeostasis in mouse retina responsive to dietary and pharmacologic treatments. J Lipid Res. 2015;56:81–97.

11. Fliesler SJ, Florman R, Rapp LM, Pittler SJ, Keller RK. In vivo biosynthesis of cholesterol in the rat retina. FEBS Lett. 1993;335:234–8.

12. Fliesler SJ, Keller RK. Metabolism of [3H]farnesol to cholesterol and cholesterogenic intermediates in the living rat eye. Biochem Biophys Res Commun. 1995;210:695–702.

13. Lin JB, Mast N, Bederman IR, et al. Cholesterol in mouse retina originates primarily from in situ de novo biosynthesis. J Lipid Res. 2016;57:258–64. https://doi.org/10.1194/jlr.M064469.

14. Elner VM. Retinal pigment epithelial acid lipase activity and lipoprotein receptors: effects of dietary omega-3 fatty acids. Trans Am Ophthalmol Soc. 2002;100:301–38.

15. Tserentsoodol N, Sztein J, Campos M, Gordiyenko NV, Fariss RN, Lee JW, Fliesler SJ, Rodriguez IR. Uptake of cholesterol by the retina occurs primarily via a low density lipoprotein receptor-mediated process. Mol Vis. 2006b;12:1306–18.

16. Wu M, Chen Y, Wilson K, Chirindel A, Ihnat MA, Yu Y, Boulton ME, Szweda LI, Ma JX, Lyons TJ. Intraretinal leakage and oxidation of LDL in diabetic retinopathy. Invest Ophthalmol Vis Sci. 2008;49:2679–85.

17. Tserentsoodol N, Gordiyenko NV, Pascual I, Lee JW, Fliesler SJ, Rodriguez IR. Intraretinal lipid transport is dependent on high density lipoprotein-like particles and class B scavenger receptors. Mol Vis. 2006a;12:1319–33.

18. Duncan KG, Hosseini K, Bailey KR, Yang H, Lowe RJ, Matthes MT, Kane JP, LaVail MM, Schwartz DM, Duncan JL. Expression of reverse cholesterol transport proteins ATP-binding cassette A1 (ABCA1) and scavenger receptor BI (SR-BI) in the retina and retinal pigment epithelium. Br J Ophthalmol. 2009;93:1116–20.

19. Curcio CA, Johnson M, Rudolf M, Huang JD. The oil spill in ageing Bruch membrane. Br J Ophthalmol. 2011;95:1638–45.

20. Mast N, Reem R, Bederman I, Huang S, DiPatre PL, Björkhem I, Pikuleva IA. Cholestenoic acid is an important elimination product of cholesterol in the retina: comparison of retinal cholesterol metabolism with that in the brain. Invest Ophthalmol Vis Sci. 2011;52:594–603.

21. El-Darzi N, Mast N, Dailey B, Denker J, Li Y, Vance J, Pikuleva IA. Characterizations of hamster retina as a model for studies of retinal cholesterol homeostasis. Biology. 2021;10:1003.

22. Liao WL, Heo GY, Dodder NG, Reem RE, Mast N, Huang S, Dipatre PL, Turko IV, Pikuleva IA. Quantification of cholesterol-metabolizing P450s CYP27A1 and CYP46A1 in neural tissues reveals a lack of enzyme-product correlations in human retina but not human brain. J Proteome Res. 2011;10:241–8.

23. Janowski BA, Grogan MJ, Jones SA, Wisely GB, Kliewer SA, Corey EJ, Mangelsdorf DJ. Structural requirements of ligands for the oxysterol liver X receptors LXRalpha and LXRbeta. Proc Natl Acad Sci U S A. 1999;96:266–71.

24. Hammer SS, Beli E, Kady N, Wang Q, Wood K, Lydic TA, Malek G, Saban DR, Wang XX, Hazra S, Levi M, Busik JV, Grant MB. The mechanism of diabetic retinopathy pathogenesis unifying key lipid regulators, sirtuin 1 and liver X receptor. EBioMed. 2017;22:181–90.

https://doi.org/10.1016/j.ebiom.2017.07.008; Epub 2017 Jul 11. PMID: 28774737; PMCID: PMC5552206.

25. Laffitte BA, Chao LC, Li J, Walczak R, Hummasti S, Joseph SB, Castrillo A, Wilpitz DC, Mangelsdorf DJ, Collins JL, Saez E, Tontonoz P. Activation of liver X receptor improves glucose tolerance through coordinate regulation of glucose metabolism in liver and adipose tissue. Proc Natl Acad Sci U S A. 2003;100:5419–24.

26. Calkin AC, Tontonoz P. Transcriptional integration of metabolism by the nuclear sterol-activated receptors LXR and FXR. Nat Rev Mol Cell Biol. 2012;13:213–24.

27. Glass CK, Ogawa S. Combinatorial roles of nuclear receptors in inflammation and immunity. Nat Rev Immunol. 2006;6:44–55.

28. Zelcer N, Tontonoz P. Liver X receptors as integrators of metabolic and inflammatory signaling. J Clin Invest. 2006;116:607–14.

29. Hong C, Tontonoz P. Coordination of inflammation and metabolism by PPAR and LXR nuclear receptors. Curr Opin Genet Dev. 2008;18:461–7.

30. Spann NJ, Garmire LX, McDonald JG, Myers DS, Milne SB, Shibata N, Reichart D, Fox JN, Shaked I, Heudobler D, Raetz CR, Wang EW, Kelly SL, Sullards MC, Murphy RC, Merrill AH Jr, Brown HA, Dennis EA, Li AC, Ley K, Tsimikas S, Fahy E, Subramaniam S, Quehenberger O, Russell DW, Glass CK. Regulated accumulation of desmosterol integrates macrophage lipid metabolism and inflammatory responses. Cell. 2012;151:138–52.

31. Spann NJ, Glass CK. Sterols and oxysterols in immune cell function. Nat Immunol. 2013;14:893–900.

32. Lund EG, Guileyardo JM, Russell DW. cDNA cloning of cholesterol 24-hydroxylase, a mediator of cholesterol homeostasis in the brain. Proc Natl Acad Sci U S A. 1999;96:7238–43.

33. Lund EG, Xie C, Kotti T, Turley SD, Dietschy JM, Russell DW. Knockout of the cholesterol 24-hydroxylase gene in mice reveals a brain-specific mechanism of cholesterol turnover. J Biol Chem. 2003;278:22980–8.

34. Omarova S, Charvet CD, Reem RE, Mast N, Zheng W, Huang S, Peachey NS, Pikuleva IA. Abnormal vascularization in mouse retina with dysregulated retinal cholesterol homeostasis. J Clin Invest. 2012;122:3012–23.

35. Saadane A, Mast N, Charvet CD, Omarova S, Zheng W, Huang SS, Kern TS, Peachey NS, Pikuleva IA. Retinal and nonocular abnormalities in Cyp27a1(−/−)Cyp46a1(−/−) mice with dysfunctional metabolism of cholesterol. Am J Pathol. 2014;184:2403–19.

36. Saadane A, Mast N, Trichonas G, Chakraborty D, Hammer S, Busik JV, Grant MB, Pikuleva IA. Retinal vascular abnormalities and microglia activation in mice with deficiency in cytochrome P450 46A1-mediated cholesterol removal. Am J Pathol. 2019;189:405–25.

37. Hammer SS, Vieira CP, McFarland D, Sandler M, Levitsky Y, Dorweiler TF, Lydic TA, Asare-Bediako B, Adu-Agyeiwaah Y, Sielski MS, Dupont M, Longhini AL, Li Calzi S, Chakraborty D, Seigel GM, Proshlyakov DA, Grant MB, Busik JV. Fasting and fasting-mimicking treatment activate SIRT1/LXRα and alleviate diabetes-induced systemic and microvascular dysfunction. Diabetologia. 2021;64(7):1674–89. https://doi.org/10.1007/s00125-021-05431-5; Epub 2021 Mar 26. PMID: 33770194; PMCID: PMC8236268.

38. Vieira CP, Fortmann SD, Hossain M, Longhini AL, Hammer SS, Asare-Bediako B, Crossman DK, Sielski MS, Adu-Agyeiwaah Y, Dupont M, Floyd JL, Li Calzi S, Lydic T, Welner RS, Blanchard GJ, Busik JV, Grant MB. Selective LXR agonist DMHCA corrects retinal and bone marrow dysfunction in type 2 diabetes. JCI Insight. 2020;5(13):e137230. https://doi.org/10.1172/jci.insight.137230; PMID: 32641586; PMCID: PMC7406260.

39. Hazra S, Rasheed A, Bhatwadekar A, Wang X, Shaw LC, Patel M, Caballero S, Magomedova L, Solis N, Yan Y, Wang W, Thinschmidt JS, Verma A, Li Q, Levi M, Cummins CL, Grant MB. Liver X receptor modulates diabetic retinopathy outcome in a mouse model of streptozotocin-induced diabetes. Diabetes. 2012;61(12):3270–9. https://doi.org/10.2337/db11-1596; Epub 2012 Aug 13. PMID: 22891211; PMCID: PMC3501845.

40. Tabas I. Consequences of cellular cholesterol accumulation: basic concepts and physiological implications. J Clin Invest. 2002;110:905–11.

41. Baumer Y, Mehta NN, Dey AK, Powell-Wiley TM, Boisvert WA. Cholesterol crystals and atherosclerosis. Eur Heart J. 2020;41:2236–9.
42. Grebe A, Latz E. Cholesterol crystals and inflammation. Curr Rheumatol Rep. 2013;15:313. https://doi.org/10.1007/s11926-012-0313-z.
43. Nasiri M, Janoudi A, Vanderberg A, et al. Role of cholesterol crystals in atherosclerosis is unmasked by altering tissue preparation methods. Microsc Res Tech. 2015;78:969–74. https://doi.org/10.1002/jemt.22560.
44. Liu L, Gardecki JA, Nadkarni SK, et al. Imaging the subcellular structure of human coronary atherosclerosis using micro-optical coherence tomography. Nat Med. 2011;17:1010–4. https://doi.org/10.1038/nm.2409.
45. Shi X, Cai H, Wang F, et al. Cholesterol crystals are associated with carotid plaque vulnerability: an optical coherence tomography study. J Stroke Cerebrovasc Dis. 2020;29:104579. https://doi.org/10.1016/j.jstrokecerebrovasdis.2019.104579.
46. Fujiyoshi K, Minami Y, Ishida K, et al. Incidence, factors, and clinical significance of cholesterol crystals in coronary plaque: an optical coherence tomography study. Atherosclerosis. 2019;283:79–84. https://doi.org/10.1016/j.atherosclerosis.2019.02.009.
47. Ong SS, Cummings TJ, Freedman SF. Cholesterol crystals in the anterior segment in coats' disease. Ophthalmol Retina. 2018;2:791. https://doi.org/10.1016/j.oret.2018.04.015.
48. Goel S, Saurabh K, Roy R. Blue light fundus autofluorescence in coats disease. Retina. 2019;39:e34–5. https://doi.org/10.1097/IAE.0000000000002598.
49. Nia S, Yu C, Chen Q, et al. Multimodality analysis of hyper-reflective foci and hard exudates in patients with diabetic retinopathy. Sci Rep. 2017;7:1568. https://doi.org/10.1038/s41598-017-01733-0.
50. Hammer SS, McFarland D, Bornemann N, et al. Cholesterol crystals promote diabetic retinopathy (DR) pathology. Invest Ophthalmol Vis Sci. 2020;61:1771a.
51. Craven BM. Crystal structure of cholesterol monohydrate. Nature. 1976;260:727–9. https://doi.org/10.1038/260727a0.
52. Shu F, Chen J, Ma X, et al. Cholesterol crystal-mediated inflammation is driven by plasma membrane destabilization. Front Immunol. 2018;9:1163. https://doi.org/10.3389/fimmu.2018.01163.
53. Janoudi A, Shamoun FE, Kalimantan JK, Abela GS. Cholesterol crystal induced arterial inflammation and destabilization of atherosclerotic plaque. Eur Heart J. 2016;37:1959–67. https://doi.org/10.1093/eurheartj/ehv653.
54. Rubs A, Parikh S, Fort PE. Role of inflammation in diabetic retinopathy. Int J Mol Sci. 2018;19:942. https://doi.org/10.3390/ijms19040942.
55. Wu H, Hwang D-K, Song X, Tao Y. Association between aqueous cytokines and diabetic retinopathy stage. J Ophthalmol. 2017;2017:9402198. https://doi.org/10.1155/2017/9402198.
56. Samstad EO, Niyonzima N, Nymo S, et al. Cholesterol crystals induce complement-dependent inflammasome activation and cytokine release. J Immunol. 2014;192:2837–45. https://doi.org/10.4049/jimmunol.1302484.
57. Quevedo-Martínez JU, Garfias Y, Jimenez J, et al. Pro-inflammatory cytokine profile is present in the serum of Mexican patients with different stages of diabetic retinopathy secondary to type 2 diabetes. BMJ Open Ophthalmol. 2021;6:e000717. https://doi.org/10.1136/bmjophth-2021-000717.
58. Niyonzima N, Halvorsen B, Sporsheim B, et al. Complement activation by cholesterol crystals triggers a subsequent cytokine response. Mol Immunol. 2017;84:43–50. https://doi.org/10.1016/j.molimm.2016.09.019.
59. Huang C, Fisher KP, Hammer SS, et al. Plasma exosomes contribute to microvascular damage in diabetic retinopathy by activating the classical complement pathway. Diabetes. 2018;67:1639–49. https://doi.org/10.2337/db17-1587.
60. Mughal MM, Khan MK, DeMarco JK, Majid A, Shamoun F, Abela GS. Symptomatic and asymptomatic carotid artery plaque. Expert Rev Cardiovasc Ther. 2011;9:1315–30. https://doi.org/10.1586/erc.11.120.

61. Jomard A, Osto E. High density lipoproteins: metabolism, function, and therapeutic potential. Front Cardiovasc Med. 2020;7:39. https://doi.org/10.3389/fcvm.2020.00039.

62. Adams CWM, Abdulla YH. The action of human high-density lipoprotein on cholesterol crystals part 1. Light-microscopic observations. Atherosclerosis. 1978;31:465–71. https://doi.org/10.1016/0021-9150(78)90142-9.

63. Farbstein D, Levy AP. HDL dysfunction in diabetes: causes and possible treatments. Expert Rev Cardiovasc Ther. 2012;10:353–61. https://doi.org/10.1586/erc.11.182.

64. Morton J, Zoungas S, Li Q, et al. Low HDL cholesterol and the risk of diabetic nephropathy and retinopathy: results of the ADVANCE study. Diabetes Care. 2012;35:2201–6. https://doi.org/10.2337/dc12-0306.

65. Tomić M, Vrabec R, Bulum T, Ljubić S. HDL cholesterol is a protective predictor in the development and progression of retinopathy in type 1 diabetes: a 15-year follow-up study. Diabetes Res Clin Pract. 2022;186:109814. https://doi.org/10.1016/j.diabres.2022.109814.

66. Pignone M, Phillips C, Mulrow C. Use of lipid lowering drugs for primary prevention of coronary heart disease: meta-analysis of randomised trials. BMJ. 2000;321:983–6. https://doi.org/10.1136/bmj.321.7267.983.

67. Pahan K. Lipid-lowering drugs. Cell Mol Life Sci. 2006;63:1165–78. https://doi.org/10.1007/s00018-005-5406-7.

68. Chang Y-C, Wu W-C. Dyslipidemia and diabetic retinopathy. Rev Diabet Stud. 2013;10:121–32. https://doi.org/10.1900/RDS.2013.10.121.

69. Scott R, Best J, Forder P, et al. Fenofibrate intervention and event lowering in diabetes (FIELD) study: baseline characteristics and short-term effects of fenofibrate [ISRCTN64783481]. Cardiovasc Diabetol. 2005;4:13. https://doi.org/10.1186/1475-2840-4-13.

70. ACCORD Study Group, ACCORD Eye Study Group, Chew EY, et al. Effects of medical therapies on retinopathy progression in type 2 diabetes. N Engl J Med. 2010;363:233–44. https://doi.org/10.1056/NEJMoa1001288.

71. Duncan LJ, Cullen JF, Ireland JT, et al. A three-year trial of atromid therapy in exudative diabetic retinopathy. Diabetes. 1968;17:458–67. https://doi.org/10.2337/diab.17.7.458.

72. Mozetic V, Pacheco RL, de OC LC, Riera R. Statins and/or fibrates for diabetic retinopathy: a systematic review and meta-analysis. Diabetol Metab Syndr. 2019;11:92. https://doi.org/10.1186/s13098-019-0488-9.

73. Tur JA, Bibiloni MM, Sureda A, Pons A. Dietary sources of omega 3 fatty acids: public health risks and benefits. Br J Nutr. 2012;107(Suppl 2):S23–52. https://doi.org/10.1017/S0007114512001456.

74. Sala-Vila A, Díaz-López A, Valls-Pedret C, et al. Dietary marine ω-3 fatty acids and incident sight-threatening retinopathy in middle-aged and older individuals with type 2 diabetes: prospective investigation from the PREDIMED trial. JAMA Ophthalmol. 2016;134(10):1142.

Cholesterol in the Central Nervous System in Health and Disease

Ryan Skowronek

1 Introduction

Cholesterol subserves a wide array of functions within the central nervous system (CNS): development, regeneration, energy storage, modification of plasma membrane fluidity and permeability via lipid rafts, synaptogenesis, maintenance of synaptic plasticity, neurotransmitter exocytosis, neurotransmitter receptor modulation, axonal elongation, and dendritic differentiation [1–5]. The human brain contains approximately 25% of the body's cholesterol, predominantly in myelin sheaths, as well as neuronal and astrocytic plasma membranes [6, 7]. However, CNS cholesterol regulation is spatiotemporally independent of dietary uptake or hepatic synthesis, as the continuous non-fenestrated vessels that comprise the blood–brain barrier are impermeable to the cholesterol-carrying lipoproteins of the peripheral corpus [8, 9]. Given that cholesterol-regulated membrane proteins function optimally at certain proportions of cholesterol, tightly regulated homeostasis in CNS cholesterol content is vital [10]. Cells sense their respective cholesterol levels through membrane-bound transcription factors (sterol-regulatory element-binding proteins), which then regulate the transcription of genes encoding for cholesterol biosynthesis and lipoprotein receptors [11–14].

The metabolism of CNS cholesterol will be elucidated here, though it will be discussed in depth further on. Newly synthesized cholesterol is loaded onto "HDL-like" lipoproteins enriched with ApoE, the major cholesterol distribution molecule of the CNS. Lipidation and secretion of ApoE are mediated by ABC transporters.

R. Skowronek (✉)
Department of Neurology and Ophthalmology, Michigan State University,
East Lansing, MI, USA
e-mail: skowro30@msu.edu

G. S. Abela, S. M. Nidorf (eds.), *Cholesterol Crystals in Atherosclerosis and Other Related Diseases*, Contemporary Cardiology,
https://doi.org/10.1007/978-3-031-41192-2_21

(For clarity, ApoE-C will refer to the complex of ApoE-enriched lipoproteins loaded with cholesterol.) The ApoE-C complex binds to LDL receptors and LDL receptor-like proteins (LRP), among others, on glia and neurons. Once endocytosed, it is processed to separate the cholesterol moiety for utilization. These liberated cholesterol molecules also induce negative feedback on cholesterol biosynthesis via a sterol-detecting mechanism. To maintain homeostasis, excess cholesterol is oxidized into oxysterols, particularly 24S-hydroxycholesterol and 27-hydroxycholesterol, which are then transported across the blood–brain barrier into systemic circulation.

Humans only develop high rates of cholesterol and myelin synthesis after birth [15]. What triggers this burst of cholesterol and myelin synthesis either in the developing fetus or in the newborn is poorly understood. During the first few weeks of life, myelination proceeds rapidly with correspondingly high rates of sterol accretion; however, sterol accretion rate diminishes as mature brain size is achieved in the following weeks [16]. Brain weight begins to diminish at 20 years of age with cortical cholesterol content decreasing linearly before diminishing more rapidly after 80 years of age [17]. In fact, by 100 years of age, brain cholesterol decreases by 20–50%, likely attributable to an age-related decrease in biosynthesis and increase in the excretion of cholesterol from the brain [18–21].

2 Normal CNS Cholesterol Metabolism

2.1 Synthesis

Cholesterol biosynthesis within the CNS takes place de novo within astrocytes, oligodendrocytes, microglia, and (to a lesser extent) neuronal perikaryon and proximal axons [6, 22]. In addition, synthesis seems to occur at different rates within functionally different CNS regions (e.g., cerebrum, cerebellum, brainstem, spinal cord) to meet the respective requirements of each region [16]. Sterols are synthesized in either the astrocytic Bloch pathway via desmosterol precursor or the neuronal Kandutsch-Russell pathway, with the primary cholesterol precursors being desmosterol in astrocytes and 7-dehydrocholesterol or lanosterol in neurons [23]. Brain-derived neurotrophic factor upregulates the neuronal pathway of cholesterol synthesis [23].

Sterol-regulatory element-binding proteins (SREBP)—inactive transcription factors anchored to the membrane of the endoplasmic reticulum—regulate cholesterol synthesis, especially SREBP2, with the aid of the sterol-detecting SREBP cleavage-activating proteins (SCAP) [11, 14, 23]. In the setting of adequate cholesterol concentration, Insulin-Induced Gene proteins (INSIG) retain the SREBP-SCAP complex to the endoplasmic reticulum membrane [23]. In the setting of cholesterol depletion, SCAP escorts SREBP to the Golgi body, where the active N-terminal domain of SREBP2 is released and translocated to the nucleus to bind sterol-regulatory elements of genetic promoter regions encoding enzymes for cholesterol biosynthesis [12, 23]. Moreover, SREBP2 downregulates low density lipoprotein receptor-related protein-1 (LRP1) expression to allow for increased cholesterol circulation for cells in need [24]. The half-life of brain cholesterol has been reported to anywhere from 6 months to 5 years, much longer than its plasma half-life [1]. For intracellular storage in the form of lipid droplets, cholesterol is esterified by acyl-coenzyme A:cholesterol acyltransferase-1 (ACAT1) within the endoplasmic reticulum [25–27].

2.2 Excretion

Given the local cholesterol biosynthesis and that neither cholesterol nor ApoE can diffuse through the blood–brain barrier, several mechanisms exist for excretion to prevent CNS cholesterol overload. (1) 24-hydroxylase is a P450 enzyme—one exclusive to cortical pyramidal cells, cerebellar Purkinje cells, and hippocampal and thalamic neurons—that serves to oxidize cholesterol to 24S-hydroxycholesterol (24-OHC), which can then be excreted across the blood–brain barrier [21, 22]. (2) Another P450 enzyme expressed in both neurons and glial cells oxidizes cholesterol to 27-hydroxycholesterol (27-OHC); however, the majority of CNS 27-OHC is delivered from the peripheral circulation [5]. Both of these oxysterols influence cholesterol synthesis and transport from glia to neurons through their interactions with nuclear Liver X Receptors (LXR)—transcription factors that regulate the synthesis of ApoE and ATP-binding cassette (ABC) transporters [5, 28]. ABC transporter expression is also regulated by the SREBP-SCAP system [29]. (3) Besides enzymatic oxidation, cholesterol auto-oxidation from other compounds (e.g., lipid peroxidases, free radical species) can result in the creation of other various oxysterols, which can diffuse bidirectionally through the blood–brain barrier [5]. (4) Another excretion pathway involves the ABC transporters, which load lipids onto vacant apolipoproteins, namely ApoE, for subsequent cholesterol efflux at the plasma membrane [14, 30]. This pathway is upregulated by elevated 24-hydroxycholesterol and in the setting of demyelination or neurodegeneration [14, 31, 32].

2.3 Transport

Several lipoprotein receptors are expressed in the CNS, which can bind to a wide variety of ligands with differing specificity [14, 33]. Interactions with these ligands enable the lipoprotein receptors to conduct a diverse set of functions in the nervous system, including lipoprotein trafficking, cell migration and development, and maintenance of synaptic plasticity [34]. Of significance are the LDL and LRP1 receptors, which are primarily responsible for lipoprotein binding and cholesterol delivery by ApoE-C to glia and neurons [22, 35, 36]. LDL receptors are most highly expressed in glia, whereas LRP1 receptors are more highly expressed in neurons [14, 22]. In fact, LDL receptors have been shown to cluster at axonal growth cones during regeneration [37]. (Other receptors, including the VLDL receptor and ApoE receptor 2, are involved in processes such as neuronal development and intracellular signaling, but have little-to-no role in cholesterol transport [22]). LRP1 receptors appear to have the highest transport capacity for ApoE-C [38]. It has been demonstrated that lipoprotein receptors—ergo lipoproteins and their associated cholesterol moieties—are necessary for proper CNS organogenesis [38]. For example, selective deletion of LRP1 receptors in forebrain neurons in mice has led to global defects in brain lipid metabolism and neurodegeneration [38]. LRP2 knockout mice develop holoprosencephaly with hemispheric fusion and the absence of olfactory bulbs, due to a reduction of sonic hedgehog expression and thereby a loss of interneurons and oligodendroglial cell populations [38].

ApoE coordinates the transportation of cholesterol for the growth, maintenance, and repair of myelin and neuronal membranes during development and after injuries [8, 39]. There are three common alleles of the ApoE gene (APOE)—APOE2, APOE3, APOE4—which allow for six genotypes. The most common genotype is homozygous APOE3. The presence of APOE4 is a major susceptibility risk factor for the development of Alzheimer Disease, which will be discussed in depth in the eponymous section. Astrocytes synthesize and secrete cholesterol via ABC transporters onto "HDL-like" lipoprotein particles that have been enriched with ApoE [1, 15, 22]. (ABCA1 deletion in mice reduces ApoE levels in the plasma, brain, and cerebrospinal fluid (CSF) by >80%; however, the importance of ABCA1 in human CNS lipid metabolism is not clear, as patients with mutations in both alleles in Tangier disease do not have CNS problems [22]. Perhaps another transporter in humans, such as ABCA7, assumes a similar role to murine ABCA1 [22]). These newly synthesized ApoE-C particles are exported via ABCG1/ABCA1 and can then redistribute cholesterol by binding to a variety of receptors—including the LDL receptor, VLDL receptor, ApoE-receptor 2, and LPR1 receptor—with subsequent endocytosis [30, 32, 38]. However, the conformation and lipidation status of ApoE-C may affect the specificity of its receptor binding [14].

In addition to ApoE production by astrocytes, neurons contain a unique splicing variant of APOE mRNA that is upregulated in the setting of neurodegeneration [22, 40]. Neuronal ApoE production is regulated to some degree by an astrocyte-secreted factor, as astrocyte-conditioned medium increases neuronal ApoE expression four- to ten-fold [40]. Therefore, the upregulation of this neuronal ApoE production may be due in part to astrocytosis—the abnormal proliferation of astrocytes in response to injury or neurodegenerative diseases [22]. (However, in Alzheimer Disease, cortical astrocytic hypertrophy predominates over proliferation [41]).

Some adult neurons do not require autonomous cholesterol synthesis as they can import cholesterol via lipoprotein receptor-mediated endocytosis [14]. After ApoE-C is endocytosed by a neuron, lysosomes process the complex to free its cholesterol moieties [42, 43]. Once cholesterol is packaged into vesicles containing NPC1 (which is inactivated in Neimann-Pick Disease) and transported to the endoplasmic reticulum, it can be incorporated into plasma membranes and their lipid raft microdomains or utilized for any number of other neuronal operations, such as synaptic remodeling and synaptic vesicle biogenesis [31, 44–47]. As previously mentioned, cholesterol elicits negative feedback on its own synthesis via the SREBP-SCAP complex bound to the endoplasmic reticulum. When not bound to cholesterol, ApoE is degraded and its level drastically decreases [28].

ApoE4 affects major pathways of neurodegeneration due to its domain interaction: decreased CNS lipid transport, direct neurotoxic fragmentation within neurons, and impaired synaptic turnover [22]. The ApoE4 isoform is less stable than that of ApoE2 and ApoE3 and assumes a pathological conformation through domain interaction, an intramolecular ionic interaction between arginine-61 and glutamic acid-255 [22]. ApoE4 exhibits lower lipid-binding capacity, lower cholesterol delivery rate, and faster degradation rate, resulting in inefficient cholesterol transportation for neuronal and synaptic maintenance [22, 40, 48]. Moreover, ApoE4 is degraded by a neuron-specific protease to a greater extent than other isoforms, generating neurotoxic carboxyl-terminal fragments that stimulate tau hyperphosphorylation and mitochondrial dysfunction (Fig. 1) [22, 40, 48].

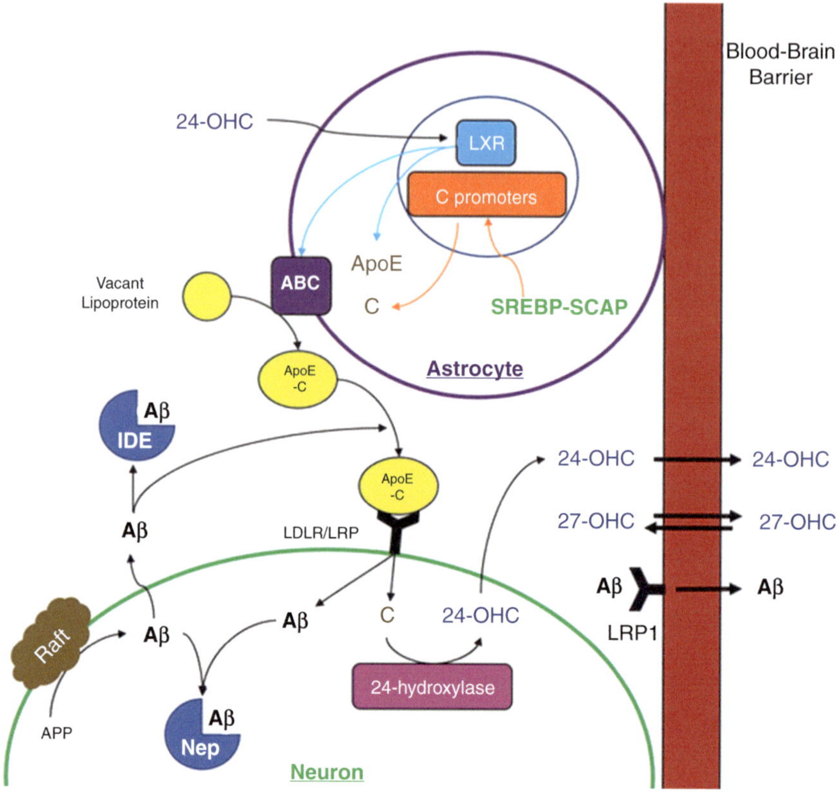

Fig. 1 Cholesterol metabolism and trafficking in the brain. When the SREBP-SCAP complex senses low intracellular cholesterol levels within astrocytes, SREBP dissociates and translocates to activate nuclear promoters of cholesterol biosynthesis. 24-OHC regulates ApoE production via nuclear LXR. ABC transporters—also regulated by LXR—enrich ApoE with cholesterol and package the complex onto vacant HDL-like lipoproteins. These lipoproteins can also carry extracellular beta-amyloid to neurons for degradation. Once bound to a neuronal lipoprotein receptor (likely LDLR or LRP1), the complex is endocytosed and cholesterol is liberated within endosome-lysosomes. Cholesterol is then utilized for any number of cellular functions. Some of the cholesterol is converted via 24-hydroxylase into 24-OHC for regulation of LXRs and excretion into peripheral circulation. APP is cleaved by secretases at lipid rafts to generate beta-amyloid. These newly generated beta-amyloid along with that which has been endocytosed can be degraded intracellularly by neprilysin, extracellularly by IDE, or loaded onto circulating lipoproteins. 27-OHC can diffuse through the blood brain barrier. LRP1 and VLDLR of the BBB endothelium also clear beta-amyloid. (Courtesy of Ryan Skowronek)

3   Role of Cholesterol in Neurologic Function

3.1   *Membrane Expansion and Regeneration*

Most biological membranes are comprised of approximately equal parts lipids and proteins [49]. Continuous addition of new membrane is required during axonal and dendritic growth and regeneration [50]. The neuronal perikaryon contains abundant rough endoplasmic reticulum (visualized as Nissl substance under light microscopy) and Golgi complexes, which together synthesize and modify lipids, proteins, and vesicular compartments [14, 51]. Membrane expansion is mediated by anterograde inter-organelle exocytosis of vesicle-bound plasmalemmal precursors from the perikaryon to the growth cone [14, 50]. Pfenninger outlined four different conditions of neurite (e.g., axonal or dendritic) growth and plasmalemmal expansion in vivo: (1) during de novo outgrowth by a growth cone; (2) during the continued elongation of axons concomitant with growth of the animal; (3) during the formation of collateral sprouts; and (4) during the regeneration of a severed neuronal process [51]. When cholesterol synthesis is inhibited in neurons, axonal elongation is supported by lipoprotein-derived cholesterol [1–3]. Upon tethering the plasma membrane via soluble N-ethylmaleimide-sensitive factor attachment protein receptor (SNARE) complexes, plasmalemmal precursor vesicles fuse with the acceptor membrane, leading to the expansion of the latter [50].

3.2   *Myelin*

As multicellular organisms continued to enlarge throughout evolution, the necessity to promptly interact with the environment required faster conduction velocities from neurons to their ever more distant targets. This was achieved by increasing the thickness of the hydrophobic sheaths surrounding axons, thereby reducing capacitance—the change in ion concentration required to initiate an action potential [15]. Myelin has interval gaps known as nodes of Ranvier that allow ionic transport along the axonal membrane. Saltatory conduction—this recurring process along the length of an axon—serves to bolster action potential propagation [34, 52].

The process of myelination is mediated in the CNS by oligodendrocytes which synthesize sheets of plasma membrane around multiple adjacent axons. Although most myelination will be completed in the peripheral nervous system (PNS) shortly after birth, myelination in the CNS is an ongoing process that continues throughout adulthood. 70% of the CNS cholesterol pool is invested in myelin [53]. Myelin is comprised of 70–85% lipids and 15–30% proteins, with the cholesterol, phospholipid, and glycolipid ratio being 40%:40%:20%, respectively [7, 49].

3.3 Synapses and Neurotransmission

Synapses are the connections between one neuron's axonal process and another's dendritic spine. Neurotransmitters are the molecules that communicate between the axon and dendrite to elicit singling cascades. They are contained within vesicles that must fuse with and undergo exocytosis from the presynaptic membrane into the synaptic cleft. These neurotransmitters can then go on to bind postsynaptic receptors to generate action potentials. Neurons have an intrinsic ability to form synapses, an ability which is enhanced considerably in the presence of cholesterol [1, 4, 46]. Cholesterol is incorporated into the lipid raft microdomains of synaptic vesicle membranes, presynaptic active zones, postsynaptic membranes, and at the edge of synapses, thus permitting synaptic vesicle biogenesis, alteration of membrane fluidity, and assembly of the fusional SNARE machinery [1, 17, 31, 44–47, 51, 54–58]. This allows for the signaling cascades enacted by neurotransmitter exocytosis from the presynaptic membrane into the synaptic cleft and subsequent binding to postsynaptic receptors. Cholesterol depletion results in a loss of synapses and dendritic spines [1].

Another important feature of synapses is synaptic plasticity, the activity-dependent modification of the strength or efficacy of synaptic transmission at pre-existing synapses [59]. In essence, it is the strengthening of specific synaptic connections in response to repeated activation. Cholesterol depletion reduces plasticity and its inherent function of long-term potentiation—closely linked to the storage of memories in the hippocampus, which is damaged in Alzheimer Disease [31, 38]. At the adult synapse, the glycoprotein Reelin has a key role in enhancing long-term potentiation, as it interacts with the both the ApoE receptor 2 and VLDL receptor [38]. The maintenance of plasticity and long-term potentiation is dependent on the proper release of neurotransmitters.

In the presynaptic region, cholesterol induces a conformational change in the transmembrane domains of vesicular SNARE proteins and vesicular membrane, allowing for fusion with the presynaptic membrane [1, 17, 45, 58]. As individuals age, cholesterol content increases within the exofacial leaflets of brain synaptic membranes—which contain the interactive lipid rafts—reducing the membrane fluidity (q.v., cholesterol's context-sensitive effects on membrane fluidity) [60]. Age-imposed and cholesterol context-sensitive rigidity may interfere with vesicle exocytosis, thus limiting synaptic transmission and thereby reducing plasticity.

Cholesterol modulates many receptors and ion functions [17]. Numerous neurotransmitter receptors have been found to be associated with the lipid raft microdomain [17, 23]. Located on the postsynaptic membrane are LRP1 and other ApoE receptors [38]. Cholesterol regulates lipid rafts and thereby regulates protein function (e.g., substrate presentation), as forming or depleting these rafts moves proteins into or out of the raft microenvironment, modulating their activity and function [61, 62].

4 Selected Neurologic Diseases Associated with Abnormal Cholesterol Handling and Cholesterol Crystallization

4.1 Alzheimer Disease

4.1.1 Introduction

Alzheimer Disease (AD) is the most common neurodegenerative disease in adults. Prevalence in the seventh decade of life is 3/1000; in the eighth, 3.2/1000; and in the ninth and above, 10.8/1000 [41]. The incidence of disease increases with age, with 125 new cases per 100,000 in persons older than 60 years of age. Major risk factors for AD include age, the presence of APOE4 alleles, mutations in either the amyloid precursor protein or presenilin genes. Modifiable risk factors include smoking, hypercholesterolemia, diabetes, and hypertension. Alzheimer Disease falls into a narrow bimodal distribution based on etiology, although both groups are clinically and pathologically indistinguishable [63]. Early-onset disease is mediated by autosomal dominant inheritance patterns of mutated APP, PSEN1, or PSEN2—all of which are directly involved in the production of amyloid-beta (Aβ). Late-onset disease is a sporadic, ostensibly multifactorial condition. There are no preventative or disease-modifying therapies.

On neuropathologic examination, there is neuronal loss in the cortex, hippocampus, parahippocampal gyri, subiculum, and the cholinergic nucleus basalis and locus coeruleus, among other locations. The remaining neurons have decreased volumes and ribonucleoproteins. Hallmarks of AD include (1) extracellular plaques of Aβ fragments from amyloid precursor proteins, (2) intracellular 'neurofibrillary tangles' of hyperphosphorylated tau (H-tau), and (3) cerebral amyloid angiopathy [5, 64].

Adams and Victor's Principles of Neurology notes that the progression of mentation changes is so insidious that neither the patient nor the family can date its onset. However, according to neuropathologic findings, the course of the disease appears to have a longer asymptomatic course preceding symptom onset. In fact, in the inherited form, biomarkers in the spinal fluid and imaging show changes that occur 15 years or longer before the clinical manifestations are apparent [65]. The initial and most prominent symptomatology is that of failures in memory—episodic (autobiographical) and retentive—after which further cerebral dysfunctions become evident and continue to deteriorate. Quantitatively demonstrable dysnomia, agnosia, and paucity of speech compromise communication and social interaction. Dyscalculia renders financial independence impossible. With visuospatial disorientation, patients may become lost in familiar places, lose the capability to dress themselves, or misunderstand directions, while ideational and ideomotor apraxia strip them of their ability to use common objects and tools such as door locks and utensils. Prosopagnosia alienates patients from their family members, alone among now unfamiliar faces. Overlaid may be sleep and behavioral disturbances, paranoias (often regarding spousal infidelity or theft), anxieties, phobias, personality changes such as increased egocentrism and indifference to others' feelings, executive dysfunction, and difficulty in locomotion that may eventually lead to a bedridden state.

4.1.2 Potential Role of CNS Amyloid Deposition in Dementia

Amyloids are misfolded protein aggregates that are found in numerous disease processes. The generation of $A\beta$ of AD is outlined here. The amyloid precursor protein (APP) undergoes sequential cleavage by secretase enzymes [38, 47]. In the pertinent amyloidogenic pathway, APP matures, becomes glycosylated, and is cleaved by beta-secretase then by gamma-secretase (encoded by PSEN1/2). Both secretases are transmembrane proteins that reside within lipid rafts; thus, cholesterol modulates their activity both by altering lipid raft fluidity and by binding to transmembrane cholesterol-binding motifs [17, 47]. Once $A\beta$ is generated, it is secreted into the interstitial fluid of the brain, where it can be cleared by a variety of mechanisms, including efflux across blood-brain barrier (BBB), cellular uptake for lysosomal degradation, and cleavage by $A\beta$-specific proteases [38]. Naturally, it follows that either accelerated generation or defective clearance of $A\beta$ may cause $A\beta$ accumulation, the former seen in familial early-onset AD and the latter in sporadic late-onset cases.

Familial cases of dementia are due to mutations in either APP or PSEN1/2, resulting in accelerated $A\beta$ generation. Mutations in APP favors beta-secretase (over alpha-secretase) cleavage to initiate the amyloidogenic pathway. In healthy brains, APP and beta-secretase are separated, but in AD the two proteins are colocalized within vastly enlarged endosome-lysosomes [38, 66]. Mutations in PSEN1/2 enhance their resultant gamma-secretase activity [24, 38].

Sporadic cases of dementia do not have any inherent defect in the enzymes of $A\beta$ generation; instead, these are attributable to inadequate clearance of $A\beta$ [24]. Approximately 70–85% of $A\beta$ undergoes efflux across BBB via ApoE-receptor-mediated transcytosis, with the rest removed through interstitial fluid bulk flow [24, 38, 67]. In both normal aging and AD, LRP1 expression decreases in brain endothelial and vascular smooth muscle cells, correlating with an increase in $A\beta$ [24]. Further dysregulation results in elevated SREBP2, decreasing LRP1 expression and thereby $A\beta$ clearance [24].

While $A\beta$ plaques and H-tau neurofibrillary tangles are found in all cortical association areas, it is the neurofibrillary tangles and quantitative neuronal loss—not the amyloid plaques—that most accurately correlate with dementia severity [5]. On the other hand, while early tau pathology in the entorhinal and limbic system can manifest without any $A\beta$, severe neocortical AD-like tau pathology in the form of neurofibrillary tangles and neuritic plaques is not seen in the absence of $A\beta$, suggesting that $A\beta$ is required in some capacity for clinically overt dementia [68]. In fact, blocking tau expression and phosphorylation completely inhibits $A\beta$ toxicity in differentiated neurons from rat culture [68]. Nevertheless, despite the amyloid hypothesis being the predominant research focus, clinical trials aimed at reducing amyloid plaques and the formation of Aβ have not been effective [22, 35, 36, 69]. Relevant to this book, the interplay of BBB compromise and cholesterol will be our focus here.

4.1.3 Potential Role of Blood–Brain Barrier Compromise in Dementia

The capillary (BBB) is comprised of endothelial cells connected by tight and adherens junction proteins, resulting in low paracellular and transcellular permeability, and its integrity is maintained by pericytes and astrocytic foot-processes [24, 70]. Hypercholesterolemia causes endothelial dysfunction, leading to increased production of adhesion molecules and cytokines, reflecting an increased inflammatory activity of the endothelium [39]. Vascular dysfunction can also influence the amyloidogenic pathway to diminish clearance and increase production of Aβ [24, 67]. A two-hit vascular hypothesis of AD has been put forth that posits cerebrovascular damage (initial hit causing BBB dysfunction) may initiate the cascade of neurodegeneration (second hit) [24, 70]. Even in the normal aging brain, BBB becomes dysfunctional [71].

Cerebrovascular dysfunction contribute to cognitive decline and neuronal loss in AD, beyond the damage caused by Aβ and tau pathology [24, 70]. In a group of 4629 patients diagnosed with AD and no evidence of mixed dementia, 80% had some form of vascular pathology, including the AD-hallmark cerebral amyloid angiopathy; moreover, those with either AD or cerebrovascular disease had a similar prevalence of vascular risk factors (e.g., coronary artery disease, hyperlipidemia, and diabetes mellitus) [70]. In preclinical AD, changes in vascular biomarkers precede both cognitive impairment and detectable alterations in amyloid and tau [70, 72]. BBB breakdown evidenced by gadolinium leakage on dynamic contrast enhanced (DCE) MRI preceded the hippocampal atrophy of early AD [70]. Susceptibility-weighted imaging MRI detects hemosiderin deposits from microhemorrhages due to BBB breakdown. High strength 7-tesla MRI has found that 78% of patients with AD have microhemorrhages; however, most studies involve lower strength 1.5- or 3-tesla MRI, so the incidence of microhemorrhages in AD is likely underestimated [70]. Recently, a large cohort autopsy found that 77% of 410 AD subjects had grossly apparent circle of Willis atherosclerosis, which occurred more often than in non-AD subjects [24, 73].

Breakdown of the BBB allows the entry of neurotoxic molecules that can elicit inflammatory and immune responses which can initiate multiple pathways of neurodegeneration [70]. ApoE4 causes BBB disruption and pericyte degeneration [74–76]. In APOE4 carriers with normal cognition or mild cognitive impairment, DCE MRI demonstrated BBB leakage prior to neural tissue loss, indicating that BBB disruption is independent of Aβ and hyperphosphorylated tau deposition [76–78]. Moreover, in APOE4 carriers, a biomarker of pericyte injury is elevated in the CSF, again independent of pathological changes in AD [76–78]. Degenerating pericytes accumulate intracellular inclusions, pinocytic vesicles, and large lipid granules [24, 79]. These microstructural changes correlate with capillary reductions, vessel dilation, and vessel tortuosity [24, 79].

ApoE4 and cholesterol crystals (CCs) activate inflammatory molecules (e.g., cytokine cyclophilin A, nuclear factor-kB, MMP-9) in pericytes and endothelial cells [71, 76, 80, 81]. ApoE2 and ApoE3 use both LRP1 and VLDLR for BBB transcytosis, leading to faster Aβ efflux, whereas ApoE4 relies primarily on the less efficient VLDLR with slower clearance [24, 38]. Moreover, ApoE4 has the weakest effect on Aβ degradation via neprilysin intracellularly and insulin degrading enzyme extracellularly [38]. ApoE4 also upregulates expression of receptor for advanced glycation end (RAGE) products [76]. Contrary to the Aβ efflux of LRP1, RAGE causes influx of peripheral Aβ, damaging pericytes and BBB [70, 75, 76]. This BBB breakdown in turn reduces P-glycoprotein and LRP1 levels as well as increased RAGE levels, resulting in further Aβ accumulation [24, 70]. In post-mortem studies, an accumulation of blood-derived proteins including fibrinogen, thrombin, plasminogen, immunoglobulin G, and albumin were found in the hippocampus and cortex of AD subjects, which was associated with pericyte degeneration [24, 79, 82]. The incidence of lobar microbleeds is positively associated with age, APOE4 carrier status, and Aβ burden, as determined by (11)C-labeled Pittsburgh Compound-B positron emission tomography [24].

4.1.4 Potential Role of Cholesterol, Cholesterol Crystals, and Oxysterols in Dementia

Endocytosis, lipoprotein signaling, and synaptic neurotransmission are all reliant on cholesterol homeostasis and are impaired in AD [38]. There is a causal relationship between hypercholesterolemia and T2DM development, oxidative stress, and insulin resistance within neural tissues [28]. Cholesterol can accumulate in a variety of manners: accelerated synthesis (e.g., SREBP dysregulation), decreased or improper transportation (e.g., ApoE4's inherent poor delivery), or impaired cellular uptake (e.g., dysfunctional receptors). Cholesterol-regulated protein clearance ability declines in normal aging [83]. Several studies have identified a link between midlife—but not late-life—hypercholesterolemia and AD development, suggesting that this process requires long-standing cholesterol excess for disease onset [39, 84]. Long-term high-cholesterol diet triggered astrocytic activation in the murine hippocampus, leading to increased cholesterol transport across cell membranes and proinflammatory cytokine IL-1B production [28, 85].

Once ApoE-C enters neurons, cholesterol and scaffolding proteins specifically traffic APP to lipid rafts, where it can be cleaved by beta- and gamma-secretases into Aβ. Elevated membrane cholesterol increases beta-secretase activity, thereby promoting the amyloidogenic pathway, whereas depletion inhibits both beta- and gamma-secretase activity [39, 47, 86]. Excess cholesterol aggregation in the endosomal-lysosomal system leads to altered APP processing, generating Aβ; in fact, in AD, endosomes exhibit volumes up to 32-fold larger than average [66, 87]. When Aβ is added to neuronal cell structure, it stimulates

ApoE-mediated internalization of cholesterol, leading to an increase in the intracellular levels of free cholesterol [39]. High level of membrane cholesterol leads to the incorporation of Aβ into the membranes and enhances cytosolic calcium which induces neuronal apoptosis [87]. Moreover, levels of free cholesterol in neurofibrillary tangle-bearing neurons are higher than those of adjacent tangle-free neurons [88].

Excess cholesterol can also form proinflammatory, membrane-piercing CCs (Fig. 2). As lipoproteins accumulate, they may either coalesce into vesicles within the interstitial space due to low clearance rates or, if cleared rapidly by macrophages, become sequestered and induce macrophage transformation into foam cells [80, 86]. In the presence of excess free unesterified cholesterol (q.v., ACAT1) and certain physiochemical environmental factors (e.g., degree of cholesterol hydration, presence of excess calcium, regional pH), these cholesterol molecules can spontaneously self-assemble into CCs [80, 89–91]. This crystallization process is also seen in amyloid crystals [80]. CCs can lead to endothelial dysfunction and

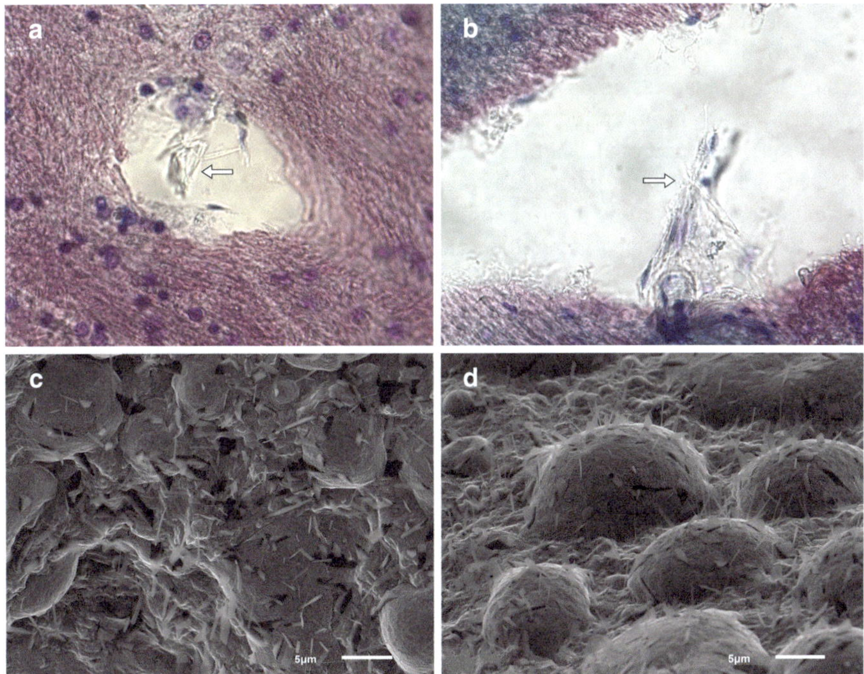

Fig. 2 Cholesterol crystal injury of blood–brain barrier and neural cells. (**a, b**) Light micrographs of cholesterol crystals piercing brain capillary endothelium (arrows). (**c**) Scanning electron micrograph of cholesterol crystals piercing through the blood–brain barrier and (**d**) brain tissue bearing multitudinous cholesterol crystals that have pierced their cellular membranes. (Courtesy of George Abela)

stimulate endothelial expression of IL-1β, which may affect cholesterol hemostasis in the endothelium by activating SREBP2, thus further exacerbating intracellular cholesterol accumulation and formation of intracellular CCs [80]. Rapid transition of quiescent metastable CCs into flat plate crystalline structures releases latent elastic energy that can be forceful enough to cause the leading edge and sharp tips of larger extracellular CCs to pierce cellular membranes or, if in vascular plaques, the vaso vasorum [80, 92]. As lipoproteins continue to accumulate within lysosomes, flat plate CCs form within them and may become large enough to disrupt the lysosomal membrane, with release of CC fragments into the cytosol [80, 92]. Once fragments of flat plate CCs overwhelm the scavenger cells in the interstitial space, they may become inflammatory foci by several different mechanisms [80]. Hence, flat plate CCs in the interstitial space promote a persistent inflammatory response.

The production of Aβ seems to correlate more closely with levels of cholesterol esters than with cholesterol [26, 39]. According to a recent meta-analysis, both 24-OHC and 27-OHC (among other non-enzymatically oxidized oxysterols) levels are elevated in the brain [5, 39, 84]. 24-OHC plasma levels are proportional to the degree of brain atrophy and the loss of active gray matter, while its CSF levels are related to the amount of Aβ and H-tau in AD subjects [93]. Although necessary for cholesterol homeostasis and prevention of neurodegeneration, 24-OHC has been demonstrated to promote inflammation, oxidative stress, Aβ production (via APP regulation), and neuronal death [5, 28, 47, 84, 94]. These contrasting effects of 24-OHC are possibly attributable to concentration-dependence and its role requires further research (for more information, read Gamba et al., 2021) [95]. The increase in 27-OHC is likely due to altered permeability of the BBB due to hypercholesterolemia and oxidative stress among other factors [5, 95]. In a positive feedback loops, oxidative stress and inflammation increase brain cholesterol conversion to 27-OHC, which in turn promotes proinflammatory molecule release [5, 94]. This allows further 27-OHC carry additional cholesterol into the CNS, linking hypercholesterolemia and AD pathogenesis. Moreover, 27-OHC upregulates RAGE in astrocytes and neurons [96]. Studies have demonstrated that 27-OHC disrupts synapses, impairs neuron morphology, and increase both Aβ and hyperphosphorylated tau levels (Fig. 3) [5, 97].

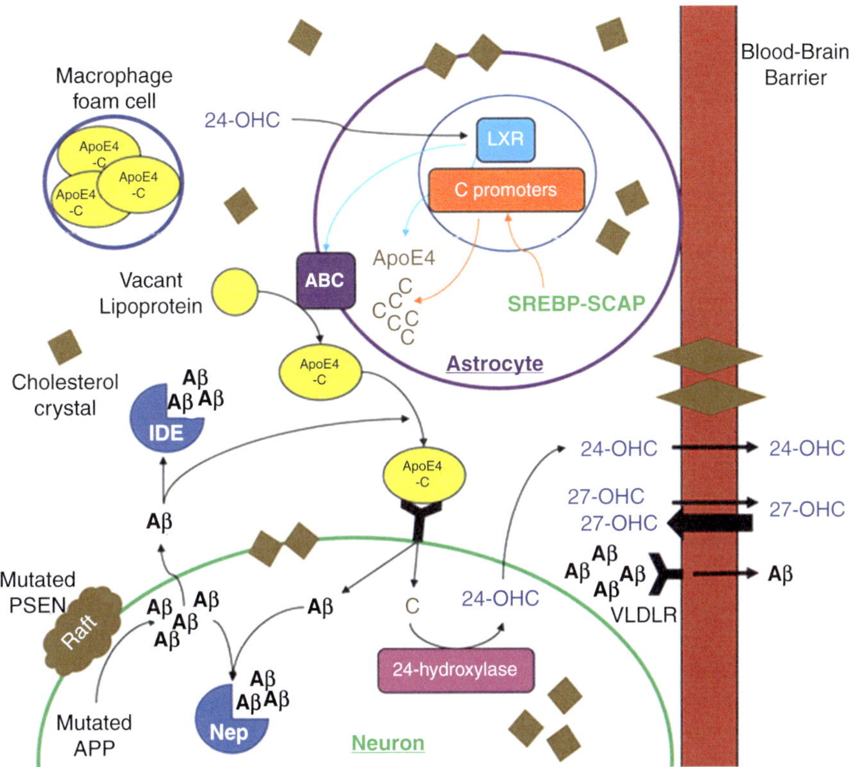

Fig. 3 How disordered handling of cholesterol may affect dementia. For ease of conception, both familial and sporadic AD will be illustrated in this figure, with delineation in this caption. In the familial form, APP and PSEN1/2 mutations favor accelerated Aβ generation. APP mutations favor beta-secretase over alpha-secretase, while PSEN1/2 mutations enhance gamma-secretase activity. (1) The presence of cholesterol increases secretase activity within lipid rafts. Excess intracellular cholesterol alters APP processing, increasing Aβ. In the sporadic form, ApoE4 exhibits faster degradation rates and lower cholesterol delivery rate than other ApoE isoforms. While other ApoE isoforms utilize both LRP1 and VLDLR for BBB transcytosis, ApoE4 primarily relies on the slower VLDLR, allowing for extracellular accumulation of Aβ. Moreover, ApoE4 induces only a weak effect from intracellular Neprilysin and extracellular IDE, resulting in further Aβ accumulation. (2) Aging, elevated cholesterol, ApoE4, and the persistent inflammation induced by central insulin resistance and cholesterol crystals all cause endothelial disruption. Insulin resistance also reduces GLUT4 expression on cell membranes, increasing insulin which saturates and thus inhibits IDE, preventing degradation of both insulin and Aβ. (3) Intracellularly cholesterol accumulation may result from accelerated cholesterol synthesis, impaired degradation via Neprilysin, and Aβ-induced internalization. Cholesterol can then be incorporated into cell structure to affect plasma membrane rigidity or as crystals with membrane-piercing potential. (4) Extracellular accumulation of cholesterol results from decreased cholesterol transport via ApoE4, impaired cellular uptake, reduced efflux from the CNS, increased influx from the periphery due to endothelial disruption, and impaired degradation result in extracellular accumulation. Thus, cholesterol can become incorporated into cell membranes or as plaques along vascular endothelium. (Courtesy of Ryan Skowronek)

4.2 Ischemic and Hemorrhagic Stroke

Low total and LDL cholesterol levels are a risk factor for intracerebral hemorrhage, whereas high total and LDL cholesterol levels are associated with cerebral infarction [98–100]. When compared to the lowest total cholesterol quintile, the highest was associated with an increased risk of ischemic stroke (OR 1.6, 95% CI 1.3–2.0), with the strongest associations of atherothrombotic (OR 3.2) and lacunar (OR 2.4), which has been replicated by several studies [99, 100]. Amarenco et al. found that LDL was associated with lacunar stroke (OR 2.71, 95% CI 1.60–4.55), while Bezerra et al. observed a similar association with larger lacunar lesions (8–20 mm on MRI) [100–103]. Larger lesions are probably attributable to microatheromata and/or plaque rupture, while smaller ones are due to lipohyalinosis [100, 103]. Elevated HDL and triglycerides have not been associated with ischemic stroke [98, 104]. By contrast, there is no association seen between cholesterol and embolic infarction [99–102, 104].

Cholesterol crystallization results in volume expansion that can tear fibrous membranes by sharp tipped crystals, which can break off into circulation (Chaps. 3 & 15 "How Innovation in Tissue Preparation and Imaging Revolutionized the Understanding of the Role of Cholesterol Crystals in Atherosclerosis" and "Role of CCs and Their Lipoprotein Precursors in NLRP3 and IL-1β Activation"). Therefore, unstable carotid plaques causing <70% stenosis may still cause events. This is the pathophysiology of Hollenhorst plaques, refractile CC emboli visualized within retinal artery branches (Chap. 17 "Omega-3 Fatty Acids Influence Membrane Cholesterol Distribution and Crystal Formation in Models of Atherosclerosis"). Carotid atherosclerotic plaques with cholesterol crystals were more likely to have concomitant macrophage and calcification accumulations. Patients with CCs plaque experienced more cerebrovascular symptoms [105]. Abela proposed a novel method for identifying unstable plaques by simultaneously compressing carotid plaques with an ultrasound probe and detecting liberated crystals via high-intensity transient signals (HITS) with a transcranial Doppler aimed at the bilateral MCAs [106, 107]. Twenty-three patients were studied with carotid stenosis ranging approximately 25–50%. Out of four patients with HITS in at least one MCA, three had concurrent neurologic symptoms. In the remaining nineteen patients, six more had neurologic symptoms without HITS detection. In a 2020 study, Shi et al. found that cholesterol crystals were significantly associated with cerebrovascular ischemic symptoms related to the ipsilateral internal carotid artery (Fig. 4) [105].

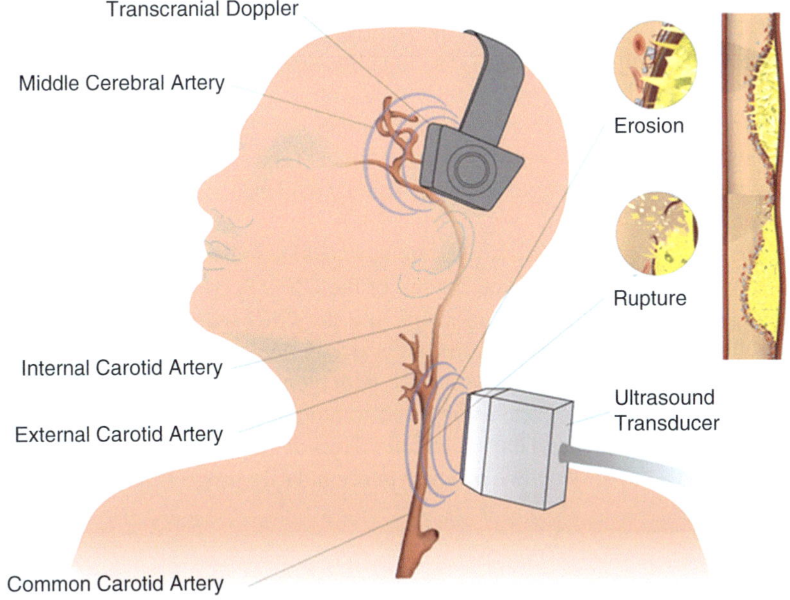

Fig. 4 Simultaneous carotid duplex and transcranial Doppler. A proposed method for the detection of plaques at higher risk for embolization and stroke. When the ultrasound transducer is placed over the carotid artery with standard pressure, it can release cholesterol crystals from a ruptured plaque that then embolize to the middle cerebral artery where they can then be readily detected by a transcranial Doppler. (Courtesy of George Abela)

4.3   Statins in Dementia and Multiple Sclerosis

There are several proposed mechanisms of statin effects on CNS autoimmune disease based on their immunomodulatory and neuroprotective properties. These mechanisms include cholesterol-dependent and cholesterol-independent effects, including inhibition of glutamate excitotoxicity and enhancement of cerebral hemodynamics [108, 109].

A recent meta-analysis found that statins are associated with decreased risk of developing dementia [110, 111]. With regard to vascular dementia, statins reduce the high levels of LDL that associated with atherothrombotic and larger lacunar infarctions [101]. Moreover, statins may reduce infarctions caused by extracranial carotid disease by limiting the formation of cholesterol crystal formation in atherosclerotic plaques [105]. A similar crystallization process takes place in microcapillaries of the brain and within neuronal cytoplasm, as shown in Figs. 2, 3 and 4. Of note, AD has been associated with mid-life but not late-life hypercholesterolemia, suggesting that long-standing cholesterol excess allows for pathology to develop and then manifest later in life in the setting of increased vascular permeability and decreased cognitive reserve [39, 84, 111]. In AD specifically, statins reduce cholesterol thereby reducing secretase activity and allowing for beta-amyloid clearance by preventing excessive beta-amyloid accumulation [112]. Patients with hypercholesterolemia and concomitant risk factors for AD may therefore benefit from early initiation of statin therapy; however, further evidence is required via randomized control trials.

Multiple sclerosis (MS) is an immune-mediated chronic inflammatory disease targeting oligodendrocytes and myelin of the CNS. Secreted molecules disrupt the BBB permitting T lymphocytes entry into the CNS where further activation and recruitment of other inflammatory cells occur. Multiple studies have shown that adverse outcomes in MS are associated with elevated circulating LDL and/or total cholesterol [113]. However, as opposed to animal studies, randomized controlled trials have not reproduced the beneficial effects of statins in patients with relapsing-remitting MS but have shown promise in secondarily progressive MS [109].

References

1. de Chaves EP, Narayanaswami V. Apolipoprotein E and cholesterol in aging and disease in the brain. Future Lipidol. 2008;3(5):505–30. https://doi.org/10.2217/17460875.3.5.505.
2. de Chaves EIP, Rusiñol AE, Vance DE, Campenot RB, Vance JE. Role of lipoproteins in the delivery of lipids to axons during axonal regeneration. J Biol Chem. 1997;272(49):30766–73. https://doi.org/10.1074/jbc.272.49.30766.
3. Posse de Chaves EI, Vance DE, Campenot RB, Kiss RS, Vance JE. Uptake of lipoproteins for axonal growth of sympathetic neurons. J Biol Chem. 2000;275(26):19883–90. https://doi.org/10.1074/jbc.275.26.19883.
4. Goritz C, Mauch DH, Pfrieger FW. Multiple mechanisms mediate cholesterol-induced synaptogenesis in a CNS neuron. Mol Cell Neurosci. 2005;29(2):190–201. https://doi.org/10.1016/j.mcn.2005.02.006.
5. Gamba P, Staurenghi E, Testa G, Giannelli S, Sottero B, Leonarduzzi G. A crosstalk between brain cholesterol oxidation and glucose metabolism in Alzheimer's disease. Front Neurosci. 2019;13:556. https://doi.org/10.3389/fnins.2019.00556.
6. Björkhem I, Meaney S. Brain cholesterol: long secret life behind a barrier. Arterioscler Thromb Vasc Biol. 2004;24(5):806–15. https://doi.org/10.1161/01.ATV.0000120374.59826.1b.
7. Poitelon Y, Kopec AM, Belin S. Myelin fat facts: an overview of lipids and fatty acid metabolism. Cell. 2020;9(4):E812. https://doi.org/10.3390/cells9040812.
8. Jurevics H, Morell P. Cholesterol for synthesis of myelin is made locally, not imported into brain. J Neurochem. 1995;64(2):895–901. https://doi.org/10.1046/j.1471-4159.1995.64020895.x.
9. Lange Y, Ye J, Rigney M, Steck TL. Regulation of endoplasmic reticulum cholesterol by plasma membrane cholesterol. J Lipid Res. 1999;40(12):2264–70.
10. Haines TH. Do sterols reduce proton and sodium leaks through lipid bilayers? Prog Lipid Res. 2001;40(4):299–324. https://doi.org/10.1016/s0163-7827(01)00009-1.
11. Brown MS, Goldstein JL. A proteolytic pathway that controls the cholesterol content of membranes, cells, and blood. Proc Natl Acad Sci U S A. 1999;96(20):11041–8. https://doi.org/10.1073/pnas.96.20.11041.

12. DeBose-Boyd RA, Brown MS, Li WP, Nohturfft A, Goldstein JL, Espenshade PJ. Transport-dependent proteolysis of SREBP: relocation of site-1 protease from Golgi to ER obviates the need for SREBP transport to Golgi. Cell. 1999;99(7):703–12. https://doi.org/10.1016/s0092-8674(00)81668-2.

13. Nohturfft A, Yabe D, Goldstein JL, Brown MS, Espenshade PJ. Regulated step in cholesterol feedback localized to budding of SCAP from ER membranes. Cell. 2000;102(3):315–23. https://doi.org/10.1016/s0092-8674(00)00037-4.

14. Zhang J, Liu Q. Cholesterol metabolism and homeostasis in the brain. Protein Cell. 2015;6(4):254–64. https://doi.org/10.1007/s13238-014-0131-3.

15. Dietschy JM, Turley SD. Thematic review series: brain lipids. Cholesterol metabolism in the central nervous system during early development and in the mature animal. J Lipid Res. 2004;45(8):1375–97. https://doi.org/10.1194/jlr.R400004-JLR200.

16. Quan G, Xie C, Dietschy JM, Turley SD. Ontogenesis and regulation of cholesterol metabolism in the central nervous system of the mouse. Brain Res Dev Brain Res. 2003;146(1–2):87–98. https://doi.org/10.1016/j.devbrainres.2003.09.015.

17. Fantini J, Yahi N. Brain lipids in synaptic function and neurological disease. 1st ed; 2015.

18. Svennerholm L, Boström K, Jungbjer B, Olsson L. Membrane lipids of adult human brain: lipid composition of frontal and temporal lobe in subjects of age 20 to 100 years. J Neurochem. 1994;63(5):1802–11. https://doi.org/10.1046/j.1471-4159.1994.63051802.x.

19. Svennerholm L, Boström K, Jungbjer B. Changes in weight and compositions of major membrane components of human brain during the span of adult human life of swedes. Acta Neuropathol. 1997;94(4):345–52. https://doi.org/10.1007/s004010050717.

20. Thelen KM, Falkai P, Bayer TA, Lütjohann D. Cholesterol synthesis rate in human hippocampus declines with aging. Neurosci Lett. 2006;403(1–2):15–9. https://doi.org/10.1016/j.neulet.2006.04.034.

21. Lütjohann D, Breuer O, Ahlborg G, et al. Cholesterol homeostasis in human brain: evidence for an age-dependent flux of 24S-hydroxycholesterol from the brain into the circulation. Proc Natl Acad Sci U S A. 1996;93(18):9799–804. https://doi.org/10.1073/pnas.93.18.9799.

22. Mahley RW. Central nervous system lipoproteins: ApoE and regulation of cholesterol metabolism. Arterioscler Thromb Vasc Biol. 2016;36(7):1305–15. https://doi.org/10.1161/ATVBAHA.116.307023.

23. Petrov AM, Kasimov MR, Zefirov AL. Brain cholesterol metabolism and its defects: linkage to neurodegenerative diseases and synaptic dysfunction. Acta Nat. 2016;8(1):58–73.

24. Nelson AR, Sweeney MD, Sagare AP, Zlokovic BV. Neurovascular dysfunction and neurodegeneration in dementia and Alzheimer's disease. Biochim Biophys Acta. 2016;1862(5):887–900. https://doi.org/10.1016/j.bbadis.2015.12.016.

25. Rudel LL, Lee RG, Cockman TL. Acyl coenzyme a: cholesterol acyltransferase types 1 and 2: structure and function in atherosclerosis. Curr Opin Lipidol. 2001;12(2):121–7. https://doi.org/10.1097/00041433-200104000-00005.

26. Puglielli L, Konopka G, Pack-Chung E, et al. Acyl-coenzyme a: cholesterol acyltransferase modulates the generation of the amyloid beta-peptide. Nat Cell Biol. 2001;3(10):905–12. https://doi.org/10.1038/ncb1001-905.

27. Bryleva EY, Rogers MA, Chang CCY, et al. ACAT1 gene ablation increases 24(S)-hydroxycholesterol content in the brain and ameliorates amyloid pathology in mice with AD. Proc Natl Acad Sci U S A. 2010;107(7):3081–6. https://doi.org/10.1073/pnas.0913828107.

28. Czuba E, Steliga A, Lietzau G, Kowiański P. Cholesterol as a modifying agent of the neurovascular unit structure and function under physiological and pathological conditions. Metab Brain Dis. 2017;32(4):935–48. https://doi.org/10.1007/s11011-017-0015-3.

29. Iwamoto N, Abe-Dohmae S, Sato R, Yokoyama S. ABCA7 expression is regulated by cellular cholesterol through the SREBP2 pathway and associated with phagocytosis. J Lipid Res. 2006;47(9):1915–27. https://doi.org/10.1194/jlr.M600127-JLR200.

30. Vaughan AM, Oram JF. ABCA1 and ABCG1 or ABCG4 act sequentially to remove cellular cholesterol and generate cholesterol-rich HDL. J Lipid Res. 2006;47(11):2433–43. https://doi.org/10.1194/jlr.M600218-JLR200.
31. Koudinov AR, Koudinova NV. Essential role for cholesterol in synaptic plasticity and neuronal degeneration. FASEB J. 2001;15(10):1858–60. https://doi.org/10.1096/fj.00-0815fje.
32. Dietschy JM. Central nervous system: cholesterol turnover, brain development and neurodegeneration. Biol Chem. 2009;390(4):287–93. https://doi.org/10.1515/BC.2009.035.
33. Pitas RE, Boyles JK, Lee SH, Foss D, Mahley RW. Astrocytes synthesize apolipoprotein E and metabolize apolipoprotein E-containing lipoproteins. Biochim Biophys Acta. 1987;917(1):148–61. https://doi.org/10.1016/0005-2760(87)90295-5.
34. Huxley AF, Stämpeli R. Evidence for saltatory conduction in peripheral myelinated nerve fibres. J Physiol. 1949;108(3):315–39. https://doi.org/10.1113/jphysiol.1949.sp004335.
35. Bu G. Apolipoprotein E and its receptors in Alzheimer's disease: pathways, pathogenesis and therapy. Nat Rev Neurosci. 2009;10(5):333–44. https://doi.org/10.1038/nrn2620.
36. Holtzman DM, Herz J, Bu G. Apolipoprotein E and apolipoprotein E receptors: normal biology and roles in Alzheimer disease. Cold Spring Harb Perspect Med. 2012;2(3):a006312. https://doi.org/10.1101/cshperspect.a006312.
37. Boyles JK, Zoellner CD, Anderson LJ, et al. A role for apolipoprotein E, apolipoprotein A-I, and low density lipoprotein receptors in cholesterol transport during regeneration and remyelination of the rat sciatic nerve. J Clin Invest. 1989;83(3):1015–31. https://doi.org/10.1172/JCI113943.
38. Lane-Donovan CE, Philips GT, Herz J. More than cholesterol transporters: lipoprotein receptors in CNS function and neurodegeneration. Neuron. 2014;83(4):771–87. https://doi.org/10.1016/j.neuron.2014.08.005.
39. Sjögren M, Mielke M, Gustafson D, Zandi P, Skoog I. Cholesterol and Alzheimer's disease—is there a relation? Mech Ageing Dev. 2006;127(2):138–47. https://doi.org/10.1016/j.mad.2005.09.020.
40. Harris FM, Tesseur I, Brecht WJ, et al. Astroglial regulation of apolipoprotein E expression in neuronal cells. Implications for Alzheimer's disease. J Biol Chem. 2004;279(5):3862–8. https://doi.org/10.1074/jbc.M309475200.
41. Ropper A, Samuels M, Klein J, Prasad S. Adams and Victor's principles of neurology. 11th ed. New York, NY: Elsevier; 2019.
42. Fagan AM, Younkin LH, Morris JC, et al. Differences in the Abeta40/Abeta42 ratio associated with cerebrospinal fluid lipoproteins as a function of apolipoprotein E genotype. Ann Neurol. 2000;48(2):201–10.
43. Ikonen E. Cellular cholesterol trafficking and compartmentalization. Nat Rev Mol Cell Biol. 2008;9(2):125–38. https://doi.org/10.1038/nrm2336.
44. Poirier J, Baccichet A, Dea D, Gauthier S. Cholesterol synthesis and lipoprotein reuptake during synaptic remodelling in hippocampus in adult rats. Neuroscience. 1993;55(1):81–90. https://doi.org/10.1016/0306-4522(93)90456-p.
45. Thiele C, Hannah MJ, Fahrenholz F, Huttner WB. Cholesterol binds to synaptophysin and is required for biogenesis of synaptic vesicles. Nat Cell Biol. 2000;2(1):42–9. https://doi.org/10.1038/71366.
46. Mauch DH, Nägler K, Schumacher S, et al. CNS synaptogenesis promoted by glia-derived cholesterol. Science. 2001;294(5545):1354–7. https://doi.org/10.1126/science.294.5545.1354.
47. Wolozin B. Cholesterol and the biology of Alzheimer's disease. Neuron. 2004;41(1):7–10. https://doi.org/10.1016/s0896-6273(03)00840-7.
48. Xu Q, Brecht WJ, Weisgraber KH, Mahley RW, Huang Y. Apolipoprotein E4 domain interaction occurs in living neuronal cells as determined by fluorescence resonance energy transfer. J Biol Chem. 2004;279(24):25511–6. https://doi.org/10.1074/jbc.M311256200.
49. Williams KA, Deber CM. The structure and function of central nervous system myelin. Crit Rev Clin Lab Sci. 1993;30(1):29–64. https://doi.org/10.3109/10408369309084665.

50. Roy D, Tedeschi A. The role of lipids, lipid metabolism and ectopic lipid accumulation in axon growth, regeneration and repair after CNS injury and disease. Cell. 2021;10(5):1078. https://doi.org/10.3390/cells10051078.

51. Pfenninger KH. Plasma membrane expansion: a neuron's herculean task. Nat Rev Neurosci. 2009;10(4):251–61. https://doi.org/10.1038/nrn2593.

52. Tasaki I, Takeuchi T. Weitere studien über den Aktionsstrom der markhaltigen nervenfaser und über die elektrosaltatorische übertragung des nervenimpulses. Pflügers Arch. 1942;245(5):764–82. https://doi.org/10.1007/BF01755237.

53. Russell DW, Halford RW, Ramirez DMO, Shah R, Kotti T. Cholesterol 24-hydroxylase: an enzyme of cholesterol turnover in the brain. Annu Rev Biochem. 2009;78:1017–40. https://doi.org/10.1146/annurev.biochem.78.072407.103859.

54. Chen Z, Rand RP. The influence of cholesterol on phospholipid membrane curvature and bending elasticity. Biophys J. 1997;73(1):267–76.

55. Tong J, Borbat PP, Freed JH, Shin YK. A scissors mechanism for stimulation of SNARE-mediated lipid mixing by cholesterol. Proc Natl Acad Sci U S A. 2009;106(13):5141–6. https://doi.org/10.1073/pnas.0813138106.

56. Wood WG, Igbavboa U, Müller WE, Eckert GP. Cholesterol asymmetry in synaptic plasma membranes. J Neurochem. 2011;116(5):684–9. https://doi.org/10.1111/j.1471-4159.2010.07017.x.

57. Pfrieger FW. Cholesterol homeostasis and function in neurons of the central nervous system. Cell Mol Life Sci. 2003;60(6):1158–71. https://doi.org/10.1007/s00018-003-3018-7.

58. Martin M, Dotti CG, Ledesma MD. Brain cholesterol in normal and pathological aging. Biochim Biophys Acta. 2010;1801(8):934–44. https://doi.org/10.1016/j.bbalip.2010.03.011.

59. Citri A, Malenka RC. Synaptic plasticity: multiple forms, functions, and mechanisms. Neuropsychopharmacology. 2008;33(1):18–41. https://doi.org/10.1038/sj.npp.1301559.

60. Igbavboa U, Avdulov NA, Schroeder F, Wood WG. Increasing age alters transbilayer fluidity and cholesterol asymmetry in synaptic plasma membranes of mice. J Neurochem. 1996;66(4):1717–25. https://doi.org/10.1046/j.1471-4159.1996.66041717.x.

61. Wang H, Kulas JA, Wang C, Holtzman DM, Ferris HA, Hansen SB. Regulation of beta-amyloid production in neurons by astrocyte-derived cholesterol. PNAS. 2021;118(33):e2102191118. https://doi.org/10.1073/pnas.2102191118.

62. Simons K, Ehehalt R. Cholesterol, lipid rafts, and disease. J Clin Invest. 2002;110(5):597–603. https://doi.org/10.1172/JCI16390.

63. Cacace R, Sleegers K, Van Broeckhoven C. Molecular genetics of early-onset Alzheimer's disease revisited. Alzheimers Dement. 2016;12(6):733–48. https://doi.org/10.1016/j.jalz.2016.01.012.

64. Querfurth HW, LaFerla FM. Alzheimer's disease. N Engl J Med. 2010;362(4):329–44. https://doi.org/10.1056/NEJMra0909142.

65. Bateman RJ, Xiong C, Benzinger TLS, et al. Clinical and biomarker changes in dominantly inherited Alzheimer's disease. N Engl J Med. 2012;367(9):795–804. https://doi.org/10.1056/NEJMoa1202753.

66. Cataldo AM, Barnett JL, Pieroni C, Nixon RA. Increased neuronal endocytosis and protease delivery to early endosomes in sporadic Alzheimer's disease: neuropathologic evidence for a mechanism of increased beta-amyloidogenesis. J Neurosci. 1997;17(16):6142–51.

67. Ramanathan A, Nelson AR, Sagare AP, Zlokovic BV. Impaired vascular-mediated clearance of brain amyloid beta in Alzheimer's disease: the role, regulation and restoration of LRP1. Front Aging Neurosci. 2015;7:136. https://doi.org/10.3389/fnagi.2015.00136.

68. Ghribi O. Potential mechanisms linking cholesterol to Alzheimer's disease-like pathology in rabbit brain, hippocampal organotypic slices, and skeletal muscle. J Alzheimers Dis. 2008;15(4):673–84. https://doi.org/10.3233/jad-2008-15412.

69. LaDu MJ, Falduto MT, Manelli AM, Reardon CA, Getz GS, Frail DE. Isoform-specific binding of apolipoprotein E to beta-amyloid. J Biol Chem. 1994;269(38):23403–6.

70. Sweeney MD, Sagare AP, Zlokovic BV. Blood-brain barrier breakdown in Alzheimer disease and other neurodegenerative disorders. Nat Rev Neurol. 2018;14(3):133–50. https://doi.org/10.1038/nrneurol.2017.188.

71. Hussain B, Fang C, Chang J. Blood-brain barrier breakdown: an emerging biomarker of cognitive impairment in normal aging and dementia. Front Neurosci. 2021;15:688090. https://doi.org/10.3389/fnins.2021.688090.

72. Iturria-Medina Y, Sotero RC, Toussaint PJ, Mateos-Pérez JM, Evans AC. Early role of vascular dysregulation on late-onset Alzheimer's disease based on multifactorial data-driven analysis. Nat Commun. 2016;7:11934. https://doi.org/10.1038/ncomms11934.

73. Yarchoan M, Xie SX, Kling MA, et al. Cerebrovascular atherosclerosis correlates with Alzheimer pathology in neurodegenerative dementias. Brain. 2012;135(12):3749–56. https://doi.org/10.1093/brain/aws271.

74. Verghese PB, Castellano JM, Holtzman DM. Apolipoprotein E in Alzheimer's disease and other neurological disorders. Lancet Neurol. 2011;10(3):241–52. https://doi.org/10.1016/S1474-4422(10)70325-2.

75. Halliday MR, Rege SV, Ma Q, et al. Accelerated pericyte degeneration and blood-brain barrier breakdown in apolipoprotein E4 carriers with Alzheimer's disease. J Cereb Blood Flow Metab. 2016;36(1):216–27. https://doi.org/10.1038/jcbfm.2015.44.

76. Xiao X, Liu X, Jiao B. Epigenetics: recent advances and its role in the treatment of Alzheimer's disease. Front Neurol. 2020;11:538301. https://doi.org/10.3389/fneur.2020.538301.

77. Montagne A, Nation DA, Sagare AP, et al. APOE4 leads to blood–brain barrier dysfunction predicting cognitive decline. Nature. 2020;581(7806):71–6. https://doi.org/10.1038/s41586-020-2247-3.

78. Ishii M, Iadecola C. Risk factor for Alzheimer's disease breaks the blood-brain barrier. Nature. 2020;581(7806):31–2. https://doi.org/10.1038/d41586-020-01152-8.

79. Baloyannis SJ, Baloyannis IS. The vascular factor in Alzheimer's disease: a study in golgi technique and electron microscopy. J Neurol Sci. 2012;322(1–2):117–21. https://doi.org/10.1016/j.jns.2012.07.010.

80. Nidorf SM, Fiolet A, Abela GS. Viewing atherosclerosis through a crystal lens: how the evolving structure of cholesterol crystals in atherosclerotic plaque alters its stability. J Clin Lipidol. 2020;14(5):619–30. https://doi.org/10.1016/j.jacl.2020.07.003.

81. Abela GS, Kalavakunta JK, Janoudi A, et al. Frequency of cholesterol crystals in culprit coronary artery aspirate during acute myocardial infarction and their relation to inflammation and myocardial injury. Am J Cardiol. 2017;120(10):1699–707. https://doi.org/10.1016/j.amjcard.2017.07.075.

82. Farkas E, Luiten PG. Cerebral microvascular pathology in aging and Alzheimer's disease. Prog Neurobiol. 2001;64(6):575–611. https://doi.org/10.1016/s0301-0082(00)00068-x.

83. Vílchez JA, Martínez-Ruiz A, Sancho-Rodríguez N, Martínez-Hernández P, Noguera-Velasco JA. The real role of prediagnostic high-density lipoprotein cholesterol and the cancer risk: a concise review. Eur J Clin Investig. 2014;44(1):103–14. https://doi.org/10.1111/eci.12185.

84. Wang HL, Wang YY, Liu XG, et al. Cholesterol, 24-hydroxycholesterol, and 27-hydroxycholesterol as surrogate biomarkers in cerebrospinal fluid in mild cognitive impairment and Alzheimer's disease: a meta-analysis. J Alzheimers Dis. 2016;51(1):45–55. https://doi.org/10.3233/JAD-150734.

85. Chen YL, Wang LM, Chen Y, et al. Changes in astrocyte functional markers and β-amyloid metabolism-related proteins in the early stages of hypercholesterolemia. Neuroscience. 2016;316:178–91. https://doi.org/10.1016/j.neuroscience.2015.12.039.

86. Wahrle S, Das P, Nyborg AC, et al. Cholesterol-dependent gamma-secretase activity in buoyant cholesterol-rich membrane microdomains. Neurobiol Dis. 2002;9(1):11–23. https://doi.org/10.1006/nbdi.2001.0470.

87. Hussain G, Wang J, Rasul A, et al. Role of cholesterol and sphingolipids in brain development and neurological diseases. Lipids Health Dis. 2019;18:26. https://doi.org/10.1186/s12944-019-0965-z.

88. Distl R, Meske V, Ohm TG. Tangle-bearing neurons contain more free cholesterol than adjacent tangle-free neurons. Acta Neuropathol. 2001;101(6):547–54. https://doi.org/10.1007/s004010000314.

89. Vedre A, Pathak DR, Crimp M, Lum C, Koochesfahani M, Abela GS. Physical factors that trigger cholesterol crystallization leading to plaque rupture. Atherosclerosis. 2009;203(1):89–96. https://doi.org/10.1016/j.atherosclerosis.2008.06.027.

90. Abela GS, Aziz K, Vedre A, Pathak DR, Talbott JD, Dejong J. Effect of cholesterol crystals on plaques and intima in arteries of patients with acute coronary and cerebrovascular syndromes. Am J Cardiol. 2009;103(7):959–68. https://doi.org/10.1016/j.amjcard.2008.12.019.

91. Janoudi A, Shamoun FE, Kalavakunta JK, Abela GS. Cholesterol crystal induced arterial inflammation and destabilization of atherosclerotic plaque. Eur Heart J. 2016;37(25):1959–67. https://doi.org/10.1093/eurheartj/ehv653.

92. Abela GS. Cholesterol crystals piercing the arterial plaque and intima trigger local and systemic inflammation. J Clin Lipidol. 2010;4(3):156–64. https://doi.org/10.1016/j.jacl.2010.03.003.

93. Leoni V, Caccia C. Potential diagnostic applications of side chain oxysterols analysis in plasma and cerebrospinal fluid. Biochem Pharmacol. 2013;86(1):26–36. https://doi.org/10.1016/j.bcp.2013.03.015.

94. Testa G, Gamba P, Badilli U, et al. Loading into nanoparticles improves Quercetin's efficacy in preventing Neuroinflammation induced by oxysterols. PLoS One. 2014;9(5):e96795. https://doi.org/10.1371/journal.pone.0096795.

95. Gamba P, Giannelli S, Staurenghi E, et al. The controversial role of 24-S-hydroxycholesterol in Alzheimer's disease. Antioxidants (Basel). 2021;10(5):740. https://doi.org/10.3390/antiox10050740.

96. Loera-Valencia R, Ismail MAM, Goikolea J, et al. Hypercholesterolemia and 27-hydroxycholesterol increase S100A8 and RAGE expression in the brain: a link between cholesterol, Alarmins, and neurodegeneration. Mol Neurobiol. 2021;58(12):6063–76. https://doi.org/10.1007/s12035-021-02521-8.

97. Gamba P, Guglielmotto M, Testa G, et al. Up-regulation of β-amyloidogenesis in neuron-like human cells by both 24- and 27-hydroxycholesterol: protective effect of N-acetyl-cysteine. Aging Cell. 2014;13(3):561–72. https://doi.org/10.1111/acel.12206.

98. Bowman TS, Sesso HD, Ma J, et al. Cholesterol and the risk of ischemic stroke. Stroke. 2003;34(12):2930–4. https://doi.org/10.1161/01.STR.0000102171.91292.DC.

99. Tirschwell DL, Smith NL, Heckbert SR, Lemaitre RN, Longstreth WT, Psaty BM. Association of cholesterol with stroke risk varies in stroke subtypes and patient subgroups. Neurology. 2004;63(10):1868–75. https://doi.org/10.1212/01.wnl.0000144282.42222.da.

100. Hackam DG, Hegele RA. Cholesterol lowering and prevention of stroke. Stroke. 2019;50(2):537–41. https://doi.org/10.1161/STROKEAHA.118.023167.

101. Amarenco P, Labreuche J, Elbaz A, et al. Blood lipids in brain infarction subtypes. Cerebrovasc Dis. 2006;22(2–3):101–8. https://doi.org/10.1159/000093237.

102. Cui R, Iso H, Yamagishi K, et al. High serum total cholesterol levels is a risk factor of ischemic stroke for general Japanese population: the JPHC study. Atherosclerosis. 2012;221(2):565–9. https://doi.org/10.1016/j.atherosclerosis.2012.01.013.

103. Bezerra DC, Sharrett AR, Matsushita K, et al. Risk factors for lacune subtypes in the atherosclerosis risk in communities (ARIC) study. Neurology. 2012;78(2):102–8. https://doi.org/10.1212/WNL.0b013e31823efc42.

104. Hindy G, Engström G, Larsson SC, et al. Role of blood lipids in the development of ischemic stroke and its subtypes. Stroke. 2018;49(4):820–7. https://doi.org/10.1161/STROKEAHA.117.019653.

105. Shi X, Cai H, Wang F, et al. Cholesterol crystals are associated with carotid plaque vulnerability: an optical coherence tomography study. J Stroke Cerebrovasc Dis. 2020;29(2):104579. https://doi.org/10.1016/j.jstrokecerebrovasdis.2019.104579.

106. Ries S, Schminke U, Daffertshofer M, Hennerici M. High intensity transient signals (HITS) in patients with carotid artery disease. Eur J Med Res. 1996;1(7):328–30.
107. Purkayastha S, Sorond F. Transcranial Doppler ultrasound: technique and application. Semin Neurol. 2012;32(4):411–20. https://doi.org/10.1055/s-0032-1331812.
108. Youssef S, Stüve O, Patarroyo JC, Ruiz PJ, Radosevich JL, Hur EM, Bravo M, Mitchell DJ, Sobel RA, Steinman L, Zamvil SS. The HMG-CoA reductase inhibitor, atorvastatin, promotes a Th2 bias and reverses paralysis in central nervous system autoimmune disease. Nature. 2002;420(6911):78. https://doi.org/10.1038/nature01158.
109. Abdalla MA, Zakhary CM, Rushdi H, et al. The effectiveness of statins as potential therapy for multiple sclerosis: a systematic review of randomized controlled trials. Cureus. 2021;13(9):e18092. https://doi.org/10.7759/cureus.18092.
110. Zhang X, Wen J, Zhang Z. Statins use and risk of dementia. Medicine (Baltimore). 2018;97(30):e11304. https://doi.org/10.1097/MD.0000000000011304.
111. Schultz BG, Patten DK, Berlau DJ. The role of statins in both cognitive impairment and protection against dementia: a tale of two mechanisms. Transl Neurodegener. 2018;7:5. https://doi.org/10.1186/s40035-018-0110-3.
112. Shinohara M, Sato N, Kurinami H, et al. Reduction of brain β-amyloid (Aβ) by Fluvastatin, a Hydroxymethylglutaryl-CoA reductase inhibitor, through increase in degradation of amyloid precursor protein C-terminal fragments (APP-CTFs) and Aβ clearance. J Biol Chem. 2010;285(29):22091–102. https://doi.org/10.1074/jbc.M110.102277.
113. Zhornitsky S, McKay KA, Metz LM, Teunissen CE, Rangachari M. Cholesterol and markers of cholesterol turnover in multiple sclerosis: relationship with disease outcomes. Mult Scler Relat Disord. 2016;5:53–65. https://doi.org/10.1016/j.msard.2015.10.005.

Interaction Between Crystals, Inflammation, and Cancer

Stefan Mark Nidorf, Abdallah Almaghraby, Yehia Saleh, Venkat R. Katkoori, Zain ul Abideen, Harvey L. Bumpers, Dorothy R. Pathak, and George S. Abela

S. M. Nidorf (✉)
The Heart and Vascular Research Institute, Sir Charles Gairdner Hospital,
Perth, WA, Australia
e-mail: smnidorf@gmail.com

A. Almaghraby
Department of Cardiology, Alexandria University, Alexandria, Egypt

Y. Saleh
Department of Cardiology, Houston Methodist DeBakey Heart and Vascular Center,
Houston, TX, USA

V. R. Katkoori
Department of Physiology, Michigan State University, East Lansing, MI, USA

Z. ul Abideen
Department of Medicine, College of Human Medicine, Michigan State University,
East Lansing, MI, USA
e-mail: fnuzain1@msu.edu

B. L. Bumpers
Department of Surgery, Michigan State University, East Lansing, MI, USA
e-mail: bumpers@msu.edu

D. R. Pathak
Department of Epidemiology and Biostatistics, Michigan State University,
East Lansing, MI, USA

G. S. Abela
Department of Medicine, Division of Cardiovascular Medicine, College of Human Medicine,
Michigan State University, East Lansing, MI, USA
e-mail: abela@msu.edu

© The Author(s), under exclusive license to Springer Nature
Switzerland AG 2023
G. S. Abela, S. M. Nidorf (eds.), *Cholesterol Crystals in Atherosclerosis and
Other Related Diseases*, Contemporary Cardiology,
https://doi.org/10.1007/978-3-031-41192-2_22

413

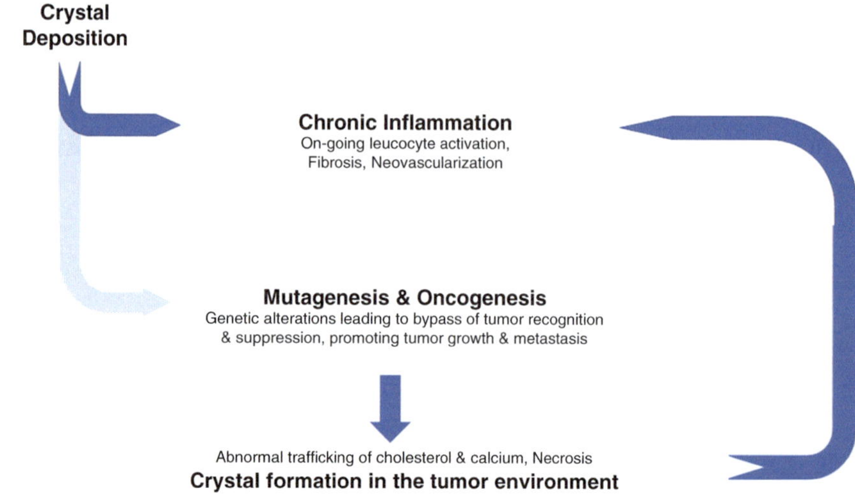

Fig. 1 Interaction between crystals and mutagenesis and oncogenesis

1 Introduction

The development and spread of cancer involve a series of complex processes. In some instances, it is believed that chronic inflammation may incite increased cellular turnover (mitogenesis) that in turn increases the risk of development of defects in DNA and DNA repair in genes (mutagenesis) that are responsible for cellular growth, division, and immune detection.

Some crystals have the ability to incite both a chronic immune response and have mutagenic effects in cells of the upper and lower airways. Separately, various crystals known to develop *de-novo* in the tumor microenvironment (TME) have the potential to enhance its pro-inflammatory inflammatory milieu that may in some instances contribute to either tumor suppression or tumor growth and spread (Fig. 1).

Herein we examine the interplay between crystals, inflammation, and cancer to provide insight into how crystals are believed to cause cancer and promote inflammation in the TME. Due to some similarities in the pathophysiologic processes that drive inflammation in atherosclerosis and the TME, the effect of therapies used for secondary prevention of atherosclerosis for the prevention and treatment of cancer are also reviewed.

2 Environmental and Endogenous Crystals That Can Cause Cancer

2.1 *Silica and Silica Fibers*

Silica is the most abundant naturally occurring substance on earth. Crystalline silica is found in quartz, sand, and thus a range of building products including concrete, brick, and cement. It is the classic exemplar of a crystal found in the environment that can cause cancer.

Several amorphous silica particles and fibers have the potential to cause a range of diseases, including silicosis, an incurable form of aggressive pulmonary fibrosis which is one of the most common occupational diseases in the world [1]. It is also classified as a definite carcinogen (Group 1) by the International Agency for Research on Cancer (IARC). Although most commonly associated with lung cancer, it has also been associated with renal, stomach, and esophageal cancers [2].

Asbestos is a naturally occurring fibrous form of silica. There are six forms of asbestos fibers each of which can be released into the atmosphere by abrasion during industrial processing. Despite recognition of the dangers of asbestos as early as 1899, it continued to be mined and used in industry until the mid-1970s. Once inhaled asbestos fibers can incite pulmonary fibrosis (asbestosis) and the development of various cancers, including small-cell cancer of the lung, mesothelioma, and less commonly laryngeal and ovarian cancer. While smaller asbestos fibers (measuring up to 5 μm) are typically associated with mesothelioma, larger fibers (measuring >10 μm) have been strongly associated with lung cancer [3]. Other sources of exposure to asbestos and silicates may come from unpurified talcum powder. This has been associated with ovarian cancer in individuals who have used it in the genital areas [4].

The inflammatory potential of silica relates to its crystalline nature. Several crystalline polymorphs as well as many kinds of amorphous forms of silica exist in nature, each with differing surface characteristics that are thought to affect their biological reactivity and pathogenicity. Although the pathogenicity of silica crystals relates in part to their size, it is notably that when silica crystals with various characteristics are exposed to macrophages and red blood cells in vitro, cellular toxicity and membranolysis only occurs in the presence of fractured crystals, suggesting that the biological activity of quartz dust requires fragmentation of the crystal structure that disorganize its surface, as may occur during industrial use [5]. Aside from these direct cellular effects, silica crystals and asbestos can induce IL-1β release via NLRP3 inflammasome activation in macrophages [6].

Numerous studies confirm that when crystalline silica is exposed to DNA strands in vitro, it causes strand breakage leading to chromosomal aberrations [7]. *Thus, silica related cancers appear to arise due to direct mutagenic effects rather than result from mitogenicity incited by chronic inflammation* [8].

2.2 *Calcium Oxalate*

There is strong evidence of an association between the formation of stones in the renal and biliary tract and cancer [9, 10]. Calcium oxalate which is commonly found in both renal and gall stones has been found to trigger epithelial-mesenchymal transition that may explain the association between oxalate stones and cancer in the urogenital and biliary tracts.

The shape of oxalate crystals as well as the shape of oxalate crystal aggregates are believed to affect their toxicity. In vitro experiments in renal epithelial cells demonstrated that a range of oxalate crystals all cause cell-membrane rupture, upgraded intracellular reactive oxygen, and decreased mitochondrial membrane potential which ultimately led to cell death [11] (Fig. 2). Crystals with a large

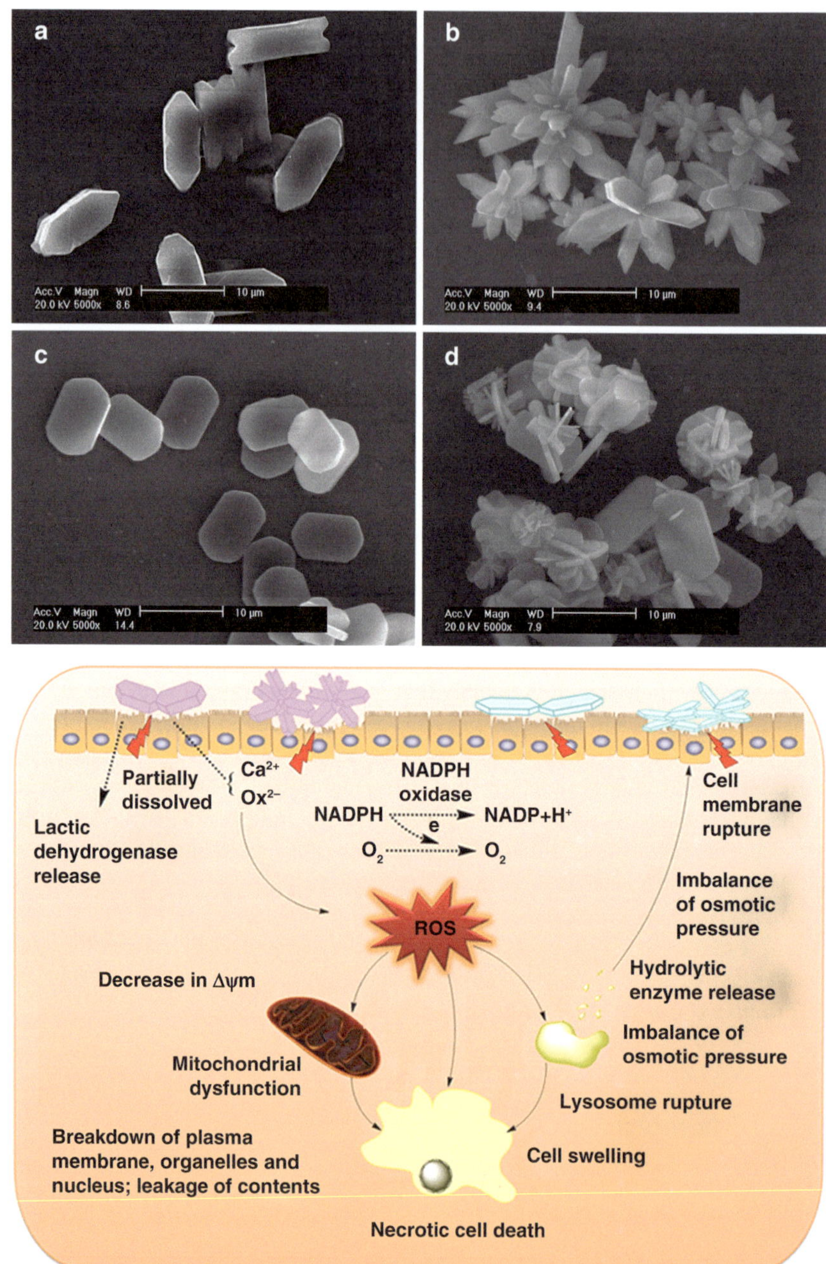

Fig. 2 Effect of crystal shape and aggregation on cell toxicity. (left) Scanning electron micrograph images (**a–d**), XRD spectra. (a) COM-HL; (b) COM-HLA; (c) COM-TL; (d) COM-TLA. Scale bars: 10 μm. (right) Renal epithelial cell injury is central to stone formation. Crystals shapes and aggregation state are important factors in cell injury. (Reproduced with permission [11])

calcium ion-rich active face show the greatest toxicity and the largest extent of adhesion to cells. Furthermore, crystal aggregates with sharp edges more readily caused cellular injury than aggregates of blunt crystals [12]. This constant irritation effect by these crystals that cannot be degraded by the body's immune system can lead to eventual mutagenic transformation.

In addition, in vitro studies have demonstrated that calcium oxalate crystals can induce morphological changes in non-cancerous renal cells from epithelial to fibroblast-like spindle shape due their ability to cause oxidative damage to DNA. In turn, this leads to an increase in the cells spindle index, an increase in mesenchymal markers (fibronectin and vimentin) and reduced expression of epithelial markers (E-cadherin and zonula occludens-1). Furthermore, calcium oxalate can downregulate ARID1A, a tumor suppressor gene with renal cancer, at both mRNA and protein levels and downregulate other renal cell tumor suppressor genes, PTEN and VHL, and upregulated oncogene TPX2. Finally, calcium oxalate crystals can enhance the ability of cells to invade, aggregate, and secrete an angiogenic factor (VEGF) [13]. *Thus, cancers associated with calcium oxalate crystals, like silica crystals, likely arise due to direct crystal induced mutagenic effects rather indirect effects resulting from their ability to incite chronic inflammation.*

2.3 *Cholesterol and Uric Acid Crystals*

Elevated serum levels of cholesterol and UA have both been associated with an increased risk of several cancers [14, 15], and both cholesterol and UA crystals can induce acute and chronic inflammation. However, while cholesterol crystals (CCs) can incite the formation of large granuloma in multiple tissues that may mimic the presence of cancer [16], and UA crystals can incite the formation of tophi, neither lesion have been demonstrated to progress to cancer.

Thus, to date the evidence suggests that the mechanism of crystal induced cancer relates to the ability of a crystal to directly damage DNA rather than their ability to incite chronic inflammation.

3 Crystals That Develop in the Tumor Microenvironment

The tumor microenvironment (TME) is highly cellular, containing cancer cells, fibroblasts, endothelial cells, and a range of leukocytes. Its non-cellular component consists of extracellular matrix that includes collagen, fibronectin, hyaluronan, and laminin. Over time the TME also becomes increasingly vascularized due to the development of a neovascular network akin to that seen in the vasa vasorum in atherosclerotic arteries (Fig. 3). Tumor cells control the function of the cellular and non-cellular components of their environment via complex signaling networks that collectively promote their growth and spread [17].

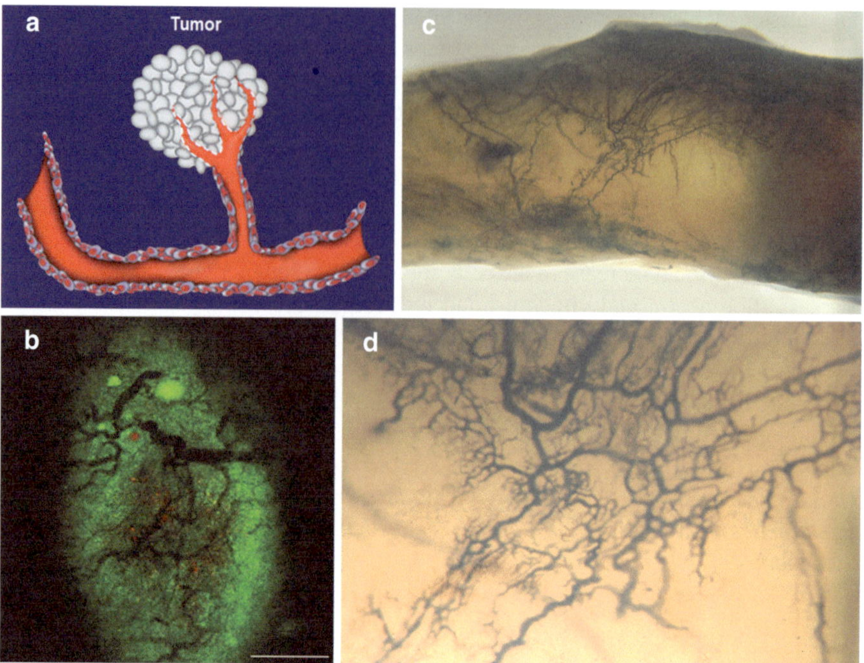

Fig. 3 Neovascularization in tumors and atherosclerosis. (**a**, **b**) neovascularization in tumor and (**c**, **d**) vasa vasorum of human arterial plaque stained by India Ink (Barberi & Abela in *Peripheral Vascular Disease: Basic Diagnostic & Therapeutic Approaches*, Ed: Abela) Lippincott, 2004; p 28

Because neoplastic cells are by nature abnormal, the way they traffic a range of molecules and metabolites is inherently dysfunctional. Notably cholesterol uptake is often enhanced, and its removal slowed leading to intracellular accumulation of cholesterol. Purines production is enhanced due to rapid tumor growth. Calcium metabolism becomes disordered. In addition, tumor cells often over express lytic enzymes such as collagenase that act to increase ability of the cancer to spread locally.

Necrosis of tumor cells due to ischemia and immune injury enriches the TME with cellular debris, which is similar to atherosclerosis and can lead to the formation of a range of organic crystals. In an environment already enriched with leukocytes, crystals can incite an immune response akin to that seen elsewhere in the body that further enhances the cellular content of the tumor and the development of its neovascular network. Furthermore, sudden enlargement of the tumor may occur due to hemorrhage caused by direct crystal induced vascular trauma (see Chap. "Molecular Pathomechanisms of Crystal-Induced Disorders").

The presence of crystals within cancers was first described more than 120 years ago, however, their exact nature and potential role in cancer development was unclear [18]. Since then, the specific nature of several crystals in solid cancers has been determined [19]. Like crystals that form elsewhere in the body, all have the potential to incite inflammation and cause local trauma, depending on their individual size and surface characteristics as well as the size and shape of their aggregates.

3.1 Calcium Crystals

The appearance of microcalcifications in solid organs is common with aging and thus, not specific for cancer. However, calcium is commonly detected in malignant and benign solid cancers, and in some instances, it may be the earliest and only sign of cancers on radiologic screening [20].

The mechanism of calcium deposition in cancers is variable. It may result from abnormal calcium hemostasis by the neoplastic cells or occur as a result of chronic inflammation as in atherosclerosis. *Hydroxyapatite* crystals are the most common form of calcium crystals found in tumors. They have been demonstrated to affect the development and growth of cancer cells and to increase metalloproteinase synthesis that may promote tumor spread [21].

Calcium oxalate has been found in several tumors including the breast, the urogenital, and biliary tract. In animal models it has been demonstrated to induce proliferation of highly malignant and undifferentiated tumors. Interestingly oxalate crystals do not induce cancer when injected into subcutaneous tissues indicating that their mutagenic effects are dependent on their cellular environment [22].

Whitlockite (calcium phosphate conjugated with magnesium) is the least common form of calcium crystals to be identified in solid tumors. When present, it is thought to reflect the avidity of tumor cells for magnesium. This form of calcium crystal deposit has only been associated with malignant breast cancers [23].

3.2 Cholesterol Crystals

Cholesterol crystals were among the first forms of crystal to be identified in-vitro in tumor cultures [24]. Their presence is not unexpected as disordered cholesterol trafficking is a common feature of cancer cells [25] (Fig. 4). Cancer and atherosclerosis share similar risk factors including aging, smoking, obesity, sedentary lifestyle, diabetes, and hormone use [26]. A related feature of neoplasia and atherosclerosis is neo-angiogenesis, a process that has been linked to cancer's ability for local and remote metastasis. The formation of neo-vessels, known as vasa vasorum, inside the atherosclerotic plaque creates one of the main entry points for lipoproteins, erythrocytes, and monocytes inside the plaques which plays a very important role in plaque growth and destabilization associated with ACS (Fig. 3) [27, 28, 29]. Neovascularization of both cancer tumors and atherosclerotic plaque provide nutrition that enhance their growth [30]. We have recently demonstrated in cell culture of breast and colon cancer that cholesterol crystals (CCs) can activate vascular endothelial growth factor (VEGF) [31]. Thus, the presence of CCs can activate neovascularization in both cancer and atherosclerosis. Moreover, we also demonstrated that CCs activate CD44 and Ubiquityl-Histone H2B (Ub-H2B) in the breast cancer cell line. These cytokines have been previously demonstrated to enhance cancer proliferation and metastasis [32, 33]. Furthermore, CCs were found to puncture the

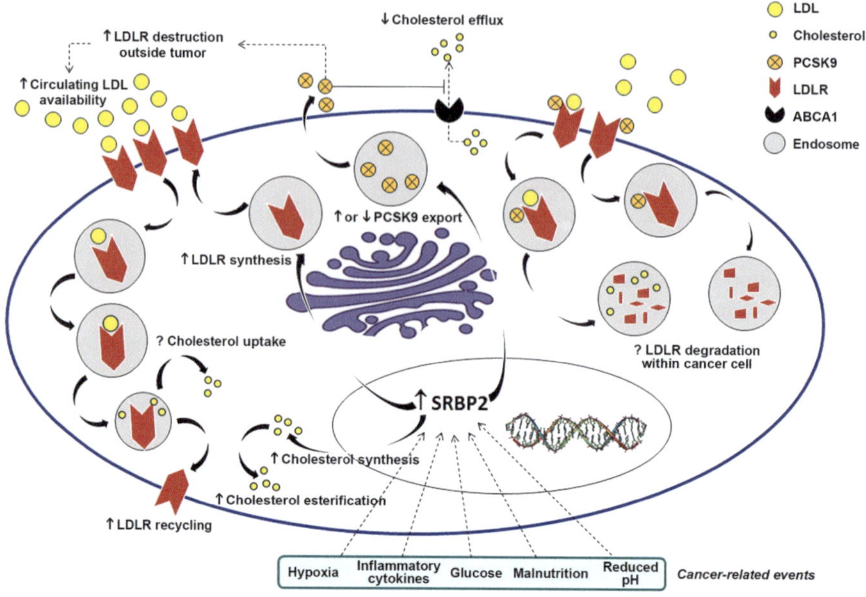

Fig. 4 Abnormalities in cholesterol trafficking in cancer cells. (Reproduced with permission [25])

tumor surfaces similar to their role in disrupting the fibrous cap to cause plaque rupture [31] (Fig. 5). Also, the sharp tipped CCs have the potential to damage the neovascular networks [34, 35], that may in some instances lead to entry of tumor cells into the circulation and enhance metastasis [36]. These findings suggest that CCs can play an important role by mechanical dissemination of cancer cells and activate inflammation similar to their effect in atherosclerosis.

Moreover, CCs content by density and distribution were significantly greater in the cancer compared to the normal marginal tissues. The source of the CCs is the free cholesterol which was also significantly greater in the cancer compared to the marginal tissues [37] (Fig. 5).

3.3 Urate Crystals

Uric acid is the end-product of purine metabolism in humans. Due to the high protein production in cancer cells, it is not unexpected that UA crystals are found in solid cancers. Although it is recognized that UA crystals can incite inflammation in solid cancers, in a mouse model of breast cancer, they were found to significantly *prevent and delay* the formation of cancer suggesting that UA crystals stimulate the release of immune mediators that dampen tumor cell activity. This is supported by evidence that UA crystals directly induce the expression of MHC class I-related chain A and B, two ligands for the immunoreceptor NKG2D, in both tumor and dendritic cells [38]. Whether this effect is unique to UA crystals is not clear,

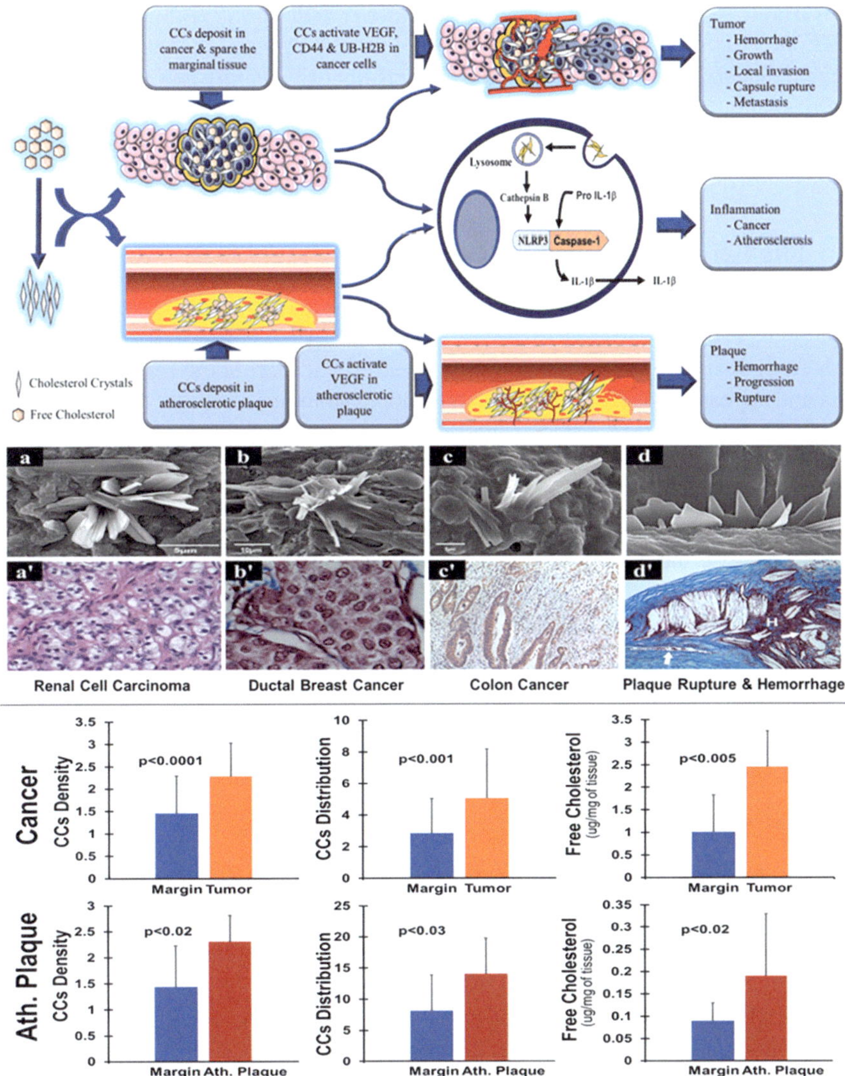

Fig. 5 Mechanisms of Cholesterol Crystal (CCs) Induced Trauma, Inflammation, and Neo-vascularization in Cancer and Atherosclerosis: (Top) There are substantial quantities of CCs in solid cancer tumors as in atherosclerosis and they were found to activate IL-1β, CD44, VB-H2B and VEGF that stimulate inflammation and neovascularization respectively. CCs can enhance tumor growth and metastasis by disruption of tissues with local spread, causing intra tumor haemorrhage with access to the circulation, activating cytokines and triggering inflammation, as in atherosclerosis. (Middle) Scanning electron microscopy of three different cancers (**a**, **b**, **c**) with their matched light microscopic images (**a'**, **b'**, **c'**) confirming their diagnosis. CCs are seen perforating the tumor surface (**a**, **b**, **c**) as noted in plaque rupture (**d**, **d'**). Haemorrhage is noted surrounding the CCs and vasa vasorum in the atherosclerotic plaque matrix. These findings support the mechanisms proposed in the cartoon image above. (Bottom) Bar graphs demonstrate a significantly greater CCs density, distribution and free cholesterol in cancers (kidney, colon, lung) and in atherosclerotic plaque compared to their marginal tissues. Ath. = atherosclerotic plaque. (Reproduced with permission [37])

however, *it suggests that the resultant immune response to crystals exposed to the TME may depend on the phase of the tumor's development. Notably, however, in animal models, UA crystals may enhance anti-tumor immunity that may prevent or delay the development of breast cancer. Thus, the effects of crystal induced inflammation on tumor cells may relate to their phase of development.*

4 The Effect of Therapies Used for 2° Prevention in Atherosclerosis on Cancer

Atherosclerosis and cancer are common diseases that share some common risk factors and appear to share some common pathophysiological features. This has led to the thesis that therapies used for the secondary prevention of atherosclerosis may have benefits in cancer [39] (Fig. 6).

While the same inflammatory cellular "players and processes" are active in the atherosclerotic bed and the TME of solid tumors, this thesis is likely an oversimplification, because these "epiphenomenon" are a consequence to different stimuli. In

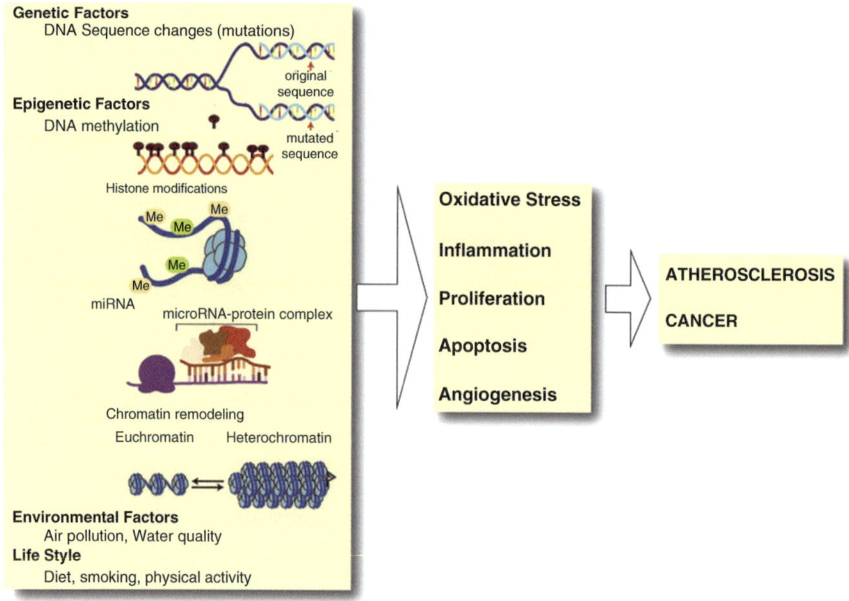

Fig. 6 Factors involved in the early stages and development of atherosclerosis and cancer. Among the important similarities found in both multifactorial diseases, the identification of changes in the DNA sequence in close correlation to epigenetic modifications can be transmitted across generations in relationship with key environmental factors. These external factors can by themselves start or potentiate anomalous processes evidenced in the long-term as oxidative stress, inflammation, aberrant apoptosis, uncontrolled cell proliferation and angiogenesis. (Reproduced with permission [39])

atherosclerotic bed the inflammatory response relates to the release of cholesterol crystals into the vascular bed from lipid rich atherosclerotic plaques. In the TME the inflammatory response occurs due to the release of cellular debris including crystals from necrotic tumor cells, as well as response to malignant cells as they attempt to evade immune detection, grow, locally invade, and begin to disseminate systemically.

None-the-less, there is intriguing albeit conflicting, laboratory and non-randomized observational clinical data, which suggests that therapies used for secondary prevention of atherosclerosis may affect tumor growth and spread [40].

4.1 Lipid Lowering Therapy

Due to defects in the trafficking of cholesterol, cancer cells tend to accumulate cholesterol via several mechanisms [25]. Although it is believed that excess intracellular cholesterol encourages tumor growth and spread [41], the mechanism by which this might occur is uncertain. It is conceivable, however, as free cholesterol accumulates in cancer cells it predisposes to the formation of CCs in the same way it leads to the formation of CCs in macrophages in the vascular wall. Once formed, they would have the capacity to cause direct cellular trauma and to activate inflammasome which in turn could incite inflammation and promote regional inflammation, tumor growth and spread.

In vitro and animal studies support the thesis that lipid lowering agents can dampen inflammation and slow the growth of several cancers lines, including cancers arising from the urogenital tract (renal cell, bladder, prostate), the gut (colonic, pancreatic hepatocellular), breast, ovaries and melanoma [25, 41].

Despite this, clinical observations have not necessarily supported the thesis that lipid lowering can prevent cancer. Early epidemiological and clinical data raised concerns that the risk of developing cancer is inversely related to serum levels of LDLc [42]. These observations significantly dampened the enthusiasm for aggressive lipid lowering therapy in patients with vascular disease. Subsequently, Mendelian randomization studies demonstrated that while low levels of LDLc were robustly associated with an increased risk of cancer, genetically determined low levels of LDLc per se were not [43]. Furthermore, post-hoc analyses of placebo-controlled lipid trials have tended to be reassuring as some suggested that the incidence of cancer is lower in those assigned to therapy. Although this later observation has not been a consistent finding, it raised hope that statins, ezetimibe and PCSK9 inhibitors may reduce mutagenesis as well as cancer growth and spread [44].

Unfortunately, no prospective placebo-controlled trials of any lipid lowering therapy either alone or in combination with chemotherapeutic agents have been conducted to answer this question. Thus, while there is no reason to cease lipid lowering therapy in patients with atherosclerosis who develop cancer, there is currently no evidence that it should be employed to prevent cancer or slow its progression.

4.2　Inflammation and Cancer

Although the etiology of many cancers has been linked to a chronic irritant causing inflammation, it appears unlikely that localized chronic crystal induced inflammation per se leads to directly to mutagenesis. Interestingly, a recent study it was demonstrated that genetic alteration in hematopoietic stem cells and their monocyte derivatives with loss of alleles in the DNMT3, TET2 and ASXL1 genes can constitute clonal hematopoiesis of intermediate potential (CHIP) that significantly increases the risk for both hematologic cancer and as well as atherosclerosis. These stem cell mutations can lead to clones of granulocytes, monocytes, and lymphocytes that can increase the risk of both cancer and coronary artery disease by increased expression of inflammation markers (i.e., IL-1β) within the plaque to cause instability (Fig. 7) [45–49]. It is estimated that individuals with CHIP have not only a risk for developing a hematologic cancer but also carry a tenfold risk for having a cardiovascular event. Moreover, in a mouse experiment, the loss of the Tet2 gene as part of CHIP demonstrated a significant increase in atherosclerotic plaque [49]. Although there appears to be a link between some pro-inflammatory pathways and the development of atherosclerosis and hematologic cancers this does not necessarily imply causality or provide a mechanism that links crystal induced inflammation with mutagenesis.

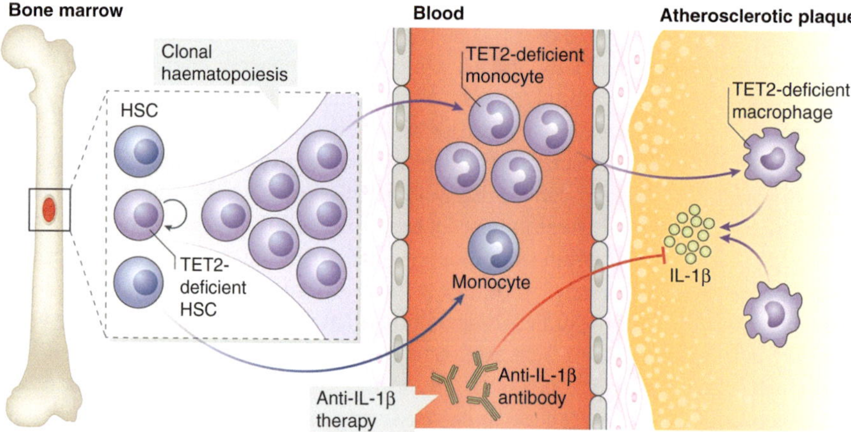

Fig. 7 Inflammation in cardiovascular disease. The bone marrow is a major site of leukocyte production. Studies have shown that some hematopoietic clones expand through a process called clonal hematopoiesis that can lead to TET-2 deficient monocytes that can infiltrate atherosclerotic lesions, where they differentiate to IL-1β-producing macrophages. Blocking the inflammatory cytokine IL-1β may lower the incidence of cardiovascular events. HSC, hematopoietic stem cell; TET2, methylcytosine dioxygenase. (Reproduced with permission [48])

4.3 Anti-Inflammatory Therapies

As expected, the TME is pro-inflammatory [50, 51] (Fig. 8) as the immune system presents a line of defense against the development and growth of cancer. As cancer develops, some cell lines may not be completely immunologically silent, and the release of debris from necrotic malignant cells will enhance the influx of pro-inflammatory cells.

Despite this, the evidence suggests that some pro-inflammatory mediators expressed as part of the immune response to cancer cells "inadvertently" promote tumor growth and spread by stimulating angiogenesis and weakening the supportive matrix within the TME. Thus, there is now increasing enthusiasm to attempt to dampen specific inflammatory pathways in the hope of slowing the progression of cancer [50].

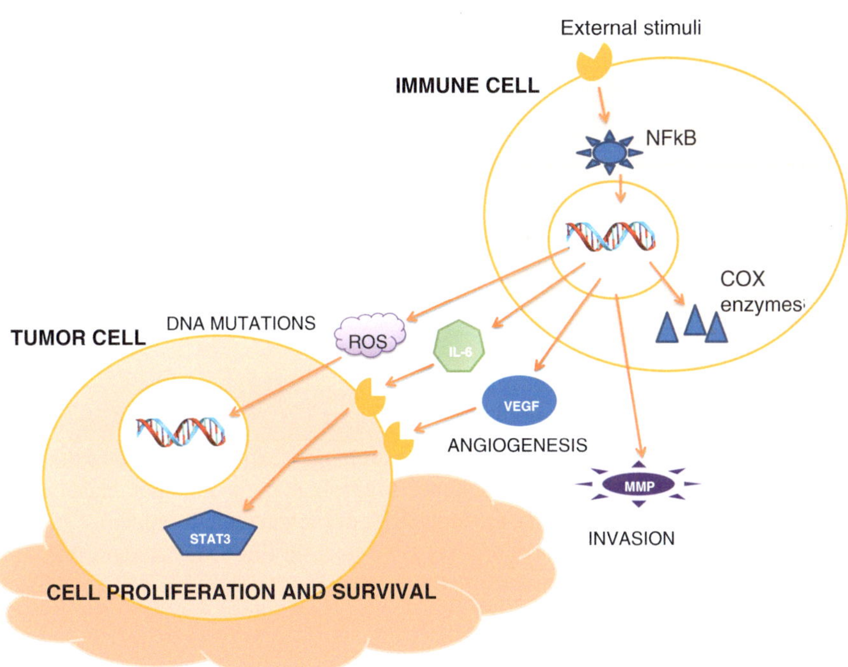

Fig. 8 Inflammation and cancer. Various inflammatory and carcinogenic agents can activate the transcription factor NFkB. Once activated, it binds to specific DNA sequences in the nucleus and induces the production of pro-inflammatory cytokines and COX enzymes. Activated immune cells produce specific cytokines (IL-6, VEGF, etc.) and metalloproteinases (MMP-2 and MMP-9). IL-6 and growth factors can induce STAT3 activation by leading to cell proliferation and survival while metalloproteases degrade the membrane basement, promoting cell invasion. Moreover, macrophages secrete a great amount of reactive oxygen species (ROS) and mutagenic agents against microbial agents that induce a persistent tissue damage and cause DNA alterations by contributing to tumorigenesis. (Reproduced with permission [50])

To date, observations from non-randomized databases have provided some evidence that non-specific anti-inflammatory agents including aspirin, colchicine (as well as NSAIDs, Allopurinol, and Diaformin) may reduce the incidence of cancer [50]. In addition, some bench studies indicate that these agents may slow the growth of some cancer cell lines, and in a post-hoc analysis of the CANTOS study it was suggested that blocking IL-1β may slow the progression of non-small cancer of the lung [51, 52].

Unfortunately, prospective studies failed to confirm the benefits of canakinumab in lung cancer [53]. Therefore, aside aspirin, no anti-inflammatory therapies have been employed for the prevention or treatment of cancer, however, recently the risk-benefit of low-dose aspirin for this purpose has been called into question [54]. Moreover, use of aspirin in the Phase III double blinded placebo control trial of aspirin (300 mg/day for 5 years) as adjuvant therapy for HER2 negative breast cancer failed to demonstrate a benefit on cancer recurrence [55].

Thus, while efforts to reduce the formation of crystals or dampen crystal induced inflammation may slow the process of atherosclerosis, and possibly reduce the size of a tumor due to a reduction in inflammatory infiltrate or prevention of hemorrhage, it is self-evident that only cytotoxic therapies can stop the inexorable growth and spread of cancer.

The observation in some studies that long term use of aspirin and statins may have beneficial effect on the incidence of certain cancers continues to raise interest [40, 37, 56]. Since these agents can dissolve CCs, this may provide a mechanism by which they could attenuate inflammation and reduce neogenesis in the TME thus delaying the onset of metastatic disease [57, 58].

5   Conclusions

Although it is believed that chronic inflammation may lead to mitogenesis that may then lead to mutagenesis, current evidence suggests that crystals that cause cancer do so due their ability to directly damage DNA or prevent strand repair.

Separately, various crystals can develop *de-novo* in the TME as abnormal trafficking of metabolites and cellular necrosis result in accumulation and crystallization of calcium, cholesterol, and UA acid. These crystals have the potential to cause cellular and tissue trauma and to enhance the inflammatory milieu of the TME. Although in some instances the response may dampen tumor growth, in other instances crystals may contribute to tumor growth, to local spread and hemorrhage within the TME.

Despite the similarity in some of the pathophysiologic processes involved with the growth of cancer and atherosclerosis, there is currently insufficient evidence to support the routine use of therapies proven useful for secondary prevention of atherosclerosis to prevent or treat cancer.

References

1. Sato T, Shimosato T, Klinman DM. Silicosis and lung cancer: current perspectives. Lung Cancer (Auckl). 2018;9:91–101.
2. Kim H-R, Kim B, Jo BS, Lee J-W. Silica exposure and work-relatedness evaluation for occupational cancer in Korea. Ann Occup Environ Med. 2018;30:4. https://doi.org/10.1186/s40557-018-0216-1.
3. Ramada Rodilla JM, Cerradab BC, Pujadas CS, Delclos GL, Benavidesa FG. Fiber burden and asbestos-related diseases: an umbrella review. Gac Sanit. 2022;36:173–83. https://doi.org/10.1016/j.gaceta.2021.04.001.
4. https://www.cancer.org/content/dam/CRC/PDF/Public/664.00.pdf.
5. Turci F, Pavan C, Leinardi R, Tomatis M, Pastero L, Garry D, Anguissola S, Lison D, Fubini B. Revisiting the paradigm of silica pathogenicity with synthetic quartz crystals: the role of crystallinity and surface disorder. Part Fibre Toxicol. 2016;13:32. https://doi.org/10.1186/s12989-016-0136-6.
6. Broz P, Dixit VM. Inflammasomes: mechanism of assembly, regulation and signaling. Nat Rev Immunol. 2016;16:407–20.
7. Wultscha G, Setayesha T, Kundib M, Kmenta M, Nersesyana A, Fenechc M, Knasmüllera S. Induction of DNA damage as a consequence of occupational exposure to crystalline silica: a review and meta-analysis. Mutat Res Rev Mutat Res. 2021;787:108349. https://doi.org/10.1016/j.mrrev.2020.108349.
8. Daniel LM, Mao Y, Williams AO, Saffiotti U. Direct interaction between crystalline silica and DNA: a proposed model for silica carcinogenesis. Scand J Work Environ Health. 1995;21(suppl 2):22–6.
9. Tsai J-L, Tsai S-f. Calcium oxalate crystal related kidney injury in a patient receiving Roux-en Y hepaticojejunostomy due to gall bladder cancer. BMC Nephrol. 2017;18:106. https://doi.org/10.1186/s12882-017-0520-y.
10. Van de Pol JAA, van Den Brandt PA, Schouten LJ. Kidney stones and the risk of renal cell carcinoma and upper tract urothelial carcinoma: the Netherlands cohort study. Br J Cancer. 2019;120:368–74. https://doi.org/10.1038/s41416-018-0356-7.
11. Sun X-Y, Xu M, Ouyang J-M. The effect of crystal shape and aggregation of calcium oxalate monohydrate on cellular toxicitiy and renal epithelial cells. ACS Omega. 2017;9:6039–52. https://doi.org/10.1021/acsomega.7b00510.
12. Werner H, Bapat S, Schobesberger M, Segets D, Scwaminger SP. Calcium oxalate crystallization: influence of pH, energy input, and supersaturation ratio on the synthesis of artificial kidney stones. ACS Omega. 2021;6:26566–74. http://pubs.acs.org/journal/acsodf.
13. Peerapen P, Boonmark W, Putpeerawit P, Thongboonkerd V. Calcium oxalate crystals trigger epithelial-mesenchymal transition and carcinogenic features in renal cells: a crossroad between kidney stone disease and renal cancer. Exp Hematol Oncol. 2022;11:62. https://doi.org/10.1186/s40164-022-00320-y.
14. Kitahara CM, Berrington de González A, Freedman ND, Huxley R, Mok Y, Jee SH, Samet JM. Total cholesterol and cancer risk in a large prospective study in Korea. J Clin Oncol. 2011;29:1592–8. https://doi.org/10.1200/JCO.2010.31.5200.
15. Rock KL, Kataoka H, Lai J-J. Uric acid as a danger signal in gout and its comorbidities. Nat Rev Rheumatol. 2013;9:13–23. https://doi.org/10.1038/nrrheum.2012.143; published online 4 September 2012.
16. Ishikawa Y, Fujio A, Tokodai K. Cholesterol granuloma of the liver mimicking malignant tumor: a case report. Tohoku J Exp Med. 2022;256:235–40. https://doi.org/10.1620/tjem.256.235.
17. Baghban R, Roshangar L, Jahaban-Esfahlan R, et al. Tumor microenvironment complexity and therapeutic implications at a glance. Cell Commun Signal. 2020;18:59. https://doi.org/10.1186/s12964-020-0530-4.

18. White CP. On the occurrence of crystals in tumours. J Pathol Bacteriol. 1909;13:1–10. https://doi.org/10.1002/path.1700130103.
19. Abela GS, Leja M, Janoudi A, Perry D, Richard J, De Feijter-Rupp H, Vanderberg A. Relationship between atherosclerosis and certain solid cancer tumors. J Am Coll Card. 2019;73(9 Suppl 1):156.
20. Scott R, Stone N, Kendall C, Geraki K, Rogers K. Relationships between pathology and crystal structure in breast calcifications: an in situ X-ray diffraction study in histological sections. NPJ Breast Cancer. 2016;2:16029. https://doi.org/10.1038/npjbcancer.2016.29; published online 14 September 2016.
21. Cheung HS, Devine TR, Hubbard W. Calcium phosphate particle induction of metalloproteinase and mitogenesis: effect of particle sizes. Osteoarthr Cartil. 1997;5:145–51.
22. Castellaro AM, Tonda A, Cejas HH, Ferreyra H, Caputto BL, Pucci OA, Gil GA. Oxalate induces breast cancer. BMC Cancer. 2015;15:761. https://doi.org/10.1186/s12885-015-1747-2.
23. Scimeca M, Giannini E, Antonacci C, Pistolese CA, Spagnoli LG, Bonanno E. Microcalcifications in breast cancer: an active phenomenon mediated by epithelial cells with mesenchymal characteristics. BMC Cancer. 2014;14:286. http://www.biomedcentral.com/1471-2407/14/286.
24. Richters A, Sherwin RP. The occurrence of biologic crystals in tumor and nontumor culture of C3H/HeJ mice. Cancer Res. 1965;25:214–9.
25. Mahboobnia K, Pirro M, Marini E, Grignani F, Bezsonov EE, Jamialahmadi T, Sahebkar A. PCSK9 and cancer: rethinking the link. Biomed Pharmacother. 2021;140:111758. https://doi.org/10.1016/j.biopha.2021.111758.
26. Koene RJ, Prizment AE, Blaes A, et al. Shared risk factors in cardiovascular disease and cancer. Circulation. 2016;133:1104–14.
27. Virmani, R, Kolodgie FD, Burke AP, et al. Atherosclerotic plaque progression and vulnerability to rupture: angiogenesis as a source of intraplaque hemorrhage. Arterioscler Thromb Vasc Biol. 2005;25:2054–61.
28. Isner JM. Cancer & atherosclerosis: broad mandate of angiogenesis. Circulation. 1999;6:1653.
29. Barger C, Beeuwkes R III, Lainey LL, Silverman KJ. Hypothesis: vasa Vasorum and neovascularization of human coronary arteries—a possible role in pathophysiology of atherosclerosis. N Engl J Med. 1984;310:175–7.
30. Xu J, Lu X, Shi GP. Vasa vasorum in atherosclerosis and clinical significance.Int J Mol Sci. 2015;16:11574–608.
31. Abela GS, Katkoori VR, Pathak DR, et al. Cholesterol crystals induce mechanical trauma, inflammation and neovascularization in solid cancers as in atherosclerosis. Am Heart J Plus. 2023;35:100317. https://doi.org/10.1016/j.ahjo.2023.100317.
32. Gao Y, Foster R, Yang X, et al. Up-regulation of CD44 in the development of metastasis, recurrence and drug resistance of ovarian cancer. Oncotarget. 2015;6(11):9313–26.
33. Espinosa JM. Histone H2B ubiquitination: the cancer connection. Genes Dev. 2008;22:2743–9.
34. Abela GS, Aziz K, Vedre A, et al. Effect of cholesterol crystals on plaques and intima in arteries of patients with acute coronary and cerebrovascular syndromes. Am J Cardiol. 2009;103:959–68.
35. Al-Handawi MB, Commins P, Karothu DP, et al. Mechanical and crystallographic analysis of cholesterol crystals puncturing biological membranes. Chem Eur J. 2018;24:11493–7.
36. Valastyan S, Weinberg RA. Tumor metastasis: molecular insights and evolving paradigms. Cell. 2011;147:275–92. https://doi.org/10.1016/j.cell.2011.09.024.
37. Cao Y, Nishihara R, Wu K, Wang M, Ogino S, Willett WC, Spiegelman D, Fuchs CS, Giovannucci EL, Chan AT. Population-wide impact of long-term use of aspirin and the risk for cancer. JAMA Oncol. 2016;2:762. https://doi.org/10.1001/jamaoncol.2015.6396.
38. Xu X, Rao G, Rinz R. Uric acid crystals as a novel adjuvant for breast cancer immunotherapy in a syngeneic and somatic mouse model. Cancer Res. 2009;69(9_Supplement):369.
39. Tapia-Vieyra JV, Delgado-Coello B, Mas-Oliva J. Atherosclerosis and cancer; a resemblance with far-reaching implications. Arch Med Res. 2017;48:12–26.

40. Demierre M-F, Higgins PDR, Gruber SB, Hawk E, Lippman SM. Statins and cancer prevention. Nat Rev Cancer. 2005;5:930–42. https://doi.org/10.1038/nrc1751.
41. Di Bello E, Zwergel C, Mai A, Valente S. The innovative potential of statins in cancer: new targets for new therapies. Front Chem. 2020;8:516. https://doi.org/10.3389/fchem.2020.00516. eCollection 2020.
42. Jacobs D, Blackburn H, Higgins M, Reed D, Iso H, McMillan G, Neaton J, Nelson J, Potter J, Rifkind B, Rossouw J, Shekelle R, Yusuf S. For participants in the conference on low cholesterol: mortality associations report of the conference on low blood cholesterol: mortality associations. Circulation. 1992;86:1046–60.
43. Benn M, Tybjærg-Hansen A, Stender S, Frikke-Schmidt R, Nordestgaard BG. Low-density lipoprotein cholesterol and the risk of cancer: a mendelian randomization study. J Natl Cancer Inst. 2011;103:508–19.
44. Barbalata CI, Tefas LR, Achim M, Tomuta I, Porfire AS. Statins in risk-reduction and treatment of cancer. World J Clin Oncol. 2020;11(8):573–88. https://doi.org/10.5306/wjco.v11.i8.573.
45. Greten FR, Grivennikov SI. Inflammation and cancer: triggers, mechanism, and consequences. Immunity. 2019;51:27i–41.
46. Libby P. Inflammation in atherosclerosis. Nature. 2002;420:868–74.
47. Düewell P, Kono H, Rayner KJ, Sirois CM, Vladimer G, Bauernfeind F, Abela GS, Franchi L, Nunez G, Schnurr M, Espevik T, Lien G, Fitzgerald KA, Rock KL, Moore KJ, Wright SD, Hornung V, Latz E. NLRP3 inflammasomes are required for atherogenesis and activated by cholesterol crystals. Nature. 2010;464:1357–61.
48. Swirski FK. From clonal haematopoiesis to the CANTOS trial. Nat Rev Cardiol. 2018;15:79–80. https://doi.org/10.1038/nrcardio.2017.208.
49. Jaiswal S, Natarajan P, Silver AJ, et al. Clonal heamtopoiesis and risk for atherosclerotic cardiovascular disease. N Engl J Med. 2017;377:111–21. https://doi.org/10.1056/NEJMoa1701719.
50. Zappavigna S, Cossu AM, Grimaldi A, et al. Anti-inflammatory drugs as anticancer agents. Int J Mol Sci. 2020;21:2605. https://doi.org/10.3390/ijms21072605./jnci/djr008.
51. Wong CC, Baum J, Silvestro A, et al. Inhibition of IL1β by canakinumab may be effective against diverse molecular subtypes of lung cancer: an exploratory analysis of the CANTOS trial. Cancer Res. 2020;80(24):5597–605. https://doi.org/10.1158/0008-5472.CAN-19-3176. Epub 2020 Oct 6.
52. Ridker PM, MacFadyen JG, Thuren T, Everett BM, Libby P, Glynn RJ. Effect of interleukin-1beta inhibition with canakinumab on incident lung cancer in patients with atherosclerosis: exploratory results from a randomised, double-blind, placebo-controlled trial. Lancet. 2017;390:1833–42. https://doi.org/10.1016/S0140-6736(17)32247-X.
53. Tan DS, Felip E, Castro G, et al. Association for Cancer Research. Canakinumab in combination with first-line (1L) pembrolizumab plus chemotherapy for advanced non-small cell lung cancer (aNSCLC): results from the CANOPY-1 phase 3 trial. Cancer Res. 2022;82(12_ Supplement):CT037. https://doi.org/10.1158/1538-7445.AM2022-CT037.
54. McNeil JJ, Wolfe R, Woods RL, ASPREE Investigator Group, et al. Effect of aspirin on cardiovascular events and bleeding in the healthy elderly. N Engl J Med. 2018;379:1509–18. https://doi.org/10.1056/NEJMoa1805819erly.
55. Chen WY, Ballman KV, Viner EP, et al. A randomized phase III, double-blinded, placebo-controlled trial of aspirin as adjuvant therapy for breast cancer (A011502): the aspirin after breast cancer (ABC). Trial J Clin Oncol. 2022;40 suppl ASCO (abstract # 360922):360922. https://doi.org/10.1200/JCO.2022.40.36_suppl.360922.
56. Nielsen SF, Nordestgaard BG, Bojesen SE. Statin use and reduced cancer-related mortality. N Engl J Med. 2012;367:1792–802.
57. Abela GS, Vedre A, Janoudi A, Huang R, Durga S, Tamhane U. Effect of statins on cholesterol crystallization and atherosclerotic plaque stabilization. Am J Cardiol. 2011;107:1710–7. https://doi.org/10.1016/j.amjcard.2011.02.336.
58. Fry L, Lee A, Khan S, Aziz K, Vedre A, Abela GS. Effect of aspirin on cholesterol crystallization: a potential mechanism for plaque stabilization. Am Heart J Plus. 2022;13:100083. https://doi.org/10.1016/j.ahjo.2021.100083.

The Interaction Between Infection, Crystals, and Cardiovascular Disease

Subhashis Mitra, Stefan Mark Nidorf, Manel Boumegouas, and George S. Abela

1 Background

The events that trigger infection of cardiac structures are often unknown, and the mechanism by which infection may lead to acute cardiovascular events remains speculative. Sterile triggers including crystals, and infectious agents including bacteria and viruses, can activate an immune response. Crystals may trigger complement and activate the NLRP3 pathway, and the surface of bacteria and viruses can be recognized by the innate and adaptive immune system via specific ligands [1–4]. In this chapter we explore how crystals may play a role in bacterial endocarditis and develop in the intra- and extracellular space of the arterial wall with the potential to trigger vasculitis, atherosclerosis, and rupture of atherosclerotic plaque.

S. Mitra (✉)
Division of Infectious Diseases, Department of Medicine, College of Human Medicine, Michigan State University, East Lansing, MI, USA
e-mail: mitrasub@msu.edu

S. M. Nidorf
The Heart and Vascular Research Institute, Sir Charles Gairdner Hospital, Perth, WA, Australia

M. Boumegouas
Division of Cardiovascular Medicine, Department of Medicine, College of Human Medicine, Michigan State University, East Lansing, MI, USA

Sparrow Hospital, Lansing, MI, USA

G. S. Abela
Department of Medicine, Division of Cardiovascular Medicine, Michigan State University, East Lansing, MI, USA
e-mail: abela@msu.edu

© The Author(s), under exclusive license to Springer Nature Switzerland AG 2023
G. S. Abela, S. M. Nidorf (eds.), *Cholesterol Crystals in Atherosclerosis and Other Related Diseases*, Contemporary Cardiology,
https://doi.org/10.1007/978-3-031-41192-2_23

2   Cholesterol Crystals Play a Role in Bacterial Endocarditis

Infective endocarditis (IE) is a complex process which occurs after a series of separate events that lead to the formation of vegetation on the valvular endothelium. Although it is more likely to develop in patients with congenital, rheumatic degenerative valve disease or a history of prosthetic valve replacement, almost half of the patients who present with IE have no obvious predisposing cause [5, 6]. In all cases, however, IE is invariably initiated by injury to the valvular endothelium that predisposes to adhesion of bacteria to valve. Once seeded, the bacteria may colonize and spread beyond the leaflet surface.

2.1   Primary Endothelial Injury

The primary endothelial injury that leads to IE may rarely relate to iatrogenic trauma during catheterization or degeneration and erosion of synthetic surfaces on cardiac devices, but most often the primary cause of injury is unidentified. In this regard, there is evidence that cholesterol crystals (CCs) are present in abundance in degenerative native and bioprosthetic valves, and that they may erode or perforate the endothelial surface of sclerotic human heart valves [7, 8] (see Chap. "Molecular Pathomechanisms of Crystal-Induced Disorders"). Thus, the growth and aggregation of CCs in the subendothelial space of valve leaflets may be a primary cause for endothelial disruption that predisposes to IE. Furthermore, in an atherosclerotic rabbit model in which a cholesterol enriched diet alternating with normal chow is provided to the animal, simvastatin and ezetimibe provided protection against CC formation which in turn may render some protection to the endothelium of the valve. However, lipid lowering after the valve was infiltrated with cholesterol was not effective in reducing CCs buried within the valve matrix and the associated macrophage infiltration [7]. These findings are consistent with the human clinical studies that evaluated the same combination of simvastatin and ezetimibe as well as other statins where there was no significant benefit found on the progression of aortic valve stenosis [9–11]. Some studies have suggested a lower embolic rate and mortality in patients with IE on statins [12, 13]. Although not as effective as lipid lowering therapy prior to CC infiltration in the valve tissue, treatment with statins may still have some potential in lowering the risk of developing IE, but that has to be further evaluated.

2.2 Initial (Non-Infectious) Response to Endothelial Injury of Valve Leaflets

No matter the cause, be it iatrogenic or crystal induced, injury to the valvular endothelial injury promotes deposition of fibrin, von Willebrand Factor (VWF), and platelets at the site of injury. This results in the formation of a nonbacterial thrombotic focus that may be associated with local inflammation that leaves the leaflet surface more susceptible to infection [6].

2.3 Bacterial Adhesion and Colonization

The bacterium inoculums necessary for the development of IE are not well defined, however, in experimental models IE typically only follows large inoculums ranging from 10^5 to 10^8 CFU/mL [14].Thus, transient low grade bacteremia that commonly occur after brushing teeth or with minor mucosal trauma seldom result in IE [15, 16].

Recently we observed in aspirates from culprit coronary arteries during acute myocardial infraction, macrophages actively engaging with and degrading CCs [17]. Since macrophages ingest CCs is in a manner akin to the scavenging activity of bacteria, we sought to evaluate whether bacteria could directly interact with CCs. Interestingly we were able to confirm that in vitro gram-positive and gram-negative bacteria do attach to CCs [18]. The observed bacterial-CC interactions raise the possibility that they may interact anywhere CCs accumulate and are exposed to specific bacteria. Thus, such interactions may explain how CCs act as a nidus for infection in the biliary tract, and how CCs that develop in degenerative valves may perforate the endothelium as they grow and act as landing sites for bacteria during bouts of bacteremia.

The ability of certain bacteria to adhere to damaged valvular endothelium, nonthrombotic foci and CCs, especially in the most inhospitable environments in the systemic circulation where high-speed flowing blood passes through the heart and across the valves, likely relates to their ability to rapidly form strong bonds between their surface and components.

Those bacterial surface components that have two adjacent IgG-like folded subdomains on their surface can recognize adhesive matrix molecules (MSCRAMMs) including integrins, cadherins or components of the extracellular matrix including collagen, fibronectin, laminin, elastin, and CCs [19]. The binding of MSCRAMMs to fibrinogen by the "dock-lock-latch" mechanism or to collagen by the "collagen hug" mechanism causes major conformational changes and is closely related to the pathogenicity of gram-positive pathogens like staphylococcus [20]. Furthermore, the mechanical stability of the bond increases when the extracellular matrix protein fibrinogen (Fn) serves as a bridging molecule between the binding of bacterial cell surface located Fn-binding proteins (FnBPA and FnBPB) and the $\alpha5\beta1$ integrin in the host cell membrane (Fig. 1) [21].

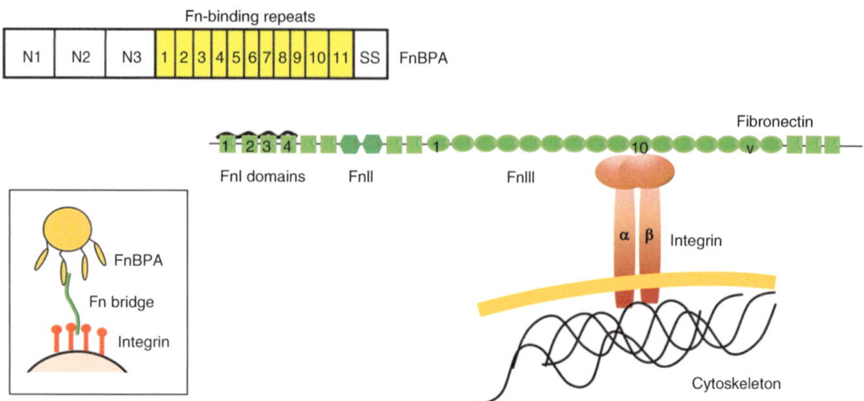

Fig. 1 Mechanism of FnBP-dependent cell invasion by *S. aureus*. The main invasion pathway of *S. aureus* involves interaction of the Fn-binding repeats of FnBPA with type I Fn modules via a tandem β-zipper structure. This triggers a conformational change in Fn, resulting in the exposure of the cryptic integrin-binding site in the tenth FnIII module, which in turn engages in a high-affinity interaction with the α5β1 integrin found in the membrane of mammalian cells. (Reproduced with permission [21])

Methicillin resistant *Staphylococcus aureus* (MRSA) that may cause fulminant IE, can adhere to endothelial cells in greater numbers in regions of (low) shear stress compared to static conditions [22]. This phenomenon, though not fully understood, may be explained by the fact that adhesins are able to form "catch-bonds" that strengthen under tension [23]. In fact, the bond between *Staphylococcus aureus* clumping factor B (ClfB) with the envelope protein loricrin was noted to be significantly enhanced by mechanical force [24]. Thus, bacterial adhesion to loricrin may be enhanced through force induced conformational changes in the ClfB molecule [25] (Fig. 2).

Streptococcus species are responsible for 20% of IE worldwide, particularly in developing countries, where rheumatic heart disease is a common predisposing condition [26]. It often presents with chronic non-specific symptoms with little or no acute prodrome. Oral streptococci are able to bind and activate platelets and adhere to host tissues. In addition, oral streptococci are able to synthesize dextran, a complex bacterial derived extracellular polysaccharide that seems important for adherence of bacteria to nonbacterial thrombotic endocarditis (NBTE) [27, 28].

Gram-negative bacteria rarely cause IE. *Pseudomonas aeruginosa* can adhere to canine aortic leaflets in vitro more easily than other gram-negative pathogens (*Escherichia coli* and *Klebsiella pneumoniae*) that are less frequent causes of IE [29]. Like *Staphylococcus aureus,* these gram-negative organisms can express a variety of adhesion molecules that allows them to attach to extracellular matrix proteins [30].

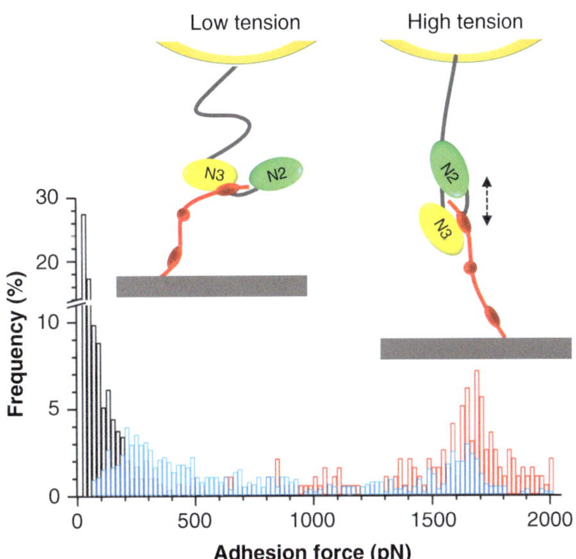

Fig. 2 Force-activated adhesion of ClfA. Under low mechanical tension, fibrinogen weakly binds to ClfA, whereas under high tension, extension and conformational changes of the ClfA N2N3 subdomains enable the formation of a fully secured DLL-like interaction. (Reproduced with permission [25])

In recent years, the role of pili, non-flagellar proteinaceous filaments found on the surface of some gram-positive and gram-negative bacteria have been demonstrated to affect their virulence. Specifically Type IV pili of *Streptococcus sanguis*, one of the most common species responsible for streptococcal IE, has been identified as an important virulence factor contributing to the pathogenesis of IE [31] and endocarditis and biofilm associated (Ebp) pilus has been found to enhance the virulence of *Enterococcus faecalis* [32].

After the initial attachment to the cardiac valve, bacteria must be further anchored to the sub endothelium by additional adhesins [33] as VWF is rapidly cleaved by the metalloproteinase ADAMTS-13 [34]. The bacterial adhesion Clfa mediates the adhesion to both fibrin and soluble fibrinogen.

2.4 Factors That Sustain the Growth of Bacteria Within the Damaged Leaflet

In our ex vivo experiments, we demonstrated that *Staphylococcus aureus* and *Pseudomonas aeruginosa* attach to CCs but not to glass shards or plastic microspheres used as controls (Figs. 3, 4 and 5) [18]. Furthermore, these organisms also dissolved CCs, raising the intriguing possibility that the organisms could utilize CCs as a source of cholesterol that may helped sustain their growth and promote colonization.

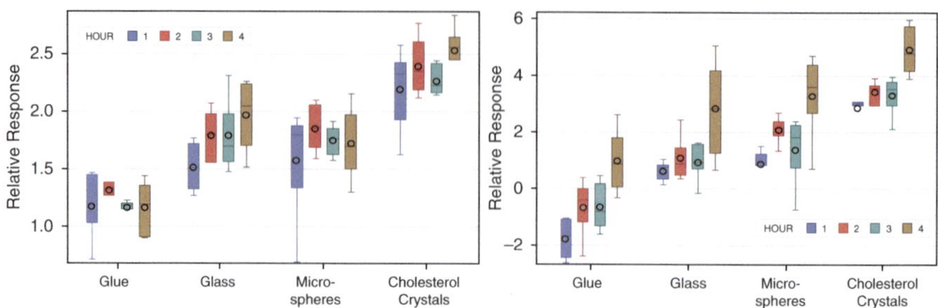

Fig. 3 In vitro bacterial adhesion. (left) Box-Cox transformed graph of S. aureus bacterial count with glue, glass, plastic microspheres, and cholesterol crystals ($p < 0.0001$). (right) Box-Cox transformed graph of P. aeruginosa bacterial count demonstrating highest count with cholesterol crystals ($p < 0.0001$). P-values were obtained from the analysis of variance and adjusted for multiplicity by the Bonferroni method. (Reproduced with permission [18])

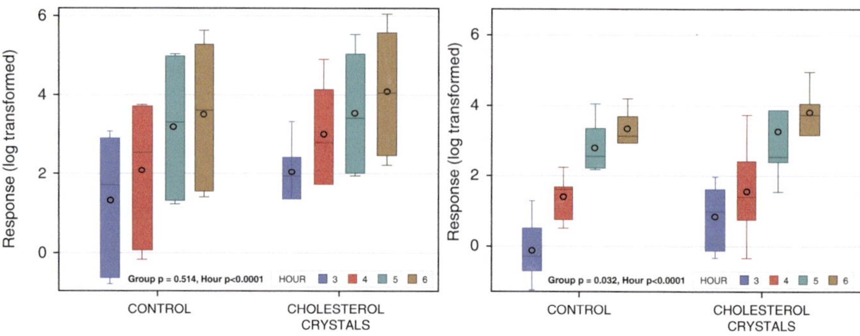

Fig. 4 In vitro bacterial growth. Log-transformed relative response of bacterial colony count with cholesterol crystals and control at 3, 4, 5, and 6 h of incubation. Left panel, S. aureus; Right panel P. aeruginosa. P-values were obtained from t-tests in repeated measures analyses. For both studies the time effect was significant ($P < 0.0001$). Group effect: $P = 0.514$ for S. aureus, and $P = 0.032$ for *P*. aeruginosa. (Reproduced with permission [18])

2.5   *Resistance to Bacterial Spread in the Leaflets*

Invading bacteria that become internalized within endothelial cells act to promote the release of pro-inflammatory cytokines including IL-6, IL-8, and monocyte chemotactic peptides [35]. Monocytes attracted to the subendothelial microenvironment cause the release of tissue thromboplastin, and if CCs are present in the interstitial space they could amplify the inflammatory process [36].

Once colonized, bacteria release lytic enzymes that promote their spread into the subendothelial space, which in some instances has already been "primed" with inflammatory cells by pre-existing CCs [34]. As with CC induced inflammation,

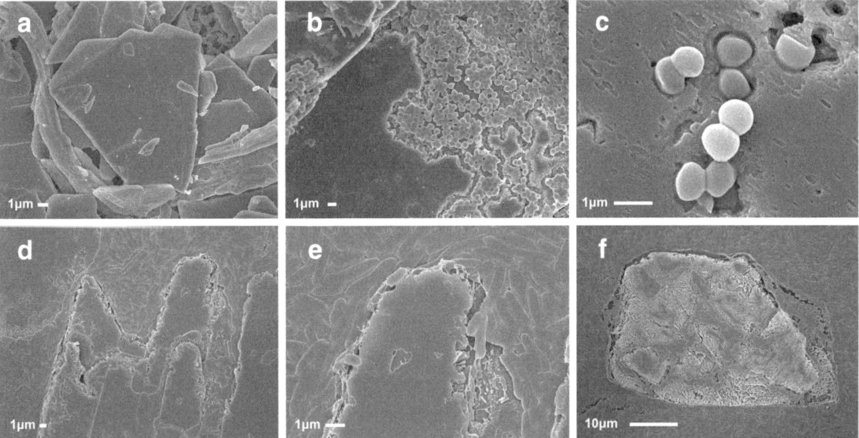

Fig. 5 Scanning electron micrograph of bacteria engaging cholesterol crystals. In vitro S. aureus incubated with cholesterol crystals (top): (**a**) Cholesterol crystals incubated in broth without bacteria as control (**b**) Staphylococcus bacteria engulfing and degrading crystal after 2.5 h incubation. (**c**) Staphylococcus bacteria noted engaging and punctuating the crystal surface at 1 h incubation. In vitro P. aeruginosa incubated with cholesterol crystals (bottom): (**d**) Pseudomonas bacteria seen engulfing and eroding crystals forming wedges into the crystal body (**e**) higher magnification demonstrates the detail of the bacterial and the crystal erosion with loss of crystal sharp edges; (**f**) another example of eroding crystal with bacteria above and around the crystal. (Reproduced with permission [18])

neutrophils play a vital role in the defense against bacteria, due in large part to the release of neutrophil extracellular traps (NETs) that can capture, neutralize, and kill microbes. NETs consist of strands of DNA extruded by activated or dying neutrophils, and release antimicrobial components such as histones, defensins, myeloperoxidase, cathepsin G, neutrophil elastase, proteinase 3, calprotectin, and cathelicidins [37]. The role of NETs in IE, therefore, is usually beneficial in the host defense [38, 39]. Under some circumstances, however, neutrophils are unable to clear bacteria entrapped in their NETS, and as these neutrophil-bacteria aggregates become entrapped in platelet-fibrin aggregates within the vegetation, the vegetation enlarges and the ongoing infection predisposes to progressive valvular injury [38, 40]. Thus, whether the invading bacteria spreads or are contained, largely depend on the ability of neutrophils to effectively ingest and neutralize them. Though the complex role that NETs play in IE needs further elucidation, at this point, it would be reasonable to hypothesize that CCs may play a role in IE by triggering the production of NETs as has been shown in atherosclerotic coronary disease during myocardial infarction. Moreover, the hypoxemia present in the vegetations could also accelerate IL-1β activation by cholesterol crystals [41].

3 Relationship Between Infection and Atherosclerosis

3.1 Bacterial Infection

A number of bacteria including *Chlamydia pneumoniae, Mycoplasma pneumoniae, Helicobacter pylori, Enterobacter hormaechei*, and multiple periodontal organisms including *Porphyromonas gingivalis, Streptococcus sanguis, and Streptococcus mutans* have been identified by nucleic acid or antigen detection methods in human atherosclerotic plaque [42–45]. In addition, several of these bacteria have been reported to accelerate atherosclerosis in animal models. Despite this, evidence to support a direct causative role for bacteria in atherogenesis remains elusive as no viable bacteria have ever been isolated from atherosclerotic plaques, and antibiotics have failed to reduce the risk of recurrent athero-thrombotic events in patients with coronary disease [46–49].

In our ex vivo experiments we demonstrated that *S. aureus* is more likely to bind to atherosclerotic arteries compared to normal vessels, and we made similar observations in the samples of fresh human carotid plaques removed at surgery compared to normal carotid arteries obtained from autopsy (Fig. 6) [18]. Although bacteria are known to adhere to the collagen and fibronectin in tissues [30], scanning electron microscopy (SEM) confirmed that the bacteria in these experiments were congregating around the CCs within the plaque. Moreover, most of the human plaque were devoid of any fibrous caps and their surfaces were lined with sheets of CCs. While these observations are consistent with our understanding that *S. aureus* can adhere to CCs, they are not sufficient to imply a causative link between *S. aureus* and atherosclerosis.

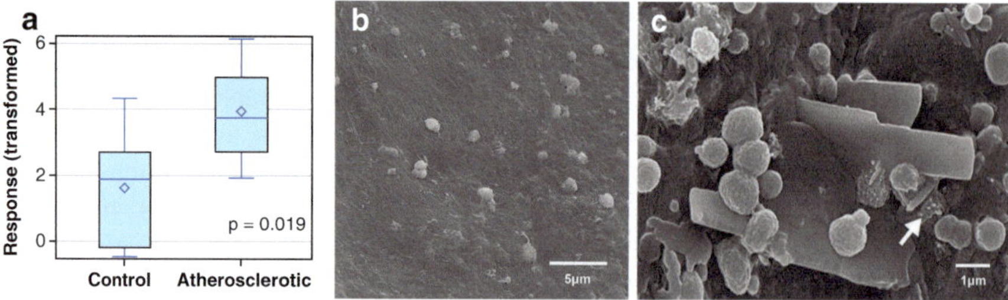

Fig. 6 Ex vivo bacterial growth in human arterial plaques. (**a**) Graphic of bacterial counts of normal control and atherosclerotic human arterial plaques using Box-Cox transformation. P-value was obtained from a two-sample t-test. (**b**) Scanning electron micrograph of normal carotid artery with few bacteria attached to intimal surface; (**c**) atherosclerotic carotid plaque with many bacteria and macrophages (white arrow) attached to cholesterol crystals. (Reproduced with permission [18])

3.2 Viral Infection

In contrast to bacterial infections, there is strong evidence that viruses may induce atherosclerosis in avian models [50, 51], however, the mechanism by which this might occur remains elusive.

Over 50 years ago, in studies on virus-induced feline urolithiasis, feline herpesvirus was isolated that produced cytopathic effects in cell cultures [52]. When the herpesvirus was cultured in cells ex vivo it was observed that after 1–16 weeks the infected cells contained numerous round refractile cytoplasmic "vacuoles" which appeared to be fat globules that contained appreciable amounts of cholesterol-like crystals. These were not seen in non-infected cells. Overtime, intracellular and extracellular crystals were observed to have formed that varied in size, shape, and structure, some of which were birefringent in polarized light and confirmed to be CCs on mass spectroscopy. Although the investigators had noted that herpesvirus could form intra- and extracellular mineral crystals [53], they believed they had previously failed to identify CCs in earlier studies due to their inherently unstable nature with processing for electron microscopy with standard techniques that dissolve CCs [54].

Upon reflection, it is possible that the extra- and intracellular vacuoles described in these cultures were exosomes and endosomes. It is known that viruses can "subvert cholesterol homeostasis" to induce host cubic membranes that form these vesicles to gain entry and release from host cells (Fig. 7) [55]. These structures vary in size, surface characteristics, and composition depending on the host. For example, it is known that in SARS-CoV-2, spike proteins may be incorporated into vesicle membrane of exosomes and thus act as decoy targets for neutralizing antibodies that thereby reduce their effectiveness in blocking viral entry into host cells [56, 57].

The formation of CCs within these lipid rich vesicles in the herpes virus model is of particular interest, as it provides a mechanism by which "viral traffic" in and out of host cells may "deliver" CCs into the intra- and extracellular space, thus providing a mechanism by which some viruses might promote the development and progression of atherosclerosis. Indeed, this possibility would support the suggestion that viral infections during childhood may cause the initial vascular injury that leads to the development of arteriosclerosis in later life [58].

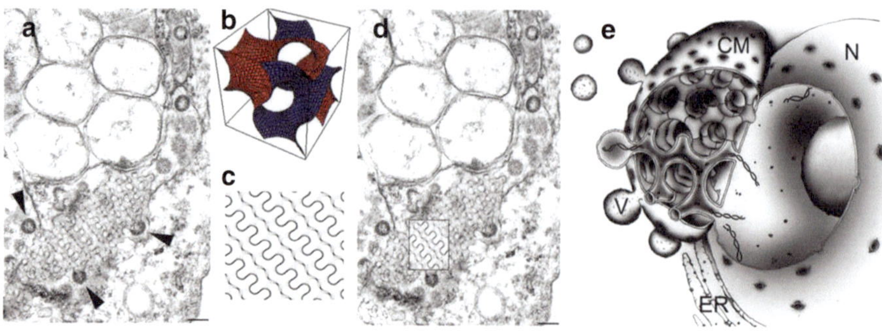

Fig. 7 SARS-CoV-induced cubic membranes in Vero cells. (**a**) The original TEM micrograph is reproduced, with permission, from Fig. 3c of Goldsmith et al. [91]. The arrow points at the regular TRS of interest; (**b**) mathematical 3D simulation to describe a gyroid (G)-based minimal surface; (**c**) a corresponding computer-simulated 2D projection map (0.4 of a unit cell thickness) derived from the 3D model in (**b**); (**d**) the theoretical projection of a slice through a G-based morphology exactly matches the TRS structure in the TEM image (see boxed area), unequivocally identifying it as "cubic membrane structure." Note the spherical virion particles budding off this cubic membrane segment (arrowheads). Scale bar, 100 nm (reproduced, with permission, from Ref (92); arrows were removed from the original image); (**e**) illustration of cubic membrane organization in a virus-infected cell and its possible function as a virus factory. The characteristic interconnected channels of the cubic membrane (CM) provide a transport conduit between the viral replication complex and the cytoplasm and/or nucleus (N). The pores at the outer surface could act as regulators that allow the entry of the essential virus precursors yet inhibit the entry of host defense proteins. The highly curved nature of cubic membranes might support viral assembly and budding. ER, endoplasmic reticulum; V, virus particle. (Reproduced with permission [55])

4 Crystallization of Inert Viral Aggregates Are Associated with Vasculitis

Vasculitis is characterized by the presence of inflammatory leukocytes in blood vessels and often associated with injury to the adjacent tissues, and is categorized by the size, type, and location of the affected vessels: *Small vessels*, (ANCA-associated and immunoglobulin A vasculitis; *Medium vessels*, (polyarteritis nodosa and Kawasaki disease; *Large vessels* (Takayasu arteritis and giant cell arteritis) [58].

Although generally classed as an "autoimmune" disease, some forms of vasculitis are due to identifiable causes [59]. Type I cryoglobulinemia vasculitis has been associated with the formation and intra-vascular deposition of immunoglobin crystals [60]. In addition, a number of studies in humans and in animal models have associated various viruses with vasculitis. Although direct infection of endothelial cells by viruses has been observed, the exact mechanism by which viruses trigger inflammation is poorly understood.

In this regard, it is of interest that several viruses, including influenza, SARS-CoV-2, and the encephalomyocarditis (EMC) virus, readily form crystals within infected cells. In studies in which newborn mice were infected with EMC, they rapidly developed patchy pathologic changes in the coronary arteries, veins, and capillaries that were not seen in shame animals. Importantly, SEM of the vascular lesions revealed the presence of viral crystals that were associated with phlebitis, capillaritis, and evidence of acute and subacute myocarditis [61]. Similar lesions in the endothelium and myocardium have been produced by other viruses including polio, Coxsackie B [62].

The SARS-CoV-2 virus uses ACE2 receptor expressed by pneumocytes in the epithelial alveolar lining to infect the host. However, the ACE2 receptor is also widely expressed on endothelium in other organs. In patients with SARS-CoV-2 infection, evidence has been found of direct viral infection of the endothelial cell and diffuse endothelial inflammation [63]. Thus, SARS-CoV-2 may cause endothelitis in several organs as a direct consequence of viral involvement and the resulting inflammatory response likely explains the systemic effects of the disease.

While the exact mechanisms by which these viruses induce endothelial injury and subsequent vascular inflammation remains uncertain, the presence of viral crystals in vascular lesions provides a mechanism by which inflammation could be triggered as a direct result of viral infection in addition to the ability of CCs to form within cholesterol rich exosomes and endosomes during viral entry and exit to and from host cells. Recent studies using X-ray free-electron laser to obtain information about the virus in the intact environment confirm the presence of viral crystals consisting of empty viral shells (procapsids) [64]. In the presence of sufficient viral load, it is possible, therefore, for these intracellular viral crystals (distinct from CCs) to enlarge and be recognized by complosome that would then trigger inflammasome and cell death. Thus, intra-cellular viral crystals, like intracellular CCs, could lead to crystal induced traumatic and inflammatory vascular injury resulting in vasculitis.

5   Relationship Between Infection and Acute Coronary Syndromes

There is good evidence that various bacterial and viral infections can increase in the risk of myocardial infarction (MI). The risk is more pronounced following lung infections, peaks at the onset of infection and returns to baseline within months following mild respiratory or urinary infections, but may persist for years after more severe infections (Fig. 8) [65]. Supporting the link between acute infection and plaque instability is the observation that influenza and pneumococcal vaccination reduces the risk of acute cardiovascular events.

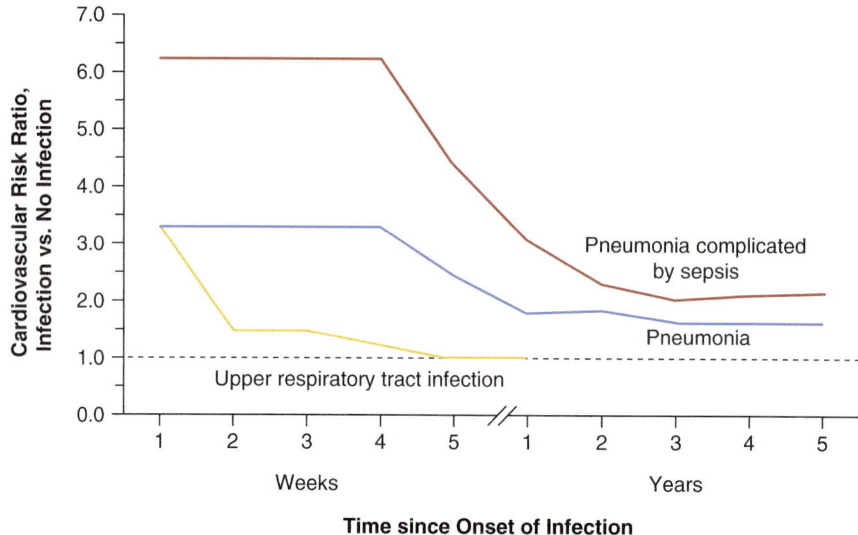

Fig. 8 Myocardial infarction following system infection. Temporal pattern of cardiovascular risk after the onset of acute infection. (Reproduced with permission [65])

Myocardial infarction in patients with viral illnesses including SARS-Cov-2 need to be distinguished from other viral cause of myocardial injury related to myocarditis, other forms of vasculitis. Collectively these forms of myocardial injury may affect up to one-quarter of patients with COVID-19 and be manifest even in the absence of previous cardiovascular disease. Most myocardial infarction associated with infections are thought to related to plaque rupture, activation of systemic triggers including priming of circulating leukocytes, increasing thromboxane synthesis, and expression of genes linked to platelet activation induced by respiratory viruses such as influenza and SARS-CoV-2.

In contrast to these systemic effects, the observation that CCs can form within lipid rich endosomes and exosomes formed when viruses enter and exit the host cell, together with the observation that crystals of inert viral capsules can form in vivo within endothelial cells, provides two plausible mechanisms by which crystals could directly destabilize atherosclerotic plaque during viral infection (Fig. 9) [66]. A recent report demonstrated the presence of SARS-CoV-2 in coronary vessels and plaque with enhanced entry into cholesterol-laden macrophages (foam cells) and robust secretion of pro-atherogenic cytokines in SARS-CoV-2 infected macrophages, providing a potential explanation for acute cardiovascular events [67].

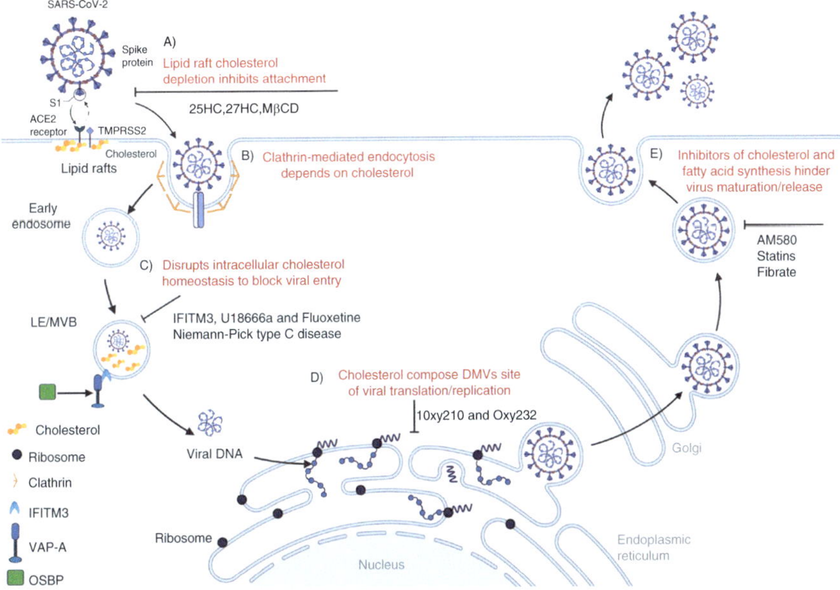

Fig. 9 Corona Virus has a lipid membrane that surrounds the capsid and this membrane is "stolen" from the infected host cells. This forms a viral envelope. This protects the virus from the host immune system but makes them vulnerable to desiccation and soaps. (Reproduced with permission [68])

6 Effect of Secondary Prevention Therapies for Atherosclerosis on the Clinical Outcome of Severe SARS-CoV-2 Infection

Statins: Cholesterol plays an important role in viral translocation/replication and maturation/release [68] and is required for the formation of syncytia which facilitate replication and evasion of the host immune response, in SARS-CoV-2 infection [68, 69].

The SARS-CoV-2 envelope differs from the host membrane as it is acquired at late stage of the virus cycle and not by coalescence of host membrane during viral entry. It comprises primarily of phospholipids (PLs) but also contains cholesterol and sphingolipids with a cholesterol/phospholipid ratio similar to that of lysosomes [70]. Additionally, the envelop exposes procoagulant lipids at levels exceeding those on activated platelets that may directly promote blood coagulation [70].

Host cell entry of coronavirus occurs either by plasma membrane fusion or endocytosis. The endocytosis-mediated process is facilitated by cholesterol rich lipid rafts that serve as a platform for SARS-CoV-2 virus entry [68]. The ratio of membrane cholesterol to fatty acid may be important for adequate viral fusion to the host cell and delivery of viral genes into the cytoplasm, an essential step for coronavirus infection.

As cholesterol is an integral part of the SARS-CoV-2 virus envelope and essential in almost every step of its life cycle, it is tempting to postulate that a greater availability of abundant cholesterol might lead to enhanced production of viral particles. Moreover, greater viral particles can pack together to form crystals (Fig. 10) [66, 71] as when they are placed in storage, thus floating viral particles, like CCs, could have the mechanical ability to scrape the arterial intima and cause vascular spam sufficient to cause ischemic injury [71]. Although unproven, this concept does seem to incorporate many of the features and behavior of the COVID-19 that

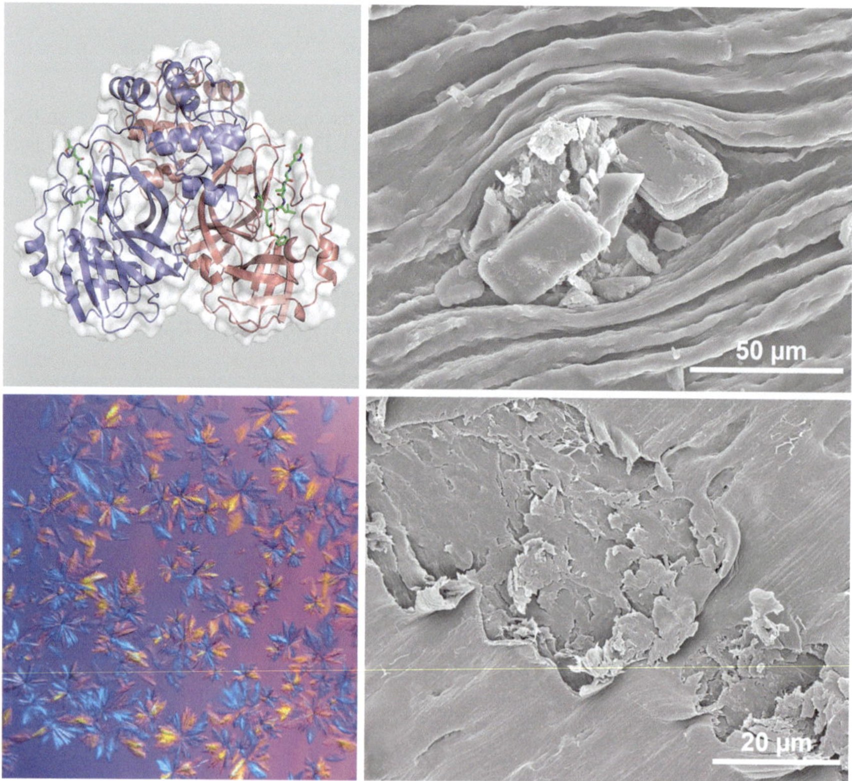

Fig. 10 COVID-19 viral crystals. (left panel) crystal formations of COVID-19 virus. (right panel) Cholesterol crystals scraping the endothelium when circulating in a rabbit artery causing vasomotor dysfunction (see Chap. "Omega-3 Fatty Acids Influence Membrane Cholesterol Distribution and Crystal Formation in Models of Atherosclerosis"). (Reproduced with permission [71, 89, 90])

involves damage to the endothelium [72]. Another line of evidence that supports this hypothesis is that statins, fenofibrate, and aspirin seem to provide protection from the more severe injury of COVID-19 [73–75] and this may be related to the effect of these agents on dissolving CCs and lower cholesterol levels on the part of statins [76, 77]. A great deal of research has focused on whether lowering cholesterol can improve the clinical outcome of patients with the disease.

Encouragingly, it was demonstrated that atorvastatin could effectively inhibit late replicative cycle steps of SARS-CoV-2 in vitro [78]. Using propensity scores, a large retrospective study including of over 20 thousand patients in each of two cohorts demonstrated that prolonged statin use was significantly more effective than short-term use in reducing the risk of viral infection and hospitalization but not intubation rate [79]. In addition, observational studies suggested that obesity and elevated serum cholesterol levels were risk factors for more severe infection, and clinical reports suggested that statins may provide clinical benefit to patients who developed the disease [80–82]. In contrast, another study that used propensity scores to match patients taking statins failed to show a consistent link between statins the risk of death after COVID-19, and a prospective controlled trial that examined the effect of atorvastatin 20 mg and aggressive anti-coagulation in patients admitted to the intensive care unit (ICU) with severe COVID infection failed to show a benefit of either therapy [83].

PCSK-9 inhibitors: In concert with the effect of lipids on severity of COVID-19 symptoms and clinical outcomes a recent double blind study of lipid lowering using evolocumab (140-mg subcutaneously) vs. placebo (1 mL 0.9% saline solution) in 60 patients hospitalized with severe COVID-19 and pneumonia revealed a significant reduction in death or need for intubation at 30 days (23.3% vs. 53.3%). Also, IL-6 levels were significantly reduced in the treatment group [84] (Fig. 11).

Aspirin: Although aspirin has a number of properties that potentially would make it useful in the treatment of SARS-CoV-2 infection, as with statin therapy, early evidence of benefits related to retrospective observations and were not borne out in several prospective placebo trials [85, 86].

Colchicine: Colchicine has been demonstrated to reduce the risk of acute cardiovascular events in patients with proven coronary atherosclerosis [87]. Since it acts to inhibit inflammasome and reduce proinflammatory cytokines that are also known to be activated in SARS-CoV-2, several prospective controlled studies have examined its effects in patients with COVID-19 pneumonia. In a meta-analysis of these trials that included 16,248 patients from eight separate trials, it was found that those who received colchicine had a lower risk of mortality-HR of 0.25 (95% CI: 0.09, 0.66) and OR of 0.22 (95% CI: 0.09, 0.57) [88].

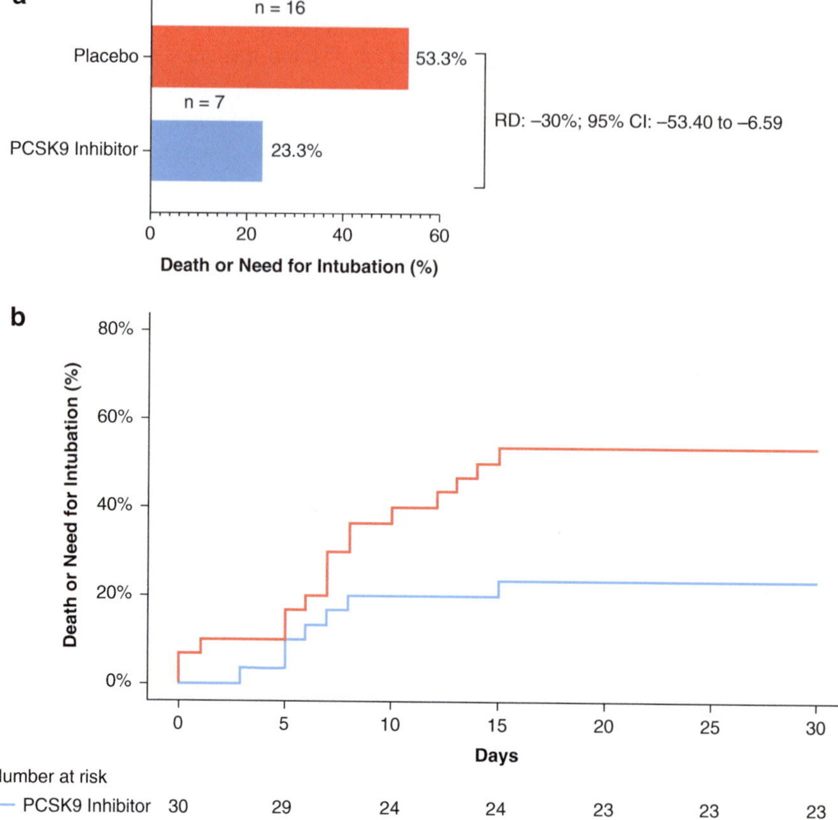

Fig. 11 Reduced Death or Intubation with PCSK9 in COVID-19. Death or need for intubation (primary endpoint) at 30 days among patients administered a proprotein convertase subtilisin/kexin type 9 (PCSK9) inhibitor or placebo. (**a**) Rates of primary endpoint in the PCSK9 inhibitor and placebo arms. (**b**) Cumulative incidence curves of 30-day death or need for intubation in the intention-to-treat population. *n* number of events, *RD* risk difference. (Reproduced with permission [84])

7   Summary

There is increasing evidence of an interplay between infection and crystals in cardiovascular disease. Specifically, it is evident that CCs likely play a role in bacterial endocarditis. In addition, some viruses may lead to the development of intracellular inert viral crystals and may promote the formation of CCs in endosomes and exosomes that together may contribute to traumatic and inflammatory injury of the arterial wall to cause vasculitis, atherosclerosis, and acute plaque rupture.

References

1. Medzhitov R. Recognition of microorganisms and activation of the immune response. Nature. 2007;449(7164):819–26.
2. Düewell P, Kono H, Rayner KJ, et al. NLRP3 inflammasomes are required for atherogenesis and activated by cholesterol crystals. Nature. 2010;464(7293):1357–61.
3. Rajamaki K, Lappalainen J, Oorni K, et al. Cholesterol crystals activate the NLRP3 inflammasome in human macrophages: a novel link between cholesterol metabolism and inflammation. PLoS One. 2010;5(7):e11765.
4. Nidorf SM, Fiolet A, Abela GS. Viewing atherosclerosis through a crystal lens: how the evolving structure of cholesterol crystals in atherosclerotic plaque alters its stability. J Clin Lipidol. 2020;14(5):619–30.
5. Olmos C, Vilacosta I, Fernandez C, et al. Comparison of clinical features of left-sided infective endocarditis involving previously normal versus previously abnormal valves. Am J Cardiol. 2014;114(2):278–83.
6. Liesenborghs L, Meyers S, Lox M, et al. Staphylococcus aureus endocarditis: distinct mechanisms of bacterial adhesion to damaged and inflamed heart valves. Eur Heart J. 2019;40(39):3248–59.
7. El-Khatib LA, De Feijter-Rupp H, Janoudi A, Fry L, Kehdi M, Abela GS. Cholesterol induced heart valve inflammation and injury: efficacy of cholesterol lowering treatment. Open Heart. 2020;7(2):e001274.
8. Price L, Sniderman A, Omerglu A, Lachapelle K. Bioprosthetic valve degeneration due to cholesterol deposition in a patient with normal lipid profile. Can J Cardiol. 2007;23:233–4.
9. Rossebo AB, Pedersen TR, Boman K, et al. Intensive lipid lowering with simvastatin and ezetimibe in aortic stenosis. N Engl J Med. 2008;359(13):1343–56.
10. Cowell SJ, Newby DE, Prescott RJ, et al. A randomized trial of intensive lipid-lowering therapy in calcific aortic stenosis. N Engl J Med. 2005;352(23):2389–97.
11. Chan KL, Teo K, Dumesnil JG, Ni A, Tam J. Effect of lipid lowering with rosuvastatin on progression of aortic stenosis: results of the aortic stenosis progression observation: measuring effects of rosuvastatin (ASTRONOMER) trial. Circulation. 2010;121(2):306–14.
12. Yang T-F, Chu H, Ou S-M, Li S-Y, Chen Y-T, Shih C-J, Tsai L-W. Effect of statin therapy on mortality in patients with infective endocarditis. Am J Cardiol. 2014;114(1):94–9.
13. Anavekar NS, Schultz JC, Correa De Sa DD, Thomas JM, Lah BD, Tleyjeh IM, Steckelberg JM, Wilson WR, Baddour LM. Modifiers of symptomatic embolic riks in infective endocarditis. Mayo Clin Proc. 2011;86(11):1068–74.
14. Veloso TR, Chaouch A, Roger T, et al. Use of a human-like low-grade bacteremia model of experimental endocarditis to study the role of Staphylococcus aureus adhesins and platelet aggregation in early endocarditis. Infect Immun. 2013;81(3):697–703.
15. Forner L, Larsen T, Kilian M, Holmstrup P. Incidence of bacteremia after chewing, tooth brushing and scaling in individuals with periodontal inflammation. J Clin Periodontol. 2006;33(6):401–7.
16. Lockhart PB. The risk for endocarditis in dental practice. Periodontol 2000. 2000;23:127–35.
17. Abela GS, Kalavakunta JK, Janoudi A, et al. Frequency of cholesterol crystals in culprit coronary artery aspirate during acute myocardial infarction and their relation to inflammation and myocardial injury. Am J Cardiol. 2017;120(10):1699–707.
18. Boumegouas M, Raju M, Gardiner J, et al. Interaction between bacteria and cholesterol crystals: implications for endocarditis and atherosclerosis. PLoS One. 2022;17(2):e0263847.
19. Foster TJ. The MSCRAMM family of cell-wall-anchored surface proteins of gram-positive cocci. Trends Microbiol. 2019;27(11):927–41.
20. Josse J, Laurent F, Diot A. Staphylococcal adhesion and host cell invasion: fibronectin-binding and other mechanisms. Front Microbiol. 2017;8:2433.
21. Prystopiuk V, Feuillie C, Herman-Bausier P, et al. Mechanical forces guiding Staphylococcus aureus cellular invasion. ACS Nano. 2018;12(4):3609–22.

22. Viegas KD, Dol SS, Salek MM, Shepherd RD, Martinuzzi RM, Rinker KD. Methicillin resistant Staphylococcus aureus adhesion to human umbilical vein endothelial cells demonstrates wall shear stress dependent behaviour. Biomed Eng Online. 2011;10:20.
23. Sokurenko EV, Vogel V, Thomas WE. Catch-bond mechanism of force-enhanced adhesion: counterintuitive, elusive, but ... Widespread? Cell Host Microbe. 2008;4(4):314–23.
24. Vitry P, Valotteau C, Feuillie C, et al. Force-induced strengthening of the interaction between Staphylococcus aureus clumping factor B and Loricrin. MBio. 2017;8(6):e01748.
25. Viela F, Mathelié-Guinle M, Viljoen A, Dufrêne YF. What makes bacterial pathogens so sticky? Mol Microbiol. 2020;113:683–90.
26. Njuguna B, Gardner A, Karwa R, Delahaye F. Infective endocarditis in low- and middle-income countries. Cardiol Clin. 2017;35(1):153–63.
27. Scheld WM, Valone JA, Sande MA. Bacterial adherence in the pathogenesis of endocarditis. Interaction of bacterial dextran, platelets, and fibrin. J Clin Invest. 1978;61(5):1394–404.
28. Pelletier LL Jr, Coyle M, Petersdorf R. Dextran production as a possible virulence factor in streptococcal endocarditis. Proc Soc Exp Biol Med. 1978;158(3):415–20.
29. Gould K, Ramirez-Ronda CH, Holmes RK, Sanford JP. Adherence of bacteria to heart valves in vitro. J Clin Invest. 1975;56(6):1364–70.
30. Vaca DJ, Thibau A, Schutz M, et al. Interaction with the host: the role of fibronectin and extracellular matrix proteins in the adhesion of gram-negative bacteria. Med Microbiol Immunol. 2020;209(3):277–99.
31. Martini AM, Moricz BS, Woods LJ, Jones BD. Type IV pili of streptococcus sanguinis contribute to pathogenesis in experimental infective endocarditis. Microbiol Spectr. 2021;9(3):e0175221.
32. Nallapareddy SR, Singh KV, Sillanpaa J, et al. Endocarditis and biofilm-associated pili of enterococcus faecalis. J Clin Invest. 2006;116(10):2799–807.
33. Claes J, Ditkowski B, Liesenborghs L, et al. Assessment of the dual role of clumping factor a in S. aureus adhesion to endothelium in absence and presence of plasma. Thromb Haemost. 2018;118(7):1230–41.
34. Turner NA, Nolasco L, Ruggeri ZM, Moake JL. Endothelial cell ADAMTS-13 and VWF: production, release, and VWF string cleavage. Blood. 2009;114(24):5102–11.
35. Yao L, Berman JW, Factor SM, Lowy FD. Correlation of histopathologic and bacteriologic changes with cytokine expression in an experimental murine model of bacteremic Staphylococcus aureus infection. Infect Immun. 1997;65(9):3889–95.
36. Bancsi MJ, Veltrop MH, Bertina RM, Thompson J. Role of phagocytosis in activation of the coagulation system in Streptococcus sanguis endocarditis. Infect Immun. 1996;64(12):5166–70.
37. Brinkmann V, Reichard U, Goosmann C, et al. Neutrophil extracellular traps kill bacteria. Science. 2004;303(5663):1532–5.
38. Jung CJ, Yeh CY, Hsu RB, Lee CM, Shun CT, Chia JS. Endocarditis pathogen promotes vegetation formation by inducing intravascular neutrophil extracellular traps through activated platelets. Circulation. 2015;131(6):571–81.
39. Hsu CC, Hsu RB, Ohniwa RL, et al. Neutrophil extracellular traps enhance Staphylococcus aureus vegetation formation through interaction with platelets in infective endocarditis. Thromb Haemost. 2019;119(5):786–96.
40. Warnatsch A, Ioannou M, Wang Q, Papayannopoulos V. Inflammation neutrophil extracellular traps license macrophages for cytokine production in atherosclerosis. Science. 2015;349(6245):316–20.
41. Folco EJ, Sukhova GK, Quillard T, Libby P. Moderate hypoxia potentiates interleukin-1β production in activated human macrophages. Circ Res. 2014;115(10):875–83.
42. Grayston JT, Kuo C-C, Coulson AS, Campbell LA, Lawrence RD, Lee MJ, Strandness ED, Wang S-P. Chlamydia pneumoniae (TWAR) in atherosclerosis of the carotid artery. Circulation. 1995;92(12):3397–400.

43. Chhibber-Goel J, Singhal V, Bhowmik D, Vivek R, Parakh N, Bhargava B, et al. Linkages between oral commensal bacteria and atherosclerotic plaques in coronary artery disease patients. NPJ Biofilms Microbiomes. 2016;2:7. https://doi.org/10.1038/s41522-016-0009-7.

44. Simon OA, Görbe A, Hegyi P, Szakó L, Oštarijaš E, Dembrovszky F, Kiss S, Czopf L, Erőss B, Szabó I. Helicobacter pylori infection is associated with carotid intima and media thickening: a systematic review and meta-analysis. J Am Heart Assoc. 2022;11(3):e022919. https://doi.org/10.1161/JAHA.121.02291.

45. Sessa R, DiPietro M, Filardo S, Turriziani O. Infectious burden and atherosclerosis: a clinical issue. World J Clin Cases. 2014;2(7):240–9 https://doi.org/10.12998/wjcc.v2.i7.240.

46. Campbell LA, Rosenfeld ME. Infection and atherosclerosis development. Arch Med Res. 2015;46(5):339–50. https://doi.org/10.1016/j.arcmed.2015.05.006; Epub 2015 May 21. PMID: 26004263; PMCID: PMC452450640.

47. Ngeh J, Anand V, Gupta S. Chlamydia pneumoniae and atherosclerosis—what we know and what we don't. Clin Microbiol Infect. 2002;8(1):2–13. https://doi.org/10.1046/j.1469-0691.2002.00382.x.

48. Epstein SE, Zhou YF, Zhu J. Infection and atherosclerosis: emerging mechanistic paradigms. Circulation. 1999;100(4):e20–8. https://doi.org/10.1161/01.cir.100.4.e20.

49. Zahn R, Schneider S, Frilling B, Seidl K, Tebbe U, Weber M, et al. Antibiotic therapy after acute myocardial infarction: a prospective randomized study. Circulation. 2003;107(9):1253–9. https://doi.org/10.1161/01.cir.0000054613.57105.06; PMID: 12628944.

50. Minick CR, Fabricant CG, Fabricant J, Litrenta MM. Atheroarteriosclerosis induced by infection with a herpesvirus. Am J Pathol. 1979;96:673–706.

51. Fabricant CG, Fabricant J, Minick CR, Litrenta MM. Herpesvirus-induced atherosclerosis in chickens. Fed Proc. 1983;42:2476–9.

52. Fabricant CG, Krook L, Gillespie JH. Virus-induced cholesterol crystals. Science. 1973;181(4099):566–7. https://doi.org/10.1126/science.181.4099.566.

53. Fabricant CG, Gillespie JH, Krook L. Intracellular and extracellular mineral crystal formation induced by viral infection of cell cultures. Infect Immun. 1971;3(3):416–9. https://doi.org/10.1128/iai.3.3.416-419.1971; PMID: 16557989; PMCID: PMC416167.

54. Nasiri M, Huang R, Janoudi A, Vanderberg A, Flegler C, Flegler S, Abela GS. Unraveling the role of cholesterol crystals in plaque rupture by altering the method of tissue preparation. Microsc Res Tech. 2015;78:969–74.

55. Deng Y, Almsherqi ZA, Ng MM, Kohlwein SD. Do viruses subvert cholesterol homeostasis to induce host cubic membranes? Trends Cell Biol. 2010;20(7):371–9. https://doi.org/10.1016/j.tcb.2010.04.001.

56. Rubio-Casillas A, Redwan EM, Uversky VN. SARS-CoV-2: a master of immune evasion. Biomedicine. 2022;10(6):1339.

57. Troyer Z, Alhusaini N, Tabler CO, Sweet T, de Carvalho KIL, Schlatzer DM, Carias L, King CL, Matreyek K, Tilton JC. Extracellular vesicles carry SARS-CoV-2 spike protein and serve as decoys for neutralizing antibodies. J Extracell Vesicles. 2021;10(8):e12112.

58. Jennette JC, Falk RJ, Bacon PA, Basu N, Cid MC, Ferrario F, Flores-Suarez LF, Gross WL, Guillevin L, Hagen EC, Hoffman GS, Jayne DR, Kallenberg CG, Lamprecht P, Langford CA, Luqmani RA, Mahr AD, Matteson EL, Merkel PA, Ozen S, Pusey CD, Rasmussen N, Rees AJ, Scott DG, Specks U, Stone JH, Takahashi K, Watts RA. 2012 revised international Chapel hill consensus conference nomenclature of vasculitides. Arthritis Rheum. 2013;65(1):1–11. https://doi.org/10.1002/art.37715; PMID: 23045170.

59. Miyabe C, Miyabe Y, Miyata R, Ishiguro N. Pathogens in vasculitis: is it really idiopathic? JMA J. 2021;4(3):216–24. https://doi.org/10.31662/jmaj.2021-0021; Epub 2021 Jul 9. PMID: 34414315; PMCID: PMC8355637.

60. Gammon B, Longmire M, DeClerck B. Intravascular crystal deposition: an early clue to the diagnosis of type 1 cryoglobulinemic vasculitis. Am J Dermatopathol. 2014;36(9):751–5. https://doi.org/10.1097/DAD.0b013e31829ff8d9; PMID: 25147987; PMCID: PMC5906036.

61. Burch GE, Rayburn P. EMC viral infection of the coronary blood vessels in newborn mice: viral vasculitis. Br J Exp Pathol. 1977;58(5):565–71; PMID: 201264; PMCID: PMC2041269.
62. Numano F. Vasa vasoritis, vasculitis and atherosclerosis. Int J Cardiol. 2000;75 Suppl 1:S1–8. https://doi.org/10.1016/s0167-5273(00)00196-0; discussion S17–9. PMID: 10980330.
63. Varga Z, Flammer AJ, Steiger P, Haberecker M, Andermatt R, Zinkernagel AS, Mehra MR, Schuepbach RA, Ruschitzka F, Moch H. Endothelial cell infection and endotheliitis in COVID-19. Lancet. 2020;395(10234):1417–8. https://doi.org/10.1016/S0140-6736(20)30937-5; Epub 2020 Apr 21. PMID: 32325026; PMCID: PMC7172722.
64. Duyvesteyn HME, Ginn HM, Pietilä MK, Wagner A, Hattne J, Grimes JM, Hirvonen E, Evans G, Parsy ML, Sauter NK, Brewster AS, Huiskonen JT, Stuart DI, Sutton G, Bamford DH. Towards in cellulo virus crystallography. Sci Rep. 2018;8(1):3771. https://doi.org/10.1038/s41598-018-21693-3; PMID: 29491457; PMCID: PMC5830620.
65. Musher DM, Abers MS, Corrales-Medina VF. Acute infection and myocardial infarction. N Engl J Med. 2019;380(2):171–6.
66. Jin Z, Du X, Xu Y, et al. Structure of M^{pro} from SARS-CoV-2 and discovery of its inhibitors. Nature. 2020;582:289–93. https://doi.org/10.1038/s41586-020-2223-y.
67. Eberhardt N, Noval M G, Kaur R, et al. SARS-CoV-2 infection triggers pro-atherogenic inflammatory responses in human coronary vessels. Nature Cardiovasc Res. 2023;2:899–916.
68. Dai J, Wang H, Liao Y, et al. Coronavirus infection and cholesterol metabolism. Front Immunol. 2022;13:791267.
69. Sanders DW, Jumper CC, Ackerman PJ, et al. SARS-CoV-2 requires cholesterol for viral entry and pathological syncytia formation. elife. 2021;10:10.
70. Saud Z, Tyrrell VJ, Zaragkoulias A, et al. The SARS-CoV2 envelope differs from host cells, exposes procoagulant lipids, and is disrupted in vivo by oral rinses. J Lipid Res. 2022;63:100208. https://doi.org/10.1016/j.jlr.2022.100208.
71. Gadeela N, Rubinstein J, Tamhane U, et al. The impact of circulating cholesterol crystals on vasomotor function: implications for no-reflow phenomenon. JACC Cardiovasc Interv. 2011;4(5):521–9.
72. Libby P, Luscher T. COVID-19 is, in the end, an endothelial disease. Eur Heart J. 2020;41(32):3038–44.
73. Kollias A, Kyriakoulis KG, Kyriakoulis IG, et al. Statin use and mortality in COVID-19 patients: updated systematic review and meta-analysis. Atherosclerosis. 2021;330:114–21.
74. Feher M, Joy M, Munro N, Hinton W, Williams J, de Lusignan S. Fenofibrate as a COVID-19 modifying drug: laboratory success versus real-world reality. Atherosclerosis. 2021;339:55–6.
75. Wijaya I, Andhika R, Huang I, Purwiga A, Budiman KY. The effects of aspirin on the outcome of COVID-19: a systematic review and meta-analysis. Clin Epidemiol Glob Health. 2021;12:100883.
76. Abela GS, Vedre A, Janoudi A, Huang R, Durga S, Tamhane U. Effect of statins on cholesterol crystallization and atherosclerotic plaque stabilization. Am J Cardiol. 2011;107(12):1710–7.
77. Fry L, Lee A, Khan S, Aziz K, Vedre A, Abela GS. Effect of aspirin on cholesterol crystallization: a potential mechanism for plaque stabilization. Am Heart J Plus. 2022;13:100083. https://doi.org/10.1016/j.ahjo.2021.100083.
78. Zapata-Cardona MI, Flórez-Álvarez L, Zapata-Builes W, Guerra-Sandoval AL, Guerra-Almonacid CM, Hincapié-García J, Rugeles MT, Hernandez JC. Atorvastatin effectively inhibits late replicative cycle steps of SARS-CoV-2 in vitro. bioRxiv. 2022;13:721103. https://doi.org/10.1101/2021.03.01.433498.
79. Wu B-R, Chen D-H, Liao W-C, Ho W-C, Yin M-C, Lin C-L, Chou C-H, Peng Y-H. Statin therapy and the risk of viral infection: a retrospective population-based cohort study. J Clin Med. 2022;11:5626. https://doi.org/10.3390/jcm11195626.
80. Zhou Y, Chi J, Lv W, Wang Y. Obesity and diabetes as high-risk factors for severe coronavirus disease 2019 (Covid-19). Diabetes Metab Res Rev. 2021;37(2):e3377. https://doi.org/10.1002/dmrr.3377.

81. Zhang K, Dong S-S, Guo Y, Tang S-H, Wu H, Yao S, Wang P-F, Zhang K, Xue H-Z, Huang W, Ding J, Yang T-L. Causal association between blood lipids and COVID-19 risk: a to-sample mendelian randomized study. Arterioscler Thromb Vasc Biol. 2021;41:2802–10. https://doi.org/10.1161/ATVBAHA.121.316324.
82. Rubin R. Could statins do more than lower cholesterol in patients with COVID-19? JAMA. 2021;325(24):2424–5. https://doi.org/10.1001/jama.2021.8201; PMID: 34081086.
83. Investigators INSPIRATION-S. Atorvastatin versus placebo in patients with covid-19 in intensive care: randomized controlled trial. BMJ. 2022;376:e068407. https://doi.org/10.1136/bmj-2021-068407; PMID: 34996756.
84. Navarese EP, Podhajski P, Gurbel PA, et al. PCSK9 inhibition during the inflammatory stage of SARS-CoV-2 infection. J Am Coll Cardiol. 2023;81:224–34. https://doi.org/10.1016/j.jacc.2022.10.030.
85. Zareef R, Diab M, Al Saleh T, Makarem A, Younis NK, Bitar F, Arabi M. Aspirin in COVID-19: pros and cons. Front Pharmacol. 2022;13:849628. https://doi.org/10.3389/fphar.2022.849628; PMID: 35370686; PMCID: PMC8965577.
86. Su W, Miao H, Guo Z, Chen Q, Huang T, Ding R. Associations between the use of aspirin or other antiplatelet drugs and all-cause mortality among patients with COVID-19: a meta-analysis. Front Pharmacol. 2022;13:989903. https://doi.org/10.3389/fphar.2022.989903; PMID: 36278186; PMCID: PMC9581252.
87. Nidorf SM, Fiolet ATL, Mosterd A, Eikelboom JW, Schut A, Opstal TSJ, The SHK, Xu XF, Ireland MA, Lenderink T, Latchem D, Hoogslag P, Jerzewski A, Nierop P, Whelan A, Hendriks R, Swart H, Schaap J, Kuijper AFM, van Hessen MWJ, Saklani P, Tan I, Thompson AG, Morton A, Judkins C, Bax WA, Dirksen M, Alings M, Hankey GJ, Budgeon CA, Tijssen JGP, Cornel JH, Thompson PL. LoDoCo2 trial Investigators. Colchicine in patients with chronic coronary disease. N Engl J Med. 2020;383(19):1838–47. https://doi.org/10.1056/NEJMoa2021372; Epub 2020 Aug 31.
88. Chiu L, Lo CH, Shen M, Chiu N, Aggarwal R, Lee J, Choi YG, Lam H, Prsic EH, Chow R, Shin HJ. Colchicine use in patients with COVID-19: a systematic review and meta-analysis. PLoS One. 2021;16(12):e0261358. https://doi.org/10.1371/journal.pone.0261358; PMID: 34962939; PMCID: PMC8714120.
89. Wang F, Chen C, Tan W, Yang K, Yan H. Structure of main protease from human coronavirus NL63: insights for wide spectrum anti-coronaryvirus drug design. Sci Rep. 2016;6:22677. https://doi.org/10.1038/srep22677.
90. https://www.ornl.gov/news/x-rays-size-protein-structure-heart-covid-19-virus.
91. Goldsmith CS, et al. Ultrastructural characterization of SARS coronavirus. Emerg Infect Dis. 2004;10:320–6.
92. Almsherqi ZA, et al. Direct template matching reveals a host subcellular membrane gyroid cubic structure that is associated with SARS virus. Redox Rep. 2005;10:167–71.

The Potential Role of Cholesterol Crystals in Preeclampsia

Robert A. Wild, Zain ul Abideen, Enhua Wang, Ayowale T. Oladeji, Nigel Paneth, Stefan Mark Nidorf, and George S. Abela

R. A. Wild (✉)
Section of Reproductive Endocrinology, Department of Obstetrics and Gynecology and Biostatistics and Clinical Epidemiology Oklahoma University Health Sciences Center, Oklahoma City, OK, USA
e-mail: Robert-Wild@ouhsc.edu

Z. u. Abideen
Division of Cardiology, Department of Medicine, Michigan State University, East Lansing, MI, USA

E. Wang
Division of Internal Medicine, Department of Medicine, Michigan State University, East Lansing, MI, USA

Sparrow Hospital, Lansing, MI, USA
e-mail: wangenhu@msu.edu

A. T. Oladeji
Division of Cardiology, Department of Medicine, Michigan State University, East Lansing, MI, USA

Sparrow Hospital, Lansing, MI, USA

N. Paneth
Department of Epidemiology and Biostatistics, Michigan State University, East Lansing, MI, USA
e-mail: paneth@msu.edu

S. M. Nidorf
The Heart and Vascular Research Institute, Sir Charles Gairdner Hospital, Perth, WA, Australia

G. S. Abela
Department of Medicine, Division of Cardiovascular Medicine, Michigan State University, East Lansing, MI, USA
e-mail: abela@msu.edu

© The Author(s), under exclusive license to Springer Nature Switzerland AG 2023
G. S. Abela, S. M. Nidorf (eds.), *Cholesterol Crystals in Atherosclerosis and Other Related Diseases*, Contemporary Cardiology, https://doi.org/10.1007/978-3-031-41192-2_24

1   Background

Preeclampsia is a major contributor to maternal morbidity and mortality for both mother and fetus. It occurs in up to 7% of pregnancies, accounts for almost 20% of maternal deaths in the USA and is the number one cause of premature birth. Early detection of preeclampsia is often elusive, but once established it is persistent and can be difficult to treat [1–4]. For the most part, delivery of the infant acutely reverses the disorder. Thus, despite the challenges of prematurity for the newborn, early delivery is often required to avoid the risk of life-threatening maternal events, including abruption of the placenta, renal failure, seizures, pulmonary edema, and hematological dyscrasia. Preeclampsia can also inhibit fetal growth, cause developmental disabilities for the child, and confer a life-long risk of cardiovascular disease for both the mother and child. These later effects appear to be triggered by placental genes expressing that involve pathways related to poor cardiometabolic traits [5].

The pathophysiology of preeclampsia centers around placental ischemia associated with inflammation, which together damage the vascular endothelium leads to "atherosis" in the maternal spiral arteries which is the pathological hallmark of the disease [6].

Recent evidence highlighting the presence of cholesterol crystals (CCs) in the placenta raises the intriguing possibility that CC-induced traumatic and inflammatory injury within the placenta may be the primary trigger of the pathophysiologic processes that lead to preeclampsia [7, 8]. Evidence that small-dense low-density lipoprotein (sd-LDL) levels become markedly elevated during the first trimester of pregnancy in women who develop preeclampsia [9] support this thesis, as sd-LDL is a potentially rich source of free cholesterol with high tissue accessibility that predisposes to CC formation . Further still, CCs associated with elevated inflammatory biomarkers have been found in the decidua/placental interface in mothers who developed preeclampsia [10, 11]. Thus, there is evidence that CCs develop in the placenta and have the potential to play a role in the development and progression of preeclampsia [12–14].

2   A Potential Mechanism for Preeclampsia

Though the exact trigger for preeclampsia is yet to be determined, it is clear that both maternal factors and placental vascular dysfunction play a role in its pathogenesis (Fig. 1). No matter the trigger, placental ischemia is believed to be central to the development of preeclampsia [1, 6]. Thus, it has been associated with impaired placentation, incomplete spiral artery remodeling, endothelial damage, propagation of immune factors, and mitochondrial stress, each of which may affect the balance of pro- and antiangiogenic substances within the placenta. As in other organs, arterial spasm induced by a range of local stimulants including CCs, can lead to regional ischemia in the placenta which in turn may lead to hypoxic and inflammatory injury [12].

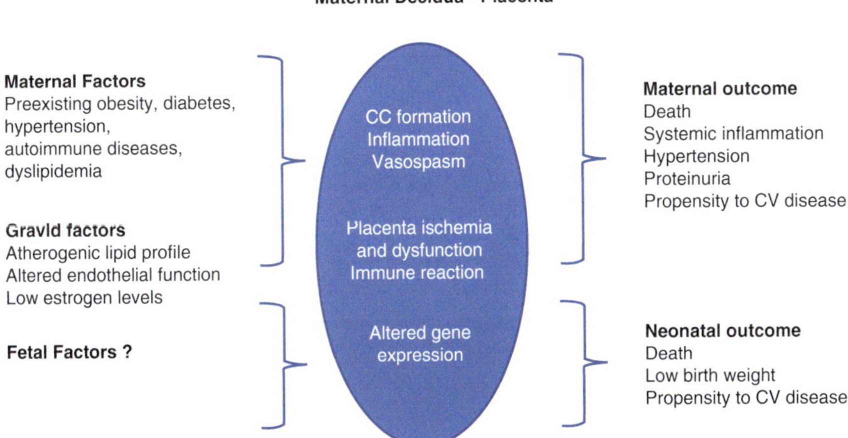

Fig. 1 Interplay between maternal, fetal factors, and decidua/placenta in preeclampsia

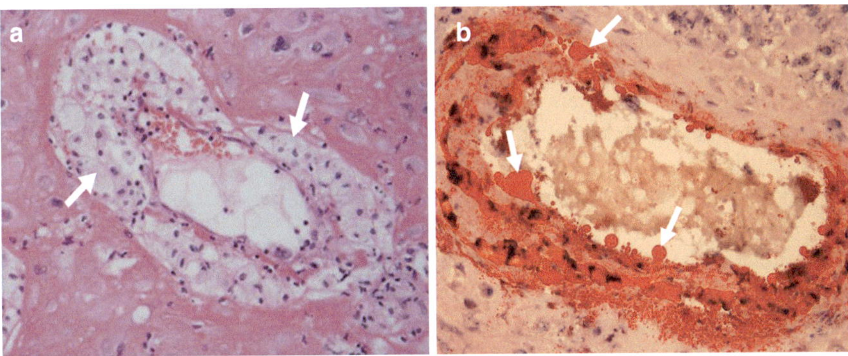

Fig. 2 Acute atherosis in decidual spiral arteries. (**a**) Many lipid-laden macrophages (arrows) are seen in the spiral arteries. (**b**) Acute atherosis on oil-red O staining. Fat droplets (arrows) in the non-transformed spiral artery are stained red. (Reproduced with permission [6])

Elevated LDL levels are strong markers of CC formation since saturated cholesterol levels in the tissues are a prerequisite for CC formation [15, 16]. Small-dense LDL and other small lipid fractions including Lp(a) pass more readily into the subendothelial space and are robust markers for the propensity for CC formation in the vasculature and cardiac valves (see Chap. "Formation of CCs in Endothelial Cells") [17]. These same highly atherogenic lipid fractions are known to become significantly elevated during pregnancy in women who develop preeclampsia [9]. Moreover, arteries from the placentas in women who developed preeclampsia display pathologic features of "atherosis," evidenced by the presence of endothelial fragmentation and detachment with fibrinoid necrosis, and the presence of lipid-laden macrophages [6] (Fig. 2). Although unproven, we suspect that the development of high levels of sd-LDL during pregnancy predispose to the development of excess amounts of CCs in the placenta that in turn predisposes to regional vaso-spasm and inflammation that then predispose to the development and progression of preeclampsia.

3 Serum Lipids in Normal Pregnancy and Preeclampsia

During a normal pregnancy, triglycerides, LDL, non-HDL cholesterol, and active total Proprotein Convertase Subtilis Kexin 9 (PCSK9) levels all increase as the pregnancy progresses towards term [18, 19]. In women who develop preeclampsia the change in lipid profile is more marked and the profile is more atherogenic as it is associated with higher levels of sd-LDL [20]. Aside from promoting uptake of cholesterol into the vascular wall, sd-LDL also stimulates the endothelium to synthesize and release thromboxane, and increases intracellular calcium in vascular smooth muscles, which together predispose to vasospasm in the placenta [21, 22]. This combined with the potential endothelial injury of spiral arteries by CCs can lead to further arterial spasm and tissue injury [12].

In the Reproductive Medicine FIT: PLESE study—for women undergoing diet and exercise prior to fertility treatment, an increase in sd-LDL became evident in the first trimester in women who later developed preeclampsia [9] (Fig. 3). This may be relevant as dysfunctional maternal endothelium can be induced by atherogenic dyslipidemia [23]. Preeclampsia has also been associated with significant elevations in other LDL fractions that have an increased susceptibility to oxidation [24, 25].

Estimates of lipid profile during the first trimester, therefore, appear to have predictive value for the development of preeclampsia. El Khouly et al. reported that among 251 pregnant women who had a lipid analysis at 4 and 12 weeks during the first trimester, those who developed preeclampsia had a greater rise in TG and LDL, and a significant decrease in HDL compared to those who did not develop preeclampsia. The changes in lipid profile were especially marked in those who developed more severe preeclampsia [26]. In the generation R study, investigators found that triglycerides and remnant cholesterol were also related to preeclampsia. These levels were not only positively associated with blood pressure during pregnancy but also associated with hypertension at 6 and 9 years after pregnancy [27]. While the lipids measured in these studies are standard and easily obtained from most pathology laboratories, these measures only allow crude inference of atherogenicity. In contrast, Ardalic et al. measured lipid oxidative indices in high-risk preeclamptic women (some diabetic) and found that they also related to preeclampsia. They then went on to develop a model that included this lipid index together with body mass index, age, and fasting glucose to improve the prediction of preeclampsia [28].

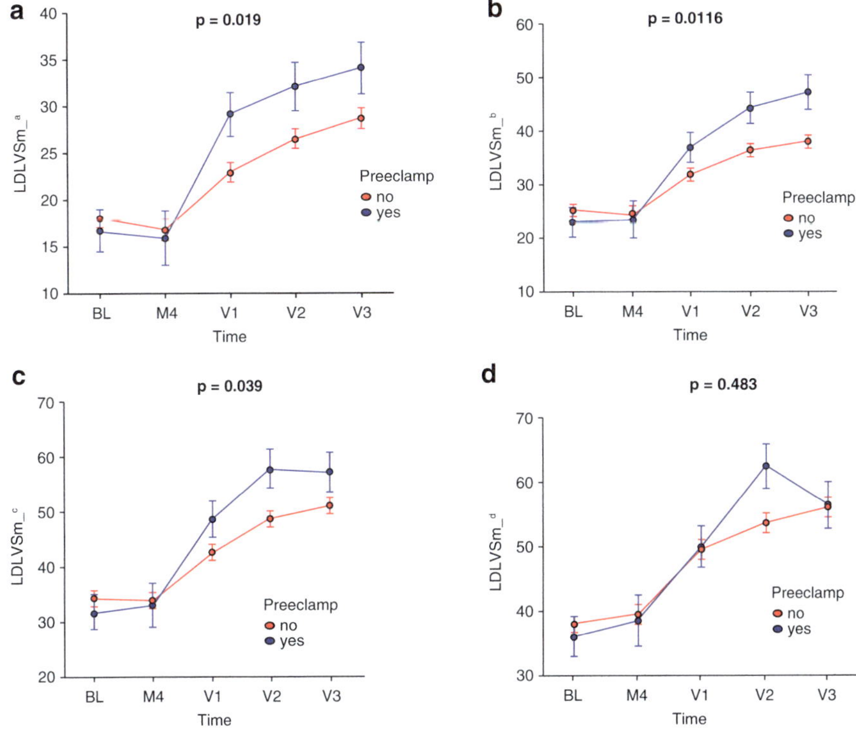

Fig. 3 Atherogenic lipid particles in preeclampsia. Graphc demonstrating that levels of very small LDL cholsterol particles are high with preeclampsia but not evident before or after 16 weeks of lifestyle intervention to lose weight before becoming pregnant. FIT: PLESE. FIT: PLESE for Preeclampsia (yes) vs. (no). (Reproduced with permission [9])

4 Small-Dense LDL Cholesterol, Cholesterol Crystals, Vascular Endothelial Damage, and Downstream Placental Inflammation

Abnormal lipid profiles are strongly related to endothelial dysfunction [29]. Elevated LDL, and sd-LDL in particular, are associated with an enhanced uptake of cholesterol by the vascular endothelium and passage of cholesterol into the sub-intimal spaces of the arterial wall. Thus, they also speed the transition of resident macrophages that clear the cholesterol into foam cells [30–32] (see Chaps. 5 & 9 "In Vivo Detection of Cholesterol Crystals in Atherosclerotic Plaque with Optical Coherence Tomography" and "Atherosclerotic Plaque Morphology and the Conundrum of the Vulnerable Plaque"). In the presence of excess free cholesterol, CCs form within endothelial membranes and macrophages. Crystallization of cholesterol in endothelial membranes leads to endothelial dysfunction, and the deposition of CCs within the cytosol of macrophages can activate inflammasome, trigger complosome, and promote cell death. As intracellular CCs are spilt into the extracellular space their sharp-tipped geometry may cause direct local tissue trauma [7, 8, 33, 34]. In addition, they can trigger innate inflammation due to their ability to activate compliment and incite macrophages to express various interleukins, including IL-1β that leads to a cascade of cytokine activation via IL-6 and then C-reactive protein (CRP) by the liver [35].

It is also known that CCs released into the circulation from atherosclerotic plaque can directly injure the vascular endothelium causing vasospasm and can promote thrombosis [12]. Ensuing distal ischemic injury can in turn trigger local production of IL1- β by resident macrophages that attract and activate circulating leukocytes [36]. Acute inflammation acts to increase the permeability of vascular channels and chronic inflammation may promote the development of a neovascular network [37]. Moreover, once CCs are deposited in tissues, they may trigger frustrated phagocytosis that leads to biochemical tissue injury related to the release of metalloproteinases and other intracellular enzymes [13].

CCs have been identified in various uteroplacental tissues and uterine vessels by scanning electron microscopy using a modified tissue preparation protocol to preserve them [10, 11, 38] (Fig. 4). In the decidua/placenta CCs usually appear as aggregates of flat plate rhomboids or spindle-shaped crystals. Rhomboid CCs are constituted from cholesterol monohydrate, whereas needle-shaped CCs are constituted from anhydrous cholesterol [8]. In preliminary work, the quantity of CCs in the decidua have been found to be more in women who developed preeclampsia [9].

In addition, nod-like receptor protein 3 (NLRP3) has been found to be expressed in the maternal decidua, in fetal trophoblasts and in maternal leukocytes. Furthermore, decidual tissue cultured in vitro has been demonstrated to express IL-1β when exposed to CCs [11]. Further still, components of the NLRP3 inflammasome and the complement system are also colocalized with IL-1β in the syncytiotrophoblast layer [39]. Thus, the inflammatory response to CCs in the syncytium of the trophoblast may be critical in the pathophysiology of preeclampsia.

Elevated syncytium expression of IL-1β and Terminal Complement Complex (TCC) and raised maternal serum cholesterol and uric acid are also found in preeclampsia. When primed with C5a/TNF-α or LPS, placental explants, and trophoblasts have been found to be responsive to cholesterol crystal-mediated activation of the NLRP3 inflammasome, resulting in the release of mature IL-1β [39]. These data support the suggestion that CC-mediated NLRP3 inflammasome activation leads to IL-1β production in the syncytium as they do in other tissues, and further support the thesis that CCs play a role in placental inflammation seen in preeclampsia.

Of further relevance is that atherosis is observed to be confined to non-transfromed spiral arteries. Atherosis is characterized by subendothelial lipid-filled form cells, fibrinoid necrosis and perivascular lymphocytic infiltration [40].

Taken together, these findings suggest that components at the syncytium surface and in maternal blood (where atherogenic dyslipidemia can lead to CC deposition

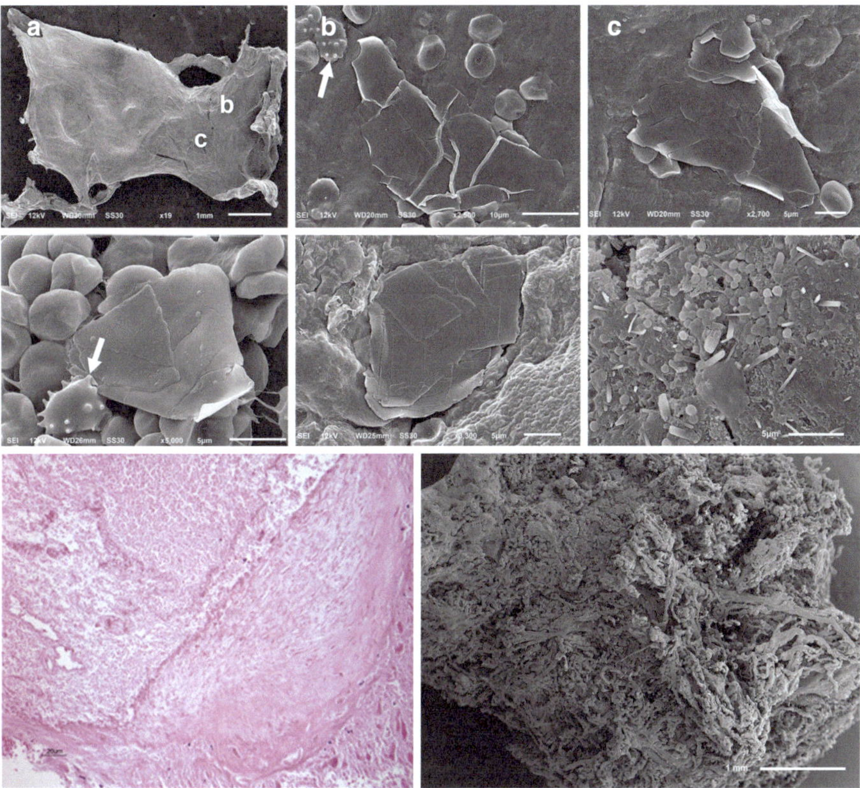

Fig. 4 Cholesterol crystals in maternal decidua. Scanning electron micrographs obtained from various placentas demonstrating both rhomboidal and needle shaped crystals (**a–c**) in the decidua. Macrophages are noted engaging the cholesterol crystals (arrows). Light micrograph and low power scanning image of the placenta. (Reproduced with permission [10] and courtesy of Dr. George Abela)

in spiral arteries leading to hypoxia) directly influence each other and may induce an escalated inflammatory response if disturbed or dysregulated. Consequently, placental dysfunction and maternal response in preeclampsia must be viewed as interdependent interactive processes.

Finally, it is also believed that antiangiogenic factor soluble fms-like tyrosine kinase1 (sFLT1) is a key factor in preeclampsia due to its ability to inhibit VEGF1 but not VEGF2. We have demonstrated that CCs can trigger VEGF expression in breast and colon cancer cell lines [41] and that they can cause breast cell lines to express CD44 and Ub-Ubiquityl-Histone (H2b). In addition, CCs can disrupt gap junctions in HUVEC cells in culture [42]. Thus, it is essential to continue to investigate the effect of CCs on VEGF1 and 2, other inflammatory cytokines, as well as hormone production that contribute to preeclampsia.

5   The Effect of Hormones on Cholesterol Crystallization

Estrogens lead to lower circualting LDL cholesterol whcih can be protective to the integrity of healthy endothelium. Progesterone opposes estrogen action, and testosterone has been implicated in an acceleration of cardiovascular events [43]. Interestingly we have found that in vitro, estrogen but not testosterone, can attenuate cholesterol crystallization in a dose-dependent manner [44]. Since women with preeclampsia have been shown to have lower estrogen levels [45–47], these findings offer yet another mechanism whereby estrogen, alongside its proven ability to promote placental angiogenesis and uterine artery vasodilation during pregnancy may protect against preeclampsia.

6   Treatment for Preeclampsia

Since CCs in placental tissue may predispose to placental ischemia and inflammation that are both central to the development and progression of preeclampsia, it would appear intuitive that inhibiting their development, dissolving them or dampening the inflammatory injury they promote may be of benefit in the prevention and treatment of preeclampsia.

Aspirin and possibly statins and metformin may reduce the risk of development of preeclampsia and reduce the risks of preeclampsia if given early in the course of pregnancy [2, 48–50]. Although the precise mechanisms by which they provide benefits are unclear, it is noteworthy that they have been shown to dissolve CCs in vitro [51–53]. Moreover, all three agents have anti-inflammatory actions that may contribute to their beneficial effects in preeclampsia. Aspirin can block the expression of MMP-9 by macrophages and enhance the efflux of cholesterol by promoting ABCA1 and SR-BI expression thus reducing potential atherogenic-like processes in the placenta [54–56]. A multicenter placebo-controlled trial by Rolnick DL et al. demonstrated that high-risk pregnant women receiving 150 mg of aspirin daily from 11 to 14 weeks through 36 weeks of gestation were less likely to develop preeclampsia compared to those taking a placebo [57]. Brownfoot FC et al. demonstrated that Pravastatin decreased the sFLT1 secretion of isolated cytotrophoblasts, HUVECs, and placental explants from patients with preeclampsia. It also increases soluble endoglin (sENG) secretion from HUVECs and stabilizes sENG secretion from placental explants from women with severe preterm preeclampsia. Additionally, pravastatin apperas to improve antiangiogenic factors (sFLT1 and sENG) through the cholesterol production pathway [58, 59]. The preeclamptic placenta's quick activation and rise in endothelial nitric-oxide synthase (eNOS), which is crucial for controlling placental blood flow, are caused by pravastatin's induction of placental microsomal arginine uptake [60].

Finally, the use of anti-inflammatory therapy to treat preeclampsia has been investigated, albeit only in animal models [61]. In this regard, it is notable that unlike NSAIDs, both colchicine and canakinumab which inhibit crystal-induced inflammation have proven safe to the fetus and the mother during pregnancy when used in women with autoinflammatory diseases including FMF, and that it may reduce the incidence of pre-eclampsia in women with FMF [62, 63]. Despite this, its potential in preventing eclampsia or affecting its clinical course in women without FMF has not been explored.

7 Summary

Preeclampsia is a common and potentially devastating complication of pregnancy. The development of preeclampsia has been associated with rising maternal levels of small-dense LDL during the first trimester of pregnancy. These lipid fractions have the potential to be a rich source of free cholesterol in the placenta that may predispose to the formation of cholesterol crystals (CCs). CCs are known to be present in the maternal decidual placenta, and to be associated with a pro-inflammatory state. Like CC found elsewhere, the formation of CCs in the placenta may promote inflammation and cause direct and indirect ischemic injury that may trigger and aggravate preeclampsia. Thus, it is possible that therapies that reduce the risk of CC formation, dissolve them or inhibit inflammatory pathways they promote may prove to be of benefit in the prevention and/or treatment of this dreaded complication of pregnancy.

References

1. Rana S, Lemoine E, Granger JP, Karumanchi SA. Preeclampsia: pathophysiology, challenges, and perspectives. Circ Res. 2019;124:1094–112.
2. Bujold E, Roberge S, Lacasse Y, et al. Prevention of preeclampsia and intrauterine growth restriction with aspirin started in early pregnancy. Obstet Gynecol. 2010;116:402–14.
3. Roberts JM, Redman CW. Pre-eclampsia: more than pregnancy-induced hypertension. Lancet. 1993;341:1447–51.
4. Chappell LC, Cluver CA, Kingdom J, Tong S. Pre-eclampsia. Lancet. 2021;398:341–98.
5. Ouidir M, Chatterjee S, Mendola P, Ahang C, Grantz KL, Tekola-Ayele F. Placental gene co-expression network for maternal plasma lipids revealed enrichment of inflammatory response pathways. Front Genet. 2021;12:681095. https://doi.org/10.3389/fgene.2021.681095.
6. Kim J-Y, Kim YM. Acute atherosis of the uterine spiral arteries: clinicopathologic implications. J Pathol Transl Med. 2015;49:462–71. https://doi.org/10.4132/jptm.2015.10.23.
7. Düewell P, Kono H, Rayner KJ, Sirois CM, Vladimer G, Bauernfeind FG, Abela GS, et al. NLRP3 inflammasomes are required for atherogenesis and activated by cholesterol crystals. Nature. 2010;464:1357–61.
8. Nidorf SM, Fiolet A, Abela GS. Viewing atherosclerosis through a crystal lens: how the evolving structure of cholesterol crystals in atherosclerotic plaque alters its stability. J Clin Lipidol. 2020;14:619–30.

9. Wild RAE, Wren D, Zhao D, Hansen KR. Highly atherogenic lipids are associated with pre-eclampsia (pre-E) in obese women with unexplained infertility who conceive after ovarian stimulation with intrauterine insemination (OS-IUI). Reprod Sci. 2021;28:1–373.

10. Salafia CM, Paneth N, Shah R, Thomas T, Abela GS, Wild R. Pregnancy-induced hypertension: the potential role of cholesterol crystals in the maternal decidua. J Clin Lipidol. 2022;16(suppl):e75. https://doi.org/10.1016/j.jacl.2022.05.062.

11. Silva GB, Gierman LM, Rakner JJ, et al. Cholesterol crystals and NLRP3 mediated inflammation in the uterine wall decidua in normal and preeclamptic pregnancies. Front Immunol. 2020;11:564712.

12. Gadeela N, Rubinstein J, Tamhane U, Huang R, Pathak DR, Hosein H-A, Rich M, Dhar G, Abela GS. The impact of circulating cholesterol crystals on vasomotor function: implications for the no-reflow phenomenon. JACC Cardiovasc Interv. 2011;4:521–9.

13. Pervaiz MH, Durga S, Janoudi A, Berger K, Abela GS. PET/CTA detection of muscle inflammation related to cholesterol crystal emboli without arterial obstruction. J Nucl Cardiol. 2018;25:433–40.

14. Ghanem F, Vodnala D, Kalavakunta JK, Durga S, Thormeier N, Subramaniyam P, Abela S, Abela GS. Cholesterol crystal embolization following plaque rupture: a systemic disease with unusual features. J Biomed Res. 2017;31:82–94. https://doi.org/10.7555/JBR.31.20160100.

15. Vedre A, Pathak DR, Crimp M, Lum C, Koochesfahani M, Abela GS. Physical factors that trigger cholesterol crystallization leading to plaque rupture. Atherosclerosis. 2008;203:89–96.

16. Janoudi A, Shamoun FE, Kalavakunta JK, Abela GS. Cholesterol crystal-induced arterial inflammation and destabilization of atherosclerotic plaque. Eur Heart J. 2016;37:1959–67.

17. Koba ST, Shinji MH, Arai T, Matsukawa N, Sakai R, Yokota Y, Sata S, Tanaka H, Masaki R, Oishi Y, Ogura K, Arai K, Nomura K, Sakai K, Tsujita H, Kondo S, Tsukamoto S, Matsumoto H, Suzuki H, Shinke T. Impact of small dense low-density lipoprotein cholesterol on cholesterol crystals in patients with acute coronary syndrome: an optical coherence tomography study. J Clin Lipidol. 2022;16:438–46.

18. Demirci O, Tugrul AS, Dolgun N, Sozen H, Eren S. Serum lipids level assessed in early pregnancy and risk of pre-eclampsia. J Obstet Gynaecol Res. 2011;37:1427–32.

19. Bansal N, Cruickshank JK, McElduff P, Durrington PN. Cord blood lipoproteins and prenatal influences. Curr Opin Lipidol. 2005;16:400–8.

20. Hoogeveen RC, Gaubatz JW, Sun W, et al. Small dense low-density lipoprotein-cholesterol concentrations predict risk for coronary heart disease. Arterioscler Thromb Vasc Biol. 2014;34:1069–77.

21. Weisser B, Locher R, de Graaf J, Moser R, Sachinidis A, Vetter W. Low-density lipoprotein subfractions increase thromboxane formation in endothelial cells. Biochem Biophys Res Commun. 1993;192:1245–50.

22. Weisser B, Locher R, de Graaf J, Vetter W. Low-density lipoprotein subfractions and [Ca2+] I in vascular smooth muscle cells. Circ Res. 1993;73:118–24.

23. Eleuterio NM, Palei AC, Rangel Machado JS, Tanus-Santos JE, Cavalli RC, Sandrim VC. Relationship between adiponectin and nitrite in healthy and preeclampsia pregnancies. Clin Chim Acta. 2013;423:112–5.

24. Kita T, Kume N, Minami M, et al. Role of oxidized LDL in atherosclerosis. Ann N Y Acad Sci. 2001;947:199–205; discussion 205–196.

25. Gratos ECE, Gomez O, et al. Increased susceptibility to low-density lipoprotein oxidation in women with a history of pre-eclampsia. BJOG. 2003;110:4.

26. El Khouly NI, Sanad ZF, Saleh SA, Shabana AA, Elhalaby AF, Badr EE. Value of first-trimester serum lipid profile in early prediction of preeclampsia and its severity: a prospective cohort study. Hypertens Pregnancy. 2016;35:73–81.

27. Adank MC, Benschop L, Peterbroers KR, et al. Is maternal lipid profile in early pregnancy associated with pregnancy complications and blood pressure in pregnancy and long-term postpartum? Am J Obstet Gynecol. 2019;221:150.e151.

28. Ardalic D, Stefanovic A, Banjac G, et al. Lipid profile and lipid oxidative modification parameters in the first trimester of high-risk pregnancies—possibilities for preeclampsia prediction. Clin Biochem. 2020;81:34–40.

29. Steinberg HO, Bayazeed B, Hook G, Johnson A, Cronin J, Baron AD. Endothelial dysfunction is associated with cholesterol levels in the high normal range in humans. Circulation. 1997;96:3287–93.

30. Hulthe J, Wiklund O, Bondjers G, Wikstrand J. LDL particle size in relation to intima-media thickness and plaque occurrence in the carotid and femoral arteries in patients with hypercholesterolemia. J Intern Med. 2000;248:42–52.

31. Baumer Y, McCurdy S, Weatherby TM, et al. Hyperlipidemia-induced cholesterol crystal production by endothelial cells promotes atherogenesis. Nat Commun. 2017;8:1129. https://doi.org/10.1038/s41467-017-01186-z.

32. Varsano N, Beghi F, Dadosh T, et al. The effect of the phospholipid bilayer environment on cholesterol crystal polymorphism. ChemPlusChem. 2019;84:338–44.

33. Abela GS, Aziz K. Cholesterol crystals rupture biological membranes and human plaques during acute cardiovascular events: a novel insight into plaque rupture by scanning electron microscopy. Scanning. 2006;28:1–10.

34. Al-Handawi MB, Commins P, Karothu DP, Raj G, Li L, Naumov P. Mechanical and crystallographic analysis of cholesterol crystals puncturing biological membranes. Chemistry. 2018;24:11493–7.

35. Samstad EO, Niyonzima N, Nymo S, et al. Cholesterol crystals induce complement-dependent inflammasome activation and cytokine release. J Immunol. 2014;192:2837–45.

36. Folco EJ, Sukhova GK, Quillard T, Libby P. Moderate hypoxia potentiates interleukin-1beta production in activated human macrophages. Circ Res. 2014;115:875–83.

37. Taqueti VR, Di Carli MF, Jerosch-Herold M, et al. Increased microvascularization and vessel permeability associated with active inflammation in human atheromata. Circ Cardiovasc Imaging. 2014;7:920–9.

38. Nasiri M, Janoudi A, Vanderberg A, Frame M, Flegler C, Flegler S, Abela GS. The role of cholesterol crystals in atherosclerosis is unmasked by altering tissue preparation methods. Microsc Res Tech. 2015;78:969–74.

39. Stødle GS, Silva GB, Tangerås LH, et al. Placental inflammation in pre-eclampsia by nod-like receptor protein (NLRP)3 inflammasome activation in trophoblasts. Clin Exp Immunol. 2018;193:84–94.

40. Kim YM, Chaemsaithong P, Romero R, et al. The frequency of acute atherosis in normal pregnancy and preterm labor, preeclampsia, small-for-gestational age, fetal death and midtrimester spontaneous abortion. J Matern Fetal Neonatal Med. 2015;28:2001–9.

41. Abela GS, Katkoori V, Bumpers H. The association between cancer and atherosclerosis: cholesterol crystal-induced neovascularization in breast cancer. J Clin Lipidol. 2020;604(207):14.

42. Fry L, DeFeijter-Rupp H, Upham B, Janoudi A, Barnaba C, Medina Meza I, Ketner A, Abela GS. Effect of cholesterol crystals on gap junction intercellular communication in human umbilical vein endothelial cells. J Clin Lipidol. 2020;564(142):14.

43. Knowlton AA, Lee AR. Estrogen and the cardiovascular system. Pharmacol Ther. 2012;135:54–70.

44. Wang E, Al-Abcha A, Osman H, Oladeji A, Boumegouas M, Abela GS. The effect of estrogen and testosterone on cholesterol crystallization. J Clin Lipidol. 2022;16(3):e75–6. https://doi.org/10.1016/j.jacl.2022.05.063.

45. Shu C, Han S, Xu P, Wang Y, Cheng T, Hu C. Estrogen and preeclampsia: potential of estrogens as therapeutic agents in preeclampsia. Drug Des Devel Ther. 2021;15:2543–50. https://doi.org/10.2147/DDDT.S304316. PMID: 34163140; PMCID: PMC8214522.

46. Jobe SO, Tyler CT, Magness RR. Aberrant synthesis, metabolism and plasma accumulation of circulating estrogens and estrogen metabolites in preeclampsia: implications for vascular dysfunction. Hypertension. 2013;61:480–7. https://doi.org/10.1161/HYPERTENSIONAHA.111.201624.

47. Pecks U, Rath W, Kleine-Eggebrecht N, et al. Maternal serum lipid, estradiol, and progesterone levels in pregnancy, and the impact of placental and hepatic pathologies. Geburtshilfe Frauenheilkd. 2016;76(7):799–808. https://doi.org/10.1055/s-0042-107078.
48. Vahedian-Azimi A, Karimi L, Reiner Z, Makvandi S, Sahebkar A. Effects of statins on preeclampsia: a systematic review. Pregnancy Hypertens. 2021;23:123–30. https://doi.org/10.1016/j.preghy.2020.11.014.
49. Brownfoot FC, Hastie R, Hannan NJ, Cannon P, Tuohey L, Parry LJ, Senadheera S, Illanes SE, Kaitu'u-Lino TJ, Tong S. Metformin as a prevention and treatment for preeclampsia: effects on soluble fms-like tyrosine kinase 1 and soluble endoglin secretion and endothelial dysfunction. Am J Obstet Gynecol. 2016;214(3):356.e1–356.e15. https://doi.org/10.1016/j.ajog.2015.12.019.
50. Cluver C, Walker SP, Mol BW, Hall D, Hiscock R, Brownfoot FC, Kaitu'u-Lino TJ, Tong S. A double blind, randomised, placebo-controlled trial to evaluate the efficacy of metformin to treat preterm pre-eclampsia (PI2 trial): study protocol. BMJ Open. 2019;9:e025809. https://doi.org/10.1136/bmjopen-2018-025809.
51. Abela GS, Vedra A, Janoudi A, Huang R, Durga S, Tamhane U. Effect of statins on cholesterol crystallization and atherosclerotic plaque stabilization. Am J Cardiol. 2011;107:1710–7.
52. Fry L, Lee A, Khan S, Aziz K, Vedre A, Abela GS. Effect of aspirin on cholesterol crystallization: a potential mechanism for plaque stabilization. Am Heart J Plus. 2022;13:100083. https://doi.org/10.1016/j.ahjo.2021.100083.
53. Boumegouas M, Grondahl B, Fry L, De Feijter-Rupp H, Janoudi A, Abela GS. Metformin inhibition of volume expansion with cholesterol crystallization may contribute to reducing plaque rupture and improved cardiac outcomes. J Clin Lipidol. 2020;579(171):14.
54. Uzui H, Harpf A, Liu M. Increased expression of membrane type 3-matrix metalloproteinase in human atherosclerotic plaque: role of activated macrophages and inflammatory cytokines. Circulation. 2002;106:3024–30.
55. Xu XP, Meisel SR, Ong JM. Oxidized low-density lipoprotein regulates matrix metalloproteinase-9 and its tissue inhibitor in human monocyte-derived macrophages. Circulation. 1999;99:993–8.
56. Lu L, Liu H, Peng J, Gan L, Shen L, Zhang Q, Li L, Zhang L, Su C, Jiang Y. Regulations of the key mediators in inflammation and atherosclerosis by aspirin in human macrophages. Lipids Health Dis. 2010;6:16. https://doi.org/10.1186/1476-511X-9-16.
57. Rolnik DL, Wright D, Poo LC, et al. Aspirin versus placebo in pregnancies at high risk for preterm preeclampsia. N Engl J Med. 2017;377:613–22.
58. Brownfoot FC, Tong S, Hannan NJ, et al. Effects of pravastatin on human placenta, endothelium, and women with severe preeclampsia. Hypertension. 2015;66:687–97.
59. Lefkou E, Mamopoulos A, Dagklis T, Vosnakis C, Rousso D, Girardi G. Pravastatin improves pregnancy outcomes in obstetric antiphospholipid syndrome refractory to antithrombotic therapy. J Clin Invest. 2016;126:2933–40.
60. Pánczél Z, Kukor Z, Supák D, et al. Pravastatin induces NO synthesis by enhancing microsomal arginine uptake in healthy and preeclamptic placentas. BMC Pregnancy Childbirth. 2019;19:426. https://doi.org/10.1186/s12884-019-2507-0.
61. Cornelius DC. Preeclampsia: from inflammation to immunoregulation. Clin Med Insights Blood Disord. 2018;10:1179545X17752325. https://doi.org/10.1177/1179545X17752325. PMID: 29371787; PMCID: PMC5772493.
62. Yasar O, Iskender C, Kaymak O, Taflan Yaman S, Uygur D, Danisman N. Retrospective evaluation of pregnancy outcomes in women with familial Mediterranean fever. J Matern Fetal Neonatal Med. 2014;27(7):733–6. https://doi.org/10.3109/14767058.2013.837446. Epub 2013 Sep 25.
63. Brien ME, Gaudreault V, Hughes K, Hayes DJL, Heazell AEP, Girard S. A systematic review of the safety of blocking the IL-1 system in human pregnancy. J Clin Med. 2021;11(1):225. https://doi.org/10.3390/jcm11010225. PMID: 35011965; PMCID: PMC8745599.

Part VIII
Treatment of Cholesterol Crystals

Agents That Affect Cholesterol Crystallization and Modify the Risk of Crystal Induced Traumatic and Inflammatory Injury

George S. Abela, Sandra Hammer, Xuefei Huang, Julia V. Busik, and Stefan Mark Nidorf

1 Introduction

The formation of cholesterol crystals (CCs) within the vascular bed is the causal link between cholesterol deposition and atherosclerosis. As CCs develop, enlarge, and aggregate within foamy macrophages and the plaque core they outgrow and traumatize their surrounding environment. CCs that spill into the interstitial space can damage the vasa-vasorum to cause intra-plaque hemorrhage and trigger an innate inflammatory response, and CCs that form within the plaque core can perforate or rupture its fibrous cap and lead to atherothrombosis and cholesterol embolism [1–5]. While most inflammatory flares induced by CCs result in progressive sequestration of CCs and the larger lipid pool to cause progressive sclerosis of the arterial wall, on occasions an inflammatory flare may predispose to plaque rupture by weakening vulnerable portions of the plaque that have been stretched and thinned due to concomitant enlargement and aggregation of CCs in its core. Thus, in order

G. S. Abela (✉)
Department of Medicine, Division of Cardiovascular Medicine, Michigan State University, East Lansing, MI, USA
e-mail: abela@msu.edu

S. Hammer · J. V. Busik
Department of Physiology, Michigan State University, East Lansing, MI, USA
e-mail: shammer@msu.edu; busik@msu.edu

X. Huang
Department of Chemistry, Michigan State University, East Lansing, MI, USA
e-mail: huangxu2@msu.edu

S. M. Nidorf
The Heart and Vascular Research Institute, Sir Charles Gairdner Hospital, Perth, WA, Australia

Table 1 Therapeutic targets of cholesterol crystals in atherosclerosis

Prevent cholesterol accumulation to reduce substrate for crystal formation
– All lipid lowering therapies
Inhibition of cholesterol crystal growth causing cellular, tissue injury, and plaque rupture
– Statins, aspirin, colchicine
Altering cholesterol crystal morphology to reduce inflammation
– Statins, aspirin
Dissolution of cholesterol crystals
– Alcohol, Cyclodextrins, HDL
Inhibition of crystal induced inflammation leading to sclerosis and plaque destabilization
– Canakinumab, colchicine, statins

to break the life-long iterative cycle of crystal induced traumatic and inflammatory injury, it is necessary to reduce the formation of CCs, alter their morphology, dissolve them, and inhibit the inflammatory processes they trigger.

This chapter details the range of agents that have displayed the potential to act on one or more of these targets, (Table 1) including some that have been proven effective for secondary prevention of atherosclerosis [6–11].

2 Agents That Inhibit Cholesterol Crystal Formation and Alter Their Growth and Morphology

2.1 Statins and Ezetimibe

The exact mechanism by which statins and ezetimibe provide their cardiovascular benefit is not fully understood. While it is likely that any means of effectively lowering LDLc reduces the concentration of free cholesterol within plaque and thereby reduces the tendency for CCs to form in situ, there is evidence that unlike ezetimibe, statins also interact directly with CCs to reduce their rate of growth and to alter their morphology which in turn reduces their potential to cause traumatic and inflammatory injury.

As outlined in Chaps. "Atherosclerosis as a Crystalloid Disease: The Discovery of the Role of Cholesterol Crystals in the Formation and Rupture of Atherosclerotic Plaques", "The Cholesterol Crystal Paradigm: Overview of How Cholesterol Crystals Evolve and Induce Traumatic and Inflammatory Vascular Injury", "How Innovation in Tissue Preparation and Imaging Revolutionized the Understanding of the Role of Cholesterol Crystals in Atherosclerosis", "Role of CCs and Their Lipoprotein Precursors in NLRP3 and IL-1β Activation", we have demonstrated that as CCs grow, they develop sharp tips that have the capacity to penetrate, perforate, and rupture fibrous tissue [3, 4]. When CCs were grown in test tubes covered with fibrous rabbit pericardium simulating the fibrous plaque cap they readily "tore it to shreds," but when pravastatin was added to the test tube, the membrane remained intact. This effect of pravastatin was dose dependent (Figs. 1 and 2) [12]. Upon

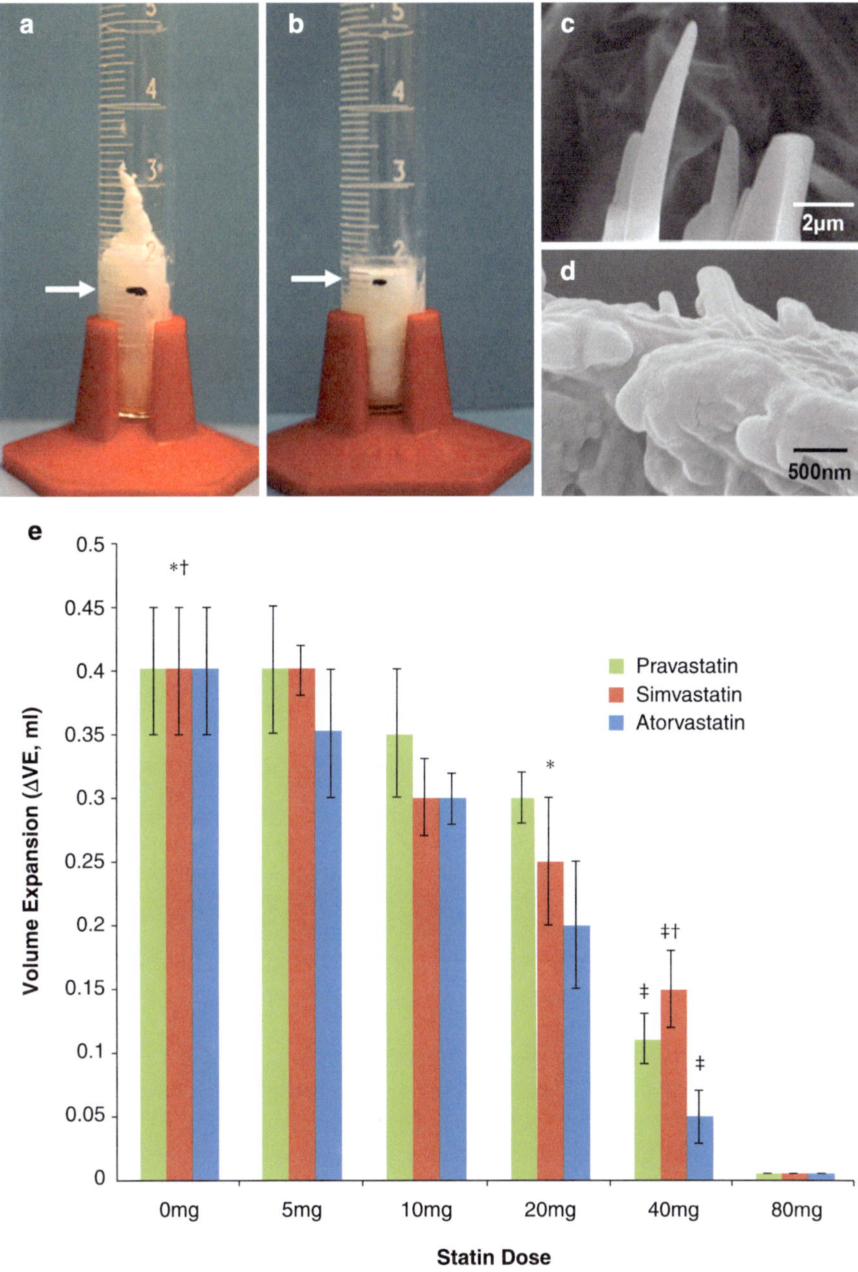

Fig. 1 Effect of statin on cholesterol crystal growth and morphology. (**a**) Test tube with cholesterol (1.5 g) expands above the meniscus. (**b**) Adding 50 mg of pravastatin inhibits volume expansion completely. (**c**) Scanning electron micrograph of normal crystal morphology with pointed tips. (**d**) Adding statin dissolves the crystals. (**e**) Bar graph demonstrating a dose related effect of atorvastatin, simvastatin, and pravastatin on volume expansion with crystallization. (Reproduced with permission [5])

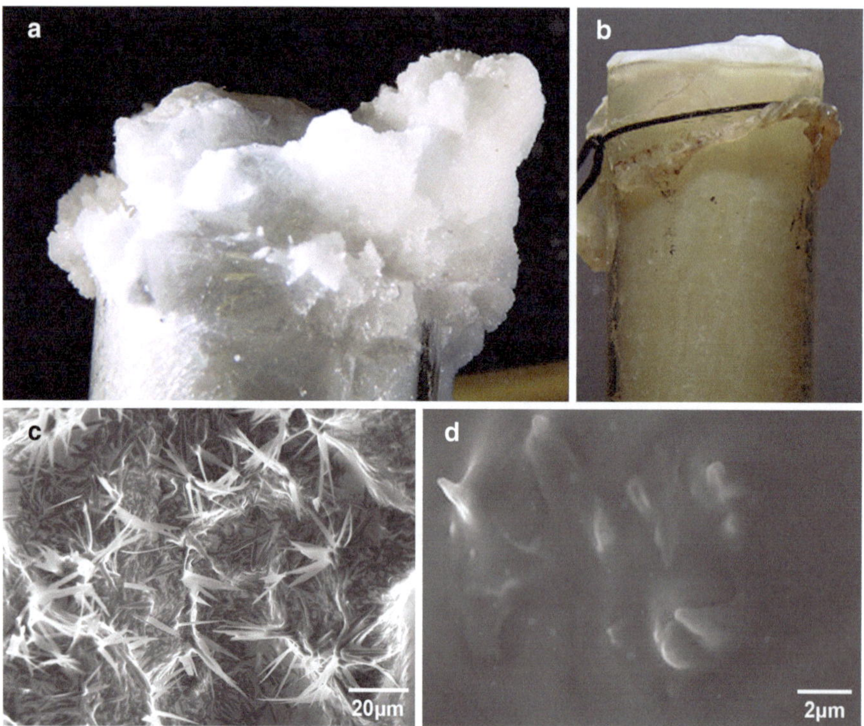

Fig. 2 Cholesterol crystal perforation of fibrous membrane. (**a**) Test tube with pure cholesterol has marked volume expansion beyond the rim of the tube and totally disrupts the membrane overlying the surface. (**b**) Test tube with cholesterol and pravastatin (90 mg) has minimal volume expansion. (**c**) Scanning electron micrograph of the membrane surface illustrates extensive cholesterol crystals perforating the membrane with pure cholesterol. (**d**) Very few crystals are seen penetrating the membrane with cholesterol and pravastatin. (Reproduced with permission [5])

further examination it became evident that pravastatin not only inhibited the development of CCs but also affected their morphology by blunting their characteristic sharp edges.

Studies in both rabbit models of atherosclerosis and in human atherosclerotic carotid plaques obtained at endarterectomy demonstrated that treatment with statins also alters the appearance of CCs in atherosclerotic plaques [13, 14] (Fig. 3), and that this effect, like the clinical benefits of statins, was dose dependent [12].

In other experiments in atherosclerotic rabbits fed a cholesterol enriched diet (1%), we found CCs protruding from the arterial wall and aortic leaflets in association with macrophage infiltration and elevated serum markers of inflammation including MMP 9 and CRP [13–15]. The appearance of CCs in plaques in this model were strikingly similar to that seen in patients who had died soon after myocardial infarction [16] (Chap. 15 "Role of CCs and Their Lipoprotein Precursors in NLRP3 and IL-1β Activation"), and their appearance in aortic leaflets was similar to human sclerotic valves obtained during valve surgery [13] (Chap. 16 "Molecular

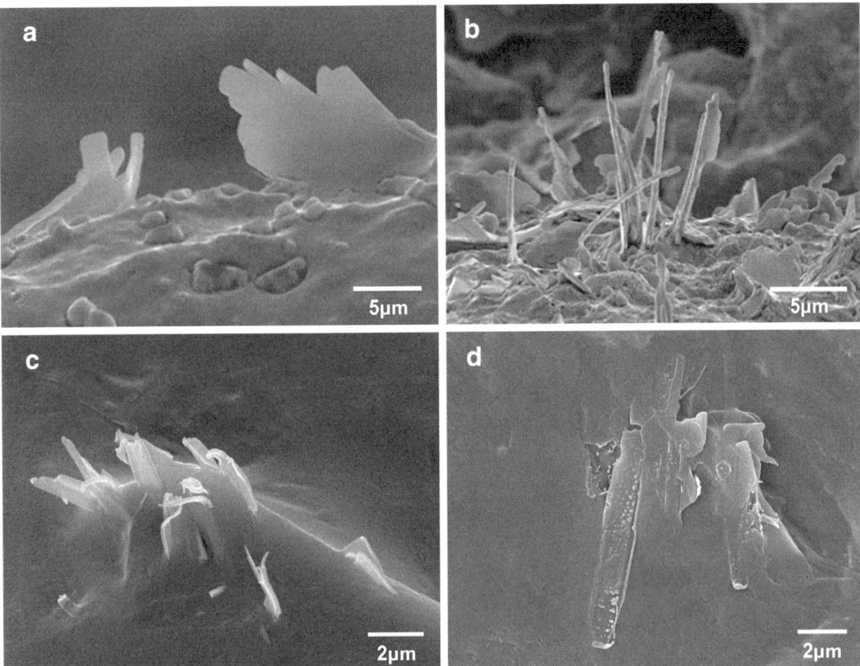

Fig. 3 In vivo cholesterol crystals from patients untreated and treated with statins. (**a**) Cholesterol crystals as commonly seen perforating the intimal surface in human carotid plaque not taking statin. (**b**) Cholesterol crystals from patient on atorvastatin treatment before carotid endarterectomy demonstrate thinning with edges that have irregular borders, and some are bent as typically seen with dissolving crystals. (**c**) Crystals from pulmonary valve from atherosclerotic rabbit (**d**) dissolving and melting crystals from mitral valve in atherosclerotic rabbit treated with simvastatin. (Reproduced with permission [5])

Pathomechanisms of Crystal-Induced Disorders"). In this model, simvastatin and ezetimibe both reduced the cholesterol content and number of CCs in the plaque core, reduced the concentration of macrophages surrounding the plaque core and reduced systemic markers of inflammation [15]. Furthermore, ruptured plaques in this model that contained less cholesterol and fewer CCs were found to induce less thrombus when exposed to pharmacological triggers [17]. Interestingly, statins and ezetimibe also reduced the level of cholesterol and macrophage infiltration in the aortic leaflets *when treatment was started with the initiation of the cholesterol enriched diet* but had no effect on these features when started *after* the initiation of the lipid rich diet.

Together these data suggest that it is the ability of effective sustained lipid lowering therapy to alter the lipid milieu within atherosclerotic plaques that reduces the likelihood of CC formation within them, leaving them less vulnerable to CC induced injury.

In addition, and unlike ezetimibe, statins have additional actions that may reduce the injurious effects of CCs. Not only is there evidenced that they reduce the expression of IL-6 and IL-18 by human retinal endothelial cells (HREC) exposed to CCs and prolong cell viability [18], but their ability to alter CC morphology provides a plausible mechanism by which they notably reduce the risk of cardiovascular events when used early after an acute coronary syndrome [19] or just prior to percutaneous coronary intervention [20] well before they could possibly decrease serum LDLc.

Thus, while all means of lowering LDLc may reduce the cholesterol content of atherosclerotic plaque and thus reduce the risk of CC formation, statins have the added ability to reduce CCs growth and alter their morphology that reduces their ability to cause traumatic and inflammatory injury. Although the mechanism by which statins alter interact with CCs as they develop and grow has yet to be elucidated, the observations support the general principle that *any agent that can interfere with CC growth or can alter their morphology can potentially affect their ability to cause injury* and thus influence the progression of atherosclerosis.

2.2 Aspirin

Aspirin has proven benefits for secondary prevention in patients with coronary disease. While the benefits are believed to relate to its anti-inflammatory and anti-platelet properties [21–24], we have found in both in vitro and ex vivo studies that aspirin also affects CC growth and morphology (Chap. 4 "Crystals in Atherosclerosis: Crystal Cholesterol Structures, Morphologies, Formation and Dissolution. What Do We Know?").

Akin to the effects of statin, bench studies confirm that at physiologic doses used in humans aspirin affects CCs morphology by blunting the development of typical sharp edges thus reducing their ability to perforate pericardial membranes (Fig. 4). In addition, CCs in ex vivo studies of human atherosclerotic plaques obtained at atherectomy incubated with aspirin at 37 °C also appeared degraded [25] (Fig. 5). Additionally, studies have also demonstrated that aspirin can reduce the size of atherosclerotic plaques and the extent of macrophage infiltration that surrounds them [26–28].

Thus, aside from its effects on cyclooxygenase-1 and platelets, aspirin, like statins, has the ability to affect the progression of atherosclerosis due to its ability to reduce the risk of CC induced traumatic and inflammatory injury by virtue of its effects on CC growth and morphology.

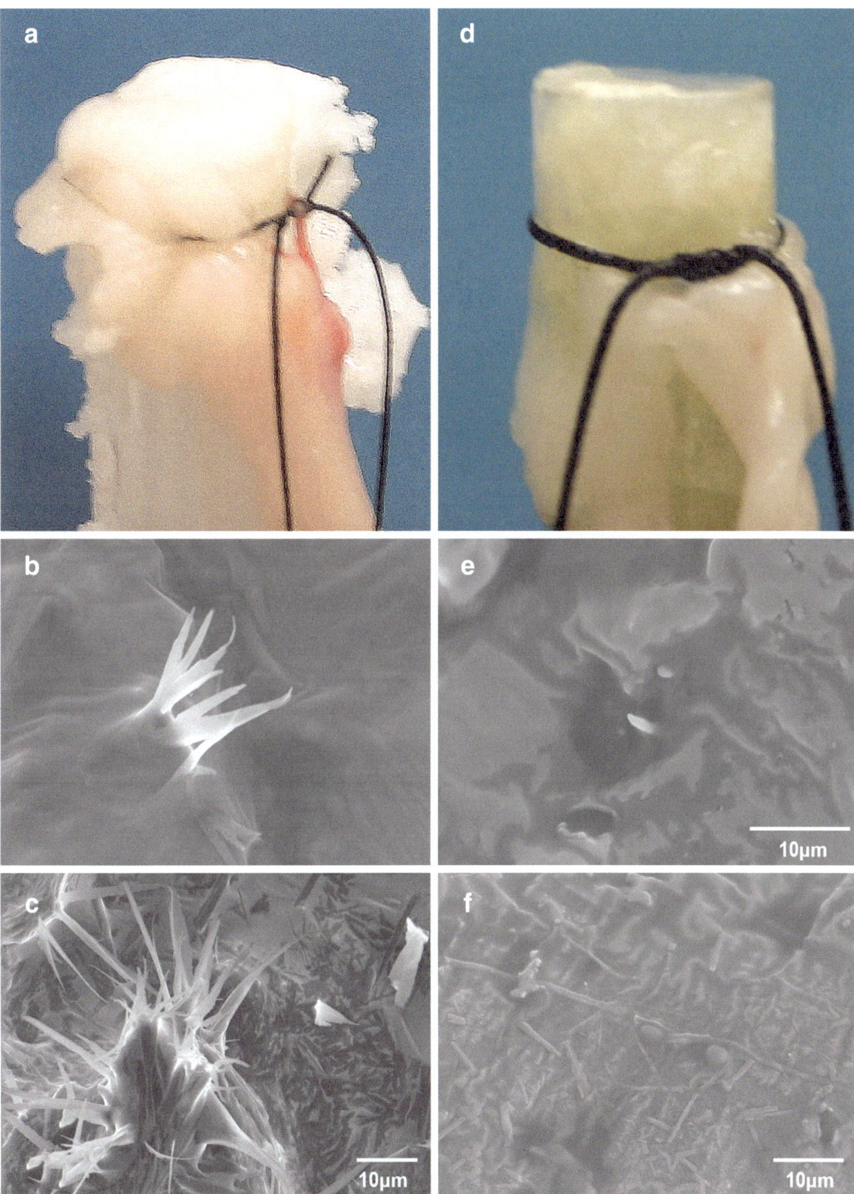

Fig. 4 Effect of aspirin on fibrous tissue injury. (**a**) Tube with cholesterol crystals expanding and disrupting pericardium during crystallization. (**b**, **c**) Scanning electron micrographs of cholesterol crystals perforating the pericardial membrane during crystallization. (**d**) Tube with cholesterol crystals and aspirin (50 mg) has minimal encroachment on the pericardial membrane. (**e**, **f**) Scanning electron micrograph of cholesterol crystals formed in the presence of aspirin demonstrating very few crystals perforating the membrane surface. (**g**) Change in volume expansion (ΔVE) at physiologic level of aspirin demonstrates reduction of ΔVE at physiologic levels of aspirin at 0.3 mg compared to higher dose at 3.0 mg. (Reproduced with permission [25])

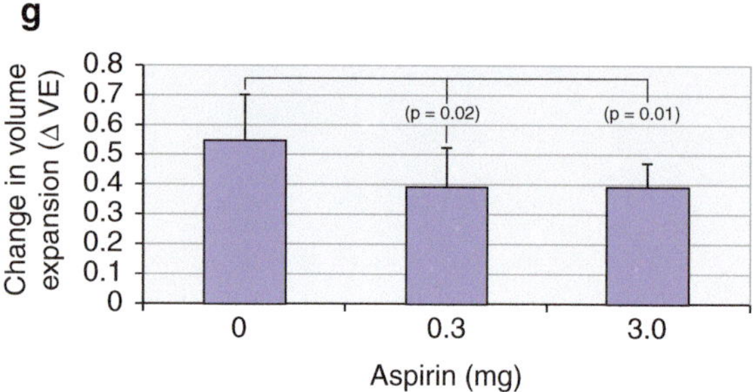

Fig. 4 (continued)

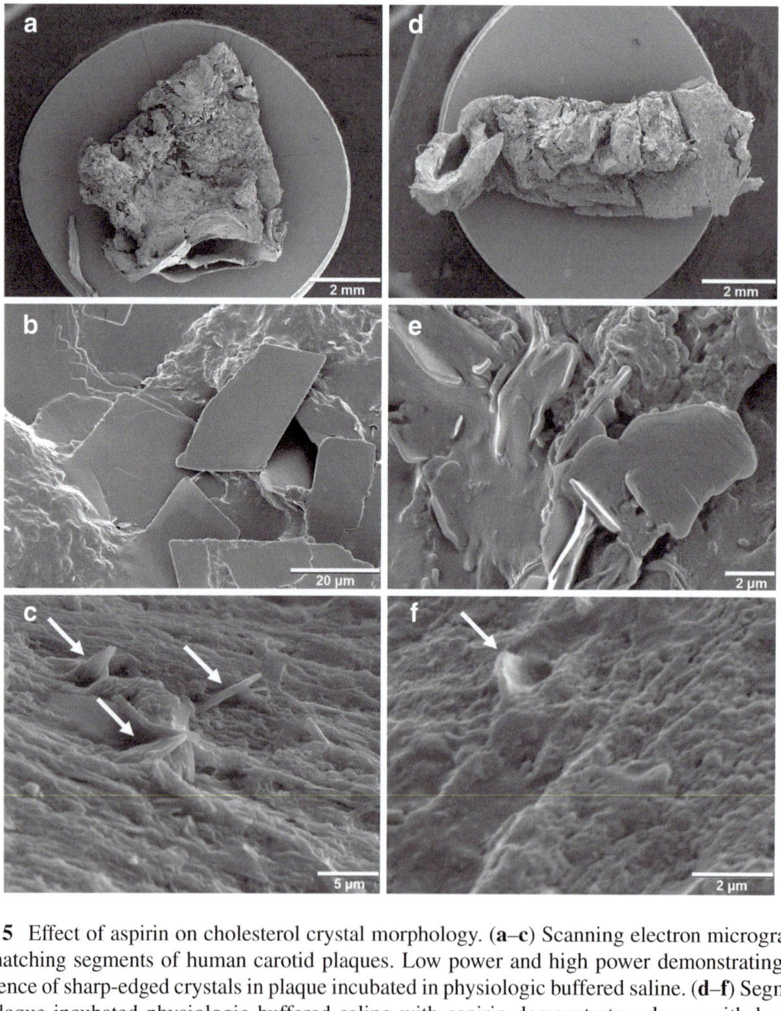

Fig. 5 Effect of aspirin on cholesterol crystal morphology. (**a–c**) Scanning electron micrographs of matching segments of human carotid plaques. Low power and high power demonstrating the presence of sharp-edged crystals in plaque incubated in physiologic buffered saline. (**d–f**) Segment of plaque incubated physiologic buffered saline with aspirin demonstrates plaque with loss of sharp edges and fewer crystals perforating the intimal surface. (Reproduced with permission [25])

3   Agents That Can Dissolve Cholesterol Crystals

Although lipid lowering drugs, aspirin, and other agents including colchicine (Abela: personal communication) may slow the growth of CCs and alter their morphology, only a few agents are known to dissolve them.

3.1   Alcohol

As highlighted in Chaps. "Atherosclerosis as a Crystalloid Disease: The Discovery of the Role of Cholesterol Crystals in the Formation and Rupture of Atherosclerotic Plaques" and "How Innovation in Tissue Preparation and Imaging Revolutionized the Understanding of the Role of Cholesterol Crystals in Atherosclerosis", it has long been appreciated that alcohol dissolves CCs when used as solvent in tissue preparation [29]. As a result, when ethanol is used in standard concentrations to dehydrate tissues and stiffen them in order to cut thin sections using a microtome for histologic examination, the existence of CCs can only be inferred by the presence of empty imprints, or "clefts," in tissue or thrombus in which they had resided in situ [30, 31]. Thus, the long-standing method of preparing histologic specimens with ethanol that dissolved CCs inadvertently delayed the recognition of their potential role in the development of atherosclerosis and plaque rupture for well over a century.

Scanning electron microscopy confirms that pretreatment of specimens with ethanol not only reduces the number of CCs, but also reduces their size and blunts their sharp edges [16, 29]. In contrast, when ethanol is excluded from tissue preparation and tissues are dehydrated using air drying or vacuum, CCs can readily be seen in and around the plaque core and can also be seen directly perforating its fibrous cap [3, 4, 16].

Many studies have demonstrated an association between moderate ethanol consumption and a reduced risk of heart attack and stroke and all-cause mortality [32, 33]. While the reason for this relationship is unknown, it is interesting to speculate that perhaps some of the cardiovascular benefits of alcohol relate to its ability to dissolve CCs at physiological serum levels and thus reduce the risk of CC induced plaque rupture (Fig. 6).

3.2   Cyclodextrins

Cyclodextrins (cyclic biocompatible oligosaccharides) have been shown to sequester CCs within their structure with high affinity and dissolve them. There are three common natural cyclodextrins, α-, β-, γ-cyclodextrin. These water-soluble complexes form cone shapes, via their six, seven or eight glucose units, respectively. Due to their hydrophobic interior, small size, and ability to access the cell membrane without internalization, low concentrations of cyclodextrins can solubilize

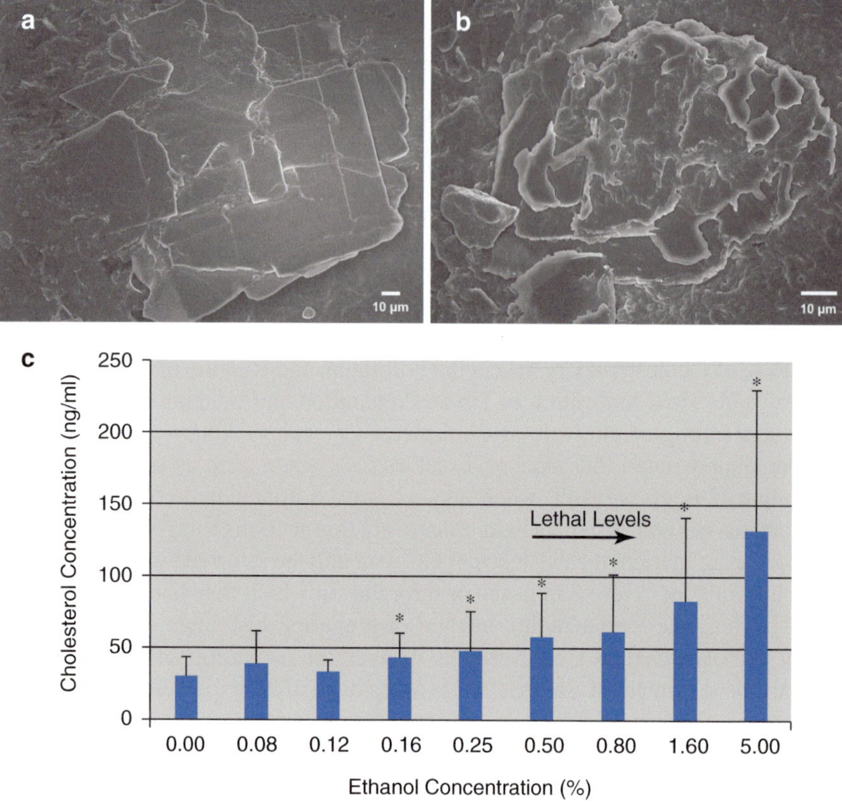

Fig. 6 Effect of ethanol on cholesterol crystals. (**a, b**) Scanning electron micrographs with an untreated cholesterol crystal cluster from human carotid plaque and (**b**) a dissolving crystal cluster with loss of architecture after exposure to ethanol (**c**) Bar graph illustrates the effect of ethanol solubility of cholesterol crystals vs. water ($p < 0.05$). (Reproduced with permission [29])

hydrophobic molecules such as free cholesterol without disrupting normal physiological cholesterol levels [34]. Mechanistically, cyclodextrins have been shown to mobilize free and esterified cholesterol in human foam cells [35, 36]. This macrophage reprogramming and activated efflux mechanisms is believed to depend on Liver X Receptor transcriptional activity [37]. The ability of cyclodextrins to trap free cholesterol has also been used to develop a non-invasive method of imaging CCs in vitro and ex vivo, by capitalizing on the superparamagnetic properties of the iron oxide core and binding properties of β-cyclodextrin and cholesterol [38].

Oral α-cyclodextrin has been shown to inhibit the untoward effects of high cholesterol in human granulocytes, monocytes, and retinal endothelial cells, including inhibiting complement activation, phagocytosis, cell death, and production of reactive oxygen species. When administered to LDLR$^{-/-}$ mice fed a western diet (high fat/high cholesterol), it decreases the level of proatherogenic lipoproteins and improves plasma lipid profiles when compared to LDLR$^{-/-}$ mice fed only a western diet [37]. Additionally, α-cyclodextrin can prevent the formation of CCs in type 2 diabetic mouse retinas, and in this animal model α- and β-cyclodextrin can significantly reduce atherogenesis and cause regression of established atherosclerosis [18, 37].

Although all three cyclodextrins are capable of dissolving CCs, α-cyclodextrin has been shown be the most potent, least toxic and best tolerated in humans. The effectiveness of oral α-cyclodextrin in preventing CC formation and CC induced pathology has been seen in dyslipidemic and obese populations, in whom it also reduces bod weight, and LDL and increases insulin sensitivity [39, 40] (Fig. 7).

The promising clinical trial results coupled with extensive preclinical studies demonstrate the potential clinical use of α-cyclodextrin in patients with diabetes and atherosclerosis. Despite these benefits, concern that it may enhance the risk of deafness have hampered its introduction but has sparked interest in determining whether lower doses can be used by delivering therapy directly to vulnerable, lipid rich plaques. Specifically, it has been suggested that it may be possible to develop a non-invasive method to detect the presence of CCs and target plaques that appear

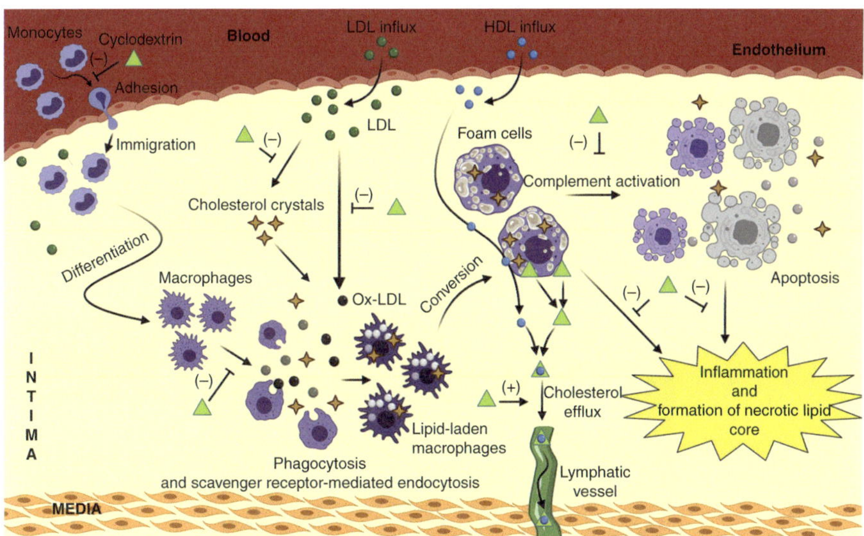

Fig. 7 Potential anti-atherogenic mechanisms of cyclodextrins in the arterial wall. The suggested mechanism derived from data obtained from experiments performed in cultured cells and/or in experimental animals. The figure shows a schematic cross-section of an advanced atherosclerotic lesion, which is formed in the subendothelial intimal layer of the arterial wall. The smooth muscle cells at the bottom denote the medial layer of the arterial wall, which is separated from the lesion by an elastic layer (not shown). The potential effects of cyclodextrins on atherosclerosis progression. Cyclodextrins (1) inhibit the entry of circulating monocytes into the lesion by inhibiting their adhesion to the endothelium; (2) stimulate cholesterol efflux, and also interact with and contribute to the dissolution of cholesterol crystals; (3) decrease the susceptibility of LDL to oxidation; (4) inhibit cholesterol crystal-induced phagocytosis; (5) inhibit cholesterol crystal-triggered complement activation; and (6) reduce inflammation and production of reactive oxygen species in atherosclerotic lesions [40]

vulnerable to rupture with lower dose of cyclodextrin. Toward this end, superparamagnetic iron oxide nanoparticles (SPIONs) have been synthesized and coated with β-cyclodextrin (β-CD) (Fig. 8a). Such β-CD-SPIONs are able to bind with CCs through the β-CD ligand on the nanoparticle surface. This in turn has enabled the

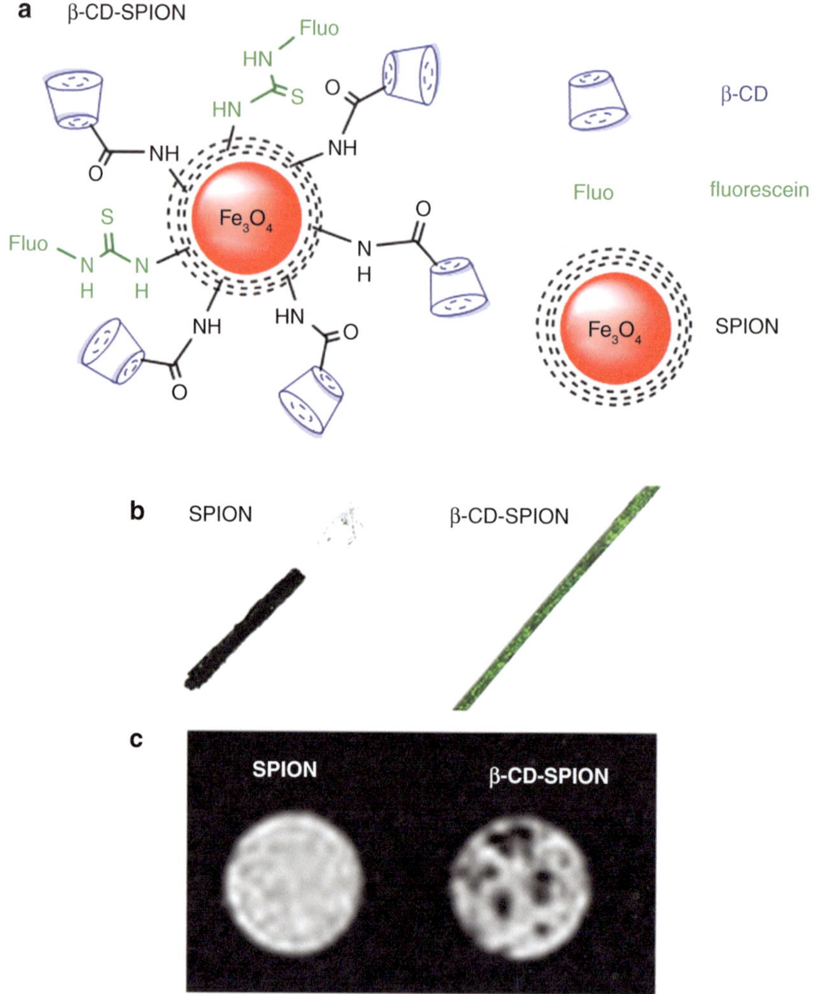

Fig. 8 Magnetic nanoparticles with conjugated β-cyclodextrin. (**a**) Schematic demonstration of the structures of β-cyclodextrin (β-CD) conjugated magnetic nanoparticles (β-CD-SPIONs) and the nonconjugated SPIONs. (**b**) Confocal microscopy images of the cholesterol crystals after incubation with unconjugated SPIONs (left) and conjugated β-CD-SPIONs (right) demonstrating the binding of β-CD-SPIONs to the crystals. (**c**) T2* weighted magnetic resonance images of the cholesterol crystals after incubation with the nonconjugated SPIONs (left) compared to conjugated β-CD-SPIONs (right) confirming the binding of β-CD-SPIONs to the crystals. (Reproduced with permission [38])

detection and imaging of CCs in vitro by both fluorescence (Fig. 8b) and MRI (Fig. 8c), paving the way for in vivo detection of CCs in the hope of delivering sufficient cyclodextrin to vulnerable plaques [38].

3.3   Biological Products

High-density lipoprotein has been demonstrated to dissolve CCs in vitro [41, 42] however it is unlikely to have an effect on CCs in vivo as it does not come into contact with CCs embedded within atherosclerotic plaques, heart valves, and other tissues (Fig. 9).

Macrophages and bacteria can both dissolve extracellular CCs in situ. In our studies we have seen macrophages attached to CCs in aspirates from culprit coronary arteries during acute myocardial infarction (Fig. 6 in Chap. 10 "The Role of Cholesterol Crystals in Plaque Rupture Leading to Acute Myocardial Infarction and Stroke") [43]. In these instances, fragments of CCs appeared to have been "etched out" by macrophages that had extended pseudo-pods onto their surface. Similarly, both gram positive and gram-negative bacteria have been seen to attach to the surface of CCs and to dissolve them (The Interaction Between Infection, Crystals and Cardiovascular Disease) [44], however, as yet the biologic products responsible for this action has not been identified.

In contrast *nor-epinephrine, epinephrine, and steroids* each *increase* CC growth in a dose-dependent manner and at serum levels seen in humans during stress [45] thus providing a potential mechanism by which emotional and physical stress may predispose to CC induced plaque rupture and acute cardiovascular events (Fig. 10).

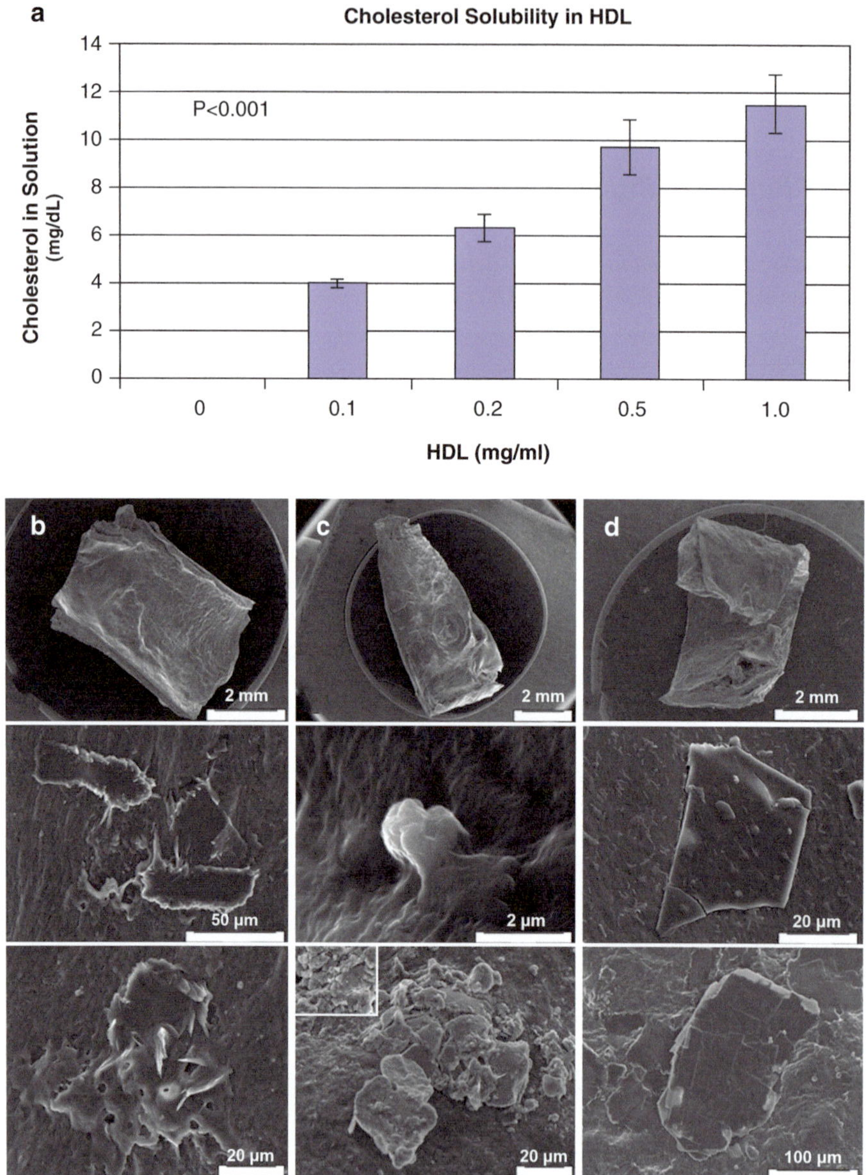

Fig. 9 Cholesterol crystal solubility in HDL. (**a**) Bar graph demonstrating increased solubility of cholesterol crystals in HDL vs. physiologic buffered saline. (**b–d**) Scanning micrographs of human carotid endarterectomy plaques. (**b, c**) Plaques incubated in HDL for 24 h demonstrating dissolving cholesterol crystals. (**d**) Plaque incubated in PBS demonstrating preserved sharp edge crystals

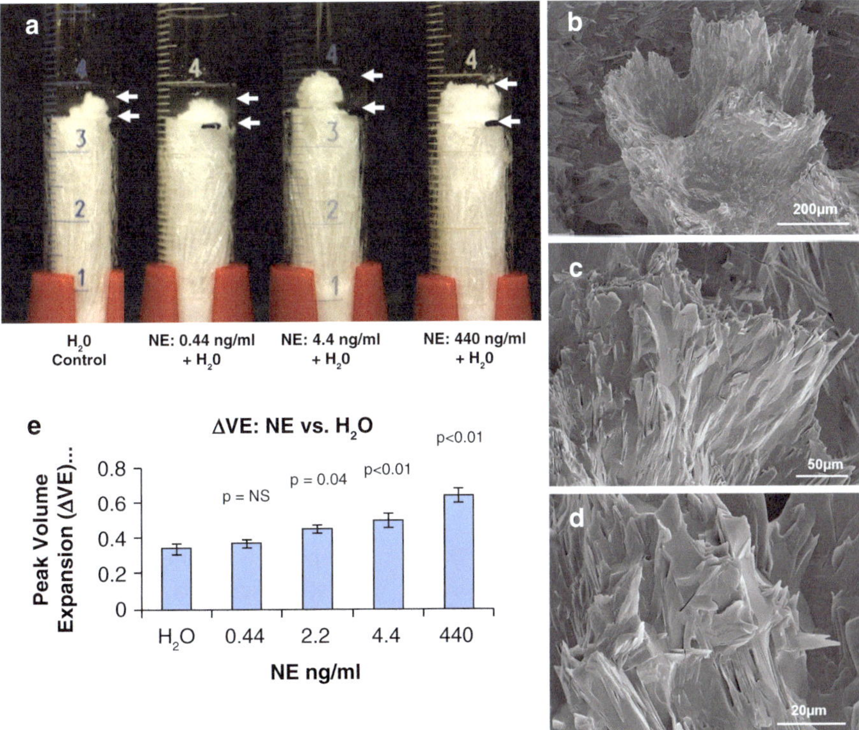

Fig. 10 Nor-epinephrine enhances cholesterol crystal growth. (**a**) Graduated cylinders with increasing concentration of nor-epinephrine demonstrating a rising peak volume expansion with cholesterol crystallization. (**e**) Bar graph illustrating an increase in crystal growth when exposed to nor-epinephrine. (**b, c, d**) Scanning electron micrographs of cholesterol crystals grown in saline with epinephrine illustrates an 'explosive' growth of crystals with a swirling pattern

4 Agents That Can Inhibit Aspects of Crystal Induced Inflammation

While reducing the risk of developing CCs or altering their growth or morphology provide attractive approaches for prevention of atherosclerosis, therapies with these properties are clearly insufficient to prevent continued formation of CCs and disease progression. Thus, inhibiting CC induced inflammation is an essential additional target for the treatment of atherosclerosis [1, 2].

As highlighted throughout the textbook, CCs released into the interstitial space surrounding atherosclerotic plaques may trigger an iterative cycle of innate inflammatory injury akin to gout (Chap. 22 "Interaction Between Crystals, Inflammation, and Cancer"), which likely explains why only those anti-inflammatory agents that inhibit aspects of crystal induced inflammation have proven to be of benefit for the secondary prevention of coronary disease.

Although CCs are by far the most common crystals to form within atherosclerotic plaque, we and others have identified a range of other crystalloids including calcium phosphate and monosodium urate crystals in the plaque core (Figs. 8 and 11 in Chap. 3 "How Innovation in Tissue Preparation and Imaging Revolutionized the Understanding of the Role of Cholesterol Crystals in Atherosclerosis") that like CCs, develop as these elements accumulate as a result of cellular senescence and necrosis [43, 46–50]. Thus, in some instances crystalloids aside CCs may promote or amplify innate inflammation in the atherosclerotic bed. Although hyperuricemia and gout have been associated with an increased risk of myocardial infarction and cardiac death, there is as yet no conclusive evidence that reducing serum uric acid reduces cardiovascular risk as is the case with cholesterol, however, an ongoing placebo-controlled trial will address this very issue [51, 52].

4.1   Canakinumab

The CANTOS trial was the first study to confirm the benefits of targeting inflammation for secondary prevention in patients with atherosclerosis. In this study, canakinumab was used to target the IL-1β inflammatory pathway. Canakinumab had already proven to be beneficial for the prevention and treatment of acute gout [6]. CANTOS confirmed that canakinumab significantly reduced the risk of MACE events and unscheduled revascularization [7]. Despite these benefits, the Food and Drug Administration chose not to approve its use for secondary prevention of coronary disease due to its cost and concerns about the small increased risk of life-threatening infection.

An early report from the CANTOS investigators raised hopes that canakinumab may also reduce the risk of development of, and survival with non-small cell cancer of the lung [7]. This is of interest, as inflammasome is believed to play a role in promoting metastatic disease. Although subsequent prospective trials including the Completely Resected Non-small Cell Lung Cancer (CANOPY-1) trial showed that when used in combination with pembrolizumab and other agents canakinumab did not improve disease free survival in these patients [53, 54], a post-hoc analysis suggested that it may have had a favorable effect in patients with elevated inflammatory markers.

4.2   Other IL-1 Inhibitors

A variety of other IL-1 inhibitors have also been evaluated in patients with cardiovascular disease. Anakinra, a recombinant human interleukin-1 receptor antagonist that inhibits both IL-1α and IL-1β as well as IL-18 has been trialed with mixed results, however, its short half-life make it ill-suited for long-term secondary prevention. Other agents include MCC950 that targets NLRP3 inflammasome assembly, and GSK1070806 a humanized antibody to IL-18 can also attenuate NLRP3 inflammasome activity are also being trialed, however, as with other biologics, their potential to suppress the immune system raises concern about the risk of infections and will require long-term safety and efficacy data to be gathered in large clinical trials before they could be considered for use in clinical practice [55].

4.3   Colchicine

Colchicine is one of the oldest medications in the pharmacopeia. Its therapeutic effects have been employed for millennia to treat and prevent gout flares. In the mid-to-late twentieth century its value was recognized for treatment and prevention of inflammatory flares and to reverse renal amyloid in patients with familial Mediterranean fever (FMF). More recently it has been used to treat other conditions including pericarditis, and Bechet's Syndrome [56].

Colchicine's action on such a broad range of conditions likely stems from its ability to dampen the innate immune response. Unlike canakinumab, colchicine effects relate to its ability to bind to tubulin. Colchicine is avidly taken up by leukocytes and endothelium. As it accumulates in macrophages it reduces the assembly of inflammasome and the expression of IL-1β and the production of several other pro-inflammatory cytokines including IL-18; accumulation in endothelium reduces expression of selectins that promote ingress of circulating leukocytes; accumulation in neutrophils affect their ability to marginate, aggregate and express cytokines, release NETs, and interact with platelets. In addition, colchicine has favorable effects on tissue healing (Fig. 11) [57, 58].

Further still, colchicine can inhibit CC growth in vitro (Abela, unpublished). Thus, unlike any other anti-inflammatory agent, its ability to concentrate within leukocytes imply that it can potentially block CC growth within foam cells. Furthermore, it may also become concentrated within the atherosclerotic bed and therefore be exposed to extracellular CCs when released from apoptotic leukocytes that become sequestered and necrose within the plaque core.

In the last decade, colchicine's potential for the secondary prevention of atherosclerosis has also been confirmed. The idea to trial it for this purpose related to the known role that inflammation plays in the chronic and acute phase of the disease, and the observation that long-term use of colchicine is safe and effective for secondary prevention of acute inflammatory flares in patients with gout and FMF [59–61].

The first study to demonstrate the potential of low-dose (0.5 mg daily) colchicine in patients with coronary disease was the low-dose colchicine (LoDoCo) pilot study [62]. Subsequently, the much larger LoDoCo2 trial, a multi-center blinded placebo-controlled trial in patients who were tolerant to colchicine confirmed its benefits on the composite of cardiovascular death, spontaneous myocardial infarction, ischemic stroke, or ischemia-driven coronary revascularization [63]. In both, the benefits of colchicine appeared early and continued to accrue over time.

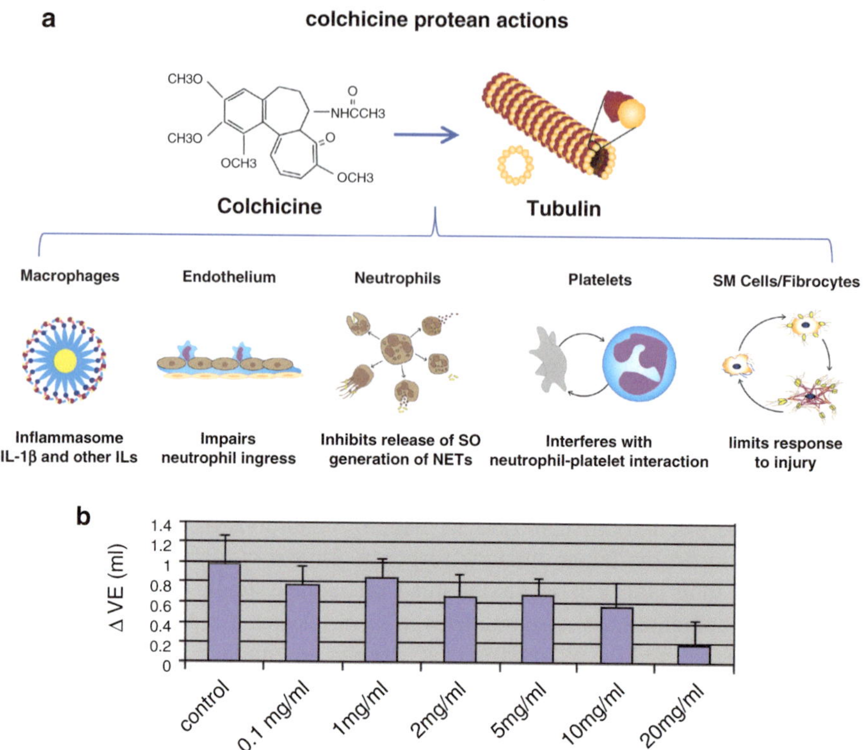

Fig. 11 (**a**) Effects of colchicine in atherosclerosis. (**b**) Colchicine inhibits cholesterol volume expansion with crystallization

Consistent with these finding is the observation that colchicine has also been demonstrated to reduce the risk of in-stent stenosis [64], and the Colchicine Cardiovascular Outcomes Trial (COLCOT) trial confirmed its long-term benefits in patients with a recent myocardial infarction [65, 66].

Meta-analysis of four independent long-term randomized controlled trials published to date now include a broad range of >11,000 patients with acute and chronic coronary disease with follow-up out to 5 years and confirm that colchicine reduces the risk of the individual outcomes of myocardial infarction, ischemic stroke, and unscheduled revascularization, and demonstrate a trend towards a reduction in cardiovascular death [67]. In addition, these trials indicate that, when used judiciously, colchicine 0.5 mg daily does not increase the risk of sepsis, cancer, neutropenia, myotoxicity, or bleeding [68].

Together these data lay the foundation supporting the repurposing colchicine as the first anti-inflammatory agent that can be widely adopted for secondary prevention in patients with CV disease atop of statins and anti-platelet therapy. In the next 3–5 years, the CLEAR SYNERGY study, the CONVINCE trial (NCT02898610), and the COLCARDIO trial (ACTRN12616000400460) will collectively recruit

>9000 patients providing further insights into the efficacy, long-term safety, and tolerability of colchicine 0.5 mg daily in various subset of patients with cardiovascular disease.

Thus, the trials of colchicine and canakinumab indicate that targeting the innate inflammatory axis slows the progression of atherosclerosis by limiting plaque growth, reducing the risk of plaque instability and the risk of in-stent stenosis, and that it favorably affects remodeling of atherosclerotic plaques following acute coronary syndrome [69]. On the tail of these trials, the ongoing Zeus trial examining the cardiovascular effects and safety of ziltivekimab, a human monoclonal antibody directed against the IL-6 ligand will be keenly awaited [70]. Based on these clinical trials, the Food and Drug Administration has recently approved colchicine for secondary prevention in patients with established coronary artery disease and those at high risk for cardiovascular events [71].

5   Summary

Understanding the central role of cholesterol crystals in the atherosclerotic process provides a useful paradigm for the treatment of the disease. Therapies that inhibit the formation of CCs, alter their morphology, dissolve them, or inhibit the inflammatory processes they (and other colloids) trigger have the potential to break the iterative cycle of crystal induced vascular injury. Some agents with proven benefits in atherosclerosis including statins, aspirin and colchicine are known to act on more than one of these targets. Undoubtedly future research will continue to focus on the development of agents that act on each of these aspects of this crystal induced disease.

References

1. Düewell P, Kono H, Rayner KJ, et al. NLRP3 inflammasomes are required for atherogenesis and activated by cholesterol crystals. Nature. 2010;464:1357–61. https://doi.org/10.1038/nature08938.
2. Rajamäki K, Lappalainen J, Öörni K, Välimäki E, Matikainen S, Kovanen PT, Eklund KK. Cholesterol crystals activate the NLRP3 inflammasome in human macrophages: a novel link between cholesterol metabolism and inflammation. PLoS One. 2010;5(7):e11765. https://doi.org/10.1371/journal.pone.0011765.
3. Abela GS. Cholesterol crystals piercing the arterial plaque and intima trigger local and systemic inflammation. J Clin Lipidol. 2010;4:156–64. https://doi.org/10.1016/j.jacl.2010.03.003.
4. Abela GS, Aziz K. Cholesterol crystals rupture biological membranes and human plaques during acute cardiovascular events: a novel insight into plaque rupture by scanning electron microscopy. Scanning. 2006;28:1–10. https://doi.org/10.1002/sca.4950280101.
5. Nidorf SM, Fiolet A, Abela GS. Viewing atherosclerosis through a crystal lens: how the evolving structure of cholesterol crystals in atherosclerotic plaque alters its stability. J Clin Lipidol. 2020;14:619. https://doi.org/10.1016/j.jacl.2020.07.003.

6. Ridker PM, Everett BM, Thuren T, McFadyen JG, CANTOS Trial Group, et al. Antiinflammatory therapy with canakinumab for atherosclerotic disease. N Engl J Med. 2017;377:1119–31. https://doi.org/10.1056/NEJMoa1707914.

7. Ridker PM, MacFadyen JG, Thuren T, et al. Effect of interleukin-1β inhibition with canakinumab on incident lung cancer in patients with atherosclerosis: exploratory results from a randomised, double-blind, placebo-controlled trial. Lancet. 2017;390:1833–42. https://doi.org/10.1016/S0140-6736(17)32247-X.

8. Demierre M-F, Higgins PDR, Gruber SB, Hawk E, Lippman SM. Statins and cancer prevention. Nat Rev. 2005;5:930–42. https://doi.org/10.1038/nrc1751.

9. Cao Y, Nishihara R, Wu K, Wang M, Ogino S, Willett WC, Spiegelman D, Fuchs CS, Giovannucci EL, Chan AT. Population-wide impact of long-term use of aspirin and the risk for cancer. JAMA Oncol. 2016;2:762. https://doi.org/10.1001/jamaoncol.2015.6396.

10. Koushki K, Shahbaz SK, Mashayekhi K, Sadeghi M, Zayeri ZD, Taba MY, Banach M, Al-Rasadi K, Johnston TP, Sahebkar A. Anti-inflammatory action of statins in cardiovascular disease: the role of inflammasome and toll-like receptor pathways. Clin Rev Allergy Immunol. 2021;60(2):175–99. https://doi.org/10.1007/s12016-020-08791-9.

11. Kuo MC, Chang SJ, Hsieh MC. Colchicine significantly reduces incident cancer in gout male patients: a 12-year cohort study. Medicine (Baltimore). 2015;94(50):e1570. https://doi.org/10.1097/MD.0000000000001570.

12. Abela GS, Vedre A, Janoudi A, Huang R, Durga S, Tamhane U. Effect of statins on cholesterol crystallization and atherosclerotic plaque stabilization. Am J Cardiol. 2011;107:1710–7. https://doi.org/10.1016/j.amjcard.2011.02.336.

13. Elkhatib L, De Feijter-Rupp H, Janoudi A, Fry L, Kehdi M, Abela GS. Cholesterol induced heart valve inflammation and injury: efficacy of cholesterol lowering treatment. Open Heart. 2020;7:e001274. https://doi.org/10.1136/openhrt-2020-001274.

14. Kotaru P, Janoudi A, Huang R, Abela GS. Cholesterol lowering with simvastatin and ezetimibe inhibits cholesterol crystal formation and associated inflammation. J Am Coll Card. 2014;63:A398.

15. Patel R, Janoudi A, Vedre A, Aziz K, Tamhane U, Rubinstein J, Abela OG, Berger K, Abela GS. Plaque rupture and thrombosis is reduced by lowering cholesterol levels and crystallization with ezetimibe and is correlated with FDG-PET. Arterioscler Thromb Vasc Biol. 2011;31:2007–14. https://doi.org/10.1161/ATVBAHA.111.226167.

16. Abela GS, Aziz K, Vedre A, Pathak DR, Talbott JD, Dejong J. Effect of cholesterol crystals on plaques and intima in arteries of patients with acute coronary and cerebrovascular syndromes. Am J Cardiol. 2009;103:959–68. https://doi.org/10.1016/j.amjcard.2008.12.019.

17. Ma H, Aziz KS, Huang R, Abela G. Arterial wall cholesterol content is a predictor of the development and severity of arterial thrombosis. J Thromb Thrombolysis. 2006;22:5–11. https://doi.org/10.1007/s11239-006-7861-x.

18. Hammer SS, McFarland D, Abela G, Calzi SL, Grant MB, Busik JV. Statins and α cyclodextrin treatments prevent cholesterol crystal-induced pathology in human retinal endothelial cells and in db/db mice. Invest Ophthalmol Vis Sci. 2021;62(8):2928.

19. Patti G, Pasceri V, Colonna G, et al. Atorvastatin pretreatment improves outcomes in patients with acute coronary syndromes undergoing early percutaneous coronary intervention: results of the ARMYDA-ACS randomized trial. J Am Coll Cardiol. 2007;49:1272–8. https://doi.org/10.1016/j.jacc.2007.02.025.

20. Pasceri V, Patti G, Nusca A, Pristipino C, Richichi G, Di Sciascio G, ARMYDA Investigators. Randomized trial of atorvastatin for reduction of myocardial damage during coronary intervention. Circulation. 2004;110:674–8. https://doi.org/10.1161/01.CIR.0000137828.06205.87.

21. Desborough MJ, Keeling DM. The aspirin story-from willow to wonder drug. Br J Haematol. 2017;177:674–83. https://doi.org/10.1111/bjh.14520.

22. Vane JR, Botting RM. The mechanism of action of aspirin. Thromb Res. 2003;110:255–8. https://doi.org/10.1016/s0049-3848(03)00379-7.

23. ISIS-2 (Second International Study of Infarct Survival) Collaborative Group. Randomised trial of intravenous streptokinase, oral aspirin, both, or neither among 17,187 cases of suspected acute myocardial infarction: ISIS-2. Lancet. 1988;2:349–60. https://doi.org/10.1016/S0140-6736(88)92833-4.

24. Antithrombotic Trialists' Collaboration. Collaborative meta-analysis of randomised trials of antiplatelet therapy for prevention of death, myocardial infarction, and stroke in high risk patients. BMJ. 2002;324:71–86. https://doi.org/10.1136/bmj.324.7329.71.

25. Fry L, Lee A, Khan S, Aziz K, Vedre A, Abela GS. Effect of aspirin on cholesterol crystallization: a potential mechanism for plaque stabilization. Am Heart J Plus. 2022;13:100083. https://doi.org/10.1016/j.ahjo.2021.100083.

26. Husain S, Andrews N, Mulcahy D, Panza J, Quyyumi A. Aspirin improves endothelial dysfunction in atherosclerosis. Circulation. 1998;97:716–20. https://doi.org/10.1161/01.CIR.97.8.716.

27. Cyrus T, Sung S, Zhao L, et al. Effect of low-dose aspirin on vascular inflammation, plaque stability, and atherogenesis in low-density lipoprotein receptor–deficient mice. Circulation. 2002;106:1282–7. https://doi.org/10.1161/01.CIR.0000027816.54430.96.

28. Ranke C, Hecker H, Creutzig A, Alexander K. Dose-dependent effect of aspirin on carotid atherosclerosis. Circulation. 1993;87:1873–9. https://doi.org/10.1161/01.cir.87.6.1873.

29. Nasiri M, Janoudi A, Vanderberg A, Frame M, Flegler C, Flegler S, Abela GS. Role of cholesterol crystals in atherosclerosis is unmasked by altering tissue preparation methods. Microsc Res Tech. 2015;78:969–74. https://doi.org/10.1002/jemt.22560.

30. Bracegridle B. A history of microtechnique: the evolution of the microtome and the development of tissue preparation. London: Heinemann; 1978. p. 64.

31. Curran RC. Colour atlas of histopathology. 3rd ed. New York, NY: Oxford University, Harvey Miller; 1985. p. 103.

32. Di Castelnuovo A, Costanzo S, Bagnardi V, Donati MB, Iacoviello L, de Gaetano G. Alcohol dosing and total mortality in men and women: an updated meta-analysis of 34 prospective studies. Arch Intern Med. 2006;166:2437–45. https://doi.org/10.1001/archinte.166.22.2437.

33. Fernandez-Jarne E, Martınez-Losa E, Serrano-Martınez M, Prado-Santamarıa M, Brugarolas-Brufau C, Martınez-Gonzalez MA. Type of alcoholic beverage and first acute myocardial infarction: a case-control study in a Mediterranean country. Clin Cardiol. 2003;26:313–8. https://doi.org/10.1002/clc.4950260704.

34. Rawyler A, Siegenthaler PA. Cyclodextrins: a new tool for the controlled lipid depletion of thylakoid membranes. Biochim Biophys Acta. 1996;1278:89–97. https://doi.org/10.1016/0005-2736(95)00190-5.

35. Liu SM, Cogny A, Kockx M, Dean RT, Gaus K, Jessup W, Kritharides L. Cyclodextrins differentially mobilize free and esterified cholesterol from primary human foam cell macrophages. J Lipid Res. 2003;44:1156–66. https://doi.org/10.1194/jlr.M200464-JLR200.

36. Janoudi A, Opreanu M, Parameswaran N, Nasiri M, Abela GS. Extracellular cholesterol crystals induce an inflammatory response in macrophages. J Am Coll Card. 2013;61(Suppl A17):E71.

37. Zimmer S, Brabe A, Bakke S, et al. Cyclodextrin promotes atherosclerosis regression via macrophage reprogramming. Sci Transl Med. 2016;8:333ra50. https://doi.org/10.1126/scitranslmed.aad6100.

38. Li H, El-Dakdouki MH, Zhu DC, Abela GS, Huang X. Synthesis of β-cyclodextrin conjugated superparamagnetic iron oxide nanoparticles for selective binding and detection of cholesterol crystals. Chem Commun (Camb). 2012;48:3385–7. https://doi.org/10.1039/c2cc17852d.

39. Comerford KB, Artiss JD, Jen K-LC, Karakas SE. The beneficial effects α-cyclodextrin on blood lipids and weight loss in healthy humans. Obesity (Silver Spring). 2012;19:1200–4. https://doi.org/10.1038/oby.2010.280.

40. Mahjoubin-Tehran M, Kovanen PT, Xu S, Jamialahmadi T, Sahebkar A. Cyclodextrins: potential therapeutics against atherosclerosis. Pharmacol Ther. 2020;214:213. https://doi.org/10.1016/j.pharmthera.2020.107620.

41. Narisetty K, Janoudi A, Abela OG, Khan SR, Huang R, Abela GS. The effect of high density lipoprotein on solubility of cholesterol crystals. J Am Coll Cardiol. 2011;57(Suppl A):E572.
42. Adams CYM, Abdullah YH. The action of human high density lipoprotein on cholesterol crystals. Part 1. Light microscopic observations. Atherosclerosis. 1978;31:465–71. https://doi.org/10.1016/0021-9150(78)90143-0.
43. Abela GS, Kalavakunta JK, Janoudi A, et al. Frequency of cholesterol crystals in culprit coronary artery aspirate during acute myocardial infarction and their relation to inflammation and myocardial injury. Am J Cardiol. 2017;120:1699–707. https://doi.org/10.1016/j.amjcard.2017.07.075.
44. Boumegouas M, Raju M, Gardiner J, Hammer N, Saleh Y, Al-Abcha KA, Abela GS. Interaction between bacteria and cholesterol crystals: implications for endocarditis and atherosclerosis. PLoS One. 2022;17:e0263847. https://doi.org/10.1371/journal.pone.0263847.
45. Durga S, Vodnala D, Xie Y, Abela GS. Effect of stress related catecholamine levels on cholesterol crystallization and plaque rupture. J Am Coll Cardiol. 2011;57(Suppl A113):E1521.
46. Gozdor J, Janoudi A, De Feijter-Rupp H, Huang R, Alsherbini A, Boumegouas M, Abela GS. The presence and potential role of monosodium urate crystals in atherosclerosis. J Am Coll Card. 2019;73(9 Suppl 1):149.
47. Feuchtner GM, Plank F, Beyer C, Schwabl C, Held J, Bellmann-Weiler R, Weiss G, Gruber J, Widmann G, Klauser AS. Monosodium urate crystal deposition in coronary artery plaque by 128-slice dual-energy computed tomography: an ex vivo phantom and in vivo study. J Comput Assist Tomogr. 2021;45(6):856–62. https://doi.org/10.1097/RCT.0000000000001222.
48. Park JJ, Roudier MP, Soman D, Mokadam NA, Simkin PA. Prevalence of birefringent crystals in cardiac and prostatic tissues, an observational study. BMJ Open. 2014;4(7):e005308. https://doi.org/10.1136/bmjopen-2014-005308. Published 2014 Jul 16.
49. Ewence AE, Bootman M, Roderick HL, Skepper JN, McCarthy G, Epple M, Neumann M, Shanahan CM, Proudfoot D. Calcium phosphate crystals induce cell death in human vascular smooth muscle cells: a potential mechanism in atherosclerotic plaque destabilization. Circ Res. 2008;103(5):e28–34. https://doi.org/10.1161/CIRCRESAHA.108.181305.
50. Pazár B, Ea H-K, Narayan S, Kolly L, Bagnoud N, Chobaz V, Roger T, Lioté F, So A, Busso N. Basic calcium phosphate crystals induce monocyte/macrophage IL-1β secretion through the NLRP3 Inflammasome in vitro. J Immunol. 2011;186:2495–502. https://doi.org/10.4049/jimmunol.1001284.
51. Muiesan ML, Agabiti-Rosei C, Paini A, Salvetti M. Uric acid and cardiovascular disease: an update. Eur Cardiol. 2016;11:54–9. https://doi.org/10.15420/ecr.2016:4:2.
52. Mackenzie IS, Ford I, Walker A, et al. Multicentre, prospective, randomised, open-label, blinded end point trial of the efficacy of allopurinol therapy in improving cardiovascular outcomes in patients with ischaemic heart disease: protocol of the ALL-HEART study. BMJ Open. 2016;6(9):e013774. https://doi.org/10.1136/bmjopen-2016-013774. Published 2016 Sep 8.
53. Tan DS, Felip E, Castro G, et al. Association for Cancer Research. Canakinumab in combination with first-line (1L) pembrolizumab plus chemotherapy for advanced non-small cell lung cancer (aNSCLC): results from the CANOPY-1 phase 3 trial. Cancer Res. 2022;82(12_Supplement):CT037. https://doi.org/10.1158/1538-7445.AM2022-CT037.
54. Lythgoe MP, Prasad V. Repositioning canakinumab for non-small cell lung cancer-important lessons for drug repurposing in oncology. Br J Cancer. 2022;127:785. https://doi.org/10.1038/s41416-022-01893-5.
55. Abbate A, Toldo S, Marchetti C, Kron J, Van Tassell BW, Dinarello CA. Interleukin-1 and inflammasome as therapeutic targets in cardiovascular disease. Circ Res. 2020;126:1260–80. https://doi.org/10.1161/CIRCRESAHA.120.315937.
56. Imazio M, Nidorf M. Colchicine and the heart. Eur Heart J. 2021;42(28):2745–60. https://doi.org/10.1093/eurheartj/ehab221.
57. Martinon F, Pétrilli V, Mayor A, Tardivel A, Tschopp J. Gout-associated uric acid crystals activate the NALP3 inflammasome. Nature. 2006;440(7081):237–41. https://doi.org/10.1038/nature04516.

58. Dalbeth N, Pool B, Gamble GD, Smith T, Callon KE, McQueen FMCJ. Cellular characterization of the gouty tophus a quantitative analysis. Arthritis Rheum. 2010;62(5):1549–62. https://doi.org/10.1002/art.27356.
59. Nidorf SM, Thompson PL. Why colchicine should be considered for secondary prevention of atherosclerosis: an overview. Clin Ther. 2019;41(1):41–8. https://doi.org/10.1016/j.clinthera.2018.11.016.
60. Robinson PC, Terkeltaub R, Pillinger MH, et al. Consensus statement regarding the efficacy and safety of long-term low-dose colchicine in gout and cardiovascular disease. Am J Med. 2021;135:32. https://doi.org/10.1016/j.amjmed.2021.07.025.
61. Khanna PP, Perez-Ruiz F, Maranian P, Khanna D. Long-term therapy for chronic gout results in clinically important improvements in the health-related quality of life: short form-36 is responsive to change in chronic gout. Rheumatology. 2011;50(4):740. https://doi.org/10.1093/rheumatology/keq346.
62. Nidorf SM, Eikelboom JWBC, PL. T. Low-dose colchicine for secondary prevention of cardiovascular disease. J Am Coll Cardiol. 2013;61(4):404–10. https://doi.org/10.1016/j.jacc.2012.10.027.
63. Nidorf SM, Fiolet ATL, Mosterd A, Eikelboom JW, Schut A, Opstal TSJ, The SHK, Xu X-F, Ireland MA, Lenderink T, Latchem D, Hoogslag P, Jerzewski A, Nierop P, Whelan A, Hendriks R, Swart H, Schaap J, Kuijper AFM, van Hessen MWJ, Saklani P, Tan I, Thompson AG, Morton A, Judkins C, Bax WA, Dirksen M, Alings M, Hankey GJ, Budgeon CA, Tijssen JGP, Cornel JH, Thompson PL, LoDoCo2 Trial Investigators. Colchicine in patients with chronic coronary disease. N Engl J Med. 2020;383(1):1838–47. https://doi.org/10.1056/NEJMoa2021372.
64. Deftereos S, Giannopoulos G, Raisakis K, et al. Colchicine treatment for the prevention of bare-metal stent restenosis in diabetic patients. J Am Coll Cardiol. 2013;61(16):1679–85. https://doi.org/10.1016/j.jacc.2013.01.055.
65. Tardif J-C, Kouz S, Waters DD, et al. Efficacy and safety of low-dose colchicine after myocardial infarction. N Engl J Med. 2019;381:2497. https://doi.org/10.1056/nejmoa1912388.
66. Bouabdallaoui N, Tardif JC, Waters DD, et al. Time-to-treatment initiation of colchicine and cardiovascular outcomes after myocardial infarction in the colchicine cardiovascular outcomes trial (COLCOT). Eur Heart J. 2020;41(42):4092–9. https://doi.org/10.1093/eurheartj/ehaa659.
67. Fiolet ATL, Opstal TSJ, Mosterd A, et al. Efficacy and safety of low-dose colchicine in patients with coronary disease: a systematic review and meta-analysis of randomized trials. Eur Heart J. 2021;42(28):2765–75. https://doi.org/10.1093/eurheartj/ehab115.
68. Robinson PC, Terkeltaub R, Pillinger MH, Shah B, Karalis V, Karatza E, Liew D, Imazio M, Cornel JH, Thompson PL, Nidorf M. Consensus statement regarding the efficacy and safety of long-term low-dose colchicine in gout and cardiovascular disease. Am J Med. 2022;135(1):32–8. https://doi.org/10.1016/j.amjmed.2021.07.025.
69. Vaidya K, Arnott C, Martínez GJ, et al. Colchicine therapy and plaque stabilization in patients with acute coronary syndrome: a CT coronary angiography study. JACC Cardiovasc Imaging. 2018;11(2):305–16. https://doi.org/10.1016/j.jcmg.2017.08.013.
70. Ridker PM, Devalaraja M, Baeres FMM, et al. IL-6 inhibition with ziltivekimab in patients at high atherosclerotic risk (RESCUE): a double-blind, randomised, placebo-controlled, phase 2 trial. Lancet. 2021;10289:2060–9. https://doi.org/10.1016/S0140-6736(21)00520-1.
71. FDA Reference ID: 5192662 - Accessdata.fda.gov.

Index

J

Janus kinase 2 (JAK2), 136

K

Kandutsch-Russel pathway, 390
Keto-cholesterol, 113
Kidney disease, 285–287, 325, 326
Kruppel-like factor 2 (KLF2), 136, 302

L

Leaflet excursion
  aortic, 221
  bioprosthetic, 222
  cholesterol crystals, 220
  endothelial and deeper layers, 222
  mineralization and calcification, 222
  surface of valve, 219
Lectin pathway (LP), 235
Left anterior descending artery (LAD), 192
Leukocytes, 204, 338
Light microscopy tissue preparation, 29
Lipid core, 77
Lipid environment, 49
Lipid lowering therapy, 279, 361, 362,
      380, 471
  anti-inflammatory therapies, 424–426
  cancer, 423
  degenerative valve disease, 226–227
  early epidemiological and clinical
      data, 423
  inflammation, 423
  in-vitro and animal studies, 423
  non-specific anti-inflammatory agents, 424
Lipid metabolites, 306
Lipid oxidation, 307, 308
Lipid rafts, 299, 301
Lipid rich plaques, 22
Lipophagy, 137
Lipopolysaccharide (LPS), 262
Lipoprotein-associated phospholipase A2
      (LpPLA2), 108
Lipoprotein modifications
  extracellular CCs, 266
  fibrous cap, 265
  intracellular CCs, 266–268
  modifications, 265
Lipoproteins, 111, 129, 299
Liposomes, 65
Lipoxygenases, 306
Liver X receptors (LXRs), 112, 377
  CYP46A1, 378

diabetes, 378
  downregulation, 377, 378
LoDoCo2 trial, 483
Low density lipoprotein (LDL), 108, 129, 262,
      264–267, 299, 338
  lipid oxidation, 301
  retention and promotes, 301, 302
  transcytosis, 129
Low-density lipoprotein cholesterol
      (LDL-c), 277
  ANGPTL3, 106
  ANGPTL4, 106
  atherosclerotic plaque, 107
  endothelial dysfunction and
      accumulation, 107
  FH, 106
  MI, 106
  oxygen free radicals, 110
  PCSK9 gene, 106
  transcytosis, 107
Low-density lipoprotein receptor (LDLR), 106
Low density lipoprotein receptor deficient
      (Ldlr$^{-/-}$) mice, 259
Low-dose colchicine (LoDoCo) trials,
      305, 483
LRP1 receptors, 392
Lung, granuloma formation in, 283, 285
Lymphocytes, 108, 322
Lymphoid follicles, 109
Lysophagy, 135
Lysosomal acidic lipase (LAL), 135
Lysosomal destabilization, 263, 286
Lysosomes, 134–136, 245

M

Macrophage (M)-colony stimulating factor
      (CSF), 277
Macrophages, 18, 66, 108, 261, 275, 286,
      333, 479
Macropinocytosis, 133
Magnesium, 356
Magnetic resonance angiography, 178
Mannose binding lectin (MBL), 240
Matrix Gla protein (MGP), 356
Matrix metalloproteinases (MMP), 108
MCC950, 482
Mediterranean fever (MEFV), 121
Membrane attack complex (MAC), 236, 380
Membrane expansion, 395
Metabolism, 239, 275
  cholesterol, 245, 249
  in macrophages, 245, 247

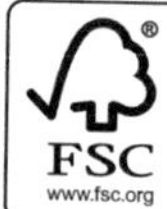

If you have any concerns about our products,
you can contact us on
ProductSafety@springernature.com

In case Publisher is established outside the EU,
the EU authorized representative is:
Springer Nature Customer Service Center GmbH
Europaplatz 3, 69115 Heidelberg, Germany

Printed by Libri Plureos GmbH
in Hamburg, Germany